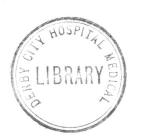

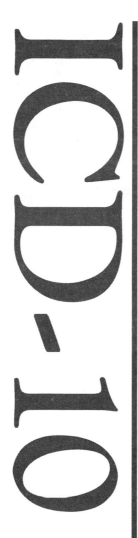

International Statistical Classification of Diseases and Related Health Problems

Tenth Revision

Volume 1

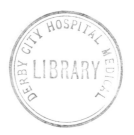

World Health Organization
Geneva
1992

Volume 1	Introduction

Volume 1 Introduction
WHO Collaborating Centres for Classification of Diseases
Report of the International Conference for the Tenth
    Revision
List of three-character categories
Tabular list of inclusions and four-character subcategories
Morphology of neoplasms
Special tabulation lists for mortality and morbidity
Definitions
Regulations

Volume 2 Instruction manual

Volume 3 Alphabetical index

WHO Library Cataloguing in Publication Data

International statistical classification of diseases and related health problems.—
    10th revision.

    Contents: v. 1. Tabular list—v. 2. Instruction manual—v. 3. Alphabetical index

    1. Classification I. Title: ICD–10

    ISBN 92 4 154419 8 (v. 1)   (NLM Classification: WB 15)
    ISBN 92 4 154420 1 (v. 2)
    ISBN 92 4 154421 X (v. 3)

Typeset in England
Printed in France
91/8833–9062—Eastern/Jouve—30000

Contents

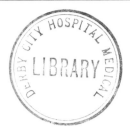

Introduction

A classification of diseases may be defined as a system of categories to which morbid entities are assigned according to established criteria. There are many possible axes of classification and the one selected will depend upon the use to be made of the statistics to be compiled. A statistical classification of diseases must encompass the entire range of morbid conditions within a manageable number of categories.

The Tenth Revision of the International Statistical Classification of Diseases and Related Health Problems is the latest in a series that was formalized in 1893 as the Bertillon Classification or International List of Causes of Death. A complete review of the historical background to the classification is given in Volume 2. While the title has been amended to make clearer the content and purpose and to reflect the progressive extension of the scope of the classification beyond diseases and injuries, the familiar abbreviation "ICD" has been retained. In the updated classification, conditions have been grouped in a way that was felt to be most suitable for general epidemiological purposes and the evaluation of health care.

Work on the Tenth Revision of the ICD started in September 1983 when a Preparatory Meeting on ICD-10 was convened in Geneva. The programme of work was guided by regular meetings of Heads of WHO Collaborating Centres for Classification of Diseases. Policy guidance was provided by a number of special meetings including those of the Expert Committee on the International Classification of Diseases—Tenth Revision, held in 1984 and 1987.

In addition to the technical contributions provided by many specialist groups and individual experts, a large number of comments and suggestions were received from WHO Member States and Regional Offices as a result of the global circulation of draft proposals for revision in 1984 and 1986. From the comments received, it was clear that many users wished the ICD to encompass types of data other than the "diagnostic information" (in the broadest sense of the term) that it has always covered. In order to accommodate the perceived needs of these users, the concept arose of a "family" of classifications centred on the traditional ICD with its familiar form and structure. The ICD itself would thus meet the requirement for diagnostic information for general purposes, while a variety of other classifications would be used in conjunction with it and would deal either

1

with different approaches to the same information or with different information (notably medical and surgical procedures and disablement).

Following suggestions at the time of development of the Ninth Revision of the classification that a different basic structure might better serve the needs of the many and varied users, several alternative models were evaluated. It became clear, however, that the traditional single-variable-axis design of the classification, and other aspects of its structure that gave emphasis to conditions that were frequent, costly or otherwise of public health importance, had withstood the test of time and that many users would be unhappy with any of the models that had been proposed as a possible replacement.

Consequently, as study of the Tenth Revision will show, the traditional ICD structure has been retained, but an alphanumeric coding scheme replaces the previous numeric one. This provides a larger coding frame and leaves room for future revision without disruption of the numbering system, as has occurred at previous revisions.

In order to make optimum use of the available space, certain disorders of the immune mechanism are included with diseases of the blood and blood-forming organs (Chapter III). New chapters have been created for diseases of the eye and adnexa and diseases of the ear and mastoid process. The former supplementary classifications of external causes and of factors influencing health status and contact with health services now form part of the main classification.

The dagger and asterisk system of dual classification for certain diagnostic statements, introduced in the Ninth Revision, has been retained and extended, with the asterisk axis being contained in homogeneous categories at the three-character level.

Content of the three volumes of ICD-10

The presentation of the classification has been changed and there are now three volumes:

Volume 1. Tabular List. This contains the report of the International Conference for the Tenth Revision, the classification itself at the three- and four-character levels, the classification of the morphology of neoplasms, special tabulation lists for mortality and morbidity, definitions, and the nomenclature regulations.

Volume 2. Instruction Manual. This brings together the notes on certification and classification formerly included in Volume 1 with a good deal of new background and instructional matter and guidance on the use of Volume 1, on tabulations, and on planning for the use of ICD, which was seen as lacking in earlier revisions. It also includes the historical material formerly presented in the introduction to Volume 1.

Volume 3. Alphabetical Index. This presents the index itself with an introduction and expanded instructions on its use.

*   *   *

The classification was approved by the International Conference for the Tenth Revision of the International Classification of Diseases in 1989 and adopted by the Forty-third World Health Assembly in the following resolution:

The Forty-third World Health Assembly,

Having considered the report of the International Conference for the Tenth Revision of the International Classification of Diseases;

1. ADOPTS the following, recommended by the Conference:

    (1) the detailed list of three-character categories and optional four-character subcategories with the Short Tabulation Lists for Mortality and Morbidity, constituting the Tenth Revision of the International Statistical Classification of Diseases and Related Health Problems, due to come into effect on 1 January 1993;
    (2) the definitions, standards and reporting requirements related to maternal, fetal, perinatal, neonatal and infant mortality;
    (3) the rules and instructions for underlying cause coding for mortality and main condition coding for morbidity;

2. REQUESTS the Director-General to issue the *Manual of the International Statistical Classification of Diseases and Related Health Problems*;

3. ENDORSES the recommendations of the Conference concerning:

    (1) the concept and implementation of the family of disease and health-related classifications, with the International Statistical Classification of Diseases and Related Health Problems as the core classification surrounded by a number of related and supplementary classifications and the International Nomenclature of Diseases;

(2) the establishment of an updating process within the ten-year revision cycle.

Acknowledgements

The periodic revision of the ICD has, since the Sixth Revision in 1948, been coordinated by the World Health Organization. As the use of the classification has increased, so, understandably, has the desire among its users to contribute to the revision process. The Tenth Revision is the product of a vast amount of international activity, cooperation and compromise. WHO acknowledges with gratitude the contributions of the numerous international and national specialist groups and individuals in many countries.

WHO Collaborating Centres for Classification of Diseases

Nine WHO Collaborating Centres for Classification of Diseases have been established to assist countries with problems encountered in the development and use of health-related classifications and, in particular, in the use of the ICD.

It is important that countries bring to the attention of the respective Centre any significant problems they might encounter in the use of the ICD and especially when a new disease for which the ICD does not provide a suitable classification is encountered frequently. Until now the ICD has not been updated between revisions but it has been proposed that, through the Centres, a mechanism will be introduced to provide suitable codes for new diseases where necessary.

In addition to the official WHO Collaborating Centres, there are a number of national reference centres and individual users should first consult these, or their appropriate national office, when they encounter problems.

There are three centres for English-language users. Communications should be addressed to the Head, WHO Collaborating Centre for Classification of Diseases at:

> Australian Institute of Health
> GPO Box 570
> Canberra ACT 2601,
> Australia
>
> Office of Population Censuses and Surveys
> St Catherine's House
> Kingsway 10
> London WC2B 6JP
> England
>
> National Center for Health Statistics
> 6525 Belcrest Road
> Hyattsville, MD 20782
> United States of America

The other six centres, each based on an individual language or group of languages, are located in the following institutions:

Peking Union Medical College Hospital
Chinese Academy of Medical Sciences
Beijing 100730
China (for Chinese)

INSERM
44 Chemin de Ronde
F-78110 Le Vésinet
France (for French)

Department of Social Medicine
University Hospital
S-751 85 Uppsala
Sweden (for the Nordic countries)

Faculdade de Saúde Publica/Universidade de São Paulo
Avenida Dr Arnaldo 715,
0255 São Paulo, SP
Brazil (for Portuguese)

The N.A. Semaško Institute,
U1. Obuha 12
Moscow B-120
Russian Federation (for Russian)

Centro Venezolano de Clasificación de Enfermedades
Edificio Sur, 9° Piso
M.S.A.S.,
Centro Simon Bolivar,
P.O. Box 6653
Caracas
Venezuela (for Spanish)

Report of the International Conference for the Tenth Revision of the International Classification of Diseases

The International Conference for the Tenth Revision of the International Classification of Diseases was convened by the World Health Organization at WHO headquarters in Geneva from 26 September to 2 October 1989. The Conference was attended by delegates from 43 Member States:

Angola
Australia
Bahamas
Belgium
Brazil
Bulgaria
Burundi
Canada
China
Cuba
Cyprus
Denmark
Finland
France
German Democratic Republic
Germany, Federal Republic of
Hungary
India
Indonesia
Israel
Japan
Kuwait

Luxembourg
Madagascar
Mali
Malta
Mozambique
Netherlands
Niger
Portugal
Republic of Korea
Senegal
Singapore
Spain
Sweden
Switzerland
Thailand
Uganda
Union of Soviet Socialist Republics
United Arab Emirates
United Kingdom of Great Britain
    and Northern Ireland
United States of America
Venezuela

The United Nations, the International Labour Organisation and the WHO Regional Offices sent representatives to participate in the Conference, as did the Council for International Organizations of Medical Sciences, and twelve other nongovernmental organizations concerned with cancer registration, the deaf, epidemiology, family medicine, gynaecology and obstetrics, hypertension, health records, preventive and social medicine, neurology, psychiatry, rehabilitation and sexually transmitted diseases.

The Conference was opened by Dr J.-P. Jardel, Assistant Director-General, on behalf of the Director-General. Dr Jardel spoke of the extensive consultations and preparatory work that had gone into the revision proposals and had necessitated a longer than usual interval between revisions. He noted that the Tenth Revision would have a new title, *International Statistical Classification of Diseases and Related Health Problems*, to emphasize its statistical purpose and reflect the widening of its scope. The convenient abbreviation ICD would, however, be retained. He also mentioned the new alphanumeric coding scheme, which had made it possible to provide a better balance between the content of the chapters and to leave room for future additions and changes, as well as the intention to produce an ICD manual of three-character categories with an alphabetical index for use where the more complex, detailed four-character version would be inappropriate.

The Conference elected the following officers:

Dr R.H.C. Wells, Australia (*Chairman*)
Dr H. Bay-Nielsen, Denmark (*Vice-Chairman*)
Dr R. Braun, German Democratic Republic (*Vice-Chairman*)
Mr R.A. Israel, United States of America (*Vice-Chairman*)
Dr R. Laurenti, Brazil (*Vice-Chairman*)
Dr P. Maguin, France (*Rapporteur*)
Ms E. Taylor, Canada (*Rapporteur*)

The secretariat of the Conference was as follows:

Dr J.-P. Jardel, Assistant Director-General, WHO, Geneva, Switzerland
Dr H.R. Hapsara, Director, Division of Epidemiological Surveillance and Health Situation and Trend Assessment, WHO, Geneva, Switzerland
Dr J.-C. Alary, Chief Medical Officer, Development of Epidemiological and Health Statistical Services, WHO, Geneva, Switzerland
Dr G.R. Brämer, Medical Officer, Development of Epidemiological and Health Statistical Services, WHO, Geneva, Switzerland (*Secretary*)
Mr A. L'Hours, Technical Officer, Development of Epidemiological and Health Statistical Services, WHO, Geneva, Switzerland
Professor W. Jänisch, German Democratic Republic (*Temporary Adviser*)
Mr T. Kruse, Denmark (*Temporary Adviser*)
Dr K. Kupka, France (*Temporary Adviser*)
Dr J. Leowski, Poland (*Temporary Adviser*)
Ms R.M. Loy, United Kingdom of Great Britain and Northern Ireland (*Temporary Adviser*)
Mr R.H. Seeman, United States of America (*Temporary Adviser*)

The secretariat of the Conference was assisted by representatives of other relevant technical units of WHO headquarters.

The Conference adopted an agenda dealing with the proposed content of the chapters of the Tenth Revision, and material to be incorporated in the published manual; the process for its introduction; and the family of classifications and related matters.

1. History and development of uses of the International Classification of Diseases (ICD)

The Conference was reminded of the impressive history of a statistical classification which dated back to the eighteenth century. While early revisions of the classification had been concerned only with causes of death, its scope had been extended at the Sixth Revision in 1948 to include non-fatal diseases. This extension had continued through the Ninth Revision, with certain innovations being made to meet the statistical needs of widely differing organizations. In addition, at the International Conference for the Ninth Revision (Geneva, 1975) (1), recommendations had been made and approved for the publication for trial purposes of supplementary classifications of procedures in medicine and of impairments, disabilities, and handicaps.

2. Review of activities in the preparation of proposals for the Tenth Revision of the ICD

The proposals before the Conference were the product of a vast amount of activity at WHO headquarters and around the world. The programme of work had been guided by regular meetings of the heads of WHO Collaborating Centres for Classification of Diseases. Policy guidance had been provided by a number of special meetings and by the Expert Committee on the International Classification of Diseases—Tenth Revision, which met in 1984 (2) and 1987 (3) to make decisions on the direction the work should take and the form of the final proposals.

Extensive preparatory activity had been devoted to a radical review of the suitability of the structure of the ICD, essentially a statistical classification of diseases and other health problems, to serve a wide variety of needs for mortality and health-care data. Ways of stabilizing the coding system to minimize disruption at successive revisions had been investigated, as had the possibility of providing a better balance between the content of the different chapters of the ICD.

Even with a new structure, it was plain that one classification could not cope with the extremes of the requirements. The concept had therefore been developed of a "family" of classifications, with the main ICD as the core, covering the centre ground of needs for traditional mortality and morbidity statistics, while needs for more detailed, less detailed or different classifications and associated matters would be dealt with by other members of the family.

Several alternative models for the structure of the ICD had been investigated by the Collaborating Centres, but it had been found that each had unsatisfactory features and none had sufficient advantages over the existing structure to justify replacing it. Special meetings held to evaluate the Ninth Revision had confirmed that, although some potential users found the existing structure of the ICD unsuitable, there was a large body of satisfied users who considered it had many inherent strengths, whatever its apparent inconsistencies, and wished it to continue in its existing form.

Various schemes involving alphanumeric notation had been examined with a view to producing a coding frame that would give a better balance to the chapters and allow sufficient space for future additions and changes without disrupting the codes.

Decisions made on these matters had paved the way for the preparation of successive drafts of chapter proposals for the Tenth Revision. These had twice been circulated to Member States for comment as well as being reviewed by other interested bodies, meetings of Centre Heads, and the Expert Committee. A large number of international professional specialist associations, individual specialists and experts, other WHO headquarters units and regional offices had given advice and guidance to the WHO unit responsible for the ICD and to the Collaborating Centres on the preparation of the proposals and the associated material placed before the Conference. WHO gratefully acknowledged this assistance.

3. General characteristics and content of the proposed Tenth Revision of the ICD

The main innovation in the proposals for the Tenth Revision was the use of an alphanumeric coding scheme of one letter followed by three numbers at the four-character level. This had the effect of more than doubling the size of the coding frame in comparison with the Ninth Revision and enabled the vast majority of chapters to be assigned a unique letter or group of letters, each capable of providing 100 three-character categories. Of the 26 available letters, 25 had been used, the letter U being left vacant for future additions and changes and for possible interim classifications to solve difficulties arising at the national and international level between revisions.

As a matter of policy, some three-character categories had been left vacant for future expansion and revision, the number varying according to the chapters: those with a primarily anatomical axis of classification had fewer vacant categories as it was considered that future changes in their content would be more limited in nature.

The Ninth Revision contained 17 chapters plus two supplementary classifications: the Supplementary Classification of External Causes of Injury and Poisoning (the E code) and the Supplementary Classification of Factors Influencing Health Status and Contact with Health Services (the V code). As recommended by the Preparatory Meeting on the Tenth Revision (Geneva, 1983) (4) and endorsed by subsequent meetings, these two chapters were no longer considered to be supplementary but were included as a part of the core classification.

The order of entry of chapters in the proposals for the Tenth Revision had originally been the same as in the Ninth Revision; however, to make effective use of the available space, disorders of the immune mechanism were later included with diseases of the blood and blood-forming organs, whereas in the Ninth Revision they had been included with endocrine, nutritional and metabolic diseases. The new chapter on "Diseases of the blood and blood-forming organs and certain disorders involving the immune mechanism" now followed the "Neoplasms" chapter, with which it shared the letter D.

During the elaboration of early drafts of the chapter on "Diseases of the nervous system and sense organs", it had soon become clear that it would not be possible to accommodate all the required detail under one letter in

100 three-character categories. It had been decided, therefore, to create three separate chapters—"Diseases of the nervous system" having the letter G, and the two chapters on "Diseases of the eye and adnexa" and on "Diseases of the ear and mastoid process" sharing the letter H.

Also, the chapters on "Diseases of the genitourinary system", on "Pregnancy, childbirth and the puerperium", on "Certain conditions originating in the perinatal period, and on "Congenital malformations, deformations and chromosomal abnormalities" had been brought together as contiguous chapters XIV to XVII.

With the inclusion of the former supplementary classifications as part of the core classification and the creation of two new chapters, the total number of chapters in the proposal for the Tenth Revision had become 21. The titles of some chapters had been amended to give a better indication of their content.

Where radical changes to the ICD had been proposed, field-testing had been appropriate. This had been the case for the following chapters:

V.   Mental and behavioural disorders
XIX. Injury, poisoning and certain other consequences of external causes
XX.   External causes of morbidity and mortality

Chapter II, "Neoplasms", had also been subject to some field-testing, although the changes in its content had been of a minor nature.

Some new features of the proposals for the Tenth Revision were as follows:
- The exclusion notes at the beginning of each chapter had been expanded to explain the relative hierarchy of chapters, and to make it clear that the "special group" chapters had priority of assignment over the organ or system chapters and that, among the special group chapters, those on "Pregnancy, childbirth and the puerperium" and on "Certain conditions originating in the perinatal period" had priority over the others.
- Also, at the beginning of each chapter an overview was given of the blocks of three-character categories and, where relevant, the asterisk categories; this had been done to clarify the structure of the chapters and to facilitate the use of the asterisk categories.
- The notes in the tabular list applied to all uses of the classification; if a note was appropriate only to morbidity or only to mortality, it was included in the special notes accompanying either the morbidity coding rules or the mortality coding rules.
- The Ninth Revision had identified a certain number of conditions as

being drug-induced; this approach had been continued in drawing up the proposals for the Tenth Revision and many such conditions were now separately identified.

An important innovation was the creation towards the end of certain chapters of categories for postprocedural disorders. These identified important conditions that constituted a medical care problem in their own right and included such examples as endocrine and metabolic diseases following ablation of an organ and other specific conditions such as postgastrectomy dumping syndrome. Postprocedural conditions that were not specific to a particular body system, including immediate complications such as air embolism and postoperative shock, continued to be classified in the chapter on "Injury, poisoning and certain other consequences of external causes".

Another change was that in the Ninth Revision, the four-digit titles had often had to be read in conjunction with the three-digit titles to ascertain the full meaning and intent of the subcategory, whereas in the draft presented to the Conference the titles were almost invariably complete and could stand alone.

The dual classification scheme for etiology and manifestation, known as the dagger and asterisk system, introduced in the Ninth Revision, had been the subject of a certain amount of criticism. This related mainly to the fact that the classification frequently contained a mixture of manifestation and other information at the three- and four-digit levels, with the same diagnostic labels sometimes appearing under both axes. Also, many considered the system to be insufficiently comprehensive. To overcome these problems, in the draft for the Tenth Revision, the asterisk information was contained in 82 homogeneous three-character categories for optional use. This approach enabled those diagnostic statements containing information about both a generalized underlying disease process and a manifestation or complication in a particular organ or site to receive two codes, allowing retrieval or tabulation according to either axis.

These characteristics of the proposed Tenth Revision were accepted by the Conference.

Each of the chapters was introduced to the Conference with a presentation on changes introduced since the Ninth Revision and some background information about certain innovations. Some issues related to changes in chapter structure and content were discussed by the Conference and agreement reached on follow-up and modification by the secretariat.

4. Standards and definitions related to maternal and child health

The Conference considered with interest the recommended definitions, standards and reporting requirements for the Tenth Revision with regard to maternal mortality and to fetal, perinatal, neonatal and infant mortality. These recommendations were the outcome of a series of special meetings and consultations and were directed towards improving the comparability of data.

The Conference agreed that it was desirable to retain the definitions of live birth and fetal death as they appeared in the Ninth Revision.

After some discussion, the Conference set up a working party on the subject of maternal mortality and, on the basis of its recommendations, also agreed to retain the definition of maternal death as it appeared in the Ninth Revision.

In order to improve the quality of maternal mortality data and provide alternative methods of collecting data on deaths during pregnancy or related to it, as well as to encourage the recording of deaths from obstetric causes occurring more than 42 days following termination of pregnancy, two additional definitions, for "pregnancy-related death" and "late maternal death", were formulated by the working party. [These are included on page 1238.]

The Conference

> RECOMMENDED that countries consider the inclusion on death certificates of questions regarding current pregnancy and pregnancy within one year preceding death.

The Conference agreed that, since the number of live births was more universally available than the number of total births (live births plus fetal deaths), it should be used as the denominator in the ratios related to maternal mortality [as contained in Volume 2].

With respect to perinatal, neonatal and infant mortality, it was strongly advised that published rates based on birth cohorts should be so identified and differentiated.

The Conference confirmed the practice of expressing age in completed units of time and thus designating the first day of life as day zero.

The Conference

> RECOMMENDED the inclusion, in the manual of the Tenth Revision of the ICD, of definitions, standards and reporting requirements related to maternal mortality and to fetal, perinatal, neonatal and infant mortality.

5. Coding and selection rules and tabulation lists

5.1 Coding and selection rules for mortality

The Conference was informed about a process for review of the selection and modification rules for underlying cause of death and the associated notes, as they appeared in the Ninth Revision, which had resulted in several recommended changes in the rules and extensive changes to the notes.

The Conference

> RECOMMENDED that the rules for selection of cause of death for primary mortality tabulation, as they appear in the Ninth Revision, be replaced in the Tenth Revision [by those contained in Volume 2].

The Conference was further informed that additional notes for use in underlying cause coding and the interpretation of entries of causes of death had been drafted and were being reviewed. As these notes were intended to improve consistency in coding, the Conference agreed that they would also be incorporated in the Tenth Revision.

The Conference noted the continued use of multiple-condition coding and analysis in relation to causes of death. It expressed encouragement for such activities, but did not recommend that the Tenth Revision should contain any particular rules or methods of analysis to be followed.

In considering the international form of medical certificate of cause of death, the Expert Committee had recognized that the situation of an aging population with a greater proportion of deaths involving multiple disease processes, and the effects of associated therapeutic interventions, tended to increase the number of possible statements between the underlying cause and the direct cause of death: this meant that an increasing number of conditions were being entered on death certificates in many countries. This led the Committee to recommend the inclusion of an additional line (d) in Part I of the certificate.

The Conference therefore

> RECOMMENDED that, where a need has been identified, countries consider the possibility of including an additional line (d) in Part I of the medical certificate of cause of death.

5.2 Coding and selection rules for morbidity

For the first time, the Ninth Revision had contained guidance on recording and coding for morbidity and specifically for the selection of a single condition for presentation of morbidity statistics. Experience gained in the use of the definitions and rules in the Ninth Revision had proved their usefulness and generated requests for their clarification, for further elaboration regarding the recording of diagnostic information by health care practitioners, and for more guidance on dealing with specific problem situations.

The Conference endorsed the recommendations of the 1975 Revision Conference about the condition to be selected for single-condition analysis of episodes of health care, and its view that, where practicable, multiple-condition coding and analysis should be undertaken to supplement routine statistics. It stressed that the Tenth Revision should make it clear that much of the guidance was applicable only when the tabulation of a "main condition" for an episode was appropriate and when the concept of an "episode" per se was relevant to the way in which data collection was organized.

The Conference accordingly

> RECOMMENDED that additional guidance on the recording and coding of morbidity should be included in the Tenth Revision, and that the definitions of "main condition" and "other conditions" should be incorporated, together with the modified rules for dealing with an obviously incorrectly reported "main condition". [These are included in Volume 2.]

The Conference also

RECOMMENDED that where the "main condition" is subject to the dual classification system provided in the ICD, both the dagger and asterisk codes should be recorded, to permit alternative tabulation by either.

The Conference agreed that extensive notes and examples should be added to provide further assistance.

5.3 Lists for tabulation of mortality and morbidity

The Conference was informed about difficulties that had arisen in the use of the Basic Tabulation List based on the Ninth Revision and about the activities that had been undertaken, particularly by WHO, to develop new lists for the tabulation and publication of mortality data. In this process it had become apparent that, in many countries, mortality up to the age of five was a more robust indicator than infant mortality, and that it would therefore be preferable to have a list that included infant deaths and deaths of children up to the age of five years, rather than a list for infants only.

Two versions of the general mortality list and of the infant and child mortality list had been prepared for consideration by the Conference, with the second version including chapter titles and residual items for chapters as necessary.

As some concerns were expressed regarding the mortality lists as presented, a small working party was convened to consider the possible inclusion of some additional items. The report of the working party was accepted by the Conference and is reflected in the mortality lists on pages 1207–1220.

On the topic of lists for the tabulation of morbidity, the Conference reviewed both a proposed tabulation list and a model publication list based on chapter titles, with selected items included as examples under each title. Considerable concern was expressed about the applicability of such lists to all morbidity in the broadest sense. There was general agreement that the lists as presented were probably more suited to inpatient morbidity, and it was felt that further efforts should be made to develop lists suitable for other morbidity applications and also that both mortality and morbidity tabulation lists should be accompanied in the Tenth Revision by appropriate explanations and instructions on their use.

In the light of the concerns raised in the Conference and the conclusions of the working party, the Conference agreed that the tabulation and publication lists should appear in the Tenth Revision, while an effort should be made to establish clearer, more descriptive titles for these lists. It was also agreed that, to facilitate the alternative tabulation of asterisk categories, a second version of the morbidity tabulation list should be developed, which included the asterisk categories.

6. Family of classifications

6.1 Concept of the family of classifications

During the preparation of the Ninth Revision it had already been realized that the ICD alone could not cover all the information required and that only a "family" of disease and health-related classifications would meet the different requirements in public health. Since the late 1970s, therefore, various possible solutions had been envisaged, one of which called for a core classification (ICD) with a series of modules, some hierarchically related and others of a supplementary nature.

After studies and discussions in cooperation with the various Collaborating Centres, a concept of a family of classifications had been elaborated and subsequently revised by the Expert Committee in 1987, which had recommended the scheme shown opposite.

The Conference

> RECOMMENDED that the concept of the family of disease and health-related classifications should be followed up by WHO.

In order to maintain the integrity of the ICD itself and this family concept, the Conference

> RECOMMENDED that, in the interests of international comparability, no changes should be made to the content (as indicated by the titles) of the three-character categories and four-character subcategories of the Tenth Revision in the preparation of translations or adaptations, except as authorized by WHO. The Secretariat of WHO is responsible for the ICD and acts as central clearing-house for any publication (except national statistical publications) or translation to be derived from it. WHO should be promptly notified about the intention to produce translations and adaptations or other ICD-related classifications.

Family of disease and health-related classifications

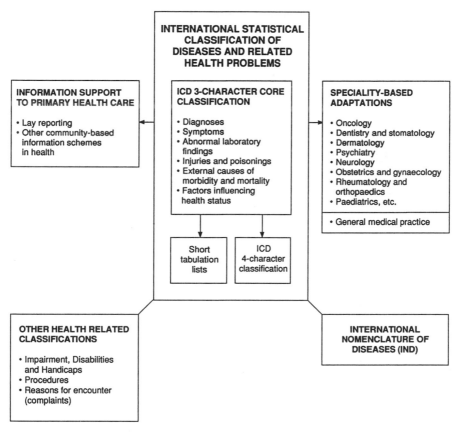

The Conference viewed with interest a presentation of the use and linkage of different members of the ICD family in the medicosocial and multidimensional assessment of the elderly in relation not only to health but also to activities of daily living as well as the social and physical environment. It was demonstrated that effective information could be obtained through use of the ICD and the International Classification of Impairments, Disabilities, and Handicaps (ICIDH), and especially through use of the codes from the proposed Chapter XXI of the Tenth Revision.

6.2 Specialty-based adaptations

The Conference was informed about plans for the development of adaptations of the Tenth Revision in the mental health programme area. Clinical guidelines would accompany a version intended for use by clinicians working in the field of psychiatry; research criteria would be proposed for use in investigations of mental health problems; and multi-axial presentations for use in dealing with childhood disorders and for the classification of adult problems would be developed as well as a version for use by general practitioners. Compilations of ICD codes relevant to psychiatry and to neurology would also be produced along the lines of previous publications on this subject.

The Conference also heard about the methods used to ensure that the basic structure and function of the ICD were preserved in the initial development of the application for medical specialists in dentistry and stomatology (ICD-DA) and was informed that a new revision of the ICD-DA linked to the Tenth Revision was in the final stages of preparation.

A presentation was given on the International Classification of Diseases for Oncology (ICD-O), Second Edition, a multi-axial classification including both the topography and morphology of neoplasms. The morphology codes of the ICD-O, which had evolved over a long period of time, had been revised and extensively field-tested. The topography codes of the second edition would be based on categories C00–C80 in the Tenth Revision and publication would, therefore, await World Health Assembly approval of the Tenth Revision.

There was agreement on the value of an adaptation in the area of general medical practice and the Conference was informed about the willingness of groups working in this area to collaborate with WHO. In respect of other specialty-based adaptations, which were likely to become more numerous, the recommended role of WHO as a clearing-house was considered to be extremely important.

6.3 Information support to primary health care

In accordance with the recommendations of the 1975 Revision Conference, a working group had been convened by the WHO Regional Office for South-East Asia in Delhi in 1976. It had drawn up a detailed list of symptom associations, and from this, two short lists were derived, one for causes of death and one for reasons for contact with health services. Field trials of this system had been carried out in countries of the Region and the results used to revise the list of symptom associations and the reporting forms. This revised version had been published by WHO in 1978 in the booklet *Lay reporting of health information* (5).

The Global Strategy for Health for All by the Year 2000, launched in 1978, had raised a number of challenges for the development of information systems in Member States. At the International Conference on Health Statistics for the Year 2000 (Bellagio, Italy, 1982) (6), the integration of "lay reporting" information with other information generated and used for health management purposes had been identified as a major problem inhibiting the wider implementation of lay reporting schemes. The Consultation on Primary Care Classifications (Geneva, 1985) (7) had stressed the need for an approach that could unify information support, health service management and community services through information based on lay reporting in the expanded sense of community-based information.

The Conference was informed about the experience of countries in developing and applying community-based health information that covered health problems and needs, related risk factors and resources. It supported the concept of developing non-conventional methods at the community level as a method of filling information gaps in individual countries and strengthening their information systems. It was stressed that, for both developed and developing countries, such methods or systems should be developed locally and that, because of factors such as morbidity patterns as well as language and cultural variations, transfer to other areas or countries should not be attempted.

6.4 Impairments, disabilities and handicaps

The International Classification of Impairments, Disabilities, and Handicaps (ICIDH) (8) had been published by WHO in English in 1980 for trial purposes, in accordance with the recommendations of the 1975 Revision Conference and resolution WHA29.35 (9) of the 1976 World Health Assembly. Since that time, research and development on the classification had followed a number of paths.

The major definitions of the three elements—impairment, disability and handicap—had undoubtedly been instrumental in changing attitudes to disablement. The definition of impairment, an area where there was considerable overlap with the terms included in the ICD, had been widely accepted. The definition of disability broadly matched the field of action of rehabilitation professionals and groups, although there was felt to be a need for more attention in the associated code to the gradation of severity, which was often a predictor of handicap. There had also been increasing requests to revise the definition of handicap so as to put more emphasis on the effect of interaction with the environment.

The rapid evolution of ideas and practices in the management of disablement had ruled out the production of a revised ICIDH in time to be submitted to the Conference. It was stated that the publication of a new version was unlikely before implementation of the Tenth Revision.

6.5 Procedures in medicine

The International Classification of Procedures in Medicine (ICPM) (*10*) had been published by WHO in 1978 for trial purposes, in accordance with the recommendations of the 1975 Revision Conference and resolution WHA29.35 (*9*) of the 1976 World Health Assembly. The classification had been adopted by a few countries and was used as a basis for national classifications of surgical operations by a number of other countries.

The Heads of WHO Collaborating Centres for Classification of Diseases had recognized that the process of drafting proposals, obtaining comments, redrafting and soliciting further comments, which WHO necessarily had to go through before finalization and publication, was inappropriate in such a rapidly advancing field as that of procedures. The Centre Heads had therefore recommended that there should be no revision of the ICPM in conjunction with the Tenth Revision of the ICD.

In 1987 the Expert Committee had asked that WHO consider updating for the Tenth Revision at least the outline of Chapter 5, "Surgical procedures", of the trial ICPM. In response to this request and the needs expressed by a number of countries, an attempt had been made by the Secretariat to prepare a tabulation list for procedures.

This list had been presented to the Centre Heads at their 1989 meeting and it had been agreed that it could serve as a guide for national presentation or publication of statistics on surgical procedures and could also facilitate intercountry comparisons. The aim of the list was to identify procedures and groups of procedures and define them as a basis for the development of national classifications, thereby improving the comparability of such classifications.

The Conference agreed that such a list was of value and that work should continue on its development, even though any publication would follow the implementation of the Tenth Revision.

6.6 International Nomenclature of Diseases

Since 1970 the Council for International Organizations of Medical Sciences (CIOMS) had been involved in the preparation of an International Nomenclature of Diseases (IND) which would serve as a complement to the ICD.

The main purpose of the IND was to provide a single recommended name for every disease entity. The main criteria for selection of that name were that it should be specific, unambiguous, as self-descriptive and simple as possible, and based on cause wherever feasible. Each disease or syndrome for which a name was recommended was defined as unambiguously, and yet briefly, as possible. A list of synonyms was appended to each definition.

At the time of the Conference, volumes had been published on diseases of the lower respiratory tract, infectious diseases (viral, bacterial and parasitic diseases and mycoses) and cardiac and vascular diseases, and work was under way on volumes for the digestive system, female genital system, urinary and male genital system, metabolic and endocrine diseases, blood and blood-forming organs, immunological system, musculoskeletal system and nervous system. Subjects proposed for future volumes included psychiatric diseases, as well as diseases of the skin, ear, nose and throat, and eye and adnexa.

The Conference recognized that an authoritative, up-to-date and international nomenclature of diseases was important in developing the ICD and improving the comparability of health information. The Conference therefore

> RECOMMENDED that WHO and CIOMS be encouraged to explore cost-efficient ways to achieve the timely completion and maintenance of such a nomenclature.

7. Implementation of the Tenth Revision of the ICD

The Conference was informed of WHO's intention to publish the detailed four-character version of the Tenth Revision in three volumes: one containing the Tabular List, a second containing all related definitions, standards, rules and instructions, and a third containing the Alphabetical Index.

The Conference was further informed that a three-character version of the Tenth Revision would be published as a single volume which would contain, in the Tabular List, all inclusion and exclusion notes. It would also contain all related definitions, standards, rules and instructions and a shortened Alphabetical Index.

Member States intending to produce national language versions of the Tenth Revision should notify WHO of their intentions. Copies of the drafts of the ICD at the three- and four-character levels would be made available from WHO both in printed form and on electronic media.

With respect to the physical appearance of the pages and type formats for both the Tabular List and the Alphabetical Index, the Conference was assured that recommendations from the Centre Heads and complaints from coders would be considered, and every attempt made to improve those aspects as compared with the Ninth Revision.

As with the Ninth Revision, it was intended to develop materials for the reorientation of trained coders, with the help of the Collaborating Centres. The actual training courses would be the responsibility of the WHO regional offices and individual countries. They would be carried out from late 1991 to the end of 1992, to finish before the implementation of the Tenth Revision.

Materials for the basic training of new users of the ICD would also be developed by WHO; it was not, however, planned to begin courses before 1993.

As noted above, WHO would be prepared to provide the Tenth Revision (both the Tabular List and the Alphabetical Index) on electronic media. In future, with the assistance of the Collaborating Centres, other software might also be made available. A key for conversion from the Ninth to the Tenth Revision, and the reverse, should be available before the implementation of the Tenth Revision.

As the development activities that had been endorsed by the Expert Committee were on schedule, the Conference

> RECOMMENDED that the Tenth Revision of the International Classification of Diseases should come into effect as from 1 January 1993.

8. Future revision of the ICD

The Conference discussed the difficulties experienced during the extended period of use of the Ninth Revision, related to the emergence of new diseases and the lack of an updating mechanism to accommodate them.

Various suggestions for mechanisms to overcome these difficulties and avoid similar problems with respect to the Tenth Revision were discussed. There was a clear feeling that there was a need for ongoing information exchange to standardize the use of the Tenth Revision between countries, but that any changes introduced during its "lifetime" should be considered very carefully in relation to their impact on analyses and trends. There was discussion on the type of forum in which such changes and the potential for use of the vacant letter "U" in new or temporary code assignments could be discussed. It was agreed that it would not be feasible to hold revision conferences more frequently than every 10 years.

On the basis of the needs expressed, and the fact that it would be inappropriate to attempt to determine or define the exact process to be used, the Conference

> RECOMMENDED that the next International Revision Conference should take place in ten years' time, and that WHO should endorse the concept of an updating process between revisions and give consideration as to how an effective updating mechanism could be put in place.

9. Adoption of the Tenth Revision of the ICD

The Conference made the following recommendation:

Having considered the proposals prepared by the Organization on the basis of the recommendations of the Expert Committee on the International Classification of Diseases—Tenth Revision,

Recognizing the need for a few further minor modifications to reflect the comments on points of detail submitted by Member States during the Conference,

> RECOMMENDED that the proposed revised chapters, with their

27

three-character categories and four-character subcategories and the Short Tabulation Lists for Morbidity and Mortality, constitute the Tenth Revision of the International Statistical Classification of Diseases and Related Health Problems.

References

1. *International Classification of Diseases, 1975 Revision*, Volume 1. Geneva, World Health Organization, 1977, pp. xiii-xxiv.
2. *Report of the Expert Committee on the International Classification of Diseases—10th Revision: First Meeting.* Geneva, World Health Organization, 1984 (unpublished document DES/EC/ICD-10/84.34).
3. *Report of the Expert Committee on the International Classification of Diseases—10th Revision: Second Meeting.* Geneva, World Health Organization. 1987 (unpublished document WHO/DES/EC/ICD-10/87.38).
4. *Report of the Preparatory Meeting on ICD-10.* Geneva, World Health Organization, 1983 (unpublished document DES/ICD-10/83.19).
5. *Lay reporting of health information.* Geneva, World Health Organization, 1978.
6. *International Conference on Health Statistics for the Year 2000.* Budapest, Statistical Publishing House, 1984.
7. *Report of the Consultation on Primary Care Classifications.* Geneva, World Health Organization, 1985 (unpublished document DES/PHC/85.7).
8. *International Classification of Impairments, Disabilities, and Handicaps.* Geneva, World Health Organization, 1980.
9. *WHO Official Records*, No. 233, 1976, p. 18.
10. *International Classification of Procedures in Medicine.* Geneva, World Health Organization, 1978.

List of
three-character
categories

Chapter I
Certain infectious and parasitic diseases
(A00–B99)

Intestinal infectious diseases (A00–A09)

A00	Cholera
A01	Typhoid and paratyphoid fevers
A02	Other salmonella infections
A03	Shigellosis
A04	Other bacterial intestinal infections
A05	Other bacterial foodborne intoxications
A06	Amoebiasis
A07	Other protozoal intestinal diseases
A08	Viral and other specified intestinal infections
A09	Diarrhoea and gastroenteritis of presumed infectious origin

Tuberculosis (A15–A19)

A15	Respiratory tuberculosis, bacteriologically and histologically confirmed
A16	Respiratory tuberculosis, not confirmed bacteriologically or histologically
A17†	Tuberculosis of nervous system
A18	Tuberculosis of other organs
A19	Miliary tuberculosis

Certain zoonotic bacterial diseases (A20–A28)

A20	Plague
A21	Tularaemia
A22	Anthrax
A23	Brucellosis
A24	Glanders and melioidosis
A25	Rat-bite fevers
A26	Erysipeloid
A27	Leptospirosis
A28	Other zoonotic bacterial diseases, not elsewhere classified

Other bacterial diseases (A30–A49)

A30	Leprosy [Hansen's disease]
A31	Infection due to other mycobacteria
A32	Listeriosis
A33	Tetanus neonatorum

A34   Obstetrical tetanus
A35   Other tetanus
A36   Diphtheria
A37   Whooping cough
A38   Scarlet fever
A39   Meningococcal infection
A40   Streptococcal septicaemia
A41   Other septicaemia
A42   Actinomycosis
A43   Nocardiosis
A44   Bartonellosis
A46   Erysipelas
A48   Other bacterial diseases, not elsewhere classified
A49   Bacterial infection of unspecified site

Infections with a predominantly sexual mode of transmission (A50–A64)

A50   Congenital syphilis
A51   Early syphilis
A52   Late syphilis
A53   Other and unspecified syphilis
A54   Gonococcal infection
A55   Chlamydial lymphogranuloma (venereum)
A56   Other sexually transmitted chlamydial diseases
A57   Chancroid
A58   Granuloma inguinale
A59   Trichomoniasis
A60   Anogenital herpesviral [herpes simplex] infections
A63   Other predominantly sexually transmitted diseases, not elsewhere classified
A64   Unspecified sexually transmitted disease

Other spirochaetal diseases (A65–A69)

A65   Nonvenereal syphilis
A66   Yaws
A67   Pinta [carate]
A68   Relapsing fevers
A69   Other spirochaetal infections

Other diseases caused by chlamydiae (A70–A74)

A70   *Chlamydia psittaci* infection
A71   Trachoma
A74   Other diseases caused by chlamydiae

Rickettsioses (A75–A79)

A75   Typhus fever
A77   Spotted fever [tick-borne rickettsioses]
A78   Q fever
A79   Other rickettsioses

Viral infections of the central nervous system (A80–A89)

A80   Acute poliomyelitis
A81   Slow virus infections of central nervous system
A82   Rabies
A83   Mosquito-borne viral encephalitis
A84   Tick-borne viral encephalitis
A85   Other viral encephalitis, not elsewhere classified
A86   Unspecified viral encephalitis
A87   Viral meningitis
A88   Other viral infections of central nervous system, not elsewhere classified
A89   Unspecified viral infection of central nervous system

Arthropod-borne viral fevers and viral haemorrhagic fevers (A90–A99)

A90   Dengue fever [classical dengue]
A91   Dengue haemorrhagic fever
A92   Other mosquito-borne viral fevers
A93   Other arthropod-borne viral fevers, not elsewhere classified
A94   Unspecified arthropod-borne viral fever
A95   Yellow fever
A96   Arenaviral haemorrhagic fever
A98   Other viral haemorrhagic fevers, not elsewhere classified
A99   Unspecified viral haemorrhagic fever

Viral infections characterized by skin and mucous membrane lesions (B00–B09)

B00   Herpesviral [herpes simplex] infections
B01   Varicella [chickenpox]
B02   Zoster [herpes zoster]
B03   Smallpox
B04   Monkeypox
B05   Measles
B06   Rubella [German measles]
B07   Viral warts
B08   Other viral infections characterized by skin and mucous membrane lesions, not elsewhere classified
B09   Unspecified viral infection characterized by skin and mucous membrane lesions

Viral hepatitis (B15–B19)
B15	Acute hepatitis A
B16	Acute hepatitis B
B17	Other acute viral hepatitis
B18	Chronic viral hepatitis
B19	Unspecified viral hepatitis

Human immunodeficiency virus [HIV] disease (B20–B24)
B20	Human immunodeficiency virus [HIV] disease resulting in infectious and parasitic diseases
B21	Human immunodeficiency virus [HIV] disease resulting in malignant neoplasms
B22	Human immunodeficiency virus [HIV] disease resulting in other specified diseases
B23	Human immunodeficiency virus [HIV] disease resulting in other conditions
B24	Unspecified human immunodeficiency virus [HIV] disease

Other viral diseases (B25–B34)
B25	Cytomegaloviral disease
B26	Mumps
B27	Infectious mononucleosis
B30	Viral conjunctivitis
B33	Other viral diseases, not elsewhere classified
B34	Viral infection of unspecified site

Mycoses (B35–B49)
B35	Dermatophytosis
B36	Other superficial mycoses
B37	Candidiasis
B38	Coccidioidomycosis
B39	Histoplasmosis
B40	Blastomycosis
B41	Paracoccidioidomycosis
B42	Sporotrichosis
B43	Chromomycosis and phaeomycotic abscess
B44	Aspergillosis
B45	Cryptococcosis
B46	Zygomycosis
B47	Mycetoma
B48	Other mycoses, not elsewhere classified
B49	Unspecified mycosis

Protozoal diseases (B50–B64)

B50	*Plasmodium falciparum* malaria
B51	*Plasmodium vivax* malaria
B52	*Plasmodium malariae* malaria
B53	Other parasitologically confirmed malaria
B54	Unspecified malaria
B55	Leishmaniasis
B56	African trypanosomiasis
B57	Chagas' disease
B58	Toxoplasmosis
B59	Pneumocystosis
B60	Other protozoal diseases, not elsewhere classified
B64	Unspecified protozoal disease

Helminthiases (B65–B83)

B65	Schistosomiasis [bilharziasis]
B66	Other fluke infections
B67	Echinococcosis
B68	Taeniasis
B69	Cysticercosis
B70	Diphyllobothriasis and sparganosis
B71	Other cestode infections
B72	Dracunculiasis
B73	Onchocerciasis
B74	Filariasis
B75	Trichinellosis
B76	Hookworm diseases
B77	Ascariasis
B78	Strongyloidiasis
B79	Trichuriasis
B80	Enterobiasis
B81	Other intestinal helminthiases, not elsewhere classified
B82	Unspecified intestinal parasitism
B83	Other helminthiases

Pediculosis, acariasis and other infestations (B85–B89)

B85	Pediculosis and phthiriasis
B86	Scabies
B87	Myiasis
B88	Other infestations
B89	Unspecified parasitic disease

Sequelae of infectious and parasitic diseases (B90–B94)

B90   Sequelae of tuberculosis

B91   Sequelae of poliomyelitis

B92   Sequelae of leprosy

B94   Sequelae of other and unspecified infectious and parasitic diseases

Bacterial, viral and other infectious agents (B95–B97)

B95   Streptococcus and staphylococcus as the cause of diseases classified to other chapters

B96   Other bacterial agents as the cause of diseases classified to other chapters

B97   Viral agents as the cause of diseases classified to other chapters

Other infectious diseases (B99)

B99   Other and unspecified infectious diseases

Chapter II
Neoplasms
(C00–D48)

Malignant neoplasms (C00–C97)

Malignant neoplasms of lip, oral cavity and pharynx (C00–C14)

C00   Malignant neoplasm of lip

C01   Malignant neoplasm of base of tongue

C02   Malignant neoplasm of other and unspecified parts of tongue

C03   Malignant neoplasm of gum

C04   Malignant neoplasm of floor of mouth

C05   Malignant neoplasm of palate

C06   Malignant neoplasm of other and unspecified parts of mouth

C07   Malignant neoplasm of parotid gland

C08   Malignant neoplasm of other and unspecified major salivary glands

C09   Malignant neoplasm of tonsil

C10   Malignant neoplasm of oropharynx

C11   Malignant neoplasm of nasopharynx

C12   Malignant neoplasm of pyriform sinus

C13   Malignant neoplasm of hypopharynx

C14   Malignant neoplasm of other and ill-defined sites in the lip, oral cavity and pharynx

Malignant neoplasms of digestive organs (C15–C26)

C15   Malignant neoplasm of oesophagus

C16   Malignant neoplasm of stomach

C17   Malignant neoplasm of small intestine

C18   Malignant neoplasm of colon

C19   Malignant neoplasm of rectosigmoid junction

C20   Malignant neoplasm of rectum

C21   Malignant neoplasm of anus and anal canal

C22   Malignant neoplasm of liver and intrahepatic bile ducts

C23   Malignant neoplasm of gallbladder

C24   Malignant neoplasm of other and unspecified parts of biliary tract

C25   Malignant neoplasm of pancreas

C26   Malignant neoplasm of other and ill-defined digestive organs

Malignant neoplasms of respiratory and intrathoracic organs (C30–C39)

C30   Malignant neoplasm of nasal cavity and middle ear

C31   Malignant neoplasm of accessory sinuses

C32   Malignant neoplasm of larynx

C33   Malignant neoplasm of trachea

C34   Malignant neoplasm of bronchus and lung

C37   Malignant neoplasm of thymus

C38   Malignant neoplasm of heart, mediastinum and pleura

C39   Malignant neoplasm of other and ill-defined sites in the respiratory system and intrathoracic organs

Malignant neoplasms of bone and articular cartilage (C40–C41)

C40   Malignant neoplasm of bone and articular cartilage of limbs

C41   Malignant neoplasm of bone and articular cartilage of other and unspecified sites

Melanoma and other malignant neoplasms of skin (C43–C44)

C43   Malignant melanoma of skin

C44   Other malignant neoplasms of skin

Malignant neoplasms of mesothelial and soft tissue (C45–C49)

C45   Mesothelioma

C46   Kaposi's sarcoma

C47   Malignant neoplasm of peripheral nerves and autonomic nervous system

C48   Malignant neoplasm of retroperitoneum and peritoneum

C49   Malignant neoplasm of other connective and soft tissue

Malignant neoplasm of breast (C50)

C50   Malignant neoplasm of breast

Malignant neoplasms of female genital organs (C51–C58)

C51   Malignant neoplasm of vulva

C52   Malignant neoplasm of vagina

C53   Malignant neoplasm of cervix uteri

C54   Malignant neoplasm of corpus uteri

C55   Malignant neoplasm of uterus, part unspecified

C56   Malignant neoplasm of ovary

C57   Malignant neoplasm of other and unspecified female genital organs

C58   Malignant neoplasm of placenta

Malignant neoplasms of male genital organs (C60–C63)

C60   Malignant neoplasm of penis

C61   Malignant neoplasm of prostate

C62   Malignant neoplasm of testis

C63   Malignant neoplasm of other and unspecified male genital organs

Malignant neoplasms of urinary tract (C64–C68)

C64   Malignant neoplasm of kidney, except renal pelvis

C65   Malignant neoplasm of renal pelvis

C66   Malignant neoplasm of ureter

C67   Malignant neoplasm of bladder

C68   Malignant neoplasm of other and unspecified urinary organs

Malignant neoplasms of eye, brain and other parts of central nervous system (C69–C72)

C69   Malignant neoplasm of eye and adnexa

C70   Malignant neoplasm of meninges

C71   Malignant neoplasm of brain

C72   Malignant neoplasm of spinal cord, cranial nerves and other parts of central nervous system

Malignant neoplasms of thyroid and other endocrine glands (C73–C75)
C73   Malignant neoplasm of thyroid gland
C74   Malignant neoplasm of adrenal gland
C75   Malignant neoplasm of other endocrine glands and related structures

Malignant neoplasms of ill-defined, secondary and unspecified sites (C76–C80)
C76   Malignant neoplasm of other and ill-defined sites
C77   Secondary and unspecified malignant neoplasm of lymph nodes
C78   Secondary malignant neoplasm of respiratory and digestive organs
C79   Secondary malignant neoplasm of other sites
C80   Malignant neoplasm without specification of site

Malignant neoplasms of lymphoid, haematopoietic and related tissue (C81–C96)
C81   Hodgkin's disease
C82   Follicular [nodular] non-Hodgkin's lymphoma
C83   Diffuse non-Hodgkin's lymphoma
C84   Peripheral and cutaneous T-cell lymphomas
C85   Other and unspecified types of non-Hodgkin's lymphoma
C88   Malignant immunoproliferative diseases
C90   Multiple myeloma and malignant plasma cell neoplasms
C91   Lymphoid leukaemia
C92   Myeloid leukaemia
C93   Monocytic leukaemia
C94   Other leukaemias of specified cell type
C95   Leukaemia of unspecified cell type
C96   Other and unspecified malignant neoplasms of lymphoid, haematopoietic and related tissue

Malignant neoplasms of independent (primary) multiple sites (C97)
C97   Malignant neoplasms of independent (primary) multiple sites

In situ neoplasms (D00–D09)
D00   Carcinoma in situ of oral cavity, oesophagus and stomach
D01   Carcinoma in situ of other and unspecified digestive organs
D02   Carcinoma in situ of middle ear and respiratory system
D03   Melanoma in situ
D04   Carcinoma in situ of skin
D05   Carcinoma in situ of breast

D06	Carcinoma in situ of cervix uteri
D07	Carcinoma in situ of other and unspecified genital organs
D09	Carcinoma in situ of other and unspecified sites

Benign neoplasms (D10–D36)

D10	Benign neoplasm of mouth and pharynx
D11	Benign neoplasm of major salivary glands
D12	Benign neoplasm of colon, rectum, anus and anal canal
D13	Benign neoplasm of other and ill-defined parts of digestive system
D14	Benign neoplasm of middle ear and respiratory system
D15	Benign neoplasm of other and unspecified intrathoracic organs
D16	Benign neoplasm of bone and articular cartilage
D17	Benign lipomatous neoplasm
D18	Haemangioma and lymphangioma, any site
D19	Benign neoplasm of mesothelial tissue
D20	Benign neoplasm of soft tissue of retroperitoneum and peritoneum
D21	Other benign neoplasms of connective and other soft tissue
D22	Melanocytic naevi
D23	Other benign neoplasms of skin
D24	Benign neoplasm of breast
D25	Leiomyoma of uterus
D26	Other benign neoplasms of uterus
D27	Benign neoplasm of ovary
D28	Benign neoplasm of other and unspecified female genital organs
D29	Benign neoplasm of male genital organs
D30	Benign neoplasm of urinary organs
D31	Benign neoplasm of eye and adnexa
D32	Benign neoplasm of meninges
D33	Benign neoplasm of brain and other parts of central nervous system
D34	Benign neoplasm of thyroid gland
D35	Benign neoplasm of other and unspecified endocrine glands
D36	Benign neoplasm of other and unspecified sites

Neoplasms of uncertain or unknown behaviour (D37–D48)

D37	Neoplasm of uncertain or unknown behaviour of oral cavity and digestive organs
D38	Neoplasm of uncertain or unknown behaviour of middle ear and respiratory and intrathoracic organs
D39	Neoplasm of uncertain or unknown behaviour of female genital organs

D40   Neoplasm of uncertain or unknown behaviour of male genital organs

D41   Neoplasm of uncertain or unknown behaviour of urinary organs

D42   Neoplasm of uncertain or unknown behaviour of meninges

D43   Neoplasm of uncertain or unknown behaviour of brain and central nervous system

D44   Neoplasm of uncertain or unknown behaviour of endocrine glands

D45   Polycythaemia vera

D46   Myelodysplastic syndromes

D47   Other neoplasms of uncertain or unknown behaviour of lymphoid, haematopoietic and related tissue

D48   Neoplasm of uncertain or unknown behaviour of other and unspecified sites

Chapter III
Diseases of the blood and blood-forming organs and certain disorders involving the immune mechanism
(D50–D89)

Nutritional anaemias (D50–D53)

D50   Iron deficiency anaemia

D51   Vitamin B_{12} deficiency anaemia

D52   Folate deficiency anaemia

D53   Other nutritional anaemias

Haemolytic anaemias (D55–D59)

D55   Anaemia due to enzyme disorders

D56   Thalassaemia

D57   Sickle-cell disorders

D58   Other hereditary haemolytic anaemias

D59   Acquired haemolytic anaemia

Aplastic and other anaemias (D60–D64)

D60   Acquired pure red cell aplasia [erythroblastopenia]

D61   Other aplastic anaemias

D62   Acute posthaemorrhagic anaemia

D63*   Anaemia in chronic diseases classified elsewhere

D64   Other anaemias

Coagulation defects, purpura and other haemorrhagic conditions (D65–D69)

D65   Disseminated intravascular coagulation [defibrination syndrome]
D66   Hereditary factor VIII deficiency
D67   Hereditary factor IX deficiency
D68   Other coagulation defects
D69   Purpura and other haemorrhagic conditions

Other diseases of blood and blood-forming organs (D70–D77)

D70   Agranulocytosis
D71   Functional disorders of polymorphonuclear neutrophils
D72   Other disorders of white blood cells
D73   Diseases of spleen
D74   Methaemoglobinaemia
D75   Other diseases of blood and blood-forming organs
D76   Certain diseases involving lymphoreticular tissue and reticulohistiocytic system
D77*   Other disorders of blood and blood-forming organs in diseases classified elsewhere

Certain disorders involving the immune mechanism (D80–D89)

D80   Immunodeficiency with predominantly antibody defects
D81   Combined immunodeficiencies
D82   Immunodeficiency associated with other major defects
D83   Common variable immunodeficiency
D84   Other immunodeficiencies
D86   Sarcoidosis
D89   Other disorders involving the immune mechanism, not elsewhere classified

Chapter IV
Endocrine, nutritional and metabolic diseases
(E00–E90)

Disorders of thyroid gland (E00–E07)

E00   Congenital iodine-deficiency syndrome
E01   Iodine-deficiency-related thyroid disorders and allied conditions
E02   Subclinical iodine-deficiency hypothyroidism
E03   Other hypothyroidism
E04   Other nontoxic goitre

E05   Thyrotoxicosis [hyperthyroidism]
E06   Thyroiditis
E07   Other disorders of thyroid

Diabetes mellitus (E10–E14)
E10   Insulin-dependent diabetes mellitus
E11   Non-insulin-dependent diabetes mellitus
E12   Malnutrition-related diabetes mellitus
E13   Other specified diabetes mellitus
E14   Unspecified diabetes mellitus

Other disorders of glucose regulation and pancreatic internal secretion (E15–E16)
E15   Nondiabetic hypoglycaemic coma
E16   Other disorders of pancreatic internal secretion

Disorders of other endocrine glands (E20–E35)
E20   Hypoparathyroidism
E21   Hyperparathyroidism and other disorders of parathyroid gland
E22   Hyperfunction of pituitary gland
E23   Hypofunction and other disorders of pituitary gland
E24   Cushing's syndrome
E25   Adrenogenital disorders
E26   Hyperaldosteronism
E27   Other disorders of adrenal gland
E28   Ovarian dysfunction
E29   Testicular dysfunction
E30   Disorders of puberty, not elsewhere classified
E31   Polyglandular dysfunction
E32   Diseases of thymus
E34   Other endocrine disorders
E35*   Disorders of endocrine glands in diseases classified elsewhere

Malnutrition (E40–E46)
E40   Kwashiorkor
E41   Nutritional marasmus
E42   Marasmic kwashiorkor
E43   Unspecified severe protein-energy malnutrition
E44   Protein-energy malnutrition of moderate and mild degree
E45   Retarded development following protein-energy malnutrition
E46   Unspecified protein-energy malnutrition

Other nutritional deficiencies (E50–E64)

E50	Vitamin A deficiency
E51	Thiamine deficiency
E52	Niacin deficiency [pellagra]
E53	Deficiency of other B group vitamins
E54	Ascorbic acid deficiency
E55	Vitamin D deficiency
E56	Other vitamin deficiencies
E58	Dietary calcium deficiency
E59	Dietary selenium deficiency
E60	Dietary zinc deficiency
E61	Deficiency of other nutrient elements
E63	Other nutritional deficiencies
E64	Sequelae of malnutrition and other nutritional deficiencies

Obesity and other hyperalimentation (E65–E68)

E65	Localized adiposity
E66	Obesity
E67	Other hyperalimentation
E68	Sequelae of hyperalimentation

Metabolic disorders (E70–E90)

E70	Disorders of aromatic amino-acid metabolism
E71	Disorders of branched-chain amino-acid metabolism and fatty-acid metabolism
E72	Other disorders of amino-acid metabolism
E73	Lactose intolerance
E74	Other disorders of carbohydrate metabolism
E75	Disorders of sphingolipid metabolism and other lipid storage disorders
E76	Disorders of glycosaminoglycan metabolism
E77	Disorders of glycoprotein metabolism
E78	Disorders of lipoprotein metabolism and other lipidaemias
E79	Disorders of purine and pyrimidine metabolism
E80	Disorders of porphyrin and bilirubin metabolism
E83	Disorders of mineral metabolism
E84	Cystic fibrosis
E85	Amyloidosis
E86	Volume depletion
E87	Other disorders of fluid, electrolyte and acid–base balance
E88	Other metabolic disorders
E89	Postprocedural endocrine and metabolic disorders, not elsewhere classified

E90*   Nutritional and metabolic disorders in diseases classified
        elsewhere

Chapter V
Mental and behavioural disorders
(F00–F99)

Organic, including symptomatic, mental disorders (F00–F09)

F00*   Dementia in Alzheimer's disease
F01   Vascular dementia
F02*   Dementia in other diseases classified elsewhere
F03   Unspecified dementia
F04   Organic amnesic syndrome, not induced by alcohol and other
        psychoactive substances
F05   Delirium, not induced by alcohol and other psychoactive
        substances
F06   Other mental disorders due to brain damage and dysfunction
        and to physical disease
F07   Personality and behavioural disorders due to brain disease,
        damage and dysfunction
F09   Unspecified organic or symptomatic mental disorder

Mental and behavioural disorders due to psychoactive substance use (F10–F19)

F10   Mental and behavioural disorders due to use of alcohol
F11   Mental and behavioural disorders due to use of opioids
F12   Mental and behavioural disorders due to use of cannabinoids
F13   Mental and behavioural disorders due to use of sedatives or
        hypnotics
F14   Mental and behavioural disorders due to use of cocaine
F15   Mental and behavioural disorders due to use of other stimulants,
        including caffeine
F16   Mental and behavioural disorders due to use of hallucinogens
F17   Mental and behavioural disorders due to use of tobacco
F18   Mental and behavioural disorders due to use of volatile solvents
F19   Mental and behavioural disorders due to multiple drug use and
        use of other psychoactive substances

Schizophrenia, schizotypal and delusional disorders (F20–F29)

F20   Schizophrenia

F21	Schizotypal disorder
F22	Persistent delusional disorders
F23	Acute and transient psychotic disorders
F24	Induced delusional disorder
F25	Schizoaffective disorders
F28	Other nonorganic psychotic disorders
F29	Unspecified nonorganic psychosis

Mood [affective] disorders (F30–F39)

F30	Manic episode
F31	Bipolar affective disorder
F32	Depressive episode
F33	Recurrent depressive disorder
F34	Persistent mood [affective] disorders
F38	Other mood [affective] disorders
F39	Unspecified mood [affective] disorder

Neurotic, stress-related and somatoform disorders (F40–F48)

F40	Phobic anxiety disorders
F41	Other anxiety disorders
F42	Obsessive–compulsive disorder
F43	Reaction to severe stress, and adjustment disorders
F44	Dissociative [conversion] disorders
F45	Somatoform disorders
F48	Other neurotic disorders

Behavioural syndromes associated with physiological disturbances and physical factors (F50–F59)

F50	Eating disorders
F51	Nonorganic sleep disorders
F52	Sexual dysfunction, not caused by organic disorder or disease
F53	Mental and behavioural disorders associated with the puerperium, not elsewhere classified
F54	Psychological and behavioural factors associated with disorders or diseases classified elsewhere
F55	Abuse of non-dependence-producing substances
F59	Unspecified behavioural syndromes associated with physiological disturbances and physical factors

Disorders of adult personality and behaviour (F60–F69)

| F60 | Specific personality disorders |
| F61 | Mixed and other personality disorders |

F62	Enduring personality changes, not attributable to brain damage and disease
F63	Habit and impulse disorders
F64	Gender identity disorders
F65	Disorders of sexual preference
F66	Psychological and behavioural disorders associated with sexual development and orientation
F68	Other disorders of adult personality and behaviour
F69	Unspecified disorder of adult personality and behaviour

Mental retardation (F70–F79)

F70	Mild mental retardation
F71	Moderate mental retardation
F72	Severe mental retardation
F73	Profound mental retardation
F78	Other mental retardation
F79	Unspecified mental retardation

Disorders of psychological development (F80–F89)

F80	Specific developmental disorders of speech and language
F81	Specific developmental disorders of scholastic skills
F82	Specific developmental disorder of motor function
F83	Mixed specific developmental disorders
F84	Pervasive developmental disorders
F88	Other disorders of psychological development
F89	Unspecified disorder of psychological development

Behavioural and emotional disorders with onset usually occurring in childhood and adolescence (F90–F98)

F90	Hyperkinetic disorders
F91	Conduct disorders
F92	Mixed disorders of conduct and emotions
F93	Emotional disorders with onset specific to childhood
F94	Disorders of social functioning with onset specific to childhood and adolescence
F95	Tic disorders
F98	Other behavioural and emotional disorders with onset usually occurring in childhood and adolescence

Unspecified mental disorder (F99)

F99	Mental disorder, not otherwise specified

Chapter VI
Diseases of the nervous system
(G00–G99)

Inflammatory diseases of the central nervous system (G00–G09)

G00 Bacterial meningitis, not elsewhere classified
G01* Meningitis in bacterial diseases classified elsewhere
G02* Meningitis in other infectious and parasitic diseases classified elsewhere
G03 Meningitis due to other and unspecified causes
G04 Encephalitis, myelitis and encephalomyelitis
G05* Encephalitis, myelitis and encephalomyelitis in diseases classified elsewhere
G06 Intracranial and intraspinal abscess and granuloma
G07* Intracranial and intraspinal abscess and granuloma in diseases classified elsewhere
G08 Intracranial and intraspinal phlebitis and thrombophlebitis
G09 Sequelae of inflammatory diseases of central nervous system

Systemic atrophies primarily affecting the central nervous system (G10–G13)

G10 Huntington's disease
G11 Hereditary ataxia
G12 Spinal muscular atrophy and related syndromes
G13* Systemic atrophies primarily affecting central nervous system in diseases classified elsewhere

Extrapyramidal and movement disorders (G20–G26)

G20 Parkinson's disease
G21 Secondary parkinsonism
G22* Parkinsonism in diseases classified elsewhere
G23 Other degenerative diseases of basal ganglia
G24 Dystonia
G25 Other extrapyramidal and movement disorders
G26* Extrapyramidal and movement disorders in diseases classified elsewhere

Other degenerative diseases of the nervous system (G30–G32)

G30 Alzheimer's disease
G31 Other degenerative diseases of nervous system, not elsewhere classified
G32* Other degenerative disorders of nervous system in diseases classified elsewhere

Demyelinating diseases of the central nervous system (G35–G37)

G35   Multiple sclerosis
G36   Other acute disseminated demyelination
G37   Other demyelinating diseases of central nervous system

Episodic and paroxysmal disorders (G40–G47)

G40   Epilepsy
G41   Status epilepticus
G43   Migraine
G44   Other headache syndromes
G45   Transient cerebral ischaemic attacks and related syndromes
G46*   Vascular syndromes of brain in cerebrovascular diseases
G47   Sleep disorders

Nerve, nerve root and plexus disorders (G50–G59)

G50   Disorders of trigeminal nerve
G51   Facial nerve disorders
G52   Disorders of other cranial nerves
G53*   Cranial nerve disorders in diseases classified elsewhere
G54   Nerve root and plexus disorders
G55*   Nerve root and plexus compressions in diseases classified elsewhere
G56   Mononeuropathies of upper limb
G57   Mononeuropathies of lower limb
G58   Other mononeuropathies
G59*   Mononeuropathy in diseases classified elsewhere

Polyneuropathies and other disorders of the peripheral nervous system (G60–G64)

G60   Hereditary and idiopathic neuropathy
G61   Inflammatory polyneuropathy
G62   Other polyneuropathies
G63*   Polyneuropathy in diseases classified elsewhere
G64   Other disorders of peripheral nervous system

Diseases of myoneural junction and muscle (G70–G73)

G70   Myasthenia gravis and other myoneural disorders
G71   Primary disorders of muscles
G72   Other myopathies
G73*   Disorders of myoneural junction and muscle in diseases classified elsewhere

Cerebral palsy and other paralytic syndromes (G80–G83)

G80   Infantile cerebral palsy
G81   Hemiplegia
G82   Paraplegia and tetraplegia
G83   Other paralytic syndromes

Other disorders of the nervous system (G90–G99)

G90   Disorders of autonomic nervous system
G91   Hydrocephalus
G92   Toxic encephalopathy
G93   Other disorders of brain
G94*   Other disorders of brain in diseases classified elsewhere
G95   Other diseases of spinal cord
G96   Other disorders of central nervous system
G97   Postprocedural disorders of nervous system, not elsewhere
        classified
G98   Other disorders of nervous system, not elsewhere classified
G99*   Other disorders of nervous system in diseases classified elsewhere

Chapter VII
Diseases of the eye and adnexa
(H00–H59)

Disorders of eyelid, lacrimal system and orbit (H00–H06)

H00   Hordeolum and chalazion
H01   Other inflammation of eyelid
H02   Other disorders of eyelid
H03*   Disorders of eyelid in diseases classified elsewhere
H04   Disorders of lacrimal system
H05   Disorders of orbit
H06*   Disorders of lacrimal system and orbit in diseases classified
        elsewhere

Disorders of conjunctiva (H10–H13)

H10   Conjunctivitis
H11   Other disorders of conjunctiva
H13*   Disorders of conjunctiva in diseases classified elsewhere

Disorders of sclera, cornea, iris and ciliary body (H15–H22)

H15	Disorders of sclera
H16	Keratitis
H17	Corneal scars and opacities
H18	Other disorders of cornea
H19*	Disorders of sclera and cornea in diseases classified elsewhere
H20	Iridocyclitis
H21	Other disorders of iris and ciliary body
H22*	Disorders of iris and ciliary body in diseases classified elsewhere

Disorders of lens (H25–H28)

H25	Senile cataract
H26	Other cataract
H27	Other disorders of lens
H28*	Cataract and other disorders of lens in diseases classified elsewhere

Disorders of choroid and retina (H30–H36)

H30	Chorioretinal inflammation
H31	Other disorders of choroid
H32*	Chorioretinal disorders in diseases classified elsewhere
H33	Retinal detachments and breaks
H34	Retinal vascular occlusions
H35	Other retinal disorders
H36*	Retinal disorders in diseases classified elsewhere

Glaucoma (H40–H42)

H40	Glaucoma
H42*	Glaucoma in diseases classified elsewhere

Disorders of vitreous body and globe (H43–H45)

H43	Disorders of vitreous body
H44	Disorders of globe
H45*	Disorders of vitreous body and globe in diseases classified elsewhere

Disorders of optic nerve and visual pathways (H46–H48)

H46	Optic neuritis
H47	Other disorders of optic [2nd] nerve and visual pathways
H48*	Disorders of optic [2nd] nerve and visual pathways in diseases classified elsewhere

Disorders of ocular muscles, binocular movement, accommodation and refraction (H49–H52)
H49   Paralytic strabismus
H50   Other strabismus
H51   Other disorders of binocular movement
H52   Disorders of refraction and accommodation

Visual disturbances and blindness (H53–H54)
H53   Visual disturbances
H54   Blindness and low vision

Other disorders of eye and adnexa (H55–H59)
H55   Nystagmus and other irregular eye movements
H57   Other disorders of eye and adnexa
H58*   Other disorders of eye and adnexa in diseases classified elsewhere
H59   Postprocedural disorders of eye and adnexa, not elsewhere classified

Chapter VIII
Diseases of the ear and mastoid process
(H60–H95)

Diseases of external ear (H60–H62)
H60   Otitis externa
H61   Other disorders of external ear
H62*   Disorders of external ear in diseases classified elsewhere

Diseases of middle ear and mastoid (H65–H75)
H65   Nonsuppurative otitis media
H66   Suppurative and unspecified otitis media
H67*   Otitis media in diseases classified elsewhere
H68   Eustachian salpingitis and obstruction
H69   Other disorders of Eustachian tube
H70   Mastoiditis and related conditions
H71   Cholesteatoma of middle ear
H72   Perforation of tympanic membrane
H73   Other disorders of tympanic membrane
H74   Other disorders of middle ear and mastoid

H75*   Other disorders of middle ear and mastoid in diseases classified
        elsewhere

Diseases of inner ear (H80–H83)
H80   Otosclerosis
H81   Disorders of vestibular function
H82*   Vertiginous syndromes in diseases classified elsewhere
H83   Other diseases of inner ear

Other disorders of ear (H90–H95)
H90   Conductive and sensorineural hearing loss
H91   Other hearing loss
H92   Otalgia and effusion of ear
H93   Other disorders of ear, not elsewhere classified
H94*   Other disorders of ear in diseases classified elsewhere
H95   Postprocedural disorders of ear and mastoid process, not
        elsewhere classified

Chapter IX
Diseases of the circulatory system
(I00–I99)

Acute rheumatic fever (I00–I02)
I00   Rheumatic fever without mention of heart involvement
I01   Rheumatic fever with heart involvement
I02   Rheumatic chorea

Chronic rheumatic heart diseases (I05–I09)
I05   Rheumatic mitral valve diseases
I06   Rheumatic aortic valve diseases
I07   Rheumatic tricuspid valve diseases
I08   Multiple valve diseases
I09   Other rheumatic heart diseases

Hypertensive diseases (I10–I15)
I10   Essential (primary) hypertension
I11   Hypertensive heart disease
I12   Hypertensive renal disease
I13   Hypertensive heart and renal disease
I15   Secondary hypertension

Ischaemic heart diseases (I20–I25)

I20	Angina pectoris
I21	Acute myocardial infarction
I22	Subsequent myocardial infarction
I23	Certain current complications following acute myocardial infarction
I24	Other acute ischaemic heart diseases
I25	Chronic ischaemic heart disease

Pulmonary heart disease and diseases of pulmonary circulation (I26–I28)

I26	Pulmonary embolism
I27	Other pulmonary heart diseases
I28	Other diseases of pulmonary vessels

Other forms of heart disease (I30–I52)

I30	Acute pericarditis
I31	Other diseases of pericardium
I32*	Pericarditis in diseases classified elsewhere
I33	Acute and subacute endocarditis
I34	Nonrheumatic mitral valve disorders
I35	Nonrheumatic aortic valve disorders
I36	Nonrheumatic tricuspid valve disorders
I37	Pulmonary valve disorders
I38	Endocarditis, valve unspecified
I39*	Endocarditis and heart valve disorders in diseases classified elsewhere
I40	Acute myocarditis
I41*	Myocarditis in diseases classified elsewhere
I42	Cardiomyopathy
I43*	Cardiomyopathy in diseases classified elsewhere
I44	Atrioventricular and left bundle-branch block
I45	Other conduction disorders
I46	Cardiac arrest
I47	Paroxysmal tachycardia
I48	Atrial fibrillation and flutter
I49	Other cardiac arrhythmias
I50	Heart failure
I51	Complications and ill-defined descriptions of heart disease
I52*	Other heart disorders in diseases classified elsewhere

Cerebrovascular diseases (I60–I69)

I60   Subarachnoid haemorrhage
I61   Intracerebral haemorrhage
I62   Other nontraumatic intracranial haemorrhage
I63   Cerebral infarction
I64   Stroke, not specified as haemorrhage or infarction
I65   Occlusion and stenosis of precerebral arteries, not resulting in cerebral infarction
I66   Occlusion and stenosis of cerebral arteries, not resulting in cerebral infarction
I67   Other cerebrovascular diseases
I68*   Cerebrovascular disorders in diseases classified elsewhere
I69   Sequelae of cerebrovascular disease

Diseases of arteries, arterioles and capillaries (I70–I79)

I70   Atherosclerosis
I71   Aortic aneurysm and dissection
I72   Other aneurysm
I73   Other peripheral vascular diseases
I74   Arterial embolism and thrombosis
I77   Other disorders of arteries and arterioles
I78   Diseases of capillaries
I79*   Disorders of arteries, arterioles and capillaries in diseases classified elsewhere

Diseases of veins, lymphatic vessels and lymph nodes, not elsewhere classified (I80–I89)

I80   Phlebitis and thrombophlebitis
I81   Portal vein thrombosis
I82   Other venous embolism and thrombosis
I83   Varicose veins of lower extremities
I84   Haemorrhoids
I85   Oesophageal varices
I86   Varicose veins of other sites
I87   Other disorders of veins
I88   Nonspecific lymphadenitis
I89   Other noninfective disorders of lymphatic vessels and lymph nodes

Other and unspecified disorders of the circulatory system (I95–I99)

I95   Hypotension
I97   Postprocedural disorders of circulatory system, not elsewhere classified

I98*   Other disorders of circulatory system in diseases classified elsewhere

I99   Other and unspecified disorders of circulatory system

Chapter X
Diseases of the respiratory system
(J00–J99)

Acute upper respiratory infections (J00–J06)

J00   Acute nasopharyngitis [common cold]

J01   Acute sinusitis

J02   Acute pharyngitis

J03   Acute tonsillitis

J04   Acute laryngitis and tracheitis

J05   Acute obstructive laryngitis [croup] and epiglottitis

J06   Acute upper respiratory infections of multiple and unspecified sites

Influenza and pneumonia (J10–J18)

J10   Influenza due to identified influenza virus

J11   Influenza, virus not identified

J12   Viral pneumonia, not elsewhere classified

J13   Pneumonia due to *Streptococcus pneumoniae*

J14   Pneumonia due to *Haemophilus influenzae*

J15   Bacterial pneumonia, not elsewhere classified

J16   Pneumonia due to other infectious organisms, not elsewhere classified

J17*   Pneumonia in diseases classified elsewhere

J18   Pneumonia, organism unspecified

Other acute lower respiratory infections (J20–J22)

J20   Acute bronchitis

J21   Acute bronchiolitis

J22   Unspecified acute lower respiratory infection

Other diseases of upper respiratory tract (J30–J39)

J30   Vasomotor and allergic rhinitis

J31   Chronic rhinitis, nasopharyngitis and pharyngitis

J32   Chronic sinusitis

J33	Nasal polyp
J34	Other disorders of nose and nasal sinuses
J35	Chronic diseases of tonsils and adenoids
J36	Peritonsillar abscess
J37	Chronic laryngitis and laryngotracheitis
J38	Diseases of vocal cords and larynx, not elsewhere classified
J39	Other diseases of upper respiratory tract

Chronic lower respiratory diseases (J40–J47)

J40	Bronchitis, not specified as acute or chronic
J41	Simple and mucopurulent chronic bronchitis
J42	Unspecified chronic bronchitis
J43	Emphysema
J44	Other chronic obstructive pulmonary disease
J45	Asthma
J46	Status asthmaticus
J47	Bronchiectasis

Lung diseases due to external agents (J60–J70)

J60	Coalworker's pneumoconiosis
J61	Pneumoconiosis due to asbestos and other mineral fibres
J62	Pneumoconiosis due to dust containing silica
J63	Pneumoconiosis due to other inorganic dusts
J64	Unspecified pneumoconiosis
J65	Pneumoconiosis associated with tuberculosis
J66	Airway disease due to specific organic dust
J67	Hypersensitivity pneumonitis due to organic dust
J68	Respiratory conditions due to inhalation of chemicals, gases, fumes and vapours
J69	Pneumonitis due to solids and liquids
J70	Respiratory conditions due to other external agents

Other respiratory diseases principally affecting the interstitium (J80–J84)

J80	Adult respiratory distress syndrome
J81	Pulmonary oedema
J82	Pulmonary eosinophilia, not elsewhere classified
J84	Other interstitial pulmonary diseases

Suppurative and necrotic conditions of lower respiratory tract (J85–J86)

J85	Abscess of lung and mediastinum
J86	Pyothorax

Other diseases of pleura (J90–J94)

J90	Pleural effusion, not elsewhere classified
J91*	Pleural effusion in conditions classified elsewhere
J92	Pleural plaque
J93	Pneumothorax
J94	Other pleural conditions

Other diseases of the respiratory system (J95–J99)

J95	Postprocedural respiratory disorders, not elsewhere classified
J96	Respiratory failure, not elsewhere classified
J98	Other respiratory disorders
J99*	Respiratory disorders in diseases classified elsewhere

Chapter XI
Diseases of the digestive system
(K00–K93)

Diseases of oral cavity, salivary glands and jaws (K00–K14)

K00	Disorders of tooth development and eruption
K01	Embedded and impacted teeth
K02	Dental caries
K03	Other diseases of hard tissues of teeth
K04	Diseases of pulp and periapical tissues
K05	Gingivitis and periodontal diseases
K06	Other disorders of gingiva and edentulous alveolar ridge
K07	Dentofacial anomalies [including malocclusion]
K08	Other disorders of teeth and supporting structures
K09	Cysts of oral region, not elsewhere classified
K10	Other diseases of jaws
K11	Diseases of salivary glands
K12	Stomatitis and related lesions
K13	Other diseases of lip and oral mucosa
K14	Diseases of tongue

Diseases of oesophagus, stomach and duodenum (K20–K31)

K20	Oesophagitis
K21	Gastro-oesophageal reflux disease
K22	Other diseases of oesophagus

K23*   Disorders of oesophagus in diseases classified elsewhere
K25   Gastric ulcer
K26   Duodenal ulcer
K27   Peptic ulcer, site unspecified
K28   Gastrojejunal ulcer
K29   Gastritis and duodenitis
K30   Dyspepsia
K31   Other diseases of stomach and duodenum

Diseases of appendix (K35–K38)
K35   Acute appendicitis
K36   Other appendicitis
K37   Unspecified appendicitis
K38   Other diseases of appendix

Hernia (K40–K46)
K40   Inguinal hernia
K41   Femoral hernia
K42   Umbilical hernia
K43   Ventral hernia
K44   Diaphragmatic hernia
K45   Other abdominal hernia
K46   Unspecified abdominal hernia

Noninfective enteritis and colitis (K50–K52)
K50   Crohn's disease [regional enteritis]
K51   Ulcerative colitis
K52   Other noninfective gastroenteritis and colitis

Other diseases of intestines (K55–K63)
K55   Vascular disorders of intestine
K56   Paralytic ileus and intestinal obstruction without hernia
K57   Diverticular disease of intestine
K58   Irritable bowel syndrome
K59   Other functional intestinal disorders
K60   Fissure and fistula of anal and rectal regions
K61   Abscess of anal and rectal regions
K62   Other diseases of anus and rectum
K63   Other diseases of intestine

Diseases of peritoneum (K65–K67)
K65   Peritonitis

K66   Other disorders of peritoneum
K67*   Disorders of peritoneum in infectious diseases classified
        elsewhere

Diseases of liver (K70–K77)
K70   Alcoholic liver disease
K71   Toxic liver disease
K72   Hepatic failure, not elsewhere classified
K73   Chronic hepatitis, not elsewhere classified
K74   Fibrosis and cirrhosis of liver
K75   Other inflammatory liver diseases
K76   Other diseases of liver
K77*   Liver disorders in diseases classified elsewhere

Disorders of gallbladder, biliary tract and pancreas (K80–K87)
K80   Cholelithiasis
K81   Cholecystitis
K82   Other diseases of gallbladder
K83   Other diseases of biliary tract
K85   Acute pancreatitis
K86   Other diseases of pancreas
K87*   Disorders of gallbladder, biliary tract and pancreas in diseases
        classified elsewhere

Other diseases of the digestive system (K90–K93)
K90   Intestinal malabsorption
K91   Postprocedural disorders of digestive system, not elsewhere
        classified
K92   Other diseases of digestive system
K93*   Disorders of other digestive organs in diseases classified
        elsewhere

Chapter XII
Diseases of the skin and subcutaneous tissue
(L00–L99)

Infections of the skin and subcutaneous tissue (L00–L08)
L00   Staphylococcal scalded skin syndrome
L01   Impetigo

L02	Cutaneous abscess, furuncle and carbuncle
L03	Cellulitis
L04	Acute lymphadenitis
L05	Pilonidal cyst
L08	Other local infections of skin and subcutaneous tissue

Bullous disorders (L10–L14)

L10	Pemphigus
L11	Other acantholytic disorders
L12	Pemphigoid
L13	Other bullous disorders
L14*	Bullous disorders in diseases classified elsewhere

Dermatitis and eczema (L20–L30)

L20	Atopic dermatitis
L21	Seborrhoeic dermatitis
L22	Diaper [napkin] dermatitis
L23	Allergic contact dermatitis
L24	Irritant contact dermatitis
L25	Unspecified contact dermatitis
L26	Exfoliative dermatitis
L27	Dermatitis due to substances taken internally
L28	Lichen simplex chronicus and prurigo
L29	Pruritus
L30	Other dermatitis

Papulosquamous disorders (L40–L45)

L40	Psoriasis
L41	Parapsoriasis
L42	Pityriasis rosea
L43	Lichen planus
L44	Other papulosquamous disorders
L45*	Papulosquamous disorders in diseases classified elsewhere

Urticaria and erythema (L50–L54)

L50	Urticaria
L51	Erythema multiforme
L52	Erythema nodosum
L53	Other erythematous conditions
L54*	Erythema in diseases classified elsewhere

Radiation-related disorders of the skin and subcutaneous tissue (L55–L59)

L55 Sunburn
L56 Other acute skin changes due to ultraviolet radiation
L57 Skin changes due to chronic exposure to nonionizing radiation
L58 Radiodermatitis
L59 Other disorders of skin and subcutaneous tissue related to radiation

Disorders of skin appendages (L60–L75)

L60 Nail disorders
L62* Nail disorders in diseases classified elsewhere
L63 Alopecia areata
L64 Androgenic alopecia
L65 Other nonscarring hair loss
L66 Cicatricial alopecia [scarring hair loss]
L67 Hair colour and hair shaft abnormalities
L68 Hypertrichosis
L70 Acne
L71 Rosacea
L72 Follicular cysts of skin and subcutaneous tissue
L73 Other follicular disorders
L74 Eccrine sweat disorders
L75 Apocrine sweat disorders

Other disorders of the skin and subcutaneous tissue (L80–L99)

L80 Vitiligo
L81 Other disorders of pigmentation
L82 Seborrhoeic keratosis
L83 Acanthosis nigricans
L84 Corns and callosities
L85 Other epidermal thickening
L86* Keratoderma in diseases classified elsewhere
L87 Transepidermal elimination disorders
L88 Pyoderma gangrenosum
L89 Decubitus ulcer
L90 Atrophic disorders of skin
L91 Hypertrophic disorders of skin
L92 Granulomatous disorders of skin and subcutaneous tissue
L93 Lupus erythematosus
L94 Other localized connective tissue disorders
L95 Vasculitis limited to skin, not elsewhere classified
L97 Ulcer of lower limb, not elsewhere classified

L98   Other disorders of skin and subcutaneous tissue, not elsewhere
            classified
L99*   Other disorders of skin and subcutaneous tissue in diseases
            classified elsewhere

Chapter XIII
Diseases of the musculoskeletal system and connective tissue
(M00–M99)

Arthropathies (M00–M25)

Infectious arthropathies (M00–M03)
M00   Pyogenic arthritis
M01*   Direct infections of joint in infectious and parasitic diseases
            classified elsewhere
M02   Reactive arthropathies
M03*   Postinfective and reactive arthropathies in diseases classified
            elsewhere

Inflammatory polyarthropathies (M05–M14)
M05   Seropositive rheumatoid arthritis
M06   Other rheumatoid arthritis
M07*   Psoriatic and enteropathic arthropathies
M08   Juvenile arthritis
M09*   Juvenile arthritis in diseases classified elsewhere
M10   Gout
M11   Other crystal arthropathies
M12   Other specific arthropathies
M13   Other arthritis
M14*   Arthropathies in other diseases classified elsewhere

Arthrosis (M15–M19)
M15   Polyarthrosis
M16   Coxarthrosis [arthrosis of hip]
M17   Gonarthrosis [arthrosis of knee]
M18   Arthrosis of first carpometacarpal joint
M19   Other arthrosis

Other joint disorders (M20–M25)
M20   Acquired deformities of fingers and toes
M21   Other acquired deformities of limbs
M22   Disorders of patella
M23   Internal derangement of knee
M24   Other specific joint derangements
M25   Other joint disorders, not elsewhere classified

Systemic connective tissue disorders (M30–M36)
M30   Polyarteritis nodosa and related conditions
M31   Other necrotizing vasculopathies
M32   Systemic lupus erythematosus
M33   Dermatopolymyositis
M34   Systemic sclerosis
M35   Other systemic involvement of connective tissue
M36*   Systemic disorders of connective tissue in diseases classified elsewhere

Dorsopathies (M40–M54)

Deforming dorsopathies (M40–M43)
M40   Kyphosis and lordosis
M41   Scoliosis
M42   Spinal osteochondrosis
M43   Other deforming dorsopathies

Spondylopathies (M45–M49)
M45   Ankylosing spondylitis
M46   Other inflammatory spondylopathies
M47   Spondylosis
M48   Other spondylopathies
M49*   Spondylopathies in diseases classified elsewhere

Other dorsopathies (M50–M54)
M50   Cervical disc disorders
M51   Other intervertebral disc disorders
M53   Other dorsopathies, not elsewhere classified
M54   Dorsalgia

Soft tissue disorders (M60–M79)

Disorders of muscles (M60–M63)
M60   Myositis
M61   Calcification and ossification of muscle
M62   Other disorders of muscle
M63*   Disorders of muscle in diseases classified elsewhere

Disorders of synovium and tendon (M65–M68)
M65   Synovitis and tenosynovitis
M66   Spontaneous rupture of synovium and tendon
M67   Other disorders of synovium and tendon
M68*   Disorders of synovium and tendon in diseases classified
        elsewhere

Other soft tissue disorders (M70–M79)
M70   Soft tissue disorders related to use, overuse and pressure
M71   Other bursopathies
M72   Fibroblastic disorders
M73*   Soft tissue disorders in diseases classified elsewhere
M75   Shoulder lesions
M76   Enthesopathies of lower limb, excluding foot
M77   Other enthesopathies
M79   Other soft tissue disorders, not elsewhere classified

Osteopathies and chondropathies (M80–M94)

Disorders of bone density and structure (M80–M85)
M80   Osteoporosis with pathological fracture
M81   Osteoporosis without pathological fracture
M82*   Osteoporosis in diseases classified elsewhere
M83   Adult osteomalacia
M84   Disorders of continuity of bone
M85   Other disorders of bone density and structure

Other osteopathies (M86–M90)
M86   Osteomyelitis
M87   Osteonecrosis
M88   Paget's disease of bone [osteitis deformans]
M89   Other disorders of bone
M90*   Osteopathies in diseases classified elsewhere

Chondropathies (M91–M94)

M91	Juvenile osteochondrosis of hip and pelvis
M92	Other juvenile osteochondrosis
M93	Other osteochondropathies
M94	Other disorders of cartilage

Other disorders of the musculoskeletal system and connective tissue (M95–M99)

M95	Other acquired deformities of musculoskeletal system and connective tissue
M96	Postprocedural musculoskeletal disorders, not elsewhere classified
M99	Biomechanical lesions, not elsewhere classified

**Chapter XIV
Diseases of the genitourinary system
(N00–N99)**

Glomerular diseases (N00–N08)

N00	Acute nephritic syndrome
N01	Rapidly progressive nephritic syndrome
N02	Recurrent and persistent haematuria
N03	Chronic nephritic syndrome
N04	Nephrotic syndrome
N05	Unspecified nephritic syndrome
N06	Isolated proteinuria with specified morphological lesion
N07	Hereditary nephropathy, not elsewhere classified
N08*	Glomerular disorders in diseases classified elsewhere

Renal tubulo-interstitial diseases (N10–N16)

N10	Acute tubulo-interstitial nephritis
N11	Chronic tubulo-interstitial nephritis
N12	Tubulo-interstitial nephritis, not specified as acute or chronic
N13	Obstructive and reflux uropathy
N14	Drug- and heavy-metal-induced tubulo-interstitial and tubular conditions
N15	Other renal tubulo-interstitial diseases
N16*	Renal tubulo-interstitial disorders in diseases classified elsewhere

Renal failure (N17–N19)

N17   Acute renal failure
N18   Chronic renal failure
N19   Unspecified renal failure

Urolithiasis (N20–N23)

N20   Calculus of kidney and ureter
N21   Calculus of lower urinary tract
N22* Calculus of urinary tract in diseases classified elsewhere
N23   Unspecified renal colic

Other disorders of kidney and ureter (N25–N29)

N25   Disorders resulting from impaired renal tubular function
N26   Unspecified contracted kidney
N27   Small kidney of unknown cause
N28   Other disorders of kidney and ureter, not elsewhere classified
N29* Other disorders of kidney and ureter in diseases classified
      elsewhere

Other diseases of the urinary system (N30–N39)

N30   Cystitis
N31   Neuromuscular dysfunction of bladder, not elsewhere classified
N32   Other disorders of bladder
N33* Bladder disorders in diseases classified elsewhere
N34   Urethritis and urethral syndrome
N35   Urethral stricture
N36   Other disorders of urethra
N37* Urethral disorders in diseases classified elsewhere
N39   Other disorders of urinary system

Diseases of male genital organs (N40–N51)

N40   Hyperplasia of prostate
N41   Inflammatory diseases of prostate
N42   Other disorders of prostate
N43   Hydrocele and spermatocele
N44   Torsion of testis
N45   Orchitis and epididymitis
N46   Male infertility
N47   Redundant prepuce, phimosis and paraphimosis
N48   Other disorders of penis
N49   Inflammatory disorders of male genital organs, not elsewhere
      classified

N50   Other disorders of male genital organs
N51*   Disorders of male genital organs in diseases classified elsewhere

Disorders of breast (N60–N64)
N60   Benign mammary dysplasia
N61   Inflammatory disorders of breast
N62   Hypertrophy of breast
N63   Unspecified lump in breast
N64   Other disorders of breast

Inflammatory diseases of female pelvic organs (N70–N77)
N70   Salpingitis and oophoritis
N71   Inflammatory disease of uterus, except cervix
N72   Inflammatory disease of cervix uteri
N73   Other female pelvic inflammatory diseases
N74*   Female pelvic inflammatory disorders in diseases classified elsewhere
N75   Diseases of Bartholin's gland
N76   Other inflammation of vagina and vulva
N77*   Vulvovaginal ulceration and inflammation in diseases classified elsewhere

Noninflammatory disorders of female genital tract (N80–N98)
N80   Endometriosis
N81   Female genital prolapse
N82   Fistulae involving female genital tract
N83   Noninflammatory disorders of ovary, fallopian tube and broad ligament
N84   Polyp of female genital tract
N85   Other noninflammatory disorders of uterus, except cervix
N86   Erosion and ectropion of cervix uteri
N87   Dysplasia of cervix uteri
N88   Other noninflammatory disorders of cervix uteri
N89   Other noninflammatory disorders of vagina
N90   Other noninflammatory disorders of vulva and perineum
N91   Absent, scanty and rare menstruation
N92   Excessive, frequent and irregular menstruation
N93   Other abnormal uterine and vaginal bleeding
N94   Pain and other conditions associated with female genital organs and menstrual cycle
N95   Menopausal and other perimenopausal disorders
N96   Habitual aborter

N97   Female infertility
N98   Complications associated with artificial fertilization

Other disorders of the genitourinary system (N99)
N99   Postprocedural disorders of genitourinary system, not elsewhere
        classified

Chapter XV
Pregnancy, childbirth and the puerperium
(O00–O99)

Pregnancy with abortive outcome (O00–O08)
O00   Ectopic pregnancy
O01   Hydatidiform mole
O02   Other abnormal products of conception
O03   Spontaneous abortion
O04   Medical abortion
O05   Other abortion
O06   Unspecified abortion
O07   Failed attempted abortion
O08   Complications following abortion and ectopic and molar
        pregnancy

Oedema, proteinuria and hypertensive disorders in pregnancy, childbirth and the puerperium (O10–O16)
O10   Pre-existing hypertension complicating pregnancy, childbirth
        and the puerperium
O11   Pre-existing hypertensive disorder with superimposed proteinuria
O12   Gestational [pregnancy-induced] oedema and proteinuria without
        hypertension
O13   Gestational [pregnancy-induced] hypertension without significant
        proteinuria
O14   Gestational [pregnancy-induced] hypertension with significant
        proteinuria
O15   Eclampsia
O16   Unspecified maternal hypertension

Other maternal disorders predominantly related to pregnancy (O20–O29)

O20	Haemorrhage in early pregnancy
O21	Excessive vomiting in pregnancy
O22	Venous complications in pregnancy
O23	Infections of genitourinary tract in pregnancy
O24	Diabetes mellitus in pregnancy
O25	Malnutrition in pregnancy
O26	Maternal care for other conditions predominantly related to pregnancy
O28	Abnormal findings on antenatal screening of mother
O29	Complications of anaesthesia during pregnancy

Maternal care related to the fetus and amniotic cavity and possible delivery problems (O30–O48)

O30	Multiple gestation
O31	Complications specific to multiple gestation
O32	Maternal care for known or suspected malpresentation of fetus
O33	Maternal care for known or suspected disproportion
O34	Maternal care for known or suspected abnormality of pelvic organs
O35	Maternal care for known or suspected fetal abnormality and damage
O36	Maternal care for other known or suspected fetal problems
O40	Polyhydramnios
O41	Other disorders of amniotic fluid and membranes
O42	Premature rupture of membranes
O43	Placental disorders
O44	Placenta praevia
O45	Premature separation of placenta [abruptio placentae]
O46	Antepartum haemorrhage, not elsewhere classified
O47	False labour
O48	Prolonged pregnancy

Complications of labour and delivery (O60–O75)

O60	Preterm delivery
O61	Failed induction of labour
O62	Abnormalities of forces of labour
O63	Long labour
O64	Obstructed labour due to malposition and malpresentation of fetus
O65	Obstructed labour due to maternal pelvic abnormality
O66	Other obstructed labour

O67	Labour and delivery complicated by intrapartum haemorrhage, not elsewhere classified
O68	Labour and delivery complicated by fetal stress [distress]
O69	Labour and delivery complicated by umbilical cord complications
O70	Perineal laceration during delivery
O71	Other obstetric trauma
O72	Postpartum haemorrhage
O73	Retained placenta and membranes, without haemorrhage
O74	Complications of anaesthesia during labour and delivery
O75	Other complications of labour and delivery, not elsewhere classified

Delivery (O80–O84)

O80	Single spontaneous delivery
O81	Single delivery by forceps and vacuum extractor
O82	Single delivery by caesarean section
O83	Other assisted single delivery
O84	Multiple delivery

Complications predominantly related to the puerperium (O85–O92)

O85	Puerperal sepsis
O86	Other puerperal infections
O87	Venous complications in the puerperium
O88	Obstetric embolism
O89	Complications of anaesthesia during the puerperium
O90	Complications of the puerperium, not elsewhere classified
O91	Infections of breast associated with childbirth
O92	Other disorders of breast and lactation associated with childbirth

Other obstetric conditions, not elsewhere classified (O95–O99)

O95	Obstetric death of unspecified cause
O96	Death from any obstetric cause occurring more than 42 days but less than one year after delivery
O97	Death from sequelae of direct obstetric causes
O98	Maternal infectious and parasitic diseases classifiable elsewhere but complicating pregnancy, childbirth and the puerperium
O99	Other maternal diseases classifiable elsewhere but complicating pregnancy, childbirth and the puerperium

Chapter XVI
Certain conditions originating in the perinatal period
(P00–P96)

Fetus and newborn affected by maternal factors and by complications of pregnancy, labour and delivery (P00–P04)

P00	Fetus and newborn affected by maternal conditions that may be unrelated to present pregnancy
P01	Fetus and newborn affected by maternal complications of pregnancy
P02	Fetus and newborn affected by complications of placenta, cord and membranes
P03	Fetus and newborn affected by other complications of labour and delivery
P04	Fetus and newborn affected by noxious influences transmitted via placenta or breast milk

Disorders related to length of gestation and fetal growth (P05–P08)

P05	Slow fetal growth and fetal malnutrition
P07	Disorders related to short gestation and low birth weight, not elsewhere classified
P08	Disorders related to long gestation and high birth weight

Birth trauma (P10–P15)

P10	Intracranial laceration and haemorrhage due to birth injury
P11	Other birth injuries to central nervous system
P12	Birth injury to scalp
P13	Birth injury to skeleton
P14	Birth injury to peripheral nervous system
P15	Other birth injuries

Respiratory and cardiovascular disorders specific to the perinatal period (P20–P29)

P20	Intrauterine hypoxia
P21	Birth asphyxia
P22	Respiratory distress of newborn
P23	Congenital pneumonia
P24	Neonatal aspiration syndromes
P25	Interstitial emphysema and related conditions originating in the perinatal period
P26	Pulmonary haemorrhage originating in the perinatal period

P27	Chronic respiratory disease originating in the perinatal period
P28	Other respiratory conditions originating in the perinatal period
P29	Cardiovascular disorders originating in the perinatal period

Infections specific to the perinatal period (P35–P39)

P35	Congenital viral diseases
P36	Bacterial sepsis of newborn
P37	Other congenital infectious and parasitic diseases
P38	Omphalitis of newborn with or without mild haemorrhage
P39	Other infections specific to the perinatal period

Haemorrhagic and haematological disorders of fetus and newborn (P50–P61)

P50	Fetal blood loss
P51	Umbilical haemorrhage of newborn
P52	Intracranial nontraumatic haemorrhage of fetus and newborn
P53	Haemorrhagic disease of fetus and newborn
P54	Other neonatal haemorrhages
P55	Haemolytic disease of fetus and newborn
P56	Hydrops fetalis due to haemolytic disease
P57	Kernicterus
P58	Neonatal jaundice due to other excessive haemolysis
P59	Neonatal jaundice from other and unspecified causes
P60	Disseminated intravascular coagulation of fetus and newborn
P61	Other perinatal haematological disorders

Transitory endocrine and metabolic disorders specific to fetus and newborn (P70–P74)

P70	Transitory disorders of carbohydrate metabolism specific to fetus and newborn
P71	Transitory neonatal disorders of calcium and magnesium metabolism
P72	Other transitory neonatal endocrine disorders
P74	Other transitory neonatal electrolyte and metabolic disturbances

Digestive system disorders of fetus and newborn (P75–P78)

P75*	Meconium ileus
P76	Other intestinal obstruction of newborn
P77	Necrotizing enterocolitis of fetus and newborn
P78	Other perinatal digestive system disorders

Conditions involving the integument and temperature regulation of fetus and newborn (P80–P83)

P80   Hypothermia of newborn
P81   Other disturbances of temperature regulation of newborn
P83   Other conditions of integument specific to fetus and newborn

Other disorders originating in the perinatal period (P90–P96)

P90   Convulsions of newborn
P91   Other disturbances of cerebral status of newborn
P92   Feeding problems of newborn
P93   Reactions and intoxications due to drugs administered to fetus and newborn
P94   Disorders of muscle tone of newborn
P95   Fetal death of unspecified cause
P96   Other conditions originating in the perinatal period

Chapter XVII
Congenital malformations, deformations and chromosomal abnormalities
(Q00–Q99)

Congenital malformations of the nervous system (Q00–Q07)

Q00   Anencephaly and similar malformations
Q01   Encephalocele
Q02   Microcephaly
Q03   Congenital hydrocephalus
Q04   Other congenital malformations of brain
Q05   Spina bifida
Q06   Other congenital malformations of spinal cord
Q07   Other congenital malformations of nervous system

Congenital malformations of eye, ear, face and neck (Q10–Q18)

Q10   Congenital malformations of eyelid, lacrimal apparatus and orbit
Q11   Anophthalmos, microphthalmos and macrophthalmos
Q12   Congenital lens malformations
Q13   Congenital malformations of anterior segment of eye
Q14   Congenital malformations of posterior segment of eye
Q15   Other congenital malformations of eye
Q16   Congenital malformations of ear causing impairment of hearing

Q17   Other congenital malformations of ear
Q18   Other congenital malformations of face and neck

Congenital malformations of the circulatory system (Q20–Q28)
Q20   Congenital malformations of cardiac chambers and connections
Q21   Congenital malformations of cardiac septa
Q22   Congenital malformations of pulmonary and tricuspid valves
Q23   Congenital malformations of aortic and mitral valves
Q24   Other congenital malformations of heart
Q25   Congenital malformations of great arteries
Q26   Congenital malformations of great veins
Q27   Other congenital malformations of peripheral vascular system
Q28   Other congenital malformations of circulatory system

Congenital malformations of the respiratory system (Q30–Q34)
Q30   Congenital malformations of nose
Q31   Congenital malformations of larynx
Q32   Congenital malformations of trachea and bronchus
Q33   Congenital malformations of lung
Q34   Other congenital malformations of respiratory system

Cleft lip and cleft palate (Q35–Q37)
Q35   Cleft palate
Q36   Cleft lip
Q37   Cleft palate with cleft lip

Other congenital malformations of the digestive system (Q38–Q45)
Q38   Other congenital malformations of tongue, mouth and pharynx
Q39   Congenital malformations of oesophagus
Q40   Other congenital malformations of upper alimentary tract
Q41   Congenital absence, atresia and stenosis of small intestine
Q42   Congenital absence, atresia and stenosis of large intestine
Q43   Other congenital malformations of intestine
Q44   Congenital malformations of gallbladder, bile ducts and liver
Q45   Other congenital malformations of digestive system

Congenital malformations of genital organs (Q50–Q56)
Q50   Congenital malformations of ovaries, fallopian tubes and broad
     ligaments
Q51   Congenital malformations of uterus and cervix
Q52   Other congenital malformations of female genitalia
Q53   Undescended testicle

Q54   Hypospadias
Q55   Other congenital malformations of male genital organs
Q56   Indeterminate sex and pseudohermaphroditism

Congenital malformations of the urinary system (Q60–Q64)
Q60   Renal agenesis and other reduction defects of kidney
Q61   Cystic kidney disease
Q62   Congenital obstructive defects of renal pelvis and congenital
       malformations of ureter
Q63   Other congenital malformations of kidney
Q64   Other congenital malformations of urinary system

**Congenital malformations and deformations of the musculoskeletal system
(Q65–Q79)**
Q65   Congenital deformities of hip
Q66   Congenital deformities of feet
Q67   Congenital musculoskeletal deformities of head, face, spine and
       chest
Q68   Other congenital musculoskeletal deformities
Q69   Polydactyly
Q70   Syndactyly
Q71   Reduction defects of upper limb
Q72   Reduction defects of lower limb
Q73   Reduction defects of unspecified limb
Q74   Other congenital malformations of limb(s)
Q75   Other congenital malformations of skull and face bones
Q76   Congenital malformations of spine and bony thorax
Q77   Osteochondrodysplasia with defects of growth of tubular bones
       and spine
Q78   Other osteochondrodysplasias
Q79   Congenital malformations of musculoskeletal system, not
       elsewhere classified

Other congenital malformations (Q80–Q89)
Q80   Congenital ichthyosis
Q81   Epidermolysis bullosa
Q82   Other congenital malformations of skin
Q83   Congenital malformations of breast
Q84   Other congenital malformations of integument
Q85   Phakomatoses, not elsewhere classified
Q86   Congenital malformation syndromes due to known exogenous
       causes, not elsewhere classified

Q87   Other specified congenital malformation syndromes affecting multiple systems
Q89   Other congenital malformations, not elsewhere classified

Chromosomal abnormalities, not elsewhere classified (Q90–Q99)
Q90   Down's syndrome
Q91   Edwards' syndrome and Patau's syndrome
Q92   Other trisomies and partial trisomies of the autosomes, not elsewhere classified
Q93   Monosomies and deletions from the autosomes, not elsewhere classified
Q95   Balanced rearrangements and structural markers, not elsewhere classified
Q96   Turner's syndrome
Q97   Other sex chromosome abnormalities, female phenotype, not elsewhere classified
Q98   Other sex chromosome abnormalities, male phenotype, not elsewhere classified
Q99   Other chromosome abnormalities, not elsewhere classified

Chapter XVIII
Symptoms, signs and abnormal clinical and laboratory findings, not elsewhere classified
(R00–R99)

Symptoms and signs involving the circulatory and respiratory systems (R00–R09)
R00   Abnormalities of heart beat
R01   Cardiac murmurs and other cardiac sounds
R02   Gangrene, not elsewhere classified
R03   Abnormal blood-pressure reading, without diagnosis
R04   Haemorrhage from respiratory passages
R05   Cough
R06   Abnormalities of breathing
R07   Pain in throat and chest
R09   Other symptoms and signs involving the circulatory and respiratory systems

Symptoms and signs involving the digestive system and abdomen (R10–R19)

R10	Abdominal and pelvic pain
R11	Nausea and vomiting
R12	Heartburn
R13	Dysphagia
R14	Flatulence and related conditions
R15	Faecal incontinence
R16	Hepatomegaly and splenomegaly, not elsewhere classified
R17	Unspecified jaundice
R18	Ascites
R19	Other symptoms and signs involving the digestive system and abdomen

Symptoms and signs involving the skin and subcutaneous tissue (R20–R23)

R20	Disturbances of skin sensation
R21	Rash and other nonspecific skin eruption
R22	Localized swelling, mass and lump of skin and subcutaneous tissue
R23	Other skin changes

Symptoms and signs involving the nervous and musculoskeletal systems (R25–R29)

R25	Abnormal involuntary movements
R26	Abnormalities of gait and mobility
R27	Other lack of coordination
R29	Other symptoms and signs involving the nervous and musculoskeletal systems

Symptoms and signs involving the urinary system (R30–R39)

R30	Pain associated with micturition
R31	Unspecified haematuria
R32	Unspecified urinary incontinence
R33	Retention of urine
R34	Anuria and oliguria
R35	Polyuria
R36	Urethral discharge
R39	Other symptoms and signs involving the urinary system

Symptoms and signs involving cognition, perception, emotional state and behaviour (R40–R46)

R40   Somnolence, stupor and coma

R41   Other symptoms and signs involving cognitive functions and awareness

R42   Dizziness and giddiness

R43   Disturbances of smell and taste

R44   Other symptoms and signs involving general sensations and perceptions

R45   Symptoms and signs involving emotional state

R46   Symptoms and signs involving appearance and behaviour

Symptoms and signs involving speech and voice (R47–R49)

R47   Speech disturbances, not elsewhere classified

R48   Dyslexia and other symbolic dysfunctions, not elsewhere classified

R49   Voice disturbances

General symptoms and signs (R50–R69)

R50   Fever of unknown origin

R51   Headache

R52   Pain, not elsewhere classified

R53   Malaise and fatigue

R54   Senility

R55   Syncope and collapse

R56   Convulsions, not elsewhere classified

R57   Shock, not elsewhere classified

R58   Haemorrhage, not elsewhere classified

R59   Enlarged lymph nodes

R60   Oedema, not elsewhere classified

R61   Hyperhidrosis

R62   Lack of expected normal physiological development

R63   Symptoms and signs concerning food and fluid intake

R64   Cachexia

R68   Other general symptoms and signs

R69   Unknown and unspecified causes of morbidity

Abnormal findings on examination of blood, without diagnosis (R70–R79)

R70   Elevated erythrocyte sedimentation rate and abnormality of plasma viscosity

R71   Abnormality of red blood cells

R72   Abnormality of white blood cells, not elsewhere classified

R73	Elevated blood glucose level
R74	Abnormal serum enzyme levels
R75	Laboratory evidence of human immunodeficiency virus [HIV]
R76	Other abnormal immunological findings in serum
R77	Other abnormalities of plasma proteins
R78	Findings of drugs and other substances, not normally found in blood
R79	Other abnormal findings of blood chemistry

Abnormal findings on examination of urine, without diagnosis (R80–R82)

R80	Isolated proteinuria
R81	Glycosuria
R82	Other abnormal findings in urine

Abnormal findings on examination of other body fluids, substances and tissues, without diagnosis (R83–R89)

R83	Abnormal findings in cerebrospinal fluid
R84	Abnormal findings in specimens from respiratory organs and thorax
R85	Abnormal findings in specimens from digestive organs and abdominal cavity
R86	Abnormal findings in specimens from male genital organs
R87	Abnormal findings in specimens from female genital organs
R89	Abnormal findings in specimens from other organs, systems and tissues

Abnormal findings on diagnostic imaging and in function studies, without diagnosis (R90–R94)

R90	Abnormal findings on diagnostic imaging of central nervous system
R91	Abnormal findings on diagnostic imaging of lung
R92	Abnormal findings on diagnostic imaging of breast
R93	Abnormal findings on diagnostic imaging of other body structures
R94	Abnormal results of function studies

Ill-defined and unknown causes of mortality (R95–R99)

R95	Sudden infant death syndrome
R96	Other sudden death, cause unknown
R98	Unattended death
R99	Other ill-defined and unspecified causes of mortality

Chapter XIX
Injury, poisoning and certain other consequences of external causes (S00–T98)

Injuries to the head (S00–S09)

S00   Superficial injury of head
S01   Open wound of head
S02   Fracture of skull and facial bones
S03   Dislocation, sprain and strain of joints and ligaments of head
S04   Injury of cranial nerves
S05   Injury of eye and orbit
S06   Intracranial injury
S07   Crushing injury of head
S08   Traumatic amputation of part of head
S09   Other and unspecified injuries of head

Injuries to the neck (S10–S19)

S10   Superficial injury of neck
S11   Open wound of neck
S12   Fracture of neck
S13   Dislocation, sprain and strain of joints and ligaments at neck level
S14   Injury of nerves and spinal cord at neck level
S15   Injury of blood vessels at neck level
S16   Injury of muscle and tendon at neck level
S17   Crushing injury of neck
S18   Traumatic amputation at neck level
S19   Other and unspecified injuries of neck

Injuries to the thorax (S20–S29)

S20   Superficial injury of thorax
S21   Open wound of thorax
S22   Fracture of rib(s), sternum and thoracic spine
S23   Dislocation, sprain and strain of joints and ligaments of thorax
S24   Injury of nerves and spinal cord at thorax level
S25   Injury of blood vessels of thorax
S26   Injury of heart
S27   Injury of other and unspecified intrathoracic organs
S28   Crushing injury of thorax and traumatic amputation of part of thorax
S29   Other and unspecified injuries of thorax

Injuries to the abdomen, lower back, lumbar spine and pelvis (S30–S39)

S30	Superficial injury of abdomen, lower back and pelvis
S31	Open wound of abdomen, lower back and pelvis
S32	Fracture of lumbar spine and pelvis
S33	Dislocation, sprain and strain of joints and ligaments of lumbar spine and pelvis
S34	Injury of nerves and lumbar spinal cord at abdomen, lower back and pelvis level
S35	Injury of blood vessels at abdomen, lower back and pelvis level
S36	Injury of intra-abdominal organs
S37	Injury of pelvic organs
S38	Crushing injury and traumatic amputation of part of abdomen, lower back and pelvis
S39	Other and unspecified injuries of abdomen, lower back and pelvis

Injuries to the shoulder and upper arm (S40–S49)

S40	Superficial injury of shoulder and upper arm
S41	Open wound of shoulder and upper arm
S42	Fracture of shoulder and upper arm
S43	Dislocation, sprain and strain of joints and ligaments of shoulder girdle
S44	Injury of nerves at shoulder and upper arm level
S45	Injury of blood vessels at shoulder and upper arm level
S46	Injury of muscle and tendon at shoulder and upper arm level
S47	Crushing injury of shoulder and upper arm
S48	Traumatic amputation of shoulder and upper arm
S49	Other and unspecified injuries of shoulder and upper arm

Injuries to the elbow and forearm (S50–S59)

S50	Superficial injury of forearm
S51	Open wound of forearm
S52	Fracture of forearm
S53	Dislocation, sprain and strain of joints and ligaments of elbow
S54	Injury of nerves at forearm level
S55	Injury of blood vessels at forearm level
S56	Injury of muscle and tendon at forearm level
S57	Crushing injury of forearm
S58	Traumatic amputation of forearm
S59	Other and unspecified injuries of forearm

Injuries to the wrist and hand (S60–S69)

S60	Superficial injury of wrist and hand
S61	Open wound of wrist and hand
S62	Fracture at wrist and hand level
S63	Dislocation, sprain and strain of joints and ligaments at wrist and hand level
S64	Injury of nerves at wrist and hand level
S65	Injury of blood vessels at wrist and hand level
S66	Injury of muscle and tendon at wrist and hand level
S67	Crushing injury of wrist and hand
S68	Traumatic amputation of wrist and hand
S69	Other and unspecified injuries of wrist and hand

Injuries to the hip and thigh (S70–S79)

S70	Superficial injury of hip and thigh
S71	Open wound of hip and thigh
S72	Fracture of femur
S73	Dislocation, sprain and strain of joint and ligaments of hip
S74	Injury of nerves at hip and thigh level
S75	Injury of blood vessels at hip and thigh level
S76	Injury of muscle and tendon at hip and thigh level
S77	Crushing injury of hip and thigh
S78	Traumatic amputation of hip and thigh
S79	Other and unspecified injuries of hip and thigh

Injuries to the knee and lower leg (S80–S89)

S80	Superficial injury of lower leg
S81	Open wound of lower leg
S82	Fracture of lower leg, including ankle
S83	Dislocation, sprain and strain of joints and ligaments of knee
S84	Injury of nerves at lower leg level
S85	Injury of blood vessels at lower leg level
S86	Injury of muscle and tendon at lower leg level
S87	Crushing injury of lower leg
S88	Traumatic amputation of lower leg
S89	Other and unspecified injuries of lower leg

Injuries to the ankle and foot (S90–S99)

S90	Superficial injury of ankle and foot
S91	Open wound of ankle and foot
S92	Fracture of foot, except ankle
S93	Dislocation, sprain and strain of joints and ligaments at ankle and foot level

S94	Injury of nerves at ankle and foot level
S95	Injury of blood vessels at ankle and foot level
S96	Injury of muscle and tendon at ankle and foot level
S97	Crushing injury of ankle and foot
S98	Traumatic amputation of ankle and foot
S99	Other and unspecified injuries of ankle and foot

Injuries involving multiple body regions (T00–T07)

T00	Superficial injuries involving multiple body regions
T01	Open wounds involving multiple body regions
T02	Fractures involving multiple body regions
T03	Dislocations, sprains and strains involving multiple body regions
T04	Crushing injuries involving multiple body regions
T05	Traumatic amputations involving multiple body regions
T06	Other injuries involving multiple body regions, not elsewhere classified
T07	Unspecified multiple injuries

Injuries to unspecified part of trunk, limb or body region (T08–T14)

T08	Fracture of spine, level unspecified
T09	Other injuries of spine and trunk, level unspecified
T10	Fracture of upper limb, level unspecified
T11	Other injuries of upper limb, level unspecified
T12	Fracture of lower limb, level unspecified
T13	Other injuries of lower limb, level unspecified
T14	Injury of unspecified body region

Effects of foreign body entering through natural orifice (T15–T19)

T15	Foreign body on external eye
T16	Foreign body in ear
T17	Foreign body in respiratory tract
T18	Foreign body in alimentary tract
T19	Foreign body in genitourinary tract

Burns and corrosions (T20–T32)

Burns and corrosions of external body surface, specified by site (T20–T25)

T20	Burn and corrosion of head and neck
T21	Burn and corrosion of trunk
T22	Burn and corrosion of shoulder and upper limb, except wrist and hand
T23	Burn and corrosion of wrist and hand

T24   Burn and corrosion of hip and lower limb, except ankle and foot

T25   Burn and corrosion of ankle and foot

Burns and corrosions confined to eye and internal organs (T26–T28)

T26   Burn and corrosion confined to eye and adnexa

T27   Burn and corrosion of respiratory tract

T28   Burn and corrosion of other internal organs

Burns and corrosions of multiple and unspecified body regions (T29–T32)

T29   Burns and corrosions of multiple body regions

T30   Burn and corrosion, body region unspecified

T31   Burns classified according to extent of body surface involved

T32   Corrosions classified according to extent of body surface involved

Frostbite (T33–T35)

T33   Superficial frostbite

T34   Frostbite with tissue necrosis

T35   Frostbite involving multiple body regions and unspecified frostbite

Poisoning by drugs, medicaments and biological substances (T36–T50)

T36   Poisoning by systemic antibiotics

T37   Poisoning by other systemic anti-infectives and antiparasitics

T38   Poisoning by hormones and their synthetic substitutes and antagonists, not elsewhere classified

T39   Poisoning by nonopioid analgesics, antipyretics and antirheumatics

T40   Poisoning by narcotics and psychodysleptics [hallucinogens]

T41   Poisoning by anaesthetics and therapeutic gases

T42   Poisoning by antiepileptic, sedative–hypnotic and antiparkinsonism drugs

T43   Poisoning by psychotropic drugs, not elsewhere classified

T44   Poisoning by drugs primarily affecting the autonomic nervous system

T45   Poisoning by primarily systemic and haematological agents, not elsewhere classified

T46   Poisoning by agents primarily affecting the cardiovascular system

T47   Poisoning by agents primarily affecting the gastrointestinal system

T48   Poisoning by agents primarily acting on smooth and skeletal muscles and the respiratory system

T49	Poisoning by topical agents primarily affecting skin and mucous membrane and by ophthalmological, otorhinolaryngological and dental drugs
T50	Poisoning by diuretics and other and unspecified drugs, medicaments and biological substances

Toxic effects of substances chiefly nonmedicinal as to source (T51–T65)

T51	Toxic effect of alcohol
T52	Toxic effect of organic solvents
T53	Toxic effect of halogen derivatives of aliphatic and aromatic hydrocarbons
T54	Toxic effect of corrosive substances
T55	Toxic effect of soaps and detergents
T56	Toxic effect of metals
T57	Toxic effect of other inorganic substances
T58	Toxic effect of carbon monoxide
T59	Toxic effect of other gases, fumes and vapours
T60	Toxic effect of pesticides
T61	Toxic effect of noxious substances eaten as seafood
T62	Toxic effect of other noxious substances eaten as food
T63	Toxic effect of contact with venomous animals
T64	Toxic effect of aflatoxin and other mycotoxin food contaminants
T65	Toxic effect of other and unspecified substances

Other and unspecified effects of external causes (T66–T78)

T66	Unspecified effects of radiation
T67	Effects of heat and light
T68	Hypothermia
T69	Other effects of reduced temperature
T70	Effects of air pressure and water pressure
T71	Asphyxiation
T73	Effects of other deprivation
T74	Maltreatment syndromes
T75	Effects of other external causes
T78	Adverse effects, not elsewhere classified

Certain early complications of trauma (T79)

T79	Certain early complications of trauma, not elsewhere classified

Complications of surgical and medical care, not elsewhere classified (T80–T88)

T80   Complications following infusion, transfusion and therapeutic injection

T81   Complications of procedures, not elsewhere classified

T82   Complications of cardiac and vascular prosthetic devices, implants and grafts

T83   Complications of genitourinary prosthetic devices, implants and grafts

T84   Complications of internal orthopaedic prosthetic devices, implants and grafts

T85   Complications of other internal prosthetic devices, implants and grafts

T86   Failure and rejection of transplanted organs and tissues

T87   Complications peculiar to reattachment and amputation

T88   Other complications of surgical and medical care, not elsewhere classified

Sequelae of injuries, of poisoning and of other consequences of external causes (T90–T98)

T90   Sequelae of injuries of head

T91   Sequelae of injuries of neck and trunk

T92   Sequelae of injuries of upper limb

T93   Sequelae of injuries of lower limb

T94   Sequelae of injuries involving multiple and unspecified body regions

T95   Sequelae of burns, corrosions and frostbite

T96   Sequelae of poisoning by drugs, medicaments and biological substances

T97   Sequelae of toxic effects of substances chiefly nonmedicinal as to source

T98   Sequelae of other and unspecified effects of external causes

Chapter XX
External causes of morbidity and mortality
(V01–Y98)

Transport accidents (V01–V99)

Pedestrian injured in transport accident (V01–V09)

V01   Pedestrian injured in collision with pedal cycle
V02   Pedestrian injured in collision with two- or three-wheeled motor vehicle
V03   Pedestrian injured in collision with car, pick-up truck or van
V04   Pedestrian injured in collision with heavy transport vehicle or bus
V05   Pedestrian injured in collision with railway train or railway vehicle
V06   Pedestrian injured in collision with other nonmotor vehicle
V09   Pedestrian injured in other and unspecified transport accidents

Pedal cyclist injured in transport accident (V10-V19)

V10   Pedal cyclist injured in collision with pedestrian or animal
V11   Pedal cyclist injured in collision with other pedal cycle
V12   Pedal cyclist injured in collision with two- or three-wheeled motor vehicle
V13   Pedal cyclist injured in collision with car, pick-up truck or van
V14   Pedal cyclist injured in collision with heavy transport vehicle or bus
Vl5   Pedal cyclist injured in collision with railway train or railway vehicle
V16   Pedal cyclist injured in collision with other nonmotor vehicle
V17   Pedal cyclist injured in collision with fixed or stationary object
V18   Pedal cyclist injured in noncollision transport accident
V19   Pedal cyclist injured in other and unspecified transport accidents

Motorcycle rider injured in transport accident (V20–V29)

V20   Motorcyle rider injured in collision with pedestrian or animal
V21   Motorcyle rider injured in collision with pedal cycle
V22   Motorcyle rider injured in collision with two- or three-wheeled motor vehicle
V23   Motorcyle rider injured in collision with car, pick-up truck or van
V24   Motorcyle rider injured in collision with heavy transport vehicle or bus

V25   Motorcyle rider injured in collision with railway train or railway vehicle
V26   Motorcyle rider injured in collision with other nonmotor vehicle
V27   Motorcyle rider injured in collision with fixed or stationary object
V28   Motorcyle rider injured in noncollision transport accident
V29   Motorcyle rider injured in other and unspecified transport accidents

Occupant of three-wheeled motor vehicle injured in transport accident (V30–V39)

V30   Occupant of three-wheeled motor vehicle injured in collision with pedestrian or animal
V31   Occupant of three-wheeled motor vehicle injured in collision with pedal cycle
V32   Occupant of three-wheeled motor vehicle injured in collision with two- or three-wheeled motor vehicle
V33   Occupant of three-wheeled motor vehicle injured in collision with car, pick-up truck or van
V34   Occupant of three-wheeled motor vehicle injured in collision with heavy transport vehicle or bus
V35   Occupant of three-wheeled motor vehicle injured in collision with railway train or railway vehicle
V36   Occupant of three-wheeled motor vehicle injured in collision with other nonmotor vehicle
V37   Occupant of three-wheeled motor vehicle injured in collision with fixed or stationary object
V38   Occupant of three-wheeled motor vehicle injured in noncollision transport accident
V39   Occupant of three-wheeled motor vehicle injured in other and unspecified transport accidents

Car occupant injured in transport accident (V40–V49)

V40   Car occupant injured in collision with pedestrian or animal
V41   Car occupant injured in collision with pedal cycle
V42   Car occupant injured in collision with two- or three-wheeled motor vehicle
V43   Car occupant injured in collision with car, pick-up truck or van
V44   Car occupant injured in collision with heavy transport vehicle or bus
V45   Car occupant injured in collision with railway train or railway vehicle

V46   Car occupant injured in collision with other nonmotor vehicle
V47   Car occupant injured in collision with fixed or stationary object
V48   Car occupant injured in noncollision transport accident
V49   Car occupant injured in other and unspecified transport accidents

Occupant of pick-up truck or van injured in transport accident (V50–V59)
V50   Occupant of pick-up truck or van injured in collision with
        pedestrian or animal
V51   Occupant of pick-up truck or van injured in collision with pedal
        cycle
V52   Occupant of pick-up truck or van injured in collision with two-
        or three-wheeled motor vehicle
V53   Occupant of pick-up truck or van injured in collision with car,
        pick-up truck or van
V54   Occupant of pick-up truck or van injured in collision with
        heavy transport vehicle or bus
V55   Occupant of pick-up truck or van injured in collision with
        railway train or railway vehicle
V56   Occupant of pick-up truck or van injured in collision with other
        nonmotor vehicle
V57   Occupant of pick-up truck or van injured in collision with fixed
        or stationary object
V58   Occupant of pick-up truck or van injured in noncollision
        transport accident
V59   Occupant of pick-up truck or van injured in other and
        unspecified transport accidents

Occupant of heavy transport vehicle injured in transport accident
(V60–V69)
V60   Occupant of heavy transport vehicle injured in collision with
        pedestrian or animal
V61   Occupant of heavy transport vehicle injured in collision with
        pedal cycle
V62   Occupant of heavy transport vehicle injured in collision with
        two- or three-wheeled motor vehicle
V63   Occupant of heavy transport vehicle injured in collision with
        car, pick-up truck or van
V64   Occupant of heavy transport vehicle injured in collision with
        heavy transport vehicle or bus
V65   Occupant of heavy transport vehicle injured in collision with
        railway train or railway vehicle
V66   Occupant of heavy transport vehicle injured in collision with
        other nonmotor vehicle

V67   Occupant of heavy transport vehicle injured in collision with fixed or stationary object

V68   Occupant of heavy transport vehicle injured in noncollision transport accident

V69   Occupant of heavy transport vehicle injured in other and unspecified transport accidents

Bus occupant injured in transport accident (V70–V79)

V70   Bus occupant injured in collision with pedestrian or animal

V71   Bus occupant injured in collision with pedal cycle

V72   Bus occupant injured in collision with two- or three-wheeled motor vehicle

V73   Bus occupant injured in collision with car, pick-up truck or van

V74   Bus occupant injured in collision with heavy transport vehicle or bus

V75   Bus occupant injured in collision with railway train or railway vehicle

V76   Bus occupant injured in collision with other nonmotor vehicle

V77   Bus occupant injured in collision with fixed or stationary object

V78   Bus occupant injured in noncollision transport accident

V79   Bus occupant injured in other and unspecified transport accidents

Other land transport accidents (V80–V89)

V80   Animal-rider or occupant of animal-drawn vehicle injured in transport accident

V81   Occupant of railway train or railway vehicle injured in transport accident

V82   Occupant of streetcar injured in transport accident

V83   Occupant of special vehicle mainly used on industrial premises injured in transport accident

V84   Occupant of special vehicle mainly used in agriculture injured in transport accident

V85   Occupant of special construction vehicle injured in transport accident

V86   Occupant of special all-terrain or other motor vehicle designed primarily for off-road use, injured in transport accident

V87   Traffic accident of specified type but victim's mode of transport unknown

V88   Nontraffic accident of specified type but victim's mode of transport unknown

V89   Motor- or nonmotor-vehicle accident, type of vehicle unspecified

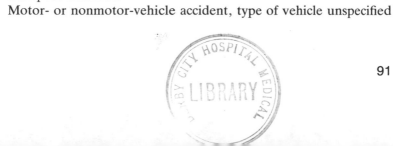

Water transport accidents (V90–V94)

V90   Accident to watercraft causing drowning and submersion
V91   Accident to watercraft causing other injury
V92   Water-transport-related drowning and submersion without accident to watercraft
V93   Accident on board watercraft without accident to watercraft, not causing drowning and submersion
V94   Other and unspecified water transport accidents

Air and space transport accidents (V95–V97)

V95   Accident to powered aircraft causing injury to occupant
V96   Accident to nonpowered aircraft causing injury to occupant
V97   Other specified air transport accidents

Other and unspecified transport accidents (V98–V99)

V98   Other specified transport accidents
V99   Unspecified transport accident

Other external causes of accidental injury (W00–X59)

Falls (W00–W19)

W00   Fall on same level involving ice and snow
W01   Fall on same level from slipping, tripping and stumbling
W02   Fall involving ice-skates, skis, roller-skates or skateboards
W03   Other fall on same level due to collision with, or pushing by, another person
W04   Fall while being carried or supported by other persons
W05   Fall involving wheelchair
W06   Fall involving bed
W07   Fall involving chair
W08   Fall involving other furniture
W09   Fall involving playground equipment
W10   Fall on and from stairs and steps
W11   Fall on and from ladder
W12   Fall on and from scaffolding
W13   Fall from, out of or through building or structure
W14   Fall from tree
W15   Fall from cliff
W16   Diving or jumping into water causing injury other than drowning or submersion
W17   Other fall from one level to another
W18   Other fall on same level
W19   Unspecified fall

Exposure to inanimate mechanical forces (W20–W49)

W20	Struck by thrown, projected or falling object
W21	Striking against or struck by sports equipment
W22	Striking against or struck by other objects
W23	Caught, crushed, jammed or pinched in or between objects
W24	Contact with lifting and transmission devices, not elsewhere classified
W25	Contact with sharp glass
W26	Contact with knife, sword or dagger
W27	Contact with nonpowered hand tool
W28	Contact with powered lawnmower
W29	Contact with other powered hand tools and household machinery
W30	Contact with agricultural machinery
W31	Contact with other and unspecified machinery
W32	Handgun discharge
W33	Rifle, shotgun and larger firearm discharge
W34	Discharge from other and unspecified firearms
W35	Explosion and rupture of boiler
W36	Explosion and rupture of gas cylinder
W37	Explosion and rupture of pressurized tyre, pipe or hose
W38	Explosion and rupture of other specified pressurized devices
W39	Discharge of firework
W40	Explosion of other materials
W41	Exposure to high-pressure jet
W42	Exposure to noise
W43	Exposure to vibration
W44	Foreign body entering into or through eye or natural orifice
W45	Foreign body or object entering through skin
W49	Exposure to other and unspecified inanimate mechanical forces

Exposure to animate mechanical forces (W50–W64)

W50	Hit, struck, kicked, twisted, bitten or scratched by another person
W51	Striking against or bumped into by another person
W52	Crushed, pushed and stepped on by crowd or human stampede
W53	Bitten by rat
W54	Bitten or struck by dog
W55	Bitten or struck by other mammals
W56	Contact with marine animal
W57	Bitten or stung by nonvenomous insect and other nonvenomous arthropods
W58	Bitten or struck by crocodile or alligator

W59   Bitten or crushed by other reptiles
W60   Contact with plant thorns and spines and sharp leaves
W64   Exposure to other and unspecified animate mechanical forces

Accidental drowning and submersion (W65–W74)
W65   Drowning and submersion while in bath-tub
W66   Drowning and submersion following fall into bath-tub
W67   Drowning and submersion while in swimming-pool
W68   Drowning and submersion following fall into swimming-pool
W69   Drowning and submersion while in natural water
W70   Drowning and submersion following fall into natural water
W73   Other specified drowning and submersion
W74   Unspecified drowning and submersion

Other accidental threats to breathing (W75–W84)
W75   Accidental suffocation and strangulation in bed
W76   Other accidental hanging and strangulation
W77   Threat to breathing due to cave-in, falling earth and other
        substances
W78   Inhalation of gastric contents
W79   Inhalation and ingestion of food causing obstruction of
        respiratory tract
W80   Inhalation and ingestion of other objects causing obstruction of
        respiratory tract
W81   Confined to or trapped in a low-oxygen environment
W83   Other specified threats to breathing
W84   Unspecified threat to breathing

*Exposure to electric current, radiation and extreme ambient air temperature
and pressure (W85–W99)*
W85   Exposure to electric transmission lines
W86   Exposure to other specified electric current
W87   Exposure to unspecified electric current
W88   Exposure to ionizing radiation
W89   Exposure to man-made visible and ultraviolet light
W90   Exposure to other nonionizing radiation
W91   Exposure to unspecified type of radiation
W92   Exposure to excessive heat of man-made origin
W93   Exposure to excessive cold of man-made origin
W94   Exposure to high and low air pressure and changes in air
        pressure
W99   Exposure to other and unspecified man-made environmental
        factors

Exposure to smoke, fire and flames (X00–X09)
X00   Exposure to uncontrolled fire in building or structure
X01   Exposure to uncontrolled fire, not in building or structure
X02   Exposure to controlled fire in building or structure
X03   Exposure to controlled fire, not in building or structure
X04   Exposure to ignition of highly flammable material
X05   Exposure to ignition or melting of nightwear
X06   Exposure to ignition or melting of other clothing and apparel
X08   Exposure to other specified smoke, fire and flames
X09   Exposure to unspecified smoke, fire and flames

Contact with heat and hot substances (X10–X19)
X10   Contact with hot drinks, food, fats and cooking oils
X11   Contact with hot tap-water
X12   Contact with other hot fluids
X13   Contact with steam and hot vapours
X14   Contact with hot air and gases
X15   Contact with hot household appliances
X16   Contact with hot heating appliances, radiators and pipes
X17   Contact with hot engines, machinery and tools
X18   Contact with other hot metals
X19   Contact with other and unspecified heat and hot substances

Contact with venomous animals and plants (X20–X29)
X20   Contact with venomous snakes and lizards
X21   Contact with venomous spiders
X22   Contact with scorpions
X23   Contact with hornets, wasps and bees
X24   Contact with centipedes and venomous millipedes (tropical)
X25   Contact with other specified venomous arthropods
X26   Contact with venomous marine animals and plants
X27   Contact with other specified venomous animals
X28   Contact with other specified venomous plants
X29   Contact with unspecified venomous animal or plant

Exposure to forces of nature (X30–X39)
X30   Exposure to excessive natural heat
X31   Exposure to excessive natural cold
X32   Exposure to sunlight
X33   Victim of lightning
X34   Victim of earthquake
X35   Victim of volcanic eruption

X36   Victim of avalanche, landslide and other earth movements
X37   Victim of cataclysmic storm
X38   Victim of flood
X39   Exposure to other and unspecified forces of nature

Accidental poisoning by and exposure to noxious substances (X40–X49)
X40   Accidental poisoning by and exposure to nonopioid analgesics,
       antipyretics and antirheumatics
X41   Accidental poisoning by and exposure to antiepileptic, sedative–
       hypnotic, antiparkinsonism and psychotropic drugs, not
       elsewhere classified
X42   Accidental poisoning by and exposure to narcotics and
       psychodysleptics [hallucinogens], not elsewhere classified
X43   Accidental poisoning by and exposure to other drugs acting on
       the autonomic nervous system
X44   Accidental poisoning by and exposure to other and unspecified
       drugs, medicaments and biological substances
X45   Accidental poisoning by and exposure to alcohol
X46   Accidental poisoning by and exposure to organic solvents and
       halogenated hydrocarbons and their vapours
X47   Accidental poisoning by and exposure to other gases and
       vapours
X48   Accidental poisoning by and exposure to pesticides
X49   Accidental poisoning by and exposure to other and unspecified
       chemicals and noxious substances

Overexertion, travel and privation (X50–X57)
X50   Overexertion and strenuous or repetitive movements
X51   Travel and motion
X52   Prolonged stay in weightless environment
X53   Lack of food
X54   Lack of water
X57   Unspecified privation

Accidental exposure to other and unspecified factors (X58–X59)
X58   Exposure to other specified factors
X59   Exposure to unspecified factor

Intentional self-harm (X60–X84)
X60   Intentional self-poisoning by and exposure to nonopioid
       analgesics, antipyretics and antirheumatics
X61   Intentional self-poisoning by and exposure to antiepileptic,
       sedative–hypnotic, antiparkinsonism and psychotropic drugs,
       not elsewhere classified

X62   Intentional self-poisoning by and exposure to narcotics and psychodysleptics [hallucinogens], not elsewhere classified
X63   Intentional self-poisoning by and exposure to other drugs acting on the autonomic nervous system
X64   Intentional self-poisoning by and exposure to other and unspecified drugs, medicaments and biological substances
X65   Intentional self-poisoning by and exposure to alcohol
X66   Intentional self-poisoning by and exposure to organic solvents and halogenated hydrocarbons and their vapours
X67   Intentional self-poisoning by and exposure to other gases and vapours
X68   Intentional self-poisoning by and exposure to pesticides
X69   Intentional self-poisoning by and exposure to other and unspecified chemicals and noxious substances
X70   Intentional self-harm by hanging, strangulation and suffocation
X71   Intentional self-harm by drowning and submersion
X72   Intentional self-harm by handgun discharge
X73   Intentional self-harm by rifle, shotgun and larger firearm discharge
X74   Intentional self-harm by other and unspecified firearm discharge
X75   Intentional self-harm by explosive material
X76   Intentional self-harm by smoke, fire and flames
X77   Intentional self-harm by steam, hot vapours and hot objects
X78   Intentional self-harm by sharp object
X79   Intentional self-harm by blunt object
X80   Intentional self-harm by jumping from a high place
X81   Intentional self-harm by jumping or lying before moving object
X82   Intentional self-harm by crashing of motor vehicle
X83   Intentional self-harm by other specified means
X84   Intentional self-harm by unspecified means

Assault (X85–Y09)
X85   Assault by drugs, medicaments and biological substances
X86   Assault by corrosive substance
X87   Assault by pesticides
X88   Assault by gases and vapours
X89   Assault by other specified chemicals and noxious substances
X90   Assault by unspecified chemical or noxious substance
X91   Assault by hanging, strangulation and suffocation
X92   Assault by drowning and submersion
X93   Assault by handgun discharge
X94   Assault by rifle, shotgun and larger firearm discharge

X95	Assault by other and unspecified firearm discharge
X96	Assault by explosive material
X97	Assault by smoke, fire and flames
X98	Assault by steam, hot vapours and hot objects
X99	Assault by sharp object
Y00	Assault by blunt object
Y01	Assault by pushing from high place
Y02	Assault by pushing or placing victim before moving object
Y03	Assault by crashing of motor vehicle
Y04	Assault by bodily force
Y05	Sexual assault by bodily force
Y06	Neglect and abandonment
Y07	Other maltreatment syndromes
Y08	Assault by other specified means
Y09	Assault by unspecified means

Event of undetermined intent (Y10–Y34)

Y10	Poisoning by and exposure to nonopioid analgesics, antipyretics and antirheumatics, undetermined intent
Y11	Poisoning by and exposure to antiepileptic, sedative–hypnotic, antiparkinsonism and psychotropic drugs, not elsewhere classified, undetermined intent
Y12	Poisoning by and exposure to narcotics and psychodysleptics [hallucinogens], not elsewhere classified, undetermined intent
Y13	Poisoning by and exposure to other drugs acting on the autonomic nervous system, undetermined intent
Y14	Poisoning by and exposure to other and unspecified drugs, medicaments and biological substances, undetermined intent
Y15	Poisoning by and exposure to alcohol, undetermined intent
Y16	Poisoning by and exposure to organic solvents and halogenated hydrocarbons and their vapours, undetermined intent
Y17	Poisoning by and exposure to other gases and vapours, undetermined intent
Y18	Poisoning by and exposure to pesticides, undetermined intent
Y19	Poisoning by and exposure to other and unspecified chemicals and noxious substances, undetermined intent
Y20	Hanging, strangulation and suffocation, undetermined intent
Y21	Drowning and submersion, undetermined intent
Y22	Handgun discharge, undetermined intent
Y23	Rifle, shotgun and larger firearm discharge, undetermined intent
Y24	Other and unspecified firearm discharge, undetermined intent

Y25   Contact with explosive material, undetermined intent

Y26   Exposure to smoke, fire and flames, undetermined intent

Y27   Contact with steam, hot vapours and hot objects, undetermined intent

Y28   Contact with sharp object, undetermined intent

Y29   Contact with blunt object, undetermined intent

Y30   Falling, jumping or pushed from a high place, undetermined intent

Y31   Falling, lying or running before or into moving object, undetermined intent

Y32   Crashing of motor vehicle, undetermined intent

Y33   Other specified events, undetermined intent

Y34   Unspecified event, undetermined intent

Legal intervention and operations of war (Y35–Y36)

Y35   Legal intervention

Y36   Operations of war

Complications of medical and surgical care (Y40–Y84)

Drugs, medicaments and biological substances causing adverse effects in therapeutic use (Y40–Y59)

Y40   Systemic antibiotics

Y41   Other systemic anti-infectives and antiparasitics

Y42   Hormones and their synthetic substitutes and antagonists, not elsewhere classified

Y43   Primarily systemic agents

Y44   Agents primarily affecting blood constituents

Y45   Analgesics, antipyretics and anti-inflammatory drugs

Y46   Antiepileptics and antiparkinsonism drugs

Y47   Sedatives, hypnotics and antianxiety drugs

Y48   Anaesthetics and therapeutic gases

Y49   Psychotropic drugs, not elsewhere classified

Y50   Central nervous system stimulants, not elsewhere classified

Y51   Drugs primarily affecting the autonomic nervous system

Y52   Agents primarily affecting the cardiovascular system

Y53   Agents primarily affecting the gastrointestinal system

Y54   Agents primarily affecting water-balance and mineral and uric acid metabolism

Y55   Agents primarily acting on smooth and skeletal muscles and the respiratory system

Y56   Topical agents primarily affecting skin and mucous membrane and ophthalmological, otorhinolaryngological and dental drugs

Y57   Other and unspecified drugs and medicaments
Y58   Bacterial vaccines
Y59   Other and unspecified vaccines and biological substances

Misadventures to patients during surgical and medical care (Y60–Y69)
Y60   Unintentional cut, puncture, perforation or haemorrhage during surgical and medical care
Y61   Foreign object accidentally left in body during surgical and medical care
Y62   Failure of sterile precautions during surgical and medical care
Y63   Failure in dosage during surgical and medical care
Y64   Contaminated medical or biological substances
Y65   Other misadventures during surgical and medical care
Y66   Nonadministration of surgical and medical care
Y69   Unspecified misadventure during surgical and medical care

Medical devices associated with adverse incidents in diagnostic and therapeutic use (Y70–Y82)
Y70   Anaesthesiology devices associated with adverse incidents
Y71   Cardiovascular devices associated with adverse incidents
Y72   Otorhinolaryngological devices associated with adverse incidents
Y73   Gastroenterology and urology devices associated with adverse incidents
Y74   General hospital and personal-use devices associated with adverse incidents
Y75   Neurological devices associated with adverse incidents
Y76   Obstetric and gynaecological devices associated with adverse incidents
Y77   Ophthalmic devices associated with adverse incidents
Y78   Radiological devices associated with adverse incidents
Y79   Orthopaedic devices associated with adverse incidents
Y80   Physical medicine devices associated with adverse incidents
Y81   General- and plastic-surgery devices associated with adverse incidents
Y82   Other and unspecified medical devices associated with adverse incidents

Surgical and other medical procedures as the cause of abnormal reaction of the patient, or of later complication, without mention of misadventure at the time of the procedure (Y83–Y84)
Y83   Surgical operation and other surgical procedures as the cause of abnormal reaction of the patient, or of later complication, without mention of misadventure at the time of the procedure

Y84   Other medical procedures as the cause of abnormal reaction of the patient, or of later complication, without mention of misadventure at the time of the procedure

Sequelae of external causes of morbidity and mortality (Y85–Y89)
Y85   Sequelae of transport accidents
Y86   Sequelae of other accidents
Y87   Sequelae of intentional self-harm, assault and events of undetermined intent
Y88   Sequelae of surgical and medical care as external cause
Y89   Sequelae of other external causes

Supplementary factors related to causes of morbidity and mortality classified elsewhere (Y90–Y98)
Y90   Evidence of alcohol involvement determined by blood alcohol level
Y91   Evidence of alcohol involvement determined by level of intoxication
Y95   Nosocomial condition
Y96   Work-related condition
Y97   Environmental-pollution-related condition
Y98   Lifestyle-related condition

Chapter XXI
Factors influencing health status and contact with health services (Z00–Z99)

Persons encountering health services for examination and investigation (Z00–Z13)
Z00   General examination and investigation of persons without complaint or reported diagnosis
Z01   Other special examinations and investigations of persons without complaint or reported diagnosis
Z02   Examination and encounter for administrative purposes
Z03   Medical observation and evaluation for suspected diseases and conditions
Z04   Examination and observation for other reasons
Z08   Follow-up examination after treatment for malignant neoplasm

Z09   Follow-up examination after treatment for conditions other than malignant neoplasms
Z10   Routine general health check-up of defined subpopulation
Z11   Special screening examination for infectious and parasitic diseases
Z12   Special screening examination for neoplasms
Z13   Special screening examination for other diseases and disorders

Persons with potential health hazards related to communicable diseases (Z20–Z29)

Z20   Contact with and exposure to communicable diseases
Z21   Asymptomatic human immunodeficiency virus [HIV] infection status
Z22   Carrier of infectious disease
Z23   Need for immunization against single bacterial diseases
Z24   Need for immunization against certain single viral diseases
Z25   Need for immunization against other single viral diseases
Z26   Need for immunization against other single infectious diseases
Z27   Need for immunization against combinations of infectious diseases
Z28   Immunization not carried out
Z29   Need for other prophylactic measures

Persons encountering health services in circumstances related to reproduction (Z30–Z39)

Z30   Contraceptive management
Z31   Procreative management
Z32   Pregnancy examination and test
Z33   Pregnant state, incidental
Z34   Supervision of normal pregnancy
Z35   Supervision of high-risk pregnancy
Z36   Antenatal screening
Z37   Outcome of delivery
Z38   Liveborn infants according to place of birth
Z39   Postpartum care and examination

Persons encountering health services for specific procedures and health care (Z40–Z54)

Z40   Prophylactic surgery
Z41   Procedures for purposes other than remedying health state
Z42   Follow-up care involving plastic surgery
Z43   Attention to artificial openings

Z44	Fitting and adjustment of external prosthetic device
Z45	Adjustment and management of implanted device
Z46	Fitting and adjustment of other devices
Z47	Other orthopaedic follow-up care
Z48	Other surgical follow-up care
Z49	Care involving dialysis
Z50	Care involving use of rehabilitation procedures
Z51	Other medical care
Z52	Donors of organs and tissues
Z53	Persons encountering health services for specific procedures, not carried out
Z54	Convalescence

Persons with potential health hazards related to socioeconomic and psychosocial circumstances (Z55–Z65)

Z55	Problems related to education and literacy
Z56	Problems related to employment and unemployment
Z57	Occupational exposure to risk-factors
Z58	Problems related to physical environment
Z59	Problems related to housing and economic circumstances
Z60	Problems related to social environment
Z61	Problems related to negative life events in childhood
Z62	Other problems related to upbringing
Z63	Other problems related to primary support group, including family circumstances
Z64	Problems related to certain psychosocial circumstances
Z65	Problems related to other psychosocial circumstances

Persons encountering health services in other circumstances (Z70–Z76)

Z70	Counselling related to sexual attitude, behaviour and orientation
Z71	Persons encountering health services for other counselling and medical advice, not elsewhere classified
Z72	Problems related to lifestyle
Z73	Problems related to life-management difficulty
Z74	Problems related to care-provider dependency
Z75	Problems related to medical facilities and other health care
Z76	Persons encountering health services in other circumstances

Persons with potential health hazards related to family and personal history and certain conditions influencing health status (Z80–Z99)

Z80	Family history of malignant neoplasm
Z81	Family history of mental and behavioural disorders

Z82	Family history of certain disabilities and chronic diseases leading to disablement
Z83	Family history of other specific disorders
Z84	Family history of other conditions
Z85	Personal history of malignant neoplasm
Z86	Personal history of certain other diseases
Z87	Personal history of other diseases and conditions
Z88	Personal history of allergy to drugs, medicaments and biological substances
Z89	Acquired absence of limb
Z90	Acquired absence of organs, not elsewhere classified
Z91	Personal history of risk-factors, not elsewhere classified
Z92	Personal history of medical treatment
Z93	Artificial opening status
Z94	Transplanted organ and tissue status
Z95	Presence of cardiac and vascular implants and grafts
Z96	Presence of other functional implants
Z97	Presence of other devices
Z98	Other postsurgical states
Z99	Dependence on enabling machines and devices, not elsewhere classified

Tabular list of inclusions and four-character subcategories

CHAPTER I

Certain infectious and parasitic diseases (A00–B99)

Includes: diseases generally recognized as communicable or transmissible

Excludes: carrier or suspected carrier of infectious disease (Z22.–)
certain localized infections—see body system-related chapters
infectious and parasitic diseases complicating pregnancy,
childbirth and the puerperium [except obstetrical tetanus
and human immunodeficiency virus [HIV] disease] (O98.–)
infectious and parasitic diseases specific to the perinatal period
[except tetanus neonatorum, congenital syphilis, perinatal
gonococcal infection and perinatal human immunodeficiency
virus [HIV] disease] (P35–P39)
influenza and other acute respiratory infections (J00–J22)

This chapter contains the following blocks:

A00–A09 Intestinal infectious diseases
A15–A19 Tuberculosis
A20–A28 Certain zoonotic bacterial diseases
A30–A49 Other bacterial diseases
A50–A64 Infections with a predominantly sexual mode of transmission
A65–A69 Other spirochaetal diseases
A70–A74 Other diseases caused by chlamydiae
A75–A79 Rickettsioses
A80–A89 Viral infections of the central nervous system
A90–A99 Arthropod-borne viral fevers and viral haemorrhagic fevers
B00–B09 Viral infections characterized by skin and mucous membrane lesions
B15–B19 Viral hepatitis
B20–B24 Human immunodeficiency virus [HIV] disease
B25–B34 Other viral diseases
B35–B49 Mycoses
B50–B64 Protozoal diseases
B65–B83 Helminthiases
B85–B89 Pediculosis, acariasis and other infestations
B90–B94 Sequelae of infectious and parasitic diseases
B95–B97 Bacterial, viral and other infectious agents
B99 Other infectious diseases

Intestinal infectious diseases (A00–A09)

A00 Cholera

A00.0 Cholera due to *Vibrio cholerae* 01, biovar cholerae
Classical cholera

A00.1 Cholera due to *Vibrio cholerae* 01, biovar eltor
Cholera eltor

A00.9 Cholera, unspecified

A01 Typhoid and paratyphoid fevers

A01.0 Typhoid fever
Infection due to *Salmonella typhi*

A01.1 Paratyphoid fever A

A01.2 Paratyphoid fever B

A01.3 Paratyphoid fever C

A01.4 Paratyphoid fever, unspecified
Infection due to *Salmonella paratyphi* NOS

A02 Other salmonella infections

Includes: infection or foodborne intoxication due to any *Salmonella* species other than *S. typhi* and *S. paratyphi*

A02.0 Salmonella enteritis
Salmonellosis

A02.1 Salmonella septicaemia

A02.2† Localized salmonella infections
Salmonella:
- arthritis (M01.3*)
- meningitis (G01*)
- osteomyelitis (M90.2*)
- pneumonia (J17.0*)
- renal tubulo-interstitial disease (N16.0*)

A02.8 Other specified salmonella infections

A02.9 Salmonella infection, unspecified

A03 Shigellosis

A03.0 Shigellosis due to *Shigella dysenteriae*
Group A shigellosis [Shiga-Kruse dysentery]

A03.1 Shigellosis due to *Shigella flexneri*
Group B shigellosis

A03.2 Shigellosis due to *Shigella boydii*
Group C shigellosis

A03.3 Shigellosis due to *Shigella sonnei*
Group D shigellosis

A03.8 Other shigellosis

A03.9 Shigellosis, unspecified
Bacillary dysentery NOS

A04 Other bacterial intestinal infections
Excludes: foodborne intoxications, bacterial (A05.–)
          tuberculous enteritis (A18.3)

A04.0 Enteropathogenic *Escherichia coli* infection

A04.1 Enterotoxigenic *Escherichia coli* infection

A04.2 Enteroinvasive *Escherichia coli* infection

A04.3 Enterohaemorrhagic *Escherichia coli* infection

A04.4 Other intestinal *Escherichia coli* infections
Escherichia coli enteritis NOS

A04.5 Campylobacter enteritis

A04.6 Enteritis due to *Yersinia enterocolitica*
Excludes: extraintestinal yersiniosis (A28.2)

A04.7 Enterocolitis due to *Clostridium difficile*

A04.8 Other specified bacterial intestinal infections

A04.9 Bacterial intestinal infection, unspecified
Bacterial enteritis NOS

A05 Other bacterial foodborne intoxications

Excludes: *Escherichia coli* infection (A04.0–A04.4)
listeriosis (A32.–)
salmonella foodborne intoxication and infection (A02.–)
toxic effect of noxious foodstuffs (T61–T62)

A05.0 Foodborne staphylococcal intoxication

A05.1 Botulism
Classical foodborne intoxication due to *Clostridium botulinum*

A05.2 Foodborne *Clostridium perfringens* [*Clostridium welchii*] intoxication
Enteritis necroticans
Pig-bel

A05.3 Foodborne *Vibrio parahaemolyticus* intoxication

A05.4 Foodborne *Bacillus cereus* intoxication

A05.8 Other specified bacterial foodborne intoxications

A05.9 Bacterial foodborne intoxication, unspecified

A06 Amoebiasis

Includes: infection due to *Entamoeba histolytica*
Excludes: other protozoal intestinal diseases (A07.–)

A06.0 Acute amoebic dysentery
Acute amoebiasis
Intestinal amoebiasis NOS

A06.1 Chronic intestinal amoebiasis

A06.2 Amoebic nondysenteric colitis

A06.3 Amoeboma of intestine
Amoeboma NOS

A06.4 Amoebic liver abscess
Hepatic amoebiasis

A06.5† Amoebic lung abscess (J99.8*)
Amoebic abscess of lung (and liver)

A06.6† Amoebic brain abscess (G07*)
Amoebic abscess of brain (and liver)(and lung)

A06.7 Cutaneous amoebiasis

A06.8   Amoebic infection of other sites
Amoebic:
- appendicitis
- balanitis† (N51.2*)

A06.9   Amoebiasis, unspecified

A07   Other protozoal intestinal diseases

A07.0   Balantidiasis
Balantidial dysentery

A07.1   Giardiasis [lambliasis]

A07.2   Cryptosporidiosis

A07.3   Isosporiasis
Infection due to *Isospora belli* and *Isospora hominis*
Intestinal coccidiosis
Isosporosis

A07.8   Other specified protozoal intestinal diseases
Intestinal trichomoniasis
Sarcocystosis
Sarcosporidiosis

A07.9   Protozoal intestinal disease, unspecified
Flagellate diarrhoea
Protozoal:
- colitis
- diarrhoea
- dysentery

A08   Viral and other specified intestinal infections

Excludes: influenza with involvement of gastrointestinal tract
(J10.8, J11.8)

A08.0   Rotaviral enteritis

A08.1   Acute gastroenteropathy due to Norwalk agent
Small round structured virus enteritis

A08.2   Adenoviral enteritis

A08.3   Other viral enteritis

A08.4   **Viral intestinal infection, unspecified**
Viral:
- enteritis NOS
- gastroenteritis NOS
- gastroenteropathy NOS

A08.5   **Other specified intestinal infections**

A09   **Diarrhoea and gastroenteritis of presumed infectious origin**

Note: In countries where any term listed in A09 without further specification can be assumed to be of noninfectious origin, the condition should be classified to K52.9.

Catarrh, enteric or intestinal

Colitis   } NOS
Enteritis   } haemorrhagic
Gastroenteritis } septic

Diarrhoea:
- NOS
- dysenteric
- epidemic

Infectious diarrhoeal disease NOS

Excludes: due to bacterial, protozoal, viral and other specified infectious agents (A00–A08)
noninfective diarrhoea (K52.9)
- neonatal (P78.3)

Tuberculosis
(A15–A19)

Includes: infections due to *Mycobacterium tuberculosis* and *Mycobacterium bovis*

Excludes: congenital tuberculosis (P37.0)
pneumoconiosis associated with tuberculosis (J65)
sequelae of tuberculosis (B90.–)
silicotuberculosis (J65)

A15 Respiratory tuberculosis, bacteriologically and histologically confirmed

A15.0 Tuberculosis of lung, confirmed by sputum microscopy with or without culture
Tuberculous:
- bronchiectasis
- fibrosis of lung } confirmed by sputum microscopy with or
- pneumonia   without culture
- pneumothorax

A15.1 Tuberculosis of lung, confirmed by culture only
Conditions listed in A15.0, confirmed by culture only

A15.2 Tuberculosis of lung, confirmed histologically
Conditions listed in A15.0, confirmed histologically

A15.3 Tuberculosis of lung, confirmed by unspecified means
Conditions listed in A15.0, confirmed but unspecified whether
    bacteriologically or histologically

A15.4 Tuberculosis of intrathoracic lymph nodes, confirmed bacteriologically and histologically
Tuberculosis of lymph nodes:
- hilar
- mediastinal   } confirmed bacteriogically and
- tracheobronchial   histologically

Excludes: specified as primary (A15.7)

A15.5 Tuberculosis of larynx, trachea and bronchus, confirmed bacteriologically and histologically
Tuberculosis of:
- bronchus
- glottis
- larynx   } confirmed bacteriologically and histologically
- trachea

A15.6 Tuberculous pleurisy, confirmed bacteriologically and histologically

Tuberculosis of pleura } confirmed bacteriologically and
Tuberculous empyema   histologically

Excludes: in primary respiratory tuberculosis, confirmed
                bacteriologically and histologically (A15.7)

A15.7 Primary respiratory tuberculosis, confirmed bacteriologically and histologically

113

A15.8   Other respiratory tuberculosis, confirmed bacteriologically and histologically

Mediastinal tuberculosis
Nasopharyngeal tuberculosis
Tuberculosis of: } confirmed bacteriologically and histologically
• nose
• sinus [any nasal]

A15.9   Respiratory tuberculosis unspecified, confirmed bacteriologically and histologically

A16   Respiratory tuberculosis, not confirmed bacteriologically or histologically

A16.0   Tuberculosis of lung, bacteriologically and histologically negative

Tuberculous:
• bronchiectasis
• fibrosis of lung } bacteriologically and histologically
• pneumonia   negative
• pneumothorax

A16.1   Tuberculosis of lung, bacteriological and histological examination not done

Conditions listed in A16.0, bacteriological and histological examination not done

A16.2   Tuberculosis of lung, without mention of bacteriological or histological confirmation

Tuberculosis of lung
Tuberculous:
• bronchiectasis } NOS (without mention of
• fibrosis of lung   bacteriological or histological
• pneumonia   confirmation)
• pneumothorax

A16.3   Tuberculosis of intrathoracic lymph nodes, without mention of bacteriological or histological confirmation

Tuberculosis of lymph nodes:
• hilar
• intrathoracic } NOS (without mention of
• mediastinal   bacteriological or histological
• tracheobronchial confirmation)

Excludes: when specified as primary (A16.7)

A16.4 **Tuberculosis of larynx, trachea and bronchus, without mention of bacteriological or histological confirmation**
Tuberculosis of:
- bronchus ⎫
- glottis ⎬ NOS (without mention of bacteriological or
- larynx ⎪ histological confirmation)
- trachea ⎭

A16.5 **Tuberculous pleurisy, without mention of bacteriological or histological confirmation**
Tuberculosis of pleura ⎫
Tuberculous: ⎪ NOS (without mention of
- empyema ⎬ bacteriological or histological
- pleurisy ⎭ confirmation)
Excludes: in primary respiratory tuberculosis (A16.7)

A16.7 **Primary respiratory tuberculosis without mention of bacteriological or histological confirmation**
Primary:
- respiratory tuberculosis NOS
- tuberculous complex

A16.8 **Other respiratory tuberculosis, without mention of bacteriological or histological confirmation**
Mediastinal tuberculosis ⎫
Nasopharyngeal tuberculosis ⎪ NOS (without mention of
Tuberculosis of: ⎬ bacteriological or
- nose ⎪ histological confirmation)
- sinus [any nasal] ⎭

A16.9 **Respiratory tuberculosis unspecified, without mention of bacteriological or histological confirmation**
Respiratory tuberculosis NOS
Tuberculosis NOS

A17† Tuberculosis of nervous system

A17.0† **Tuberculous meningitis (G01*)**
Tuberculosis of meninges (cerebral)(spinal)
Tuberculous leptomeningitis

A17.1† **Meningeal tuberculoma (G07*)**
Tuberculoma of meninges

A17.8† **Other tuberculosis of nervous system**

Tuberculoma ⎫ of ⎧ brain (G07*)
Tuberculosis ⎭   ⎩ spinal cord (G07*)
Tuberculous:
- abscess of brain (G07*)
- meningoencephalitis (G05.0*)
- myelitis (G05.0*)
- polyneuropathy (G63.0*)

A17.9† **Tuberculosis of nervous system, unspecified (G99.8*)**

A18 Tuberculosis of other organs

A18.0† **Tuberculosis of bones and joints**
Tuberculosis of:
- hip (M01.1*)
- knee (M01.1*)
- vertebral column (M49.0*)
Tuberculous:
- arthritis (M01.1*)
- mastoiditis (H75.0*)
- necrosis of bone (M90.0*)
- osteitis (M90.0*)
- osteomyelitis (M90.0*)
- synovitis (M68.0*)
- tenosynovitis (M68.0*)

A18.1† **Tuberculosis of genitourinary system**
Tuberculosis of:
- bladder (N33.0*)
- cervix (N74.0*)
- kidney (N29.1*)
- male genital organs (N51.–*)
- ureter (N29.1*)
Tuberculous female pelvic inflammatory disease (N74.1*)

A18.2 **Tuberculous peripheral lymphadenopathy**
Tuberculous adenitis

Excludes: tuberculosis of lymph nodes:
- intrathoracic (A15.4, A16.3)
- mesenteric and retroperitoneal (A18.3)
tuberculous tracheobronchial adenopathy (A15.4, A16.3)

A18.3   **Tuberculosis of intestines, peritoneum and mesenteric glands**
Tuberculosis (of):
- anus and rectum† (K93.0*)
- intestine (large)(small)† (K93.0*)
- retroperitoneal (lymph nodes)
Tuberculous:
- ascites
- enteritis† (K93.0*)
- peritonitis† (K67.3*)

A18.4   **Tuberculosis of skin and subcutaneous tissue**
Erythema induratum, tuberculous
Lupus:
- exedens
- vulgaris:
  - NOS
  - of eyelid† (H03.1*)
Scrofuloderma

Excludes: lupus erythematosus (L93.–)
  - systemic (M32.–)

A18.5†   **Tuberculosis of eye**
Tuberculous:
- chorioretinitis (H32.0*)
- episcleritis (H19.0*)
- interstitial keratitis (H19.2*)
- iridocyclitis (H22.0*)
- keratoconjunctivitis (interstitial)(phlyctenular) (H19.2*)

Excludes: lupus vulgaris of eyelid (A18.4)

A18.6†   **Tuberculosis of ear**
Tuberculous otitis media (H67.0*)

Excludes: tuberculous mastoiditis (A18.0†)

A18.7†   **Tuberculosis of adrenal glands (E35.1*)**
Addison's disease, tuberculous

A18.8†   **Tuberculosis of other specified organs**
Tuberculosis of:
- endocardium (I39.8*)
- myocardium (I41.0*)
- oesophagus (K23.0*)
- pericardium (I32.0*)
- thyroid gland (E35.0*)
Tuberculous cerebral arteritis (I68.1*)

117

A19 Miliary tuberculosis

Includes: tuberculosis:
- disseminated
- generalized
tuberculous polyserositis

A19.0   **Acute miliary tuberculosis of a single specified site**

A19.1   **Acute miliary tuberculosis of multiple sites**

A19.2   **Acute miliary tuberculosis, unspecified**

A19.8   **Other miliary tuberculosis**

A19.9   **Miliary tuberculosis, unspecified**

Certain zoonotic bacterial diseases (A20–A28)

A20 Plague

Includes: infection due to *Yersinia pestis*

A20.0   **Bubonic plague**

A20.1   **Cellulocutaneous plague**

A20.2   **Pneumonic plague**

A20.3   **Plague meningitis**

A20.7   **Septicaemic plague**

A20.8   **Other forms of plague**
Abortive plague
Asymptomatic plague
Pestis minor

A20.9   **Plague, unspecified**

A21 Tularaemia

Includes: deer-fly fever
infection due to *Francisella tularensis*
rabbit fever

A21.0   **Ulceroglandular tularaemia**

A21.1   **Oculoglandular tularaemia**
Ophthalmic tularaemia

A21.2   **Pulmonary tularaemia**

A21.3   **Gastrointestinal tularaemia**
Abdominal tularaemia

A21.7   **Generalized tularaemia**

A21.8   **Other forms of tularaemia**

A21.9   **Tularaemia, unspecified**

A22   Anthrax

Includes: infection due to *Bacillus anthracis*

A22.0   **Cutaneous anthrax**
Malignant:
- carbuncle
- pustule

A22.1   **Pulmonary anthrax**
Inhalation anthrax
Ragpicker's disease
Woolsorter's disease

A22.2   **Gastrointestinal anthrax**

A22.7   **Anthrax septicaemia**

A22.8   **Other forms of anthrax**
Anthrax meningitis† (G01*)

A22.9   **Anthrax, unspecified**

A23   Brucellosis

Includes: fever:
- Malta
- Mediterranean
- undulant

A23.0   **Brucellosis due to *Brucella melitensis***

A23.1   **Brucellosis due to *Brucella abortus***

A23.2   **Brucellosis due to *Brucella suis***

A23.3   **Brucellosis due to *Brucella canis***

A23.8   **Other brucellosis**

A23.9   **Brucellosis, unspecified**

A24   Glanders and melioidosis

A24.0   **Glanders**
Infection due to *Pseudomonas mallei*
Malleus

A24.1   **Acute and fulminating melioidosis**
Melioidosis:
- pneumonia
- septicaemia

A24.2   **Subacute and chronic melioidosis**

A24.3   **Other melioidosis**

A24.4   **Melioidosis, unspecified**
Infection due to *Pseudomonas pseudomallei* NOS
Whitmore's disease

A25   Rat-bite fevers

A25.0   **Spirillosis**
Sodoku

A25.1   **Streptobacillosis**
Epidemic arthritic erythema
Haverhill fever
Streptobacillary rat-bite fever

A25.9   **Rat-bite fever, unspecified**

A26   Erysipeloid

A26.0   **Cutaneous erysipeloid**
Erythema migrans

A26.7   ***Erysipelothrix* septicaemia**

A26.8   **Other forms of erysipeloid**

A26.9   Erysipeloid, unspecified

A27   Leptospirosis

A27.0   Leptospirosis icterohaemorrhagica
Leptospirosis due to *Leptospira interrogans* serovar icterohaemor-
rhagiae

A27.8   Other forms of leptospirosis

A27.9   Leptospirosis, unspecified

A28   Other zoonotic bacterial diseases, not elsewhere classified

A28.0   Pasteurellosis

A28.1   Cat-scratch disease
Cat-scratch fever

A28.2   Extraintestinal yersiniosis
Excludes: enteritis due to *Yersinia enterocolitica* (A04.6)
plague (A20.–)

A28.8   Other specified zoonotic bacterial diseases, not elsewhere classified

A28.9   Zoonotic bacterial disease, unspecified

Other bacterial diseases
(A30–A49)

A30   Leprosy [Hansen's disease]
Includes: infection due to *Mycobacterium leprae*
Excludes: sequelae of leprosy (B92)

A30.0   Indeterminate leprosy
I leprosy

A30.1   Tuberculoid leprosy
TT leprosy

A30.2   Borderline tuberculoid leprosy
BT leprosy

A30.3   Borderline leprosy
BB leprosy

A30.4   Borderline lepromatous leprosy
BL leprosy

A30.5   Lepromatous leprosy
LL leprosy

A30.8   Other forms of leprosy

A30.9   Leprosy, unspecified

A31 Infection due to other mycobacteria

Excludes: leprosy (A30.–)
              tuberculosis (A15–A19)

A31.0   Pulmonary mycobacterial infection
Infection due to *Mycobacterium*:
- *avium*
- *intracellulare* [Battey bacillus]
- *kansasii*

A31.1   Cutaneous mycobacterial infection
Buruli ulcer
Infection due to *Mycobacterium*:
- *marinum*
- *ulcerans*

A31.8   Other mycobacterial infections

A31.9   Mycobacterial infection, unspecified
Atypical mycobacterial infection NOS
Mycobacteriosis NOS

A32 Listeriosis

Includes: listerial foodborne infection
Excludes: neonatal (disseminated) listeriosis (P37.2)

A32.0   Cutaneous listeriosis

A32.1† **Listerial meningitis and meningoencephalitis**
Listerial:
- meningitis (G01*)
- meningoencephalitis (G05.0*)

A32.7 **Listerial septicaemia**

A32.8 **Other forms of listeriosis**
Listerial:
- cerebral arteritis† (I68.1*)
- endocarditis† (I39.8*)
Oculoglandular listeriosis

A32.9 **Listeriosis, unspecified**

A33 **Tetanus neonatorum**

A34 **Obstetrical tetanus**

A35 **Other tetanus**
Tetanus NOS
Excludes: tetanus:
- neonatorum (A33)
- obstetrical (A34)

A36 **Diphtheria**

A36.0 **Pharyngeal diphtheria**
Diphtheritic membranous angina
Tonsillar diphtheria

A36.1 **Nasopharyngeal diphtheria**

A36.2 **Laryngeal diphtheria**
Diphtheritic laryngotracheitis

A36.3 **Cutaneous diphtheria**
Excludes: erythrasma (L08.1)

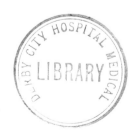

A36.8 **Other diphtheria**
Diphtheritic:
- conjunctivitis† (H13.1*)
- myocarditis† (I41.0*)
- polyneuritis† (G63.0*)

A36.9 **Diphtheria, unspecified**

A37 Whooping cough

A37.0 **Whooping cough due to *Bordetella pertussis***

A37.1 **Whooping cough due to *Bordetella parapertussis***

A37.8 **Whooping cough due to other *Bordetella* species**

A37.9 **Whooping cough, unspecified**

A38 Scarlet fever
Scarlatina
Excludes: streptococcal sore throat (J02.0)

A39 Meningococcal infection

A39.0† **Meningococcal meningitis (G01*)**

A39.1† **Waterhouse-Friderichsen syndrome (E35.1*)**
Meningococcal haemorrhagic adrenalitis
Meningococcic adrenal syndrome

A39.2 **Acute meningococcaemia**

A39.3 **Chronic meningococcaemia**

A39.4 **Meningococcaemia, unspecified**
Meningococcal bacteraemia NOS

A39.5† **Meningococcal heart disease**
Meningococcal:
- carditis NOS (I52.0*)
- endocarditis (I39.8*)
- myocarditis (I41.0*)
- pericarditis (I32.0*)

A39.8 **Other meningococcal infections**
Meningococcal:
- arthritis† (M01.0*)
- conjunctivitis† (H13.1*)
- encephalitis† (G05.0*)
- retrobulbar neuritis† (H48.1*)
Postmeningococcal arthritis† (M03.0*)

A39.9 **Meningococcal infection, unspecified**
Meningococcal disease NOS

A40 Streptococcal septicaemia

Excludes: during labour (O75.3)
following:
- abortion or ectopic or molar pregnancy (O03–O07, O08.0)
- immunization (T88.0)
- infusion, transfusion or therapeutic injection (T80.2)
neonatal (P36.0–P36.1)
postprocedural (T81.4)
puerperal (O85)

A40.0 **Septicaemia due to streptococcus, group A**

A40.1 **Septicaemia due to streptococcus, group B**

A40.2 **Septicaemia due to streptococcus, group D**

A40.3 **Septicaemia due to *Streptococcus pneumoniae***
Pneumococcal septicaemia

A40.8 **Other streptococcal septicaemia**

A40.9 **Streptococcal septicaemia, unspecified**

A41 Other septicaemia

Excludes: bacteraemia NOS (A49.9)
during labour (O75.3)
following:
- abortion or ectopic or molar pregnancy (O03–O07, O08.0)
- immunization (T88.0)
- infusion, transfusion or therapeutic injection (T80.2)
septicaemia (due to)(in):
- actinomycotic (A42.7)
- anthrax (A22.7)
- candidal (B37.7)
- *Erysipelothrix* (A26.7)
- extraintestinal yersiniosis (A28.2)
- gonococcal (A54.8)
- herpesviral (B00.7)
- listerial (A32.7)
- meningococcal (A39.2–A39.4)
- neonatal (P36.–)
- postprocedural (T81.4)
- puerperal (O85)
- streptococcal (A40.–)
- tularaemia (A21.7)
septicaemic:
- melioidosis (A24.1)
- plague (A20.7)
toxic shock syndrome (A48.3)

A41.0 Septicaemia due to *Staphylococcus aureus*

A41.1 Septicaemia due to other specified staphylococcus
Septicaemia due to coagulase-negative staphylococcus

A41.2 Septicaemia due to unspecified staphylococcus

A41.3 Septicaemia due to *Haemophilus influenzae*

A41.4 Septicaemia due to anaerobes
Excludes: gas gangrene (A48.0)

A41.5 Septicaemia due to other Gram-negative organisms
Gram-negative septicaemia NOS

A41.8 Other specified septicaemia

A41.9 Septicaemia, unspecified
Septic shock

A42 Actinomycosis

Excludes: actinomycetoma (B47.1)

A42.0	Pulmonary actinomycosis
A42.1	Abdominal actinomycosis
A42.2	Cervicofacial actinomycosis
A42.7	Actinomycotic septicaemia
A42.8	Other forms of actinomycosis
A42.9	Actinomycosis, unspecified

A43 Nocardiosis

A43.0	Pulmonary nocardiosis
A43.1	Cutaneous nocardiosis
A43.8	Other forms of nocardiosis
A43.9	Nocardiosis, unspecified

A44 Bartonellosis

A44.0	Systemic bartonellosis Oroya fever
A44.1	Cutaneous and mucocutaneous bartonellosis Verruga peruana
A44.8	Other forms of bartonellosis
A44.9	Bartonellosis, unspecified

A46 Erysipelas

Excludes: postpartum or puerperal erysipelas (O86.8)

A48 Other bacterial diseases, not elsewhere classified

Excludes: actinomycetoma (B47.1)

A48.0	Gas gangrene Clostridial: • cellulitis • myonecrosis

A48.1   Legionnaires' disease

A48.2   Nonpneumonic Legionnaires' disease [Pontiac fever]

A48.3   Toxic shock syndrome
Excludes: endotoxic shock NOS (R57.8)
septicaemia NOS (A41.9)

A48.4   Brazilian purpuric fever
Systemic *Haemophilus aegyptius* infection

A48.8   Other specified bacterial diseases

A49   Bacterial infection of unspecified site
Excludes: bacterial agents as the cause of diseases classified to
other chapters (B95–B96)
chlamydial infection NOS (A74.9)
meningococcal infection NOS (A39.9)
rickettsial infection NOS (A79.9)
spirochaetal infection NOS (A69.9)

A49.0   Staphylococcal infection, unspecified

A49.1   Streptococcal infection, unspecified

A49.2   *Haemophilus influenzae* infection, unspecified

A49.3   Mycoplasma infection, unspecified

A49.8   Other bacterial infections of unspecified site

A49.9   Bacterial infection, unspecified
Bacteraemia NOS

Infections with a predominantly sexual mode of transmission
(A50–A64)

Excludes: human immunodeficiency virus [HIV] disease
(B20–B24)
nonspecific and nongonococcal urethritis (N34.1)
Reiter's disease (M02.3)

A50 Congenital syphilis

A50.0 Early congenital syphilis, symptomatic
Any congenital syphilitic condition specified as early or manifest less than two years after birth.

Early congenital syphilis:
- cutaneous
- mucocutaneous
- visceral

Early congenital syphilitic:
- laryngitis
- oculopathy
- osteochondropathy
- pharyngitis
- pneumonia
- rhinitis

A50.1 Early congenital syphilis, latent
Congenital syphilis without clinical manifestations, with positive serological reaction and negative spinal fluid test, less than two years after birth.

A50.2 Early congenital syphilis, unspecified
Congenital syphilis NOS less than two years after birth.

A50.3 Late congenital syphilitic oculopathy
Late congenital syphilitic interstitial keratitis† (H19.2*)
Late congenital syphilitic oculopathy NEC (H58.8*)
Excludes: Hutchinson's triad (A50.5)

A50.4 Late congenital neurosyphilis [juvenile neurosyphilis]
Dementia paralytica juvenilis
Juvenile:
- general paresis
- tabes dorsalis
- taboparetic neurosyphilis

Late congenital syphilitic:
- encephalitis† (G05.0*)
- meningitis† (G01*)
- polyneuropathy† (G63.0*)

Use additional code, if desired, to identify any associated mental disorder.
Excludes: Hutchinson's triad (A50.5)

129

A50.5   Other late congenital syphilis, symptomatic
Any congenital syphilitic condition specified as late or manifest two years or more after birth.

Clutton's joints† (M03.1*)
Hutchinson's:
- teeth
- triad

Late congenital:
- cardiovascular syphilis† (I98.0*)
- syphilitic:
  - arthropathy† (M03.1*)
  - osteochondropathy† (M90.2*)

Syphilitic saddle nose

A50.6   Late congenital syphilis, latent
Congenital syphilis without clinical manifestations, with positive serological reaction and negative spinal fluid test, two years or more after birth.

A50.7   Late congenital syphilis, unspecified
Congenital syphilis NOS two years or more after birth.

A50.9   Congenital syphilis, unspecified

A51   Early syphilis

A51.0   Primary genital syphilis
Syphilitic chancre NOS

A51.1   Primary anal syphilis

A51.2   Primary syphilis of other sites

A51.3   Secondary syphilis of skin and mucous membranes
Condyloma latum
Syphilitic:
- alopecia† (L99.8*)
- leukoderma† (L99.8*)
- mucous patch

A51.4   Other secondary syphilis
Secondary syphilitic:
- female pelvic inflammatory disease† (N74.2*)
- iridocyclitis† (H22.0*)
- lymphadenopathy
- meningitis† (G01*)
- myositis† (M63.0*)
- oculopathy NEC† (H58.8*)
- periostitis† (M90.1*)

A51.5   Early syphilis, latent
Syphilis (acquired) without clinical manifestations, with positive serological reaction and negative spinal fluid test, less than two years after infection.

A51.9   Early syphilis, unspecified

A52   Late syphilis

A52.0†   Cardiovascular syphilis
Cardiovascular syphilis NOS (I98.0*)
Syphilitic:
- aneurysm of aorta (I79.0*)
- aortic incompetence (I39.1*)
- aortitis (I79.1*)
- arteritis, cerebral (I68.1*)
- endocarditis NOS (I39.8*)
- myocarditis (I41.0*)
- pericarditis (I32.0*)
- pulmonary regurgitation (I39.3*)

A52.1   Symptomatic neurosyphilis
Charcot's arthropathy (M14.6*)
Late syphilitic:
- acoustic neuritis† (H94.0*)
- encephalitis† (G05.0*)
- meningitis† (G01*)
- optic atrophy† (H48.0*)
- polyneuropathy† (G63.0*)
- retrobulbar neuritis† (H48.1*)
Syphilitic parkinsonism† (G22*)
Tabes dorsalis

A52.2   Asymptomatic neurosyphilis

131

A52.3   **Neurosyphilis, unspecified**

Gumma (syphilitic)
Syphilis (late)   } of central nervous system NOS
Syphiloma

A52.7   **Other symptomatic late syphilis**

Glomerular disease in syphilis† (N08.0*)

Gumma (syphilitic)   } any sites, except those classified to
Late or tertiary syphilis }   A52.0–A52.3
Late syphilitic:
- bursitis† (M73.1*)
- chorioretinitis† (H32.0*)
- episcleritis† (H19.0*)
- female pelvic inflammatory disease† (N74.2*)
- leukoderma† (L99.8*)
- oculopathy NEC† (H58.8*)
- peritonitis† (K67.2*)
Syphilis [stage unspecified] of:
- bone† (M90.2*)
- liver† (K77.0*)
- lung† (J99.8*)
- muscle† (M63.0*)
- synovium† (M68.0*)

A52.8   **Late syphilis, latent**

Syphilis (acquired) without clinical manifestations, with positive serological reaction and negative spinal fluid test, two years or more after infection.

A52.9   **Late syphilis, unspecified**

A53   Other and unspecified syphilis

A53.0   **Latent syphilis, unspecified as early or late**

Latent syphilis NOS
Positive serological reaction for syphilis

A53.9   **Syphilis, unspecified**

Infection due to *Treponema pallidum* NOS
Syphilis (acquired) NOS

Excludes: syphilis NOS causing death under two years of age
(A50.2)

A54 Gonococcal infection

A54.0 **Gonococcal infection of lower genitourinary tract without periurethral or accessory gland abscess**
Gonococcal:
- cervicitis NOS
- cystitis NOS
- urethritis NOS
- vulvovaginitis NOS

Excludes: with:
- genitourinary gland abscess (A54.1)
- periurethral abscess (A54.1)

A54.1 **Gonococcal infection of lower genitourinary tract with periurethral and accessory gland abscess**
Gonococcal Bartholin's gland abscess

A54.2† **Gonococcal pelviperitonitis and other gonococcal genitourinary infections**
Gonococcal:
- epididymitis (N51.1*)
- female pelvic inflammatory disease (N74.3*)
- orchitis (N51.1*)
- prostatitis (N51.0*)

Excludes: gonococcal peritonitis (A54.8)

A54.3 **Gonococcal infection of eye**
Gonococcal:
- conjunctivitis† (H13.1*)
- iridocyclitis† (H22.0*)
Ophthalmia neonatorum due to gonococcus

A54.4† **Gonococcal infection of musculoskeletal system**
Gonococcal:
- arthritis (M01.3*)
- bursitis (M73.0*)
- osteomyelitis (M90.2*)
- synovitis (M68.0*)
- tenosynovitis (M68.0*)

A54.5 **Gonococcal pharyngitis**

A54.6 **Gonococcal infection of anus and rectum**

A54.8   **Other gonococcal infections**
Gonococcal:
- brain abscess† (G07*)
- endocarditis† (I39.8*)
- meningitis† (G01*)
- myocarditis† (I41.0*)
- pericarditis† (I32.0*)
- peritonitis† (K67.1*)
- pneumonia† (J17.0*)
- septicaemia
- skin lesions

Excludes: gonococcal pelviperitonitis (A54.2)

A54.9   **Gonococcal infection, unspecified**

A55   Chlamydial lymphogranuloma (venereum)
Climatic or tropical bubo
Durand-Nicolas-Favre disease
Esthiomene
Lymphogranuloma inguinale

A56   Other sexually transmitted chlamydial diseases
Includes: sexually transmitted diseases due to *Chlamydia trachomatis*

Excludes: chlamydial:
- lymphogranuloma (A55)
- neonatal:
  - conjunctivitis (P39.1)
  - pneumonia (P23.1)

conditions classified to A74.–

A56.0   **Chlamydial infection of lower genitourinary tract**
Chlamydial:
- cervicitis
- cystitis
- urethritis
- vulvovaginitis

A56.1† **Chlamydial infection of pelviperitoneum and other genitourinary organs**
Chlamydial:
- epididymitis (N51.1*)
- female pelvic inflammatory disease (N74.4*)
- orchitis (N51.1*)

A56.2 **Chlamydial infection of genitourinary tract, unspecified**

A56.3 **Chlamydial infection of anus and rectum**

A56.4 **Chlamydial infection of pharynx**

A56.8 **Sexually transmitted chlamydial infection of other sites**

A57 **Chancroid**
Ulcus molle

A58 **Granuloma inguinale**
Donovanosis

A59 **Trichomoniasis**
Excludes: intestinal trichomoniasis (A07.8)

A59.0 **Urogenital trichomoniasis**
Leukorrhoea (vaginalis)
Prostatitis† (N51.0*) $\Big\}$ due to *Trichomonas (vaginalis)*

A59.8 **Trichomoniasis of other sites**

A59.9 **Trichomoniasis, unspecified**

A60 **Anogenital herpesviral [herpes simplex] infection**

A60.0 **Herpesviral infection of genitalia and urogenital tract**
Herpesviral infection of genital tract:
- female† (N77.0–N77.1*)
- male† (N51.–*)

A60.1 **Herpesviral infection of perianal skin and rectum**

A60.9 **Anogenital herpesviral infection, unspecified**

A63 Other predominantly sexually transmitted diseases, not elsewhere classified

Excludes: molluscum contagiosum (B08.1)
papilloma of cervix (D26.0)

A63.0 **Anogenital (venereal) warts**

A63.8 **Other specified predominantly sexually transmitted diseases**

A64 Unspecified sexually transmitted disease
Venereal disease NOS

Other spirochaetal diseases (A65–A69)

Excludes: leptospirosis (A27.–)
syphilis (A50–A53)

A65 Nonvenereal syphilis
Bejel
Endemic syphilis
Njovera

A66 Yaws
Includes: bouba
framboesia (tropica)
pian

A66.0 **Initial lesions of yaws**
Chancre of yaws
Framboesia, initial or primary
Initial framboesial ulcer
Mother yaw

A66.1 **Multiple papillomata and wet crab yaws**
Framboesioma
Pianoma
Plantar or palmar papilloma of yaws

A66.2 **Other early skin lesions of yaws**
Cutaneous yaws, less than five years after infection
Early yaws (cutaneous) (macular) (maculopapular) (micropapular)
    (papular)
Framboeside of early yaws

A66.3 **Hyperkeratosis of yaws**
Ghoul hand
Hyperkeratosis, palmar or plantar (early)(late) due to yaws
Worm-eaten soles

A66.4 **Gummata and ulcers of yaws**
Gummatous framboeside
Nodular late yaws (ulcerated)

A66.5 **Gangosa**
Rhinopharyngitis mutilans

A66.6 **Bone and joint lesions of yaws**
Ganglion
Hydrarthrosis
Osteitis } of yaws (early)(late)
Periostitis (hypertrophic)
Goundou
Gumma, bone } of yaws (late)
Gummatous osteitis or periostitis

A66.7 **Other manifestations of yaws**
Juxta-articular nodules of yaws
Mucosal yaws

A66.8 **Latent yaws**
Yaws without clinical manifestations, with positive serology

A66.9 **Yaws, unspecified**

A67 Pinta [carate]

A67.0 **Primary lesions of pinta**
Chancre (primary) } of pinta [carate]
Papule (primary)

A67.1 **Intermediate lesions of pinta**

Erythematous plaques ⎫
Hyperchromic lesions ⎬ of pinta [carate]
Hyperkeratosis ⎭
Pintids

A67.2 **Late lesions of pinta**

Cardiovascular lesions† (I98.1*) ⎫
Skin lesions: ⎪
• achromic ⎬ of pinta [carate]
• cicatricial ⎪
• dyschromic ⎭

A67.3 **Mixed lesions of pinta**
Achromic with hyperchromic skin lesions of pinta [carate]

A67.9 **Pinta, unspecified**

A68 Relapsing fevers

Includes: recurrent fever

Excludes: Lyme disease (A69.2)

A68.0 **Louse-borne relapsing fever**
Relapsing fever due to *Borrelia recurrentis*

A68.1 **Tick-borne relapsing fever**
Relapsing fever due to any *Borrelia* species other than *Borrelia recurrentis*

A68.9 **Relapsing fever, unspecified**

A69 Other spirochaetal infections

A69.0 **Necrotizing ulcerative stomatitis**
Cancrum oris
Fusospirochaetal gangrene
Noma
Stomatitis gangrenosa

A69.1 **Other Vincent's infections**
Fusospirochaetal pharyngitis
Necrotizing ulcerative (acute):
• gingivitis
• gingivostomatitis
Spirochaetal stomatitis
Trench mouth
Vincent's:
• angina
• gingivitis

A69.2 **Lyme disease**
Erythema chronicum migrans due to *Borrelia burgdorferi*

A69.8 **Other specified spirochaetal infections**

A69.9 **Spirochaetal infection, unspecified**

Other diseases caused by chlamydiae (A70–A74)

A70 *Chlamydia psittaci* **infection**
Ornithosis
Parrot fever
Psittacosis

A71 **Trachoma**
Excludes: sequelae of trachoma (B94.0)

A71.0 **Initial stage of trachoma**
Trachoma dubium

A71.1 **Active stage of trachoma**
Granular conjunctivitis (trachomatous)
Trachomatous:
• follicular conjunctivitis
• pannus

A71.9 **Trachoma, unspecified**

A74 Other diseases caused by chlamydiae

Excludes: chlamydial pneumonia (J16.0)
neonatal chlamydial:
- conjunctivitis (P39.1)
- pneumonia (P23.1)
sexually transmitted chlamydial diseases (A55–A56)

A74.0†   Chlamydial conjunctivitis (H13.1*)
Paratrachoma

A74.8   Other chlamydial diseases
Chlamydial peritonitis† (K67.0*)

A74.9   Chlamydial infection, unspecified
Chlamydiosis NOS

Rickettsioses
(A75–A79)

A75 Typhus fever

Excludes: rickettsiosis due to *Ehrlichia sennetsu* (A79.8)

A75.0   Epidemic louse-borne typhus fever due to *Rickettsia prowazekii*
Classical typhus (fever)
Epidemic (louse-borne) typhus

A75.1   Recrudescent typhus [Brill's disease]
Brill-Zinsser disease

A75.2   Typhus fever due to *Rickettsia typhi*
Murine (flea-borne) typhus

A75.3   Typhus fever due to *Rickettsia tsutsugamushi*
Scrub (mite-borne) typhus
Tsutsugamushi fever

A75.9   Typhus fever, unspecified
Typhus (fever) NOS

A77 Spotted fever [tick-borne rickettsioses]

A77.0 Spotted fever due to *Rickettsia rickettsii*
Rocky Mountain spotted fever
Sao Paulo fever

A77.1 Spotted fever due to *Rickettsia conorii*
African tick typhus
Boutonneuse fever
India tick typhus
Kenya tick typhus
Marseilles fever
Mediterranean tick fever

A77.2 Spotted fever due to *Rickettsia siberica*
North Asian tick fever
Siberian tick typhus

A77.3 Spotted fever due to *Rickettsia australis*
Queensland tick typhus

A77.8 Other spotted fevers

A77.9 Spotted fever, unspecified
Tick-borne typhus NOS

A78 Q fever
Infection due to *Coxiella burnetii*
Nine Mile fever
Quadrilateral fever

A79 Other rickettsioses

A79.0 Trench fever
Quintan fever
Wolhynian fever

A79.1 Rickettsialpox due to *Rickettsia akari*
Kew Garden fever
Vesicular rickettsiosis

A79.8 Other specified rickettsioses
Rickettsiosis due to *Ehrlichia sennetsu*

A79.9 Rickettsiosis, unspecified
Rickettsial infection NOS

Viral infections of the central nervous system (A80–A89)

Excludes: sequelae of:
- poliomyelitis (B91)
- viral encephalitis (B94.1)

A80 Acute poliomyelitis

A80.0 Acute paralytic poliomyelitis, vaccine-associated

A80.1 Acute paralytic poliomyelitis, wild virus, imported

A80.2 Acute paralytic poliomyelitis, wild virus, indigenous

A80.3 Acute paralytic poliomyelitis, other and unspecified

A80.4 Acute nonparalytic poliomyelitis

A80.9 Acute poliomyelitis, unspecified

A81 Slow virus infections of central nervous system

A81.0 Creutzfeldt-Jakob disease
Subacute spongiform encephalopathy

A81.1 Subacute sclerosing panencephalitis
Dawson's inclusion body encephalitis
Van Bogaert's sclerosing leukoencephalopathy

A81.2 Progressive multifocal leukoencephalopathy
Multifocal leukoencephalopathy NOS

A81.8 Other slow virus infections of central nervous system
Kuru

A81.9 Slow virus infection of central nervous system, unspecified
Slow virus infection NOS

A82 Rabies

A82.0 Sylvatic rabies

A82.1 Urban rabies

A82.9 Rabies, unspecified

A83   Mosquito-borne viral encephalitis

Includes: mosquito-borne viral meningoencephalitis
Excludes: Venezuelan equine encephalitis (A92.2)

A83.0   **Japanese encephalitis**

A83.1   **Western equine encephalitis**

A83.2   **Eastern equine encephalitis**

A83.3   **St Louis encephalitis**

A83.4   **Australian encephalitis**
Kunjin virus disease

A83.5   **California encephalitis**
California meningoencephalitis
La Crosse encephalitis

A83.6   **Rocio virus disease**

A83.8   **Other mosquito-borne viral encephalitis**

A83.9   **Mosquito-borne viral encephalitis, unspecified**

A84   Tick-borne viral encephalitis

Includes: tick-borne viral meningoencephalitis

A84.0   **Far Eastern tick-borne encephalitis [Russian spring-summer encephalitis]**

A84.1   **Central European tick-borne encephalitis**

A84.8   **Other tick-borne viral encephalitis**
Louping ill
Powassan virus disease

A84.9   **Tick-borne viral encephalitis, unspecified**

A85   Other viral encephalitis, not elsewhere classified

Includes: specified viral:
- encephalomyelitis NEC
- meningoencephalitis NEC

Excludes: benign myalgic encephalomyelitis (G93.3)
encephalitis due to:
- herpesvirus [herpes simplex] (B00.4)
- measles virus (B05.0)
- mumps virus (B26.2)
- poliomyelitis virus (A80.–)
- zoster (B02.0)
lymphocytic choriomeningitis (A87.2)

A85.0†   **Enteroviral encephalitis (G05.1*)**
Enteroviral encephalomyelitis

A85.1†   **Adenoviral encephalitis (G05.1*)**
Adenoviral meningoencephalitis

A85.2   **Arthropod-borne viral encephalitis, unspecified**

A85.8   **Other specified viral encephalitis**
Encephalitis lethargica
Von Economo-Cruchet disease

A86   Unspecified viral encephalitis

Viral:
- encephalomyelitis NOS
- meningoencephalitis NOS

A87   Viral meningitis

Excludes: meningitis due to:
- herpesvirus [herpes simplex] (B00.3)
- measles virus (B05.1)
- mumps virus (B26.1)
- poliomyelitis virus (A80.–)
- zoster (B02.1)

A87.0†   **Enteroviral meningitis (G02.0*)**
Coxsackievirus meningitis
Echovirus meningitis

A87.1† **Adenoviral meningitis (G02.0*)**

A87.2 **Lymphocytic choriomeningitis**
Lymphocytic meningoencephalitis

A87.8 **Other viral meningitis**

A87.9 **Viral meningitis, unspecified**

A88 Other viral infections of central nervous system, not elsewhere classified
Excludes: viral:
 • encephalitis NOS (A86)
 • meningitis NOS (A87.9)

A88.0 **Enteroviral exanthematous fever [Boston exanthem]**

A88.1 **Epidemic vertigo**

A88.8 **Other specified viral infections of central nervous system**

A89 Unspecified viral infection of central nervous system

Arthropod-borne viral fevers and viral haemorrhagic fevers (A90–A99)

A90 Dengue fever [classical dengue]
Excludes: dengue haemorrhagic fever (A91)

A91 Dengue haemorrhagic fever

A92 Other mosquito-borne viral fevers
Excludes: Ross River disease (B33.1)

A92.0 **Chikungunya virus disease**
Chikungunya (haemorrhagic) fever

A92.1   **O'nyong-nyong fever**

A92.2   **Venezuelan equine fever**
Venezuelan equine:
- encephalitis
- encephalomyelitis virus disease

A92.3   **West Nile fever**

A92.4   **Rift Valley fever**

A92.8   **Other specified mosquito-borne viral fevers**

A92.9   **Mosquito-borne viral fever, unspecified**

A93   Other arthropod-borne viral fevers, not elsewhere classified

A93.0   **Oropouche virus disease**
Oropouche fever

A93.1   **Sandfly fever**
Pappataci fever
Phlebotomus fever

A93.2   **Colorado tick fever**

A93.8   **Other specified arthropod-borne viral fevers**
Piry virus disease
Vesicular stomatitis virus disease [Indiana fever]

A94   Unspecified arthropod-borne viral fever
Arboviral fever NOS
Arbovirus infection NOS

A95   Yellow fever

A95.0   **Sylvatic yellow fever**
Jungle yellow fever

A95.1   **Urban yellow fever**

A95.9   **Yellow fever, unspecified**

A96 Arenaviral haemorrhagic fever

A96.0 Junin haemorrhagic fever
Argentinian haemorrhagic fever

A96.1 Machupo haemorrhagic fever
Bolivian haemorrhagic fever

A96.2 Lassa fever

A96.8 Other arenaviral haemorrhagic fevers

A96.9 Arenaviral haemorrhagic fever, unspecified

A98 Other viral haemorrhagic fevers, not elsewhere classified
Excludes: chikungunya haemorrhagic fever (A92.0)
dengue haemorrhagic fever (A91)

A98.0 Crimean-Congo haemorrhagic fever
Central Asian haemorrhagic fever

A98.1 Omsk haemorrhagic fever

A98.2 Kyasanur Forest disease

A98.3 Marburg virus disease

A98.4 Ebola virus disease

A98.5 Haemorrhagic fever with renal syndrome
Haemorrhagic fever:
- epidemic
- Korean
- Russian
Hantaan virus disease
Nephropathia epidemica

A98.8 Other specified viral haemorrhagic fevers

A99 Unspecified viral haemorrhagic fever

Viral infections characterized by skin and mucous membrane lesions (B00–B09)

B00 Herpesviral [herpes simplex] infections

Excludes: anogenital herpesviral infection (A60.–)
congenital herpesviral infection (P35.2)
gammaherpesviral mononucleosis (B27.0)
herpangina (B08.5)

B00.0 **Eczema herpeticum**
Kaposi's varicelliform eruption

B00.1 **Herpesviral vesicular dermatitis**
Herpes simplex:
• facialis
• labialis
Vesicular dermatitis of:
• ear ⎱
• lip ⎰ due to human (alpha) herpesvirus 2

B00.2 **Herpesviral gingivostomatitis and pharyngotonsillitis**
Herpesviral pharyngitis

B00.3† **Herpesviral meningitis (G02.0*)**

B00.4† **Herpesviral encephalitis (G05.1*)**
Herpesviral meningoencephalitis
Simian B disease

B00.5† **Herpesviral ocular disease**
Herpesviral:
• conjunctivitis (H13.1*)
• dermatitis of eyelid (H03.1*)
• iridocyclitis (H22.0*)
• iritis (H22.0*)
• keratitis (H19.1*)
• keratoconjunctivitis (H19.1*)
• uveitis, anterior (H22.0*)

B00.7 **Disseminated herpesviral disease**
Herpesviral septicaemia

B00.8 **Other forms of herpesviral infection**
Herpesviral:
- hepatitis† (K77.0*)
- whitlow

B00.9 **Herpesviral infection, unspecified**
Herpes simplex infection NOS

B01 Varicella [chickenpox]

B01.0† **Varicella meningitis (G02.0*)**

B01.1† **Varicella encephalitis (G05.1*)**
Postchickenpox encephalitis
Varicella encephalomyelitis

B01.2† **Varicella pneumonia (J17.1*)**

B01.8 **Varicella with other complications**

B01.9 **Varicella without complication**
Varicella NOS

B02 Zoster [herpes zoster]

Includes: shingles
zona

B02.0† **Zoster encephalitis (G05.1*)**
Zoster meningoencephalitis

B02.1† **Zoster meningitis (G02.0*)**

B02.2† **Zoster with other nervous system involvement**
Postherpetic:
- geniculate ganglionitis (G53.0*)
- polyneuropathy (G63.0*)
- trigeminal neuralgia (G53.0*)

B02.3† **Zoster ocular disease**
Zoster:
- blepharitis (H03.1*)
- conjunctivitis (H13.1*)
- iridocyclitis (H22.0*)
- iritis (H22.0*)
- keratitis (H19.2*)
- keratoconjunctivitis (H19.2*)
- scleritis (H19.0*)

B02.7   **Disseminated zoster**

B02.8   **Zoster with other complications**

B02.9   **Zoster without complication**
Zoster NOS

B03   Smallpox[1]

B04   Monkeypox

B05   Measles
Includes: morbilli
Excludes: subacute sclerosing panencephalitis (A81.1)

B05.0†   **Measles complicated by encephalitis (G05.1*)**
Postmeasles encephalitis

B05.1†   **Measles complicated by meningitis (G02.0*)**
Postmeasles meningitis

B05.2†   **Measles complicated by pneumonia (J17.1*)**
Postmeasles pneumonia

B05.3†   **Measles complicated by otitis media (H67.1*)**
Postmeasles otitis media

B05.4   **Measles with intestinal complications**

B05.8   **Measles with other complications**
Measles keratitis and keratoconjunctivitis† (H19.2*)

B05.9   **Measles without complication**
Measles NOS

B06   Rubella [German measles]
Excludes: congenital rubella (P35.0)

---

[1] In 1980 the 33rd World Health Assembly declared that smallpox had been eradicated. The classification is maintained for surveillance purposes.

B06.0† **Rubella with neurological complications**
Rubella:
- encephalitis (G05.1*)
- meningitis (G02.0*)
- meningoencephalitis (G05.1*)

B06.8 **Rubella with other complications**
Rubella:
- arthritis† (M01.4*)
- pneumonia† (J17.1*)

B06.9 **Rubella without complication**
Rubella NOS

B07 Viral warts
Verruca:
- simplex
- vulgaris

Excludes: anogenital (venereal) warts (A63.0)
papilloma of:
- bladder (D30.3)
- cervix (D26.0)
- larynx (D14.1)

B08 Other viral infections characterized by skin and mucous membrane lesions, not elsewhere classified
Excludes: vesicular stomatitis virus disease (A93.8)

B08.0 **Other orthopoxvirus infections**
Cowpox
Orf virus disease
Pseudocowpox [milker's node]
Vaccinia
Excludes: monkeypox (B04)

B08.1 **Molluscum contagiosum**

B08.2 **Exanthema subitum [sixth disease]**

B08.3 **Erythema infectiosum [fifth disease]**

B08.4 **Enteroviral vesicular stomatitis with exanthem**
Hand, foot and mouth disease

B08.5 **Enteroviral vesicular pharyngitis**
Herpangina

B08.8 **Other specified viral infections characterized by skin and mucous membrane lesions**
Enteroviral lymphonodular pharyngitis
Foot-and-mouth disease
Tanapox virus disease
Yaba pox virus disease

B09 **Unspecified viral infection characterized by skin and mucous membrane lesions**
Viral:
- enanthema NOS
- exanthema NOS

Viral hepatitis
(B15–B19)

Excludes: cytomegaloviral hepatitis (B25.1)
herpesviral [herpes simplex] hepatitis (B00.8)
sequelae of viral hepatitis (B94.2)

B15 **Acute hepatitis A**

B15.0 **Hepatitis A with hepatic coma**

B15.9 **Hepatitis A without hepatic coma**
Hepatitis A (acute)(viral) NOS

B16 **Acute hepatitis B**

B16.0 **Acute hepatitis B with delta-agent (coinfection) with hepatic coma**

B16.1 **Acute hepatitis B with delta-agent (coinfection) without hepatic coma**

B16.2 **Acute hepatitis B without delta-agent with hepatic coma**

B16.9 **Acute hepatitis B without delta-agent and without hepatic coma**
Hepatitis B (acute)(viral) NOS

B17 Other acute viral hepatitis

B17.0 **Acute delta-(super)infection of hepatitis B carrier**

B17.1 **Acute hepatitis C**

B17.2 **Acute hepatitis E**

B17.8 **Other specified acute viral hepatitis**
Hepatitis non-A non-B (acute)(viral) NEC

B18 Chronic viral hepatitis

B18.0 **Chronic viral hepatitis B with delta-agent**

B18.1 **Chronic viral hepatitis B without delta-agent**
Chronic (viral) hepatitis B

B18.2 **Chronic viral hepatitis C**

B18.8 **Other chronic viral hepatitis**

B18.9 **Chronic viral hepatitis, unspecified**

B19 Unspecified viral hepatitis

B19.0 **Unspecified viral hepatitis with coma**

B19.9 **Unspecified viral hepatitis without coma**
Viral hepatitis NOS

Human immunodeficiency virus [HIV] disease (B20–B24)

Note: The fourth-character subcategories of B20–B23 are provided for optional use where it is not possible or not desired to use multiple coding to identify the specific conditions.

Excludes: asymptomatic human immunodeficiency virus [HIV] infection status (Z21)

B20 Human immunodeficiency virus [HIV] disease resulting in infectious and parasitic diseases

Excludes: acute HIV infection syndrome (B23.0)

B20.0 **HIV disease resulting in mycobacterial infection**
HIV disease resulting in tuberculosis

B20.1 **HIV disease resulting in other bacterial infections**

B20.2 **HIV disease resulting in cytomegaloviral disease**

B20.3 **HIV disease resulting in other viral infections**

B20.4 **HIV disease resulting in candidiasis**

B20.5 **HIV disease resulting in other mycoses**

B20.6 **HIV disease resulting in *Pneumocystis carinii* pneumonia**

B20.7 **HIV disease resulting in multiple infections**

B20.8 **HIV disease resulting in other infectious and parasitic diseases**

B20.9 **HIV disease resulting in unspecified infectious or parasitic disease**
HIV disease resulting in infection NOS

B21 Human immunodeficiency virus [HIV] disease resulting in malignant neoplasms

B21.0 **HIV disease resulting in Kaposi's sarcoma**

B21.1 **HIV disease resulting in Burkitt's lymphoma**

B21.2 **HIV disease resulting in other types of non-Hodgkin's lymphoma**

B21.3 **HIV disease resulting in other malignant neoplasms of lymphoid, haematopoietic and related tissue**

B21.7 **HIV disease resulting in multiple malignant neoplasms**

B21.8 **HIV disease resulting in other malignant neoplasms**

B21.9 **HIV disease resulting in unspecified malignant neoplasm**

B22 Human immunodeficiency virus [HIV] disease resulting in other specified diseases

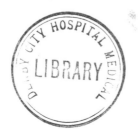

B22.0 **HIV disease resulting in encephalopathy**
HIV dementia

B22.1 **HIV disease resulting in lymphoid interstitial pneumonitis**

B22.2 **HIV disease resulting in wasting syndrome**
HIV disease resulting in failure to thrive
Slim disease

B22.7 **HIV disease resulting in multiple diseases classified elsewhere**
Note: For use of this category, reference should be made to the morbidity or mortality coding rules and guidelines in Volume 2.

B23 Human immunodeficiency virus [HIV] disease resulting in other conditions

B23.0 **Acute HIV infection syndrome**

B23.1 **HIV disease resulting in (persistent) generalized lymphadenopathy**

B23.2 **HIV disease resulting in haematological and immunological abnormalities, not elsewhere classified**

B23.8 **HIV disease resulting in other specified conditions**

B24 Unspecified human immunodeficiency virus [HIV] disease

Acquired immunodeficiency syndrome [AIDS] NOS
AIDS-related complex [ARC] NOS

Other viral diseases
(B25–B34)

B25 Cytomegaloviral disease

Excludes: congenital cytomegalovirus infection (P35.1)
cytomegaloviral mononucleosis (B27.1)

B25.0† **Cytomegaloviral pneumonitis (J17.1*)**

B25.1†   **Cytomegaloviral hepatitis (K77.0*)**

B25.2†   **Cytomegaloviral pancreatitis (K87.1*)**

B25.8   **Other cytomegaloviral diseases**

B25.9   **Cytomegaloviral disease, unspecified**

B26   Mumps

Includes: parotitis:
- epidemic
- infectious

B26.0†   **Mumps orchitis (N51.1*)**

B26.1†   **Mumps meningitis (G02.0*)**

B26.2†   **Mumps encephalitis (G05.1*)**

B26.3†   **Mumps pancreatitis (K87.1*)**

B26.8   **Mumps with other complications**
Mumps:
- arthritis† (M01.5*)
- myocarditis† (I41.1*)
- nephritis† (N08.0*)
- polyneuropathy† (G63.0*)

B26.9   **Mumps without complication**
Mumps:
- NOS
- parotitis NOS

B27   Infectious mononucleosis

Includes: glandular fever
monocytic angina
Pfeiffer's disease

B27.0   **Gammaherpesviral mononucleosis**
Mononucleosis due to Epstein-Barr virus

B27.1   **Cytomegaloviral mononucleosis**

B27.8   **Other infectious mononucleosis**

B27.9   **Infectious mononucleosis, unspecified**

B30 Viral conjunctivitis

Excludes: ocular disease:
- herpesviral [herpes simplex] (B00.5)
- zoster (B02.3)

B30.0† **Keratoconjunctivitis due to adenovirus (H19.2*)**
Epidemic keratoconjunctivitis
Shipyard eye

B30.1† **Conjunctivitis due to adenovirus (H13.1*)**
Acute adenoviral follicular conjunctivitis
Swimming-pool conjunctivitis

B30.2 **Viral pharyngoconjunctivitis**

B30.3† **Acute epidemic haemorrhagic conjunctivitis (enteroviral) (H13.1*)**
Conjunctivitis due to:
- coxsackievirus 24
- enterovirus 70
Haemorrhagic conjunctivitis (acute)(epidemic)

B30.8† **Other viral conjunctivitis (H13.1*)**
Newcastle conjunctivitis

B30.9 **Viral conjunctivitis, unspecified**

B33 Other viral diseases, not elsewhere classified

B33.0 **Epidemic myalgia**
Bornholm disease

B33.1 **Ross River disease**
Epidemic polyarthritis and exanthema
Ross River fever

B33.2 **Viral carditis**

B33.3 **Retrovirus infections, not elsewhere classified**
Retrovirus infection NOS

B33.8 **Other specified viral diseases**

B34 Viral infection of unspecified site

Excludes: cytomegaloviral disease NOS (B25.9)
   herpesvirus [herpes simplex] infection NOS (B00.9)
   retrovirus infection NOS (B33.3)
   viral agents as the cause of diseases classified to
      other chapters (B97.–)

B34.0 Adenovirus infection, unspecified

B34.1 Enterovirus infection, unspecified
Coxsackievirus infection NOS
Echovirus infection NOS

B34.2 Coronavirus infection, unspecified

B34.3 Parvovirus infection, unspecified

B34.4 Papovavirus infection, unspecified

B34.8 Other viral infections of unspecified site

B34.9 Viral infection, unspecified
Viraemia NOS

Mycoses
(B35–B49)

Excludes: hypersensitivity pneumonitis due to organic dust (J67.–)
   mycosis fungoides (C84.0)

B35 Dermatophytosis

Includes: favus
   infections due to species of *Epidermophyton, Micro-*
      sporum and *Trichophyton*
   tinea, any type except those in B36.–

B35.0 Tinea barbae and tinea capitis
Beard ringworm
Kerion
Scalp ringworm
Sycosis, mycotic

B35.1 **Tinea unguium**
Dermatophytic onychia
Dermatophytosis of nail
Onychomycosis
Ringworm of nails

B35.2 **Tinea manuum**
Dermatophytosis of hand
Hand ringworm

B35.3 **Tinea pedis**
Athlete's foot
Dermatophytosis of foot
Foot ringworm

B35.4 **Tinea corporis**
Ringworm of the body

B35.5 **Tinea imbricata**
Tokelau

B35.6 **Tinea cruris**
Dhobi itch
Groin ringworm
Jock itch

B35.8 **Other dermatophytoses**
Dermatophytosis:
• disseminated
• granulomatous

B35.9 **Dermatophytosis, unspecified**
Ringworm NOS

B36 Other superficial mycoses

B36.0 **Pityriasis versicolor**
Tinea:
• flava
• versicolor

B36.1 **Tinea nigra**
Keratomycosis nigricans palmaris
Microsporosis nigra
Pityriasis nigra

B36.2 **White piedra**
Tinea blanca

B36.3   **Black piedra**

B36.8   **Other specified superficial mycoses**

B36.9   **Superficial mycosis, unspecified**

B37   Candidiasis

Includes: candidosis
moniliasis

Excludes: neonatal candidiasis (P37.5)

B37.0   **Candidal stomatitis**
Oral thrush

B37.1   **Pulmonary candidiasis**

B37.2   **Candidiasis of skin and nail**
Candidal:
• onychia
• paronychia
Excludes: diaper [napkin] dermatitis (L22)

B37.3†   **Candidiasis of vulva and vagina (N77.1*)**
Candidal vulvovaginitis
Monilial vulvovaginitis
Vaginal thrush

B37.4†   **Candidiasis of other urogenital sites**
Candidal:
• balanitis (N51.2*)
• urethritis (N37.0*)

B37.5†   **Candidal meningitis (G02.1*)**

B37.6†   **Candidal endocarditis (I39.8*)**

B37.7   **Candidal septicaemia**

B37.8   **Candidiasis of other sites**
Candidal:
• cheilitis
• enteritis

B37.9   **Candidiasis, unspecified**
Thrush NOS

B38   Coccidioidomycosis

B38.0   **Acute pulmonary coccidioidomycosis**

B38.1   **Chronic pulmonary coccidioidomycosis**

B38.2   **Pulmonary coccidioidomycosis, unspecified**

B38.3   **Cutaneous coccidioidomycosis**

B38.4†   **Coccidioidomycosis meningitis (G02.1*)**

B38.7   **Disseminated coccidioidomycosis**
Generalized coccidioidomycosis

B38.8   **Other forms of coccidioidomycosis**

B38.9   **Coccidioidomycosis, unspecified**

B39   Histoplasmosis

B39.0   **Acute pulmonary histoplasmosis capsulati**

B39.1   **Chronic pulmonary histoplasmosis capsulati**

B39.2   **Pulmonary histoplasmosis capsulati, unspecified**

B39.3   **Disseminated histoplasmosis capsulati**
Generalized histoplasmosis capsulati

B39.4   **Histoplasmosis capsulati, unspecified**
American histoplasmosis

B39.5   **Histoplasmosis duboisii**
African histoplasmosis

B39.9   **Histoplasmosis, unspecified**

B40   Blastomycosis

Excludes: Brazilian blastomycosis (B41.–)
         keloidal blastomycosis (B48.0)

B40.0   **Acute pulmonary blastomycosis**

B40.1   **Chronic pulmonary blastomycosis**

B40.2   **Pulmonary blastomycosis, unspecified**

B40.3   **Cutaneous blastomycosis**

B40.7   **Disseminated blastomycosis**
Generalized blastomycosis

B40.8   **Other forms of blastomycosis**

B40.9   Blastomycosis, unspecified

B41   Paracoccidioidomycosis
Includes: Brazilian blastomycosis
             Lutz' disease

B41.0   Pulmonary paracoccidioidomycosis

B41.7   Disseminated paracoccidioidomycosis
Generalized paracoccidioidomycosis

B41.8   Other forms of paracoccidioidomycosis

B41.9   Paracoccidioidomycosis, unspecified

B42   Sporotrichosis

B42.0†   Pulmonary sporotrichosis (J99.8*)

B42.1   Lymphocutaneous sporotrichosis

B42.7   Disseminated sporotrichosis
Generalized sporotrichosis

B42.8   Other forms of sporotrichosis

B42.9   Sporotrichosis, unspecified

B43   Chromomycosis and phaeomycotic abscess

B43.0   Cutaneous chromomycosis
Dermatitis verrucosa

B43.1   Phaeomycotic brain abscess
Cerebral chromomycosis

B43.2   Subcutaneous phaeomycotic abscess and cyst

B43.8   Other forms of chromomycosis

B43.9   Chromomycosis, unspecified

B44   Aspergillosis
Includes: aspergilloma

B44.0   **Invasive pulmonary aspergillosis**

B44.1   **Other pulmonary aspergillosis**

B44.2   **Tonsillar aspergillosis**

B44.7   **Disseminated aspergillosis**
Generalized aspergillosis

B44.8   **Other forms of aspergillosis**

B44.9   **Aspergillosis, unspecified**

B45   Cryptococcosis

B45.0   **Pulmonary cryptococcosis**

B45.1   **Cerebral cryptococcosis**
Cryptococcal meningitis† (G02.1*)
Cryptococcosis meningocerebralis

B45.2   **Cutaneous cryptococcosis**

B45.3   **Osseous cryptococcosis**

B45.7   **Disseminated cryptococcosis**
Generalized cryptococcosis

B45.8   **Other forms of cryptococcosis**

B45.9   **Cryptococcosis, unspecified**

B46   Zygomycosis

B46.0   **Pulmonary mucormycosis**

B46.1   **Rhinocerebral mucormycosis**

B46.2   **Gastrointestinal mucormycosis**

B46.3   **Cutaneous mucormycosis**
Subcutaneous mucormycosis

B46.4   **Disseminated mucormycosis**
Generalized mucormycosis

B46.5   **Mucormycosis, unspecified**

B46.8   **Other zygomycoses**
Entomophthoromycosis

B46.9   **Zygomycosis, unspecified**
Phycomycosis NOS

B47 Mycetoma

B47.0 **Eumycetoma**
Madura foot, mycotic
Maduromycosis

B47.1 **Actinomycetoma**

B47.9 **Mycetoma, unspecified**
Madura foot NOS

B48 Other mycoses, not elsewhere classified

B48.0 **Lobomycosis**
Keloidal blastomycosis
Lobo's disease

B48.1 **Rhinosporidiosis**

B48.2 **Allescheriasis**
Infection due to *Pseudallescheria boydii*
Excludes: eumycetoma (B47.0)

B48.3 **Geotrichosis**
Geotrichum stomatitis

B48.4 **Penicillosis**

B48.7 **Opportunistic mycoses**
Mycoses caused by fungi of low virulence that can establish an infection only as a consequence of factors such as the presence of debilitating disease or the administration of immunosuppressive and other therapeutic agents or radiation therapy. Most of the causal fungi are normally saprophytic in soil and decaying vegetation.

B48.8 **Other specified mycoses**
Adiaspiromycosis

B49 Unspecified mycosis
Fungaemia NOS

Protozoal diseases
(B50–B64)

Excludes: amoebiasis (A06.–)
other protozoal intestinal diseases (A07.–)

B50   *Plasmodium falciparum* malaria

Includes: mixed infections of *Plasmodium falciparum* with any
other *Plasmodium* species

B50.0   *Plasmodium falciparum* **malaria with cerebral complications**
Cerebral malaria NOS

B50.8   **Other severe and complicated *Plasmodium falciparum*
malaria**
Severe or complicated *Plasmodium falciparum* malaria NOS

B50.9   *Plasmodium falciparum* **malaria, unspecified**

B51   *Plasmodium vivax* malaria

Includes: mixed infections of *Plasmodium vivax* with other
Plasmodium species, except *Plasmodium
falciparum*
Excludes: when mixed with *Plasmodium falciparum* (B50.–)

B51.0   *Plasmodium vivax* **malaria with rupture of spleen**
B51.8   *Plasmodium vivax* **malaria with other complications**
B51.9   *Plasmodium vivax* **malaria without complication**
Plasmodium vivax malaria NOS

B52   *Plasmodium malariae* malaria

Includes: mixed infections of *Plasmodium malariae* with other
Plasmodium species, except *Plasmodium
falciparum* and *Plasmodium vivax*
Excludes: when mixed with *Plasmodium*:
• *falciparum* (B50.–)
• *vivax* (B51.–)

B52.0   *Plasmodium malariae* **malaria with nephropathy**

B52.8 *Plasmodium malariae* malaria with other complications

B52.9 *Plasmodium malariae* malaria without complication
Plasmodium malariae malaria NOS

B53 Other parasitologically confirmed malaria

B53.0 *Plasmodium ovale* malaria
Excludes: when mixed with *Plasmodium*:
- *falciparum* (B50.–)
- *malariae* (B52.–)
- *vivax* (B51.–)

B53.1 Malaria due to simian plasmodia
Excludes: when mixed with *Plasmodium*:
- *falciparum* (B50.–)
- *malariae* (B52.–)
- *ovale* (B53.0)
- *vivax* (B51.–)

B53.8 Other parasitologically confirmed malaria, not elsewhere classified
Parasitologically confirmed malaria NOS

B54 Unspecified malaria
Clinically diagnosed malaria without parasitological confirmation.

B55 Leishmaniasis

B55.0 Visceral leishmaniasis
Kala-azar
Post-kala-azar dermal leishmaniasis

B55.1 Cutaneous leishmaniasis

B55.2 Mucocutaneous leishmaniasis

B55.9 Leishmaniasis, unspecified

B56 African trypanosomiasis

B56.0 **Gambiense trypanosomiasis**
Infection due to *Trypanosoma brucei gambiense*
West African sleeping sickness

B56.1 **Rhodesiense trypanosomiasis**
East African sleeping sickness
Infection due to *Trypanosoma brucei rhodesiense*

B56.9 **African trypanosomiasis, unspecified**
Sleeping sickness NOS
Trypanosomiasis NOS, in places where African trypanosomiasis
is prevalent

B57 Chagas' disease

Includes: American trypanosomiasis
infection due to *Trypanosoma cruzi*

B57.0† **Acute Chagas' disease with heart involvement (I41.2*, I98.1*)**
Acute Chagas' disease with:
- cardiovascular involvement NEC (I98.1*)
- myocarditis (I41.2*)

B57.1 **Acute Chagas' disease without heart involvement**
Acute Chagas' disease NOS

B57.2† **Chagas' disease (chronic) with heart involvement (I41.2*, I98.1*)**
American trypanosomiasis NOS
Chagas' disease (chronic) (with):
- NOS
- cardiovascular involvement NEC (I98.1*)
- myocarditis (I41.2*)
Trypanosomiasis NOS, in places where Chagas' disease is
prevalent

B57.3 **Chagas' disease (chronic) with digestive system involvement**

B57.4 **Chagas' disease (chronic) with nervous system involvement**

B57.5 **Chagas' disease (chronic) with other organ involvement**

B58 Toxoplasmosis

Includes: infection due to *Toxoplasma gondii*
Excludes: congenital toxoplasmosis (P37.1)

B58.0† **Toxoplasma oculopathy**
Toxoplasma chorioretinitis (H32.0*)

B58.1† **Toxoplasma hepatitis (K77.0*)**

B58.2† **Toxoplasma meningoencephalitis (G05.2*)**

B58.3† **Pulmonary toxoplasmosis (J17.3*)**

B58.8 **Toxoplasmosis with other organ involvement**
Toxoplasma:
• myocarditis† (I41.2*)
• myositis† (M63.1*)

B58.9 **Toxoplasmosis, unspecified**

B59 Pneumocystosis

Pneumonia due to *Pneumocystis carinii*

B60 Other protozoal diseases, not elsewhere classified

Excludes: cryptosporidiosis (A07.2)
isosporiasis (A07.3)

B60.0 **Babesiosis**
Piroplasmosis

B60.1 **Acanthamoebiasis**
Conjunctivitis due to *Acanthamoeba*† (H13.1*)
Keratoconjunctivitis due to *Acanthamoeba*† (H19.2*)

B60.2 **Naegleriasis**
Primary amoebic meningoencephalitis† (G05.2*)

B60.8 **Other specified protozoal diseases**
Microsporidiosis

B64 Unspecified protozoal disease

Helminthiases
(B65–B83)

B65 Schistosomiasis [bilharziasis]

Includes: snail fever

B65.0 **Schistosomiasis due to *Schistosoma haematobium* [urinary schistosomiasis]**

B65.1 **Schistosomiasis due to *Schistosoma mansoni* [intestinal schistosomiasis]**

B65.2 **Schistosomiasis due to *Schistosoma japonicum***

Asiatic schistosomiasis

B65.3 **Cercarial dermatitis**

Swimmer's itch

B65.8 **Other schistosomiases**

Infection due to *Schistosoma*:
- *intercalatum*
- *mattheei*
- *mekongi*

B65.9 **Schistosomiasis, unspecified**

B66 Other fluke infections

B66.0 **Opisthorchiasis**

Infection due to:
- cat liver fluke
- *Opisthorchis* (*felineus*)(*viverrini*)

B66.1 **Clonorchiasis**

Chinese liver fluke disease
Infection due to *Clonorchis sinensis*
Oriental liver fluke disease

B66.2 **Dicrocoeliasis**

Infection due to *Dicrocoelium dendriticum*
Lancet fluke infection

B66.3 **Fascioliasis**
Infection due to *Fasciola*:
- *gigantica*
- *hepatica*
- *indica*
Sheep liver fluke disease

B66.4 **Paragonimiasis**
Infection due to *Paragonimus* species
Lung fluke disease
Pulmonary distomiasis

B66.5 **Fasciolopsiasis**
Infection due to *Fasciolopsis buski*
Intestinal distomiasis

B66.8 **Other specified fluke infections**
Echinostomiasis
Heterophyiasis
Metagonimiasis
Nanophyetiasis
Watsoniasis

B66.9 **Fluke infection, unspecified**

B67 Echinococcosis
Includes: hydatidosis

B67.0 *Echinococcus granulosus* **infection of liver**

B67.1 *Echinococcus granulosus* **infection of lung**

B67.2 *Echinococcus granulosus* **infection of bone**

B67.3 *Echinococcus granulosus* **infection, other and multiple sites**

B67.4 *Echinococcus granulosus* **infection, unspecified**

B67.5 *Echinococcus multilocularis* **infection of liver**

B67.6 *Echinococcus multilocularis* **infection, other and multiple sites**

B67.7 *Echinococcus multilocularis* **infection, unspecified**

B67.8 **Echinococcosis, unspecified, of liver**

B67.9 **Echinococcosis, other and unspecified**
Echinococcosis NOS

B68 Taeniasis

Excludes: cysticercosis (B69.–)

B68.0 ***Taenia solium* taeniasis**
Pork tapeworm (infection)

B68.1 ***Taenia saginata* taeniasis**
Beef tapeworm (infection)
Infection due to adult tapeworm *Taenia saginata*

B68.9 **Taeniasis, unspecified**

B69 Cysticercosis

Includes: cysticerciasis infection due to larval form of *Taenia solium*

B69.0 **Cysticercosis of central nervous system**

B69.1 **Cysticercosis of eye**

B69.8 **Cysticercosis of other sites**

B69.9 **Cysticercosis, unspecified**

B70 Diphyllobothriasis and sparganosis

B70.0 **Diphyllobothriasis**
Diphyllobothrium (adult)(*latum*)(*pacificum*) infection
Fish tapeworm (infection)
Excludes: larval diphyllobothriasis (B70.1)

B70.1 **Sparganosis**
Infection due to:
- *Sparganum* (*mansoni*)(*proliferum*)
- *Spirometra* larvae
Larval diphyllobothriasis
Spirometrosis

B71 Other cestode infections

B71.0 **Hymenolepiasis**
Dwarf tapeworm (infection)
Rat tapeworm (infection)

B71.1 **Dipylidiasis**
Dog tapeworm (infection)

B71.8 **Other specified cestode infections**
Coenurosis

B71.9 **Cestode infection, unspecified**
Tapeworm (infection) NOS

B72 Dracunculiasis
Guinea worm infection
Infection due to *Dracunculus medinensis*

B73 Onchocerciasis
Onchocerca volvulus infection
Onchocercosis
River blindness

B74 Filariasis
Excludes: onchocerciasis (B73)
tropical (pulmonary) eosinophilia NOS (J82)

B74.0 **Filariasis due to *Wuchereria bancrofti***
Bancroftian:
• elephantiasis
• filariasis

B74.1 **Filariasis due to *Brugia malayi***

B74.2 **Filariasis due to *Brugia timori***

B74.3 **Loiasis**
Calabar swelling
Eyeworm disease of Africa
Loa loa infection

B74.4 **Mansonelliasis**
Infection due to *Mansonella*:
• *ozzardi*
• *perstans*
• *streptocerca*

B74.8 **Other filariases**
Dirofilariasis

B74.9 **Filariasis, unspecified**

B75 Trichinellosis
Infection due to *Trichinella* species
Trichiniasis

B76 Hookworm diseases
Includes: uncinariasis

B76.0 **Ancylostomiasis**
Infection due to *Ancylostoma* species

B76.1 **Necatoriasis**
Infection due to *Necator americanus*

B76.8 **Other hookworm diseases**

B76.9 **Hookworm disease, unspecified**
Cutaneous larva migrans NOS

B77 Ascariasis
Includes: ascaridiasis
roundworm infection

B77.0 **Ascariasis with intestinal complications**

B77.8 **Ascariasis with other complications**

B77.9 **Ascariasis, unspecified**

B78 Strongyloidiasis
Excludes: trichostrongyliasis (B81.2)

B78.0 **Intestinal strongyloidiasis**

B78.1 **Cutaneous strongyloidiasis**

B78.7 **Disseminated strongyloidiasis**

B78.9 **Strongyloidiasis, unspecified**

B79 Trichuriasis

Trichocephaliasis
Whipworm (disease)(infection)

B80 Enterobiasis

Oxyuriasis
Pinworm infection
Threadworm infection

B81 Other intestinal helminthiases, not elsewhere classified

Excludes: angiostrongyliasis due to *Parastrongylus cantonensis*
(B83.2)

B81.0 Anisakiasis
Infection due to *Anisakis* larvae

B81.1 Intestinal capillariasis
Capillariasis NOS
Infection due to *Capillaria philippinensis*
Excludes: hepatic capillariasis (B83.8)

B81.2 Trichostrongyliasis

B81.3 Intestinal angiostrongyliasis
Angiostrongyliasis due to *Parastrongylus costaricensis*

B81.4 Mixed intestinal helminthiases
Infection due to intestinal helminths classifiable to more than
one of the categories B65.0–B81.3 and B81.8
Mixed helminthiasis NOS

B81.8 Other specified intestinal helminthiases
Infection due to:
• *Oesophagostomum* species [oesophagostomiasis]
• *Ternidens diminutus* [ternidensiasis]

B82 Unspecified intestinal parasitism

B82.0 Intestinal helminthiasis, unspecified

B82.9 Intestinal parasitism, unspecified

B83   Other helminthiases

Excludes: capillariasis:
- NOS (B81.1)
- intestinal (B81.1)

B83.0   Visceral larva migrans
Toxocariasis

B83.1   Gnathostomiasis
Wandering swelling

B83.2   Angiostrongyliasis due to *Parastrongylus cantonensis*
Eosinophilic meningoencephalitis† (G05.2*)
Excludes: intestinal angiostrongyliasis (B81.3)

B83.3   Syngamiasis
Syngamosis

B83.4   Internal hirudiniasis
Excludes: external hirudiniasis (B88.3)

B83.8   Other specified helminthiases
Acanthocephaliasis
Gongylonemiasis
Hepatic capillariasis
Metastrongyliasis
Thelaziasis

B83.9   Helminthiasis, unspecified
Worms NOS
Excludes: intestinal helminthiasis NOS (B82.0)

Pediculosis, acariasis and other infestations (B85–B89)

B85   Pediculosis and phthiriasis

B85.0   Pediculosis due to *Pediculus humanus capitis*
Head-louse infestation

B85.1   Pediculosis due to *Pediculus humanus corporis*
Body-louse infestation

B85.2   Pediculosis, unspecified

B85.3 **Phthiriasis**
Infestation by:
- crab-louse
- *Phthirus pubis*

B85.4 **Mixed pediculosis and phthiriasis**
Infestation classifiable to more than one of the categories B85.0–B85.3

B86 **Scabies**
Sarcoptic itch

B87 **Myiasis**
Includes: infestation by larvae of flies

B87.0 **Cutaneous myiasis**
Creeping myiasis

B87.1 **Wound myiasis**
Traumatic myiasis

B87.2 **Ocular myiasis**

B87.3 **Nasopharyngeal myiasis**
Laryngeal myiasis

B87.4 **Aural myiasis**

B87.8 **Myiasis of other sites**
Genitourinary myiasis
Intestinal myiasis

B87.9 **Myiasis, unspecified**

B88 **Other infestations**

B88.0 **Other acariasis**
Acarine dermatitis
Dermatitis due to:
- *Demodex* species
- *Dermanyssus gallinae*
- *Liponyssoides sanguineus*
Trombiculosis
Excludes: scabies (B86)

B88.1   **Tungiasis [sandflea infestation]**

B88.2   **Other arthropod infestations**
Scarabiasis

B88.3   **External hirudiniasis**
Leech infestation NOS
Excludes: internal hirudiniasis (B83.4)

B88.8   **Other specified infestations**
Ichthyoparasitism due to *Vandellia cirrhosa*
Linguatulosis
Porocephaliasis

B88.9   **Infestation, unspecified**
Infestation (skin) NOS
Infestation by mites NOS
Skin parasites NOS

B89   Unspecified parasitic disease

Sequelae of infectious and parasitic diseases (B90–B94)

Note: These categories are to be used to indicate conditions in categories A00–B89 as the cause of sequelae, which are themselves classified elsewhere. The "sequelae" include conditions specified as such; they also include late effects of diseases classifiable to the above categories if there is evidence that the disease itself is no longer present. For use of these categories, reference should be made to the morbidity or mortality coding rules and guidelines in Volume 2.

B90   Sequelae of tuberculosis

B90.0   **Sequelae of central nervous system tuberculosis**

B90.1   **Sequelae of genitourinary tuberculosis**

B90.2   **Sequelae of tuberculosis of bones and joints**

B90.8   **Sequelae of tuberculosis of other organs**

B90.9 **Sequelae of respiratory and unspecified tuberculosis**
Sequelae of tuberculosis NOS

B91 Sequelae of poliomyelitis

B92 Sequelae of leprosy

B94 Sequelae of other and unspecified infectious and parasitic diseases

B94.0 **Sequelae of trachoma**

B94.1 **Sequelae of viral encephalitis**

B94.2 **Sequelae of viral hepatitis**

B94.8 **Sequelae of other specified infectious and parasitic diseases**

B94.9 **Sequelae of unspecified infectious or parasitic disease**

Bacterial, viral and other infectious agents (B95–B97)

Note: These categories should never be used in primary coding. They are provided for use as supplementary or additional codes when it is desired to identify the infectious agent(s) in diseases classified elsewhere.

B95 Streptococcus and staphylococcus as the cause of diseases classified to other chapters

B95.0 **Streptococcus, group A, as the cause of diseases classified to other chapters**

B95.1 **Streptococcus, group B, as the cause of diseases classified to other chapters**

B95.2 **Streptococcus, group D, as the cause of diseases classified to other chapters**

B95.3   *Streptococcus pneumoniae* as the cause of diseases classified to other chapters

B95.4   Other streptococcus as the cause of diseases classified to other chapters

B95.5   Unspecified streptococcus as the cause of diseases classified to other chapters

B95.6   *Staphylococcus aureus* as the cause of diseases classified to other chapters

B95.7   Other staphylococcus as the cause of diseases classified to other chapters

B95.8   Unspecified staphylococcus as the cause of diseases classified to other chapters

B96   Other bacterial agents as the cause of diseases classified to other chapters

B96.0   *Mycoplasma pneumoniae [M. pneumoniae]* as the cause of diseases classified to other chapters
Pleuro-pneumonia-like-organism [PPLO]

B96.1   *Klebsiella pneumoniae [K. pneumoniae]* as the cause of diseases classified to other chapters

B96.2   *Escherichia coli [E. coli]* as the cause of diseases classified to other chapters

B96.3   *Haemophilus influenzae [H. influenzae]* as the cause of diseases classified to other chapters

B96.4   *Proteus (mirabilis)(morganii)* as the cause of diseases classified to other chapters

B96.5   *Pseudomonas (aeruginosa)(mallei)(pseudomallei)* as the cause of diseases classified to other chapters

B96.6   *Bacillus fragilis [B. fragilis]* as the cause of diseases classified to other chapters

B96.7   *Clostridium perfringens [C. perfringens]* as the cause of diseases classified to other chapters

B96.8   Other specified bacterial agents as the cause of diseases classified to other chapters

B97 Viral agents as the cause of diseases classified to other chapters

B97.0 **Adenovirus as the cause of diseases classified to other chapters**

B97.1 **Enterovirus as the cause of diseases classified to other chapters**
Coxsackievirus
Echovirus

B97.2 **Coronavirus as the cause of diseases classified to other chapters**

B97.3 **Retrovirus as the cause of diseases classified to other chapters**
Lentivirus
Oncovirus

B97.4 **Respiratory syncytial virus as the cause of diseases classified to other chapters**

B97.5 **Reovirus as the cause of diseases classified to other chapters**

B97.6 **Parvovirus as the cause of diseases classified to other chapters**

B97.7 **Papillomavirus as the cause of diseases classified to other chapters**

B97.8 **Other viral agents as the cause of diseases classified to other chapters**

Other infectious diseases
(B99)

B99 Other and unspecified infectious diseases

CHAPTER II

Neoplasms
(C00–D48)

This chapter contains the following broad groups of neoplasms:

C00–C75   Malignant neoplasms, stated or presumed to be primary, of specified sites, except of lymphoid, haematopoietic and related tissue

C00–C14	Lip, oral cavity and pharynx
C15–C26	Digestive organs
C30–C39	Respiratory and intrathoracic organs
C40–C41	Bone and articular cartilage
C43–C44	Skin
C45–C49	Mesothelial and soft tissue
C50	Breast
C51–C58	Female genital organs
C60–C63	Male genital organs
C64–C68	Urinary tract
C69–C72	Eye, brain and other parts of central nervous system
C73–C75	Thyroid and other endocrine glands

C76–C80   Malignant neoplasms of ill-defined, secondary and unspecified sites

C81–C96   Malignant neoplasms, stated or presumed to be primary, of lymphoid, haematopoietic and related tissue

C97   Malignant neoplasms of independent (primary) multiple sites

D00–D09   In situ neoplasms

D10–D36   Benign neoplasms

D37–D48   Neoplasms of uncertain or unknown behaviour [see note, page 240]

Notes

1. Primary, ill-defined, secondary and unspecified sites of malignant neoplasms

Categories C76–C80 include malignant neoplasms for which there is no clear indication of the original site of the cancer or the cancer is stated to be "disseminated", "scattered" or "spread" without mention of the primary site. In both cases the primary site is considered to be unknown.

2. Functional activity

All neoplasms are classified in this chapter, whether they are functionally active or not. An additional code from Chapter IV may be used, if desired, to identify functional activity associated with any neoplasm. For example, catecholamine-producing malignant phaeochromocytoma of adrenal gland should be coded to C74 with additional code E27.5; basophil adenoma of pituitary gland with Cushing's syndrome should be coded to D35.2 with additional code E24.0.

3. Morphology

There are a number of major morphological (histological) groups of malignant neoplasms: carcinomas including squamous (cell) and adeno-carcinomas; sarcomas; other soft tissue tumours including mesotheliomas; lymphomas (Hodgkin's and non-Hodgkin's); leukaemia; other specified and site-specific types; and unspecified cancers. Cancer is a generic term and may be used for any of the above groups, although it is rarely applied to the malignant neoplasms of lymphatic, haematopoietic and related tissue. "Carcinoma" is sometimes used incorrectly as a synonym for "cancer".

In Chapter II neoplasms are classified predominantly by site within broad groupings for behaviour. In a few exceptional cases morphology is indicated in the category and subcategory titles.

For those wishing to identify the histological type of neoplasm, com-prehensive separate morphology codes are provided on pages 1177–1204. These morphology codes are derived from the second edition of International Classification of Diseases for Oncology (ICD-O), which is a dual-axis classification providing independent coding systems for topography and morphology. Morphology codes have six digits: the first four digits identify the histological type; the fifth digit is the behaviour code (malignant primary, malignant secondary (metastatic), in situ, benign, uncertain whether malignant or benign); and the sixth digit is a grading code (differentiation) for solid tumours, and is also used as a special code for lymphomas and leukaemias.

4. Use of subcategories in Chapter II

Attention is drawn to the special use of subcategory .8 in this chapter [see note 5]. Where it has been necessary to provide subcategories for "other", these have generally been designated as subcategory .7.

5. Malignant neoplasms overlapping site boundaries and the use of sub-category .8 (overlapping lesion)

Categories C00–C75 classify primary malignant neoplasms according to their point of origin. Many three-character categories are further divided into named parts or subcategories of the organ in question. A neoplasm that overlaps two or more contiguous sites within a three-character category and whose point of origin cannot be determined should be classified to the subcategory .8 ("overlapping lesion"), unless the combination is specifically indexed elsewhere. For example, carcinoma of oesophagus and stomach is specifically indexed to C16.0 (cardia), while carcinoma of the tip and ventral surface of the tongue should be assigned to C02.8. On the other hand, carcinoma of the tip of the tongue extending to involve the ventral surface should be coded to C02.1 as the point of origin, the tip, is known. "Overlapping" implies that the sites involved are contiguous (next to each other). Numerically consecutive subcategories are frequently anatomically contiguous, but this is not invariably so (e.g. bladder C67.–) and the coder may need to consult anatomical texts to determine the topographical relationships.

Sometimes a neoplasm overlaps the boundaries of three-character categories within certain systems. To take care of this the following subcategories have been designated:

C02.8	Overlapping lesion of tongue
C08.8	Overlapping lesion of major salivary glands
C14.8	Overlapping lesion of lip, oral cavity and pharynx
C21.8	Overlapping lesion of rectum, anus and anal canal
C24.8	Overlapping lesion of biliary tract
C26.8	Overlapping lesion of digestive system
C39.8	Overlapping lesion of respiratory and intrathoracic organs
C41.8	Overlapping lesion of bone and articular cartilage
C49.8	Overlapping lesion of connective and soft tissue
C57.8	Overlapping lesion of female genital organs
C63.8	Overlapping lesion of male genital organs
C68.8	Overlapping lesion of urinary organs
C72.8	Overlapping lesion of central nervous system

An example of this is a carcinoma of the stomach and small intestine, which should be coded to C26.8 (Overlapping lesion of digestive system).

6. Malignant neoplasms of ectopic tissue

Malignant neoplasms of ectopic tissue are to be coded to the site mentioned, e.g. ectopic pancreatic malignant neoplasms are coded to pancreas, unspecified (C25.9).

7. Use of the Alphabetical Index in coding neoplasms

In addition to site, morphology and behaviour must also be taken into consideration when coding neoplasms, and reference should always be made first to the Alphabetical Index entry for the morphological description.

The introductory pages of Volume 3 include general instructions about the correct use of the Alphabetical Index. The specific instructions and examples pertaining to neoplasms should be consulted to ensure correct use of the categories and subcategories in Chapter II.

8. Use of the second edition of International Classification of Diseases for Oncology (ICD-O)

For certain morphological types, Chapter II provides a rather restricted topographical classification, or none at all. The topography codes of ICD-O use for all neoplasms essentially the same three- and four-character categories that Chapter II uses for malignant neoplasms (C00–C77, C80), thus providing increased specificity of site for other neoplasms (malignant secondary (metastatic), benign, in situ and uncertain or unknown).

It is therefore recommended that agencies interested in identifying both the site and morphology of tumours, e.g. cancer registries, cancer hospitals, pathology departments and other agencies specializing in cancer, use ICD-O.

Malignant neoplasms
(C00–C97)

Malignant neoplasms of lip, oral cavity and pharynx (C00–C14)

C00 Malignant neoplasm of lip
Excludes: skin of lip (C43.0, C44.0)

C00.0 External upper lip
Upper lip:
• NOS
• lipstick area
• vermilion border

C00.1 External lower lip
Lower lip:
• NOS
• lipstick area
• vermilion border

C00.2 External lip, unspecified
Vermilion border NOS

C00.3 Upper lip, inner aspect
Upper lip:
- buccal aspect
- frenulum
- mucosa
- oral aspect

C00.4 Lower lip, inner aspect
Lower lip:
- buccal aspect
- frenulum
- mucosa
- oral aspect

C00.5 Lip, unspecified, inner aspect
Lip, not specified whether upper or lower:
- buccal aspect
- frenulum
- mucosa
- oral aspect

C00.6 Commissure of lip

C00.8 Overlapping lesion of lip
[See note 5 on page 182]

C00.9 Lip, unspecified

C01 **Malignant neoplasm of base of tongue**
Dorsal surface of base of tongue
Fixed part of tongue NOS
Posterior third of tongue

C02 **Malignant neoplasm of other and unspecified parts of tongue**

C02.0 Dorsal surface of tongue
Anterior two-thirds of tongue, dorsal surface
Excludes: dorsal surface of base of tongue (C01)

C02.1 Border of tongue
Tip of tongue

C02.2 Ventral surface of tongue
Anterior two-thirds of tongue, ventral surface
Frenulum linguae

C02.3 **Anterior two-thirds of tongue, part unspecified**
Middle third of tongue NOS
Mobile part of tongue NOS

C02.4 **Lingual tonsil**
Excludes: tonsil NOS (C09.9)

C02.8 **Overlapping lesion of tongue**
[See note 5 on page 182]
Malignant neoplasm of tongue whose point of origin cannot be
classified to any one of the categories C01–C02.4

C02.9 **Tongue, unspecified**

C03 Malignant neoplasm of gum
Includes: alveolar (ridge) mucosa
gingiva
Excludes: malignant odontogenic neoplasms (C41.0–C41.1)

C03.0 **Upper gum**

C03.1 **Lower gum**

C03.9 **Gum, unspecified**

C04 Malignant neoplasm of floor of mouth

C04.0 **Anterior floor of mouth**
Anterior to the premolar–canine junction

C04.1 **Lateral floor of mouth**

C04.8 **Overlapping lesion of floor of mouth**
[See note 5 on page 182]

C04.9 **Floor of mouth, unspecified**

C05 Malignant neoplasm of palate

C05.0 **Hard palate**

C05.1 **Soft palate**
Excludes: nasopharyngeal surface of soft palate (C11.3)

C05.2 **Uvula**

C05.8 **Overlapping lesion of palate**
[See note 5 on page 182]

C05.9 **Palate, unspecified**
Roof of mouth

C06 Malignant neoplasm of other and unspecified parts of mouth

C06.0 **Cheek mucosa**
Buccal mucosa NOS
Internal cheek

C06.1 **Vestibule of mouth**
Buccal sulcus (upper)(lower)
Labial sulcus (upper)(lower)

C06.2 **Retromolar area**

C06.8 **Overlapping lesion of other and unspecified parts of mouth**
[See note 5 on page 182]

C06.9 **Mouth, unspecified**
Minor salivary gland, unspecified site
Oral cavity NOS

C07 Malignant neoplasm of parotid gland

C08 Malignant neoplasm of other and unspecified major salivary glands

Excludes: malignant neoplasms of specified minor salivary glands
which are classified according to their anatomical
location
malignant neoplasms of minor salivary glands NOS
(C06.9)
parotid gland (C07)

C08.0 **Submandibular gland**
Submaxillary gland

C08.1 **Sublingual gland**

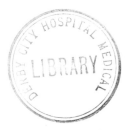

C08.8   Overlapping lesion of major salivary glands
[See note 5 on page 182]
Malignant neoplasm of major salivary glands whose point of origin cannot be classified to any one of the categories C07–C08.1

C08.9   Major salivary gland, unspecified
Salivary gland (major) NOS

C09 Malignant neoplasm of tonsil
Excludes: lingual tonsil (C02.4)
          pharyngeal tonsil (C11.1)

C09.0   Tonsillar fossa

C09.1   Tonsillar pillar (anterior)(posterior)

C09.8   Overlapping lesion of tonsil
[See note 5 on page 182]

C09.9   Tonsil, unspecified
Tonsil:
• NOS
• faucial
• palatine

C10 Malignant neoplasm of oropharynx
Excludes: tonsil (C09.–)

C10.0   Vallecula

C10.1   Anterior surface of epiglottis
Epiglottis, free border [margin]
Glossoepiglottic fold(s)
Excludes: epiglottis (suprahyoid portion) NOS (C32.1)

C10.2   Lateral wall of oropharynx

C10.3   Posterior wall of oropharynx

C10.4   Branchial cleft
Branchial cyst [site of neoplasm]

C10.8   Overlapping lesion of oropharynx
[See note 5 on page 182]
Junctional region of oropharynx

C10.9   Oropharynx, unspecified

C11 Malignant neoplasm of nasopharynx

C11.0 Superior wall of nasopharynx
Roof of nasopharynx

C11.1 Posterior wall of nasopharynx
Adenoid
Pharyngeal tonsil

C11.2 Lateral wall of nasopharynx
Fossa of Rosenmüller
Opening of auditory tube
Pharyngeal recess

C11.3 Anterior wall of nasopharynx
Floor of nasopharynx
Nasopharyngeal (anterior)(posterior) surface of soft palate
Posterior margin of nasal:
• choana
• septum

C11.8 Overlapping lesion of nasopharynx
[See note 5 on page 182]

C11.9 Nasopharynx, unspecified
Nasopharyngeal wall NOS

C12 Malignant neoplasm of pyriform sinus
Pyriform fossa

C13 Malignant neoplasm of hypopharynx
Excludes: pyriform sinus (C12)

C13.0 Postcricoid region

C13.1 Aryepiglottic fold, hypopharyngeal aspect
Aryepiglottic fold:
• NOS
• marginal zone
Excludes: aryepiglottic fold, laryngeal aspect (C32.1)

C13.2 Posterior wall of hypopharynx

C13.8 Overlapping lesion of hypopharynx
[See note 5 on page 182]

C13.9 **Hypopharynx, unspecified**
Hypopharyngeal wall NOS

C14 **Malignant neoplasm of other and ill-defined sites in the lip, oral cavity and pharynx**
Excludes: oral cavity NOS (C06.9)

C14.0 **Pharynx, unspecified**

C14.1 **Laryngopharynx**

C14.2 **Waldeyer's ring**

C14.8 **Overlapping lesion of lip, oral cavity and pharynx**
[See note 5 on page 182]
Malignant neoplasm of lip, oral cavity and pharynx whose point of origin cannot be classified to any one of the categories C00–C14.2

Malignant neoplasms of digestive organs (C15–C26)

C15 **Malignant neoplasm of oesophagus**
Note: Two alternative subclassifications are given:
.0–.2 by anatomical description
.3–.5 by thirds
This departure from the principle that categories should be mutually exclusive is deliberate, since both forms of terminology are in use but the resulting anatomical divisions are not analogous.

C15.0 **Cervical part of oesophagus**

C15.1 **Thoracic part of oesophagus**

C15.2 **Abdominal part of oesophagus**

C15.3 **Upper third of oesophagus**

C15.4 **Middle third of oesophagus**

C15.5 **Lower third of oesophagus**

C15.8 **Overlapping lesion of oesophagus**
[See note 5 on page 182]

C15.9   Oesophagus, unspecified

C16 Malignant neoplasm of stomach

C16.0   **Cardia**
Cardiac orifice
Cardio-oesophageal junction
Gastro-oesophageal junction
Oesophagus and stomach

C16.1   **Fundus of stomach**

C16.2   **Body of stomach**

C16.3   **Pyloric antrum**
Gastric antrum

C16.4   **Pylorus**
Prepylorus
Pyloric canal

C16.5   **Lesser curvature of stomach, unspecified**
Lesser curvature of stomach, not classifiable to C16.1–C16.4

C16.6   **Greater curvature of stomach, unspecified**
Greater curvature of stomach, not classifiable to C16.0–C16.4

C16.8   **Overlapping lesion of stomach**
[See note 5 on page 182]

C16.9   **Stomach, unspecified**
Gastric cancer NOS

C17 Malignant neoplasm of small intestine

C17.0   **Duodenum**

C17.1   **Jejunum**

C17.2   **Ileum**
Excludes: ileocaecal valve (C18.0)

C17.3   **Meckel's diverticulum**

C17.8   **Overlapping lesion of small intestine**
[See note 5 on page 182]

C17.9   **Small intestine, unspecified**

C18   Malignant neoplasm of colon

C18.0   **Caecum**
Ileocaecal valve

C18.1   **Appendix**

C18.2   **Ascending colon**

C18.3   **Hepatic flexure**

C18.4   **Transverse colon**

C18.5   **Splenic flexure**

C18.6   **Descending colon**

C18.7   **Sigmoid colon**
Sigmoid (flexure)
Excludes: rectosigmoid junction (C19)

C18.8   **Overlapping lesion of colon**
[See note 5 on page 182]

C18.9   **Colon, unspecified**
Large intestine NOS

C19   Malignant neoplasm of rectosigmoid junction
Colon with rectum
Rectosigmoid (colon)

C20   Malignant neoplasm of rectum
Rectal ampulla

C21   Malignant neoplasm of anus and anal canal

C21.0   **Anus, unspecified**
Excludes: anal:
• margin (C43.5, C44.5)
• skin (C43.5, C44.5)
perianal skin (C43.5, C44.5)

C21.1   **Anal canal**
Anal sphincter

C21.2   **Cloacogenic zone**

C21.8   Overlapping lesion of rectum, anus and anal canal
[See note 5 on page 182]
Anorectal junction
Anorectum
Malignant neoplasm of rectum, anus and anal canal whose point
    of origin cannot be classified to any one of the categories
    C20–C21.2

C22   Malignant neoplasm of liver and intrahepatic bile ducts
Excludes: biliary tract NOS (C24.9)
              secondary malignant neoplasm of liver (C78.7)

C22.0   Liver cell carcinoma
Hepatocellular carcinoma
Hepatoma

C22.1   Intrahepatic bile duct carcinoma
Cholangiocarcinoma

C22.2   Hepatoblastoma

C22.3   Angiosarcoma of liver
Kupffer cell sarcoma

C22.4   Other sarcomas of liver

C22.7   Other specified carcinomas of liver

C22.9   Liver, unspecified

C23   Malignant neoplasm of gallbladder

C24   Malignant neoplasm of other and unspecified parts of biliary tract
Excludes: intrahepatic bile duct (C22.1)

C24.0   Extrahepatic bile duct
Biliary duct or passage NOS
Common bile duct
Cystic duct
Hepatic duct

C24.1   Ampulla of Vater

C24.8   **Overlapping lesion of biliary tract**
[See note 5 on page 182]
Malignant neoplasm involving both intrahepatic and extrahepatic
bile ducts
Malignant neoplasm of biliary tract whose point of origin cannot
be classified to any one of the categories C22.0–C24.1

C24.9   **Biliary tract, unspecified**

C25 Malignant neoplasm of pancreas

C25.0   **Head of pancreas**

C25.1   **Body of pancreas**

C25.2   **Tail of pancreas**

C25.3   **Pancreatic duct**

C25.4   **Endocrine pancreas**
Islets of Langerhans

C25.7   **Other parts of pancreas**
Neck of pancreas

C25.8   **Overlapping lesion of pancreas**
[See note 5 on page 182]

C25.9   **Pancreas, unspecified**

C26 Malignant neoplasm of other and ill-defined digestive organs

Excludes: peritoneum and retroperitoneum (C48.–)

C26.0   **Intestinal tract, part unspecified**
Intestine NOS

C26.1   **Spleen**

Excludes: Hodgkin's disease (C81.–)
non-Hodgkin's lymphoma (C82–C85)

C26.8   **Overlapping lesion of digestive system**
[See note 5 on page 182]
Malignant neoplasm of digestive organs whose point of origin
cannot be classified to any one of the categories C15–C26.1

Excludes: cardio-oesophageal junction (C16.0)

C26.9   Ill-defined sites within the digestive system
Alimentary canal or tract NOS
Gastrointestinal tract NOS

Malignant neoplasms of respiratory and intrathoracic organs (C30–C39)

Includes: middle ear
Excludes: mesothelioma (C45.–)

C30   Malignant neoplasm of nasal cavity and middle ear

C30.0   Nasal cavity
Cartilage of nose
Concha, nasal
Internal nose
Septum of nose
Vestibule of nose
Excludes: nasal bone (C41.0)
nose NOS (C76.0)
olfactory bulb (C72.2)
posterior margin of nasal septum and choana (C11.3)
skin of nose (C43.3, C44.3)

C30.1   Middle ear
Eustachian tube
Inner ear
Mastoid air cells
Excludes: auricular canal (external) (C43.2, C44.2)
bone of ear (meatus) (C41.0)
cartilage of ear (C49.0)
skin of (external) ear (C43.2, C44.2)

C31   Malignant neoplasm of accessory sinuses

C31.0   Maxillary sinus
Antrum (Highmore)(maxillary)

C31.1   **Ethmoidal sinus**

C31.2   **Frontal sinus**

C31.3   **Sphenoidal sinus**

C31.8   **Overlapping lesion of accessory sinuses**
[See note 5 on page 182]

C31.9   **Accessory sinus, unspecified**

C32   Malignant neoplasm of larynx

C32.0   **Glottis**
Intrinsic larynx
Vocal cord (true) NOS

C32.1   **Supraglottis**
Aryepiglottic fold, laryngeal aspect
Epiglottis (suprahyoid portion) NOS
Extrinsic larynx
False vocal cord
Posterior (laryngeal) surface of epiglottis
Ventricular bands
Excludes: anterior surface of epiglottis (C10.1)
            aryepiglottic fold:
            • NOS (C13.1)
            • hypopharyngeal aspect (C13.1)
            • marginal zone (C13.1)

C32.2   **Subglottis**

C32.3   **Laryngeal cartilage**

C32.8   **Overlapping lesion of larynx**
[See note 5 on page 182]

C32.9   **Larynx, unspecified**

C33   Malignant neoplasm of trachea

C34   Malignant neoplasm of bronchus and lung

C34.0   **Main bronchus**
Carina
Hilus (of lung)

C34.1   Upper lobe, bronchus or lung

C34.2   Middle lobe, bronchus or lung

C34.3   Lower lobe, bronchus or lung

C34.8   Overlapping lesion of bronchus and lung
[See note 5 on page 182]

C34.9   Bronchus or lung, unspecified

C37   Malignant neoplasm of thymus

C38   Malignant neoplasm of heart, mediastinum and pleura
Excludes: mesothelioma (C45.–)

C38.0   Heart
Pericardium
Excludes: great vessels (C49.3)

C38.1   Anterior mediastinum

C38.2   Posterior mediastinum

C38.3   Mediastinum, part unspecified

C38.4   Pleura

C38.8   Overlapping lesion of heart, mediastinum and pleura
[See note 5 on page 182]

C39   Malignant neoplasm of other and ill-defined sites in the respiratory system and intrathoracic organs
Excludes: intrathoracic NOS (C76.1)
thoracic NOS (C76.1)

C39.0   Upper respiratory tract, part unspecified

C39.8   Overlapping lesion of respiratory and intrathoracic organs
[See note 5 on page 182]
Malignant neoplasm of respiratory and intrathoracic organs whose point of origin cannot be classified to any one of the categories C30–C39.0

C39.9   Ill-defined sites within the respiratory system
Respiratory tract NOS

Malignant neoplasms of bone and articular cartilage (C40–C41)

Excludes: bone marrow NOS (C96.7)
synovia (C49.–)

C40   Malignant neoplasm of bone and articular cartilage of limbs

C40.0   Scapula and long bones of upper limb

C40.1   Short bones of upper limb

C40.2   Long bones of lower limb

C40.3   Short bones of lower limb

C40.8   Overlapping lesion of bone and articular cartilage of limbs
[See note 5 on page 182]

C40.9   Bone and articular cartilage of limb, unspecified

C41   Malignant neoplasm of bone and articular cartilage of other and unspecified sites

Excludes: bones of limbs (C40.–)
cartilage of:
• ear (C49.0)
• larynx (C32.3)
• limbs (C40.–)
• nose (C30.0)

C41.0   Bones of skull and face
Maxilla (superior)
Orbital bone

Excludes: carcinoma, any type except intraosseous or
odontogenic of:
• maxillary sinus (C31.0)
• upper jaw (C03.0)
jaw bone (lower) (C41.1)

C41.1 **Mandible**

Lower jaw bone

Excludes: carcinoma, any type except intraosseous or
odontogenic of:
- jaw NOS (C03.9)
  - lower (C03.1)

upper jaw bone (C41.0)

C41.2 **Vertebral column**

Excludes: sacrum and coccyx (C41.4)

C41.3 **Ribs, sternum and clavicle**

C41.4 **Pelvic bones, sacrum and coccyx**

C41.8 **Overlapping lesion of bone and articular cartilage**

[See note 5 on page 182]

Malignant neoplasm of bone and articular cartilage whose point
of origin cannot be classified to any one of the categories
C40–C41.4

C41.9 **Bone and articular cartilage, unspecified**

Melanoma and other malignant neoplasms of skin (C43–C44)

C43 **Malignant melanoma of skin**

Includes: morphology codes M872–M879 with behaviour
code /3

Excludes: malignant melanoma of skin of genital organs
(C51–C52, C60.–, C63.–)

C43.0 **Malignant melanoma of lip**

Excludes: vermilion border of lip (C00.0–C00.2)

C43.1 **Malignant melanoma of eyelid, including canthus**

C43.2 **Malignant melanoma of ear and external auricular canal**

C43.3 **Malignant melanoma of other and unspecified parts of face**

C43.4 **Malignant melanoma of scalp and neck**

C43.5   **Malignant melanoma of trunk**
Anal:
• margin
• skin
Perianal skin
Skin of breast
Excludes: anus NOS (C21.0)

C43.6   **Malignant melanoma of upper limb, including shoulder**

C43.7   **Malignant melanoma of lower limb, including hip**

C43.8   **Overlapping malignant melanoma of skin**
[See note 5 on page 182]

C43.9   **Malignant melanoma of skin, unspecified**
Melanoma (malignant) NOS

C44   Other malignant neoplasms of skin
Includes: malignant neoplasm of:
• sebaceous glands
• sweat glands
Excludes: Kaposi's sarcoma (C46.–)
malignant melanoma of skin (C43.–)
skin of genital organs (C51–C52, C60.–, C63.–)

C44.0   **Skin of lip**
Basal cell carcinoma of lip
Excludes: malignant neoplasm of lip (C00.–)

C44.1   **Skin of eyelid, including canthus**
Excludes: connective tissue of eyelid (C49.0)

C44.2   **Skin of ear and external auricular canal**
Excludes: connective tissue of ear (C49.0)

C44.3   **Skin of other and unspecified parts of face**

C44.4   **Skin of scalp and neck**

C44.5   **Skin of trunk**
Anal:
• margin
• skin
Perianal skin
Skin of breast
Excludes: anus NOS (C21.0)

C44.6	**Skin of upper limb, including shoulder**
C44.7	**Skin of lower limb, including hip**
C44.8	**Overlapping lesion of skin** [See note 5 on page 182]
C44.9	**Malignant neoplasm of skin, unspecified**

Malignant neoplasms of mesothelial and soft tissue (C45–C49)

C45 Mesothelioma
Includes: morphology code M905 with behaviour code /3

C45.0	**Mesothelioma of pleura** *Excludes:* other malignant neoplasms of pleura (C38.4)
C45.1	**Mesothelioma of peritoneum** Mesentery Mesocolon Omentum Peritoneum (parietal)(pelvic) *Excludes:* other malignant neoplasms of peritoneum (C48.–)
C45.2	**Mesothelioma of pericardium** *Excludes:* other malignant neoplasms of pericardium (C38.0)
C45.7	**Mesothelioma of other sites**
C45.9	**Mesothelioma, unspecified**

C46 Kaposi's sarcoma
Includes: morphology code M9140 with behaviour code /3

C46.0	**Kaposi's sarcoma of skin**
C46.1	**Kaposi's sarcoma of soft tissue**
C46.2	**Kaposi's sarcoma of palate**
C46.3	**Kaposi's sarcoma of lymph nodes**
C46.7	**Kaposi's sarcoma of other sites**

C46.8   Kaposi's sarcoma of multiple organs

C46.9   Kaposi's sarcoma, unspecified

C47   Malignant neoplasm of peripheral nerves and autonomic nervous system

Includes: sympathetic and parasympathetic nerves and ganglia

C47.0   Peripheral nerves of head, face and neck
Excludes: peripheral nerves of orbit (C69.6)

C47.1   Peripheral nerves of upper limb, including shoulder

C47.2   Peripheral nerves of lower limb, including hip

C47.3   Peripheral nerves of thorax

C47.4   Peripheral nerves of abdomen

C47.5   Peripheral nerves of pelvis

C47.6   Peripheral nerves of trunk, unspecified

C47.8   Overlapping lesion of peripheral nerves and autonomic nervous system
[See note 5 on page 182]

C47.9   Peripheral nerves and autonomic nervous system, unspecified

C48   Malignant neoplasm of retroperitoneum and peritoneum

Excludes: Kaposi's sarcoma (C46.1)
        mesothelioma (C45.–)

C48.0   Retroperitoneum

C48.1   Specified parts of peritoneum
Mesentery
Mesocolon
Omentum
Peritoneum:
• parietal
• pelvic

C48.2   Peritoneum, unspecified

C48.8   Overlapping lesion of retroperitoneum and peritoneum
[See note 5 on page 182]

C49 Malignant neoplasm of other connective and soft tissue

Includes: blood vessel
bursa
cartilage
fascia
fat
ligament, except uterine
lymphatic vessel
muscle
synovia
tendon (sheath)

Excludes: cartilage (of):
- articular (C40–C41)
- larynx (C32.3)
- nose (C30.0)

connective tissue of breast (C50.–)
Kaposi's sarcoma (C46.–)
mesothelioma (C45.–)
peripheral nerves and autonomic nervous system (C47.–)
peritoneum (C48.–)
retroperitoneum (C48.0)

C49.0 Connective and soft tissue of head, face and neck

Connective tissue of:
- ear
- eyelid

Excludes: connective tissue of orbit (C69.6)

C49.1 Connective and soft tissue of upper limb, including shoulder

C49.2 Connective and soft tissue of lower limb, including hip

C49.3 Connective and soft tissue of thorax

Axilla
Diaphragm
Great vessels

Excludes: breast (C50.–)
heart (C38.0)
mediastinum (C38.1–C38.3)
thymus (C37)

C49.4 **Connective and soft tissue of abdomen**
Abdominal wall
Hypochondrium

C49.5 **Connective and soft tissue of pelvis**
Buttock
Groin
Perineum

C49.6 **Connective and soft tissue of trunk, unspecified**
Back NOS

C49.8 **Overlapping lesion of connective and soft tissue**
[See note 5 on page 182]
Malignant neoplasm of connective and soft tissue whose point
of origin cannot be classified to any one of the categories
C47–C49.6

C49.9 **Connective and soft tissue, unspecified**

Malignant neoplasm of breast (C50)

C50 Malignant neoplasm of breast
Includes: connective tissue of breast
Excludes: skin of breast (C43.5, C44.5)

C50.0 **Nipple and areola**

C50.1 **Central portion of breast**

C50.2 **Upper-inner quadrant of breast**

C50.3 **Lower-inner quadrant of breast**

C50.4 **Upper-outer quadrant of breast**

C50.5 **Lower-outer quadrant of breast**

C50.6 **Axillary tail of breast**

C50.8 **Overlapping lesion of breast**
[See note 5 on page 182]

C50.9 **Breast, unspecified**

Malignant neoplasms of female genital organs (C51–C58)

Includes: skin of female genital organs

C51 Malignant neoplasm of vulva

C51.0 Labium majus
Bartholin's [greater vestibular] gland

C51.1 Labium minus

C51.2 Clitoris

C51.8 Overlapping lesion of vulva
[See note 5 on page 182]

C51.9 Vulva, unspecified
External female genitalia NOS
Pudendum

C52 Malignant neoplasm of vagina

C53 Malignant neoplasm of cervix uteri

C53.0 Endocervix

C53.1 Exocervix

C53.8 Overlapping lesion of cervix uteri
[See note 5 on page 182]

C53.9 Cervix uteri, unspecified

C54 Malignant neoplasm of corpus uteri

C54.0 Isthmus uteri
Lower uterine segment

C54.1 Endometrium

C54.2 Myometrium

C54.3 Fundus uteri

C54.8 Overlapping lesion of corpus uteri
[See note 5 on page 182]

C54.9   Corpus uteri, unspecified

C55   Malignant neoplasm of uterus, part unspecified

C56   Malignant neoplasm of ovary

C57   Malignant neoplasm of other and unspecified female genital organs

C57.0   Fallopian tube
Oviduct
Uterine tube

C57.1   Broad ligament

C57.2   Round ligament

C57.3   Parametrium
Uterine ligament NOS

C57.4   Uterine adnexa, unspecified

C57.7   Other specified female genital organs
Wolffian body or duct

C57.8   Overlapping lesion of female genital organs
[See note 5 on page 182]
Malignant neoplasm of female genital organs whose point
   of origin cannot be classified to any one of the categories
   C51–C57.7, C58
Tubo-ovarian
Utero-ovarian

C57.9   Female genital organ, unspecified
Female genitourinary tract NOS

C58   Malignant neoplasm of placenta
Choriocarcinoma NOS
Chorionepithelioma NOS

Excludes: chorioadenoma (destruens) (D39.2)
              hydatidiform mole:
              • NOS (O01.9)
              • invasive (D39.2)
              • malignant (D39.2)

Malignant neoplasms of male genital organs (C60–C63)

Includes: skin of male genital organs

C60 Malignant neoplasm of penis

C60.0 Prepuce
Foreskin

C60.1 Glans penis

C60.2 Body of penis
Corpus cavernosum

C60.8 Overlapping lesion of penis
[See note 5 on page 182]

C60.9 Penis, unspecified
Skin of penis NOS

C61 Malignant neoplasm of prostate

C62 Malignant neoplasm of testis

C62.0 Undescended testis
Ectopic testis [site of neoplasm]
Retained testis [site of neoplasm]

C62.1 Descended testis
Scrotal testis

C62.9 Testis, unspecified

C63 Malignant neoplasm of other and unspecified male genital organs

C63.0 Epididymis

C63.1 Spermatic cord

C63.2 Scrotum
Skin of scrotum

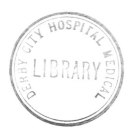

C63.7   Other specified male genital organs
Seminal vesicle
Tunica vaginalis

C63.8   Overlapping lesion of male genital organs
[See note 5 on page 182]
Malignant neoplasm of male genital organs whose point of origin cannot be classified to any one of the categories C60–C63.7

C63.9   Male genital organ, unspecified
Male genitourinary tract NOS

Malignant neoplasms of urinary tract (C64–C68)

C64   Malignant neoplasm of kidney, except renal pelvis
Excludes: renal:
- calyces (C65)
- pelvis (C65)

C65   Malignant neoplasm of renal pelvis
Pelviureteric junction
Renal calyces

C66   Malignant neoplasm of ureter
Excludes: ureteric orifice of bladder (C67.6)

C67   Malignant neoplasm of bladder

C67.0   Trigone of bladder

C67.1   Dome of bladder

C67.2   Lateral wall of bladder

C67.3   Anterior wall of bladder

C67.4   Posterior wall of bladder

C67.5 **Bladder neck**
Internal urethral orifice

C67.6 **Ureteric orifice**

C67.7 **Urachus**

C67.8 **Overlapping lesion of bladder**
[See note 5 on page 182]

C67.9 **Bladder, unspecified**

C68 **Malignant neoplasm of other and unspecified urinary organs**
Excludes: genitourinary tract NOS:
  • female (C57.9)
  • male (C63.9)

C68.0 **Urethra**
Excludes: urethral orifice of bladder (C67.5)

C68.1 **Paraurethral gland**

C68.8 **Overlapping lesion of urinary organs**
[See note 5 on page 182]
Malignant neoplasm of urinary organs whose point of origin cannot be classified to any one of the categories C64–C68.1

C68.9 **Urinary organ, unspecified**
Urinary system NOS

Malignant neoplasms of eye, brain and other parts of central nervous system (C69–C72)

C69 **Malignant neoplasm of eye and adnexa**
Excludes: connective tissue of eyelid (C49.0)
    eyelid (skin) (C43.1, C44.1)
    optic nerve (C72.3)

C69.0 **Conjunctiva**

C69.1 **Cornea**

C69.2   **Retina**

C69.3   **Choroid**

C69.4   **Ciliary body**
Eyeball

C69.5   **Lacrimal gland and duct**
Lacrimal sac
Nasolacrimal duct

C69.6   **Orbit**
Connective tissue of orbit
Extraocular muscle
Peripheral nerves of orbit
Retrobulbar tissue
Retro-ocular tissue
Excludes: orbital bone (C41.0)

C69.8   **Overlapping lesion of eye and adnexa**
[See note 5 on page 182]

C69.9   **Eye, unspecified**

C70   Malignant neoplasm of meninges

C70.0   **Cerebral meninges**

C70.1   **Spinal meninges**

C70.9   **Meninges, unspecified**

C71   Malignant neoplasm of brain
Excludes: cranial nerves (C72.2–C72.5)
          retrobulbar tissue (C69.6)

C71.0   **Cerebrum, except lobes and ventricles**
Corpus callosum
Supratentorial NOS

C71.1   **Frontal lobe**

C71.2   **Temporal lobe**

C71.3   **Parietal lobe**

C71.4   **Occipital lobe**

C71.5   **Cerebral ventricle**
Excludes: fourth ventricle (C71.7)

C71.6   **Cerebellum**

C71.7   **Brain stem**
Fourth ventricle
Infratentorial NOS

C71.8   **Overlapping lesion of brain**
[See note 5 on page 182]

C71.9   **Brain, unspecified**

C72   Malignant neoplasm of spinal cord, cranial nerves and other parts of central nervous system

Excludes: meninges (C70.–)
peripheral nerves and autonomic nervous system (C47.–)

C72.0   **Spinal cord**

C72.1   **Cauda equina**

C72.2   **Olfactory nerve**
Olfactory bulb

C72.3   **Optic nerve**

C72.4   **Acoustic nerve**

C72.5   **Other and unspecified cranial nerves**
Cranial nerve NOS

C72.8   **Overlapping lesion of brain and other parts of central nervous system**
[See note 5 on page 182]
Malignant neoplasm of brain and other parts of central nervous system whose point of origin cannot be classified to any one of the categories C70–C72.5

C72.9   **Central nervous system, unspecified**
Nervous system NOS

Malignant neoplasms of thyroid and other endocrine glands (C73–C75)

C73 Malignant neoplasm of thyroid gland

C74 Malignant neoplasm of adrenal gland

C74.0 Cortex of adrenal gland

C74.1 Medulla of adrenal gland

C74.9 Adrenal gland, unspecified

C75 Malignant neoplasm of other endocrine glands and related structures

Excludes: adrenal gland (C74.–)
endocrine pancreas (C25.4)
ovary (C56)
testis (C62.–)
thymus (C37)
thyroid gland (C73)

C75.0 Parathyroid gland

C75.1 Pituitary gland

C75.2 Craniopharyngeal duct

C75.3 Pineal gland

C75.4 Carotid body

C75.5 Aortic body and other paraganglia

C75.8 Pluriglandular involvement, unspecified
Note: If the sites of multiple involvement are known, they should be coded separately.

C75.9 Endocrine gland, unspecified

Malignant neoplasms of ill-defined, secondary and unspecified sites (C76–C80)

C76 Malignant neoplasm of other and ill-defined sites

Excludes: malignant neoplasm of:
- genitourinary tract NOS:
  - female (C57.9)
  - male (C63.9)
- lymphoid, haematopoietic and related tissue (C81–C96)
- unspecified site (C80)

C76.0 **Head, face and neck**
Cheek NOS
Nose NOS

C76.1 **Thorax**
Axilla NOS
Intrathoracic NOS
Thoracic NOS

C76.2 **Abdomen**

C76.3 **Pelvis**
Groin NOS
Sites overlapping systems within the pelvis, such as:
- rectovaginal (septum)
- rectovesical (septum)

C76.4 **Upper limb**

C76.5 **Lower limb**

C76.7 **Other ill-defined sites**

C76.8 **Overlapping lesion of other and ill-defined sites**
[See note 5 on page 182]

C77 Secondary and unspecified malignant neoplasm of lymph nodes

Excludes: malignant neoplasm of lymph nodes, specified as primary (C81–C88, C96.–)

213

C77.0 **Lymph nodes of head, face and neck**
Supraclavicular lymph nodes

C77.1 **Intrathoracic lymph nodes**

C77.2 **Intra-abdominal lymph nodes**

C77.3 **Axillary and upper limb lymph nodes**
Pectoral lymph nodes

C77.4 **Inguinal and lower limb lymph nodes**

C77.5 **Intrapelvic lymph nodes**

C77.8 **Lymph nodes of multiple regions**

C77.9 **Lymph node, unspecified**

C78 Secondary malignant neoplasm of respiratory and digestive organs

C78.0 **Secondary malignant neoplasm of lung**

C78.1 **Secondary malignant neoplasm of mediastinum**

C78.2 **Secondary malignant neoplasm of pleura**

C78.3 **Secondary malignant neoplasm of other and unspecified respiratory organs**

C78.4 **Secondary malignant neoplasm of small intestine**

C78.5 **Secondary malignant neoplasm of large intestine and rectum**

C78.6 **Secondary malignant neoplasm of retroperitoneum and peritoneum**
Malignant ascites NOS

C78.7 **Secondary malignant neoplasm of liver**

C78.8 **Secondary malignant neoplasm of other and unspecified digestive organs**

C79 Secondary malignant neoplasm of other sites

C79.0 **Secondary malignant neoplasm of kidney and renal pelvis**

C79.1 **Secondary malignant neoplasm of bladder and other and unspecified urinary organs**

C79.2 **Secondary malignant neoplasm of skin**

C79.3 Secondary malignant neoplasm of brain and cerebral meninges

C79.4 Secondary malignant neoplasm of other and unspecified parts of nervous system

C79.5 Secondary malignant neoplasm of bone and bone marrow

C79.6 Secondary malignant neoplasm of ovary

C79.7 Secondary malignant neoplasm of adrenal gland

C79.8 Secondary malignant neoplasm of other specified sites

C80 Malignant neoplasm without specification of site

Cancer
Carcinoma
Carcinomatosis
Generalized:
• cancer
• malignancy
Malignancy
Multiple cancer
Malignant cachexia
Primary site unknown

} unspecified site (primary)(secondary)

Malignant neoplasms of lymphoid, haematopoietic and related tissue (C81–C96)

Note: The terms used in categories C82–C85 for non-Hodgkin's lymphomas are those of the Working Formulation, which attempted to find common ground among several major classification schemes. The terms used in these schemes are not given in the Tabular List but appear in the Alphabetical Index; exact equivalence with the terms appearing in the Tabular List is not always possible.

Includes: morphology codes M959–M994 with behaviour code /3

Excludes: secondary and unspecified neoplasm of lymph nodes (C77.–)

C81 Hodgkin's disease

Includes: morphology codes M965–M966 with behaviour
code /3

C81.0 **Lymphocytic predominance**
Lymphocytic-histiocytic predominance

C81.1 **Nodular sclerosis**

C81.2 **Mixed cellularity**

C81.3 **Lymphocytic depletion**

C81.7 **Other Hodgkin's disease**

C81.9 **Hodgkin's disease, unspecified**

C82 Follicular [nodular] non-Hodgkin's lymphoma

Includes: follicular non-Hodgkin's lymphoma with or without
diffuse areas
morphology code M969 with behaviour code /3

C82.0 **Small cleaved cell, follicular**

C82.1 **Mixed small cleaved and large cell, follicular**

C82.2 **Large cell, follicular**

C82.7 **Other types of follicular non-Hodgkin's lymphoma**

C82.9 **Follicular non-Hodgkin's lymphoma, unspecified**
Nodular non-Hodgkin's lymphoma NOS

C83 Diffuse non-Hodgkin's lymphoma

Includes: morphology codes M9593, M9595, M967–M968 with
behaviour code /3

C83.0 **Small cell (diffuse)**

C83.1 **Small cleaved cell (diffuse)**

C83.2 **Mixed small and large cell (diffuse)**

C83.3 **Large cell (diffuse)**
Reticulum cell sarcoma

C83.4 **Immunoblastic (diffuse)**

C83.5 **Lymphoblastic (diffuse)**

C83.6   **Undifferentiated (diffuse)**

C83.7   **Burkitt's tumour**

C83.8   **Other types of diffuse non-Hodgkin's lymphoma**

C83.9   **Diffuse non-Hodgkin's lymphoma, unspecified**

C84   Peripheral and cutaneous T-cell lymphomas

Includes: morphology code M970 with behaviour code /3

C84.0   **Mycosis fungoides**

C84.1   **Sézary's disease**

C84.2   **T-zone lymphoma**

C84.3   **Lymphoepithelioid lymphoma**
Lennert's lymphoma

C84.4   **Peripheral T-cell lymphoma**

C84.5   **Other and unspecified T-cell lymphomas**
Note: If T-cell lineage or involvement is mentioned in conjunction with a specific lymphoma, code to the more specific description.

C85   Other and unspecified types of non-Hodgkin's lymphoma

Includes: morphology codes M9590–M9592, M9594, M971 with behaviour code /3

C85.0   **Lymphosarcoma**

C85.1   **B-cell lymphoma, unspecified**
Note: If B-cell lineage or involvement is mentioned in conjunction with a specific lymphoma, code to the more specific description.

C85.7   **Other specified types of non-Hodgkin's lymphoma**
Malignant:
• reticuloendotheliosis
• reticulosis
Microglioma

C85.9   **Non-Hodgkin's lymphoma, unspecified type**
Lymphoma NOS
Malignant lymphoma NOS
Non-Hodgkin's lymphoma NOS

C88 Malignant immunoproliferative diseases

Includes: morphology code M976 with behaviour code /3

C88.0 Waldenström's macroglobulinaemia

C88.1 Alpha heavy chain disease

C88.2 Gamma heavy chain disease
Franklin's disease

C88.3 Immunoproliferative small intestinal disease
Mediterranean lymphoma

C88.7 Other malignant immunoproliferative diseases

C88.9 Malignant immunoproliferative disease, unspecified
Immunoproliferative disease NOS

C90 Multiple myeloma and malignant plasma cell neoplasms

Includes: morphology codes M973, M9830 with behaviour code /3

C90.0 Multiple myeloma
Kahler's disease
Myelomatosis
Excludes: solitary myeloma (C90.2)

C90.1 Plasma cell leukaemia

C90.2 Plasmacytoma, extramedullary
Malignant plasma cell tumour NOS
Plasmacytoma NOS
Solitary myeloma

C91 Lymphoid leukaemia

Includes: morphology codes M982, M9940–M9941 with behaviour code /3

C91.0 Acute lymphoblastic leukaemia

Excludes: acute exacerbation of chronic lymphocytic leukaemia (C91.1)

C91.1 Chronic lymphocytic leukaemia

C91.2   **Subacute lymphocytic leukaemia**

C91.3   **Prolymphocytic leukaemia**

C91.4   **Hairy-cell leukaemia**
Leukaemic reticuloendotheliosis

C91.5   **Adult T-cell leukaemia**

C91.7   **Other lymphoid leukaemia**

C91.9   **Lymphoid leukaemia, unspecified**

C92   Myeloid leukaemia

Includes: leukaemia:
- granulocytic
- myelogenous
  morphology codes M986–M988, M9930 with behaviour
  code /3

C92.0   **Acute myeloid leukaemia**
Excludes: acute exacerbation of chronic myeloid leukaemia
(C92.1)

C92.1   **Chronic myeloid leukaemia**

C92.2   **Subacute myeloid leukaemia**

C92.3   **Myeloid sarcoma**
Chloroma
Granulocytic sarcoma

C92.4   **Acute promyelocytic leukaemia**

C92.5   **Acute myelomonocytic leukaemia**

C92.7   **Other myeloid leukaemia**

C92.9   **Myeloid leukaemia, unspecified**

C93   Monocytic leukaemia

Includes: monocytoid leukaemia
morphology code M989 with behaviour code /3

C93.0   **Acute monocytic leukaemia**
Excludes: acute exacerbation of chronic monocytic leukaemia
(C93.1)

C93.1   **Chronic monocytic leukaemia**

C93.2   Subacute monocytic leukaemia

C93.7   Other monocytic leukaemia

C93.9   Monocytic leukaemia, unspecified

C94 Other leukaemias of specified cell type

Includes: morphology codes M984, M9850, M9900, M9910,
M9931–M9932 with behaviour code /3

Excludes: leukaemic reticuloendotheliosis (C91.4)
plasma cell leukaemia (C90.1)

C94.0   Acute erythraemia and erythroleukaemia
Acute erythraemic myelosis
Di Guglielmo's disease

C94.1   Chronic erythraemia
Heilmeyer-Schöner disease

C94.2   Acute megakaryoblastic leukaemia
Leukaemia:
• megakaryoblastic (acute)
• megakaryocytic (acute)

C94.3   Mast cell leukaemia

C94.4   Acute panmyelosis

C94.5   Acute myelofibrosis

C94.7   Other specified leukaemias
Lymphosarcoma cell leukaemia

C95 Leukaemia of unspecified cell type

Includes: morphology code M980 with behaviour code /3

C95.0   Acute leukaemia of unspecified cell type
Blast cell leukaemia
Stem cell leukaemia

Excludes: acute exacerbation of unspecified chronic leukaemia
(C95.1)

C95.1   Chronic leukaemia of unspecified cell type

C95.2   Subacute leukaemia of unspecified cell type

C95.7   Other leukaemia of unspecified cell type

C95.9   **Leukaemia, unspecified**

C96   **Other and unspecified malignant neoplasms of lymphoid, haematopoietic and related tissue**
Includes: morphology codes M972, M974 with behaviour code /3

C96.0   **Letterer-Siwe disease**
Nonlipid:
- reticuloendotheliosis
- reticulosis

C96.1   **Malignant histiocytosis**
Histiocytic medullary reticulosis

C96.2   **Malignant mast cell tumour**
Malignant:
- mastocytoma
- mastocytosis
Mast cell sarcoma

Excludes: mast cell leukaemia (C94.3)
mastocytosis (cutaneous) (Q82.2)

C96.3   **True histiocytic lymphoma**

C96.7   **Other specified malignant neoplasms of lymphoid, haematopoietic and related tissue**

C96.9   **Malignant neoplasm of lymphoid, haematopoietic and related tissue, unspecified**

Malignant neoplasms of independent (primary) multiple sites (C97)

C97   **Malignant neoplasms of independent (primary) multiple sites**
Note: For use of this category, reference should be made to the mortality coding rules and guidelines in Volume 2.

In situ neoplasms
(D00–D09)

Note: Many in situ neoplasms are regarded as being located within a continuum of morphological change between dysplasia and invasive cancer. For example, for cervical intraepithelial neoplasia (CIN) three grades are recognized, the third of which (CIN III) includes both severe dysplasia and carcinoma in situ. This system of grading has been extended to other organs, such as vulva and vagina. Descriptions of grade III intraepithelial neoplasia, with or without mention of severe dysplasia, are assigned to this section; grades I and II are classified as dysplasia of the organ system involved and should be coded to the relevant body system chapter.

Includes: Bowen's disease
erythroplasia
morphology codes with behaviour code /2
Queyrat's erythroplasia

D00 Carcinoma in situ of oral cavity, oesophagus and stomach
Excludes: melanoma in situ (D03.–)

D00.0 Lip, oral cavity and pharynx
Aryepiglottic fold:
- NOS
- hypopharyngeal aspect
- marginal zone

Vermilion border of lip

Excludes: aryepiglottic fold, laryngeal aspect (D02.0)
epiglottis:
- NOS (D02.0)
- suprahyoid portion (D02.0)
skin of lip (D03.0, D04.0)

D00.1 Oesophagus

D00.2 Stomach

D01 Carcinoma in situ of other and unspecified digestive organs

Excludes: melanoma in situ (D03.–)

D01.0 **Colon**
Excludes: rectosigmoid junction (D01.1)

D01.1 **Rectosigmoid junction**

D01.2 **Rectum**

D01.3 **Anus and anal canal**
Excludes: anal:
- margin (D03.5, D04.5)
- skin (D03.5, D04.5)
perianal skin (D03.5, D04.5)

D01.4 **Other and unspecified parts of intestine**
Excludes: ampulla of Vater (D01.5)

D01.5 **Liver, gallbladder and bile ducts**
Ampulla of Vater

D01.7 **Other specified digestive organs**
Pancreas

D01.9 **Digestive organ, unspecified**

D02 Carcinoma in situ of middle ear and respiratory system

Excludes: melanoma in situ (D03.–)

D02.0 **Larynx**
Aryepiglottic fold, laryngeal aspect
Epiglottis (suprahyoid portion)
Excludes: aryepiglottic fold:
- NOS (D00.0)
- hypopharyngeal aspect (D00.0)
- marginal zone (D00.0)

D02.1 **Trachea**

D02.2 **Bronchus and lung**

D02.3 **Other parts of respiratory system**
Accessory sinuses
Middle ear
Nasal cavities
Excludes: ear (external)(skin) (D03.2, D04.2)
nose:
- NOS (D09.7)
- skin (D03.3, D04.3)

D02.4 **Respiratory system, unspecified**

D03 Melanoma in situ
Includes: morphology codes M872–M879 with behaviour code /2

D03.0 **Melanoma in situ of lip**

D03.1 **Melanoma in situ of eyelid, including canthus**

D03.2 **Melanoma in situ of ear and external auricular canal**

D03.3 **Melanoma in situ of other and unspecified parts of face**

D03.4 **Melanoma in situ of scalp and neck**

D03.5 **Melanoma in situ of trunk**
Anal:
- margin
- skin
Breast (skin)(soft tissue)
Perianal skin

D03.6 **Melanoma in situ of upper limb, including shoulder**

D03.7 **Melanoma in situ of lower limb, including hip**

D03.8 **Melanoma In situ of other sites**

D03.9 **Melanoma in situ, unspecified**

D04 Carcinoma in situ of skin
Excludes: erythroplasia of Queyrat (penis) NOS (D07.4)
melanoma in situ (D03.–)

D04.0 **Skin of lip**
Excludes: vermilion border of lip (D00.0)

D04.1 **Skin of eyelid, including canthus**

D04.2   **Skin of ear and external auricular canal**

D04.3   **Skin of other and unspecified parts of face**

D04.4   **Skin of scalp and neck**

D04.5   **Skin of trunk**
Anal:
- margin
- skin

Perianal skin
Skin of breast
Excludes: anus NOS (D01.3)
              skin of genital organs (D07.–)

D04.6   **Skin of upper limb, including shoulder**

D04.7   **Skin of lower limb, including hip**

D04.8   **Skin of other sites**

D04.9   **Skin, unspecified**

D05   Carcinoma in situ of breast

Excludes: carcinoma in situ of skin of breast (D04.5)
             melanoma in situ of breast (skin) (D03.5)

D05.0   **Lobular carcinoma in situ**

D05.1   **Intraductal carcinoma in situ**

D05.7   **Other carcinoma in situ of breast**

D05.9   **Carcinoma in situ of breast, unspecified**

D06   Carcinoma in situ of cervix uteri

Includes: cervical intraepithelial neoplasia [CIN], grade III,
             with or without mention of severe dysplasia
Excludes: melanoma in situ of cervix (D03.5)
             severe dysplasia of cervix NOS (N87.2)

D06.0   **Endocervix**

D06.1   **Exocervix**

D06.7   **Other parts of cervix**

D06.9   **Cervix, unspecified**

D07 Carcinoma in situ of other and unspecified genital organs

Excludes: melanoma in situ (D03.5)

D07.0 **Endometrium**

D07.1 **Vulva**
Vulvar intraepithelial neoplasia [VIN], grade III, with or without mention of severe dysplasia
Excludes: severe dysplasia of vulva NOS (N90.2)

D07.2 **Vagina**
Vaginal intraepithelial neoplasia [VAIN], grade III, with or without mention of severe dysplasia
Excludes: severe dysplasia of vagina NOS (N89.2)

D07.3 **Other and unspecified female genital organs**

D07.4 **Penis**
Erythroplasia of Queyrat NOS

D07.5 **Prostate**

D07.6 **Other and unspecified male genital organs**

D09 Carcinoma in situ of other and unspecified sites

Excludes: melanoma in situ (D03.–)

D09.0 **Bladder**

D09.1 **Other and unspecified urinary organs**

D09.2 **Eye**
Excludes: skin of eyelid (D04.1)

D09.3 **Thyroid and other endocrine glands**
Excludes: endocrine pancreas (D01.7)
ovary (D07.3)
testis (D07.6)

D09.7 **Carcinoma in situ of other specified sites**

D09.9 **Carcinoma in situ, unspecified**

Benign neoplasms
(D10–D36)

Includes: morphology codes with behaviour code /0

D10 Benign neoplasm of mouth and pharynx

D10.0 Lip
Lip (frenulum)(inner aspect)(mucosa)(vermilion border)
Excludes: skin of lip (D22.0, D23.0)

D10.1 Tongue
Lingual tonsil

D10.2 Floor of mouth

D10.3 Other and unspecified parts of mouth
Minor salivary gland NOS
Excludes: benign odontogenic neoplasms (D16.4–D16.5)
mucosa of lip (D10.0)
nasopharyngeal surface of soft palate (D10.6)

D10.4 Tonsil
Tonsil (faucial)(palatine)
Excludes: lingual tonsil (D10.1)
pharyngeal tonsil (D10.6)
tonsillar:
• fossa (D10.5)
• pillars (D10.5)

D10.5 Other parts of oropharynx
Epiglottis, anterior aspect
Tonsillar:
• fossa
• pillars
Vallecula
Excludes: epiglottis:
• NOS (D14.1)
• suprahyoid portion (D14.1)

D10.6 Nasopharynx
Pharyngeal tonsil
Posterior margin of septum and choanae

D10.7 Hypopharynx

D10.9 Pharynx, unspecified

D11 Benign neoplasm of major salivary glands

Excludes: benign neoplasms of specified minor salivary glands which are classified according to their anatomical location

benign neoplasms of minor salivary glands NOS (D10.3)

D11.0 **Parotid gland**

D11.7 **Other major salivary glands**
Gland:
- sublingual
- submandibular

D11.9 **Major salivary gland, unspecified**

D12 Benign neoplasm of colon, rectum, anus and anal canal

D12.0 **Caecum**
Ileocaecal valve

D12.1 **Appendix**

D12.2 **Ascending colon**

D12.3 **Transverse colon**
Hepatic flexure
Splenic flexure

D12.4 **Descending colon**

D12.5 **Sigmoid colon**

D12.6 **Colon, unspecified**
Adenomatosis of colon
Large intestine NOS
Polyposis (hereditary) of colon

D12.7 **Rectosigmoid junction**

D12.8 **Rectum**

D12.9 **Anus and anal canal**
Excludes: anal:
- margin (D22.5, D23.5)
- skin (D22.5, D23.5)
perianal skin (D22.5, D23.5)

D13 Benign neoplasm of other and ill-defined parts of digestive system

D13.0 **Oesophagus**

D13.1 **Stomach**

D13.2 **Duodenum**

D13.3 **Other and unspecified parts of small intestine**

D13.4 **Liver**
Intrahepatic bile ducts

D13.5 **Extrahepatic bile ducts**

D13.6 **Pancreas**
Excludes: endocrine pancreas (D13.7)

D13.7 **Endocrine pancreas**
Islet cell tumour
Islets of Langerhans

D13.9 **Ill-defined sites within the digestive system**
Digestive system NOS
Intestine NOS
Spleen

D14   Benign neoplasm of middle ear and respiratory system

D14.0   **Middle ear, nasal cavity and accessory sinuses**
Cartilage of nose
Excludes: auricular canal (external) (D22.2, D23.2)
        bone of:
          • ear (D16.4)
          • nose (D16.4)
        cartilage of ear (D21.0)
        ear (external)(skin) (D22.2, D23.2)
        nose:
          • NOS (D36.7)
          • skin (D22.3, D23.3)
        olfactory bulb (D33.3)
        polyp (of):
          • accessory sinus (J33.8)
          • ear (middle) (H74.4)
          • nasal (cavity) (J33.–)
        posterior margin of septum and choanae (D10.6)

D14.1   **Larynx**
Epiglottis (suprahyoid portion)
Excludes: epiglottis, anterior aspect (D10.5)
        polyp of vocal cord and larynx (J38.1)

D14.2   **Trachea**

D14.3   **Bronchus and lung**

D14.4   **Respiratory system, unspecified**

D15   Benign neoplasm of other and unspecified intrathoracic organs
Excludes: mesothelial tissue (D19.–)

D15.0   **Thymus**

D15.1   **Heart**
Excludes: great vessels (D21.3)

D15.2   **Mediastinum**

D15.7   **Other specified intrathoracic organs**

D15.9   **Intrathoracic organ, unspecified**

D16   Benign neoplasm of bone and articular cartilage

Excludes: connective tissue of:
- ear (D21.0)
- eyelid (D21.0)
- larynx (D14.1)
- nose (D14.0)

synovia (D21.–)

D16.0   **Scapula and long bones of upper limb**

D16.1   **Short bones of upper limb**

D16.2   **Long bones of lower limb**

D16.3   **Short bones of lower limb**

D16.4   **Bones of skull and face**
Maxilla (superior)
Orbital bone
Excludes: lower jaw bone (D16.5)

D16.5   **Lower jaw bone**

D16.6   **Vertebral column**
Excludes: sacrum and coccyx (D16.8)

D16.7   **Ribs, sternum and clavicle**

D16.8   **Pelvic bones, sacrum and coccyx**

D16.9   **Bone and articular cartilage, unspecified**

D17   Benign lipomatous neoplasm

Includes: morphology codes M885–M888 with behaviour code /0

D17.0   **Benign lipomatous neoplasm of skin and subcutaneous tissue of head, face and neck**

D17.1   **Benign lipomatous neoplasm of skin and subcutaneous tissue of trunk**

D17.2   **Benign lipomatous neoplasm of skin and subcutaneous tissue of limbs**

D17.3   **Benign lipomatous neoplasm of skin and subcutaneous tissue of other and unspecified sites**

D17.4   **Benign lipomatous neoplasm of intrathoracic organs**

D17.5   **Benign lipomatous neoplasm of intra-abdominal organs**
Excludes: peritoneum and retroperitoneum (D17.7)

D17.6   **Benign lipomatous neoplasm of spermatic cord**

D17.7   **Benign lipomatous neoplasm of other sites**
Peritoneum
Retroperitoneum

D17.9   **Benign lipomatous neoplasm, unspecified**
Lipoma NOS

D18   Haemangioma and lymphangioma, any site
Includes: morphology codes M912–M917 with behaviour code /0
Excludes: blue or pigmented naevus (D22.–)

D18.0   **Haemangioma, any site**
Angioma NOS

D18.1   **Lymphangioma, any site**

D19   Benign neoplasm of mesothelial tissue
Includes: morphology code M905 with behaviour code /0

D19.0   **Mesothelial tissue of pleura**

D19.1   **Mesothelial tissue of peritoneum**

D19.7   **Mesothelial tissue of other sites**

D19.9   **Mesothelial tissue, unspecified**
Benign mesothelioma NOS

D20   Benign neoplasm of soft tissue of retroperitoneum and peritoneum
Excludes: benign lipomatous neoplasm of peritoneum and retroperitoneum (D17.7)
mesothelial tissue (D19.–)

D20.0   **Retroperitoneum**

D20.1   **Peritoneum**

D21   Other benign neoplasms of connective and other soft tissue

Includes: blood vessel
bursa
cartilage
fascia
fat
ligament, except uterine
lymphatic channel
muscle
synovia
tendon (sheath)

Excludes: cartilage:
- articular (D16.–)
- larynx (D14.1)
- nose (D14.0)

connective tissue of breast (D24)
haemangioma (D18.0)
lipomatous neoplasm (D17.–)
lymphangioma (D18.1)
peripheral nerves and autonomic nervous system
(D36.1)
peritoneum (D20.1)
retroperitoneum (D20.0)
uterine:
- leiomyoma (D25.–)
- ligament, any (D28.2)

vascular tissue (D18.–)

D21.0   **Connective and other soft tissue of head, face and neck**
Connective tissue of:
- ear
- eyelid

Excludes: connective tissue of orbit (D31.6)

D21.1   **Connective and other soft tissue of upper limb, including shoulder**

D21.2   **Connective and other soft tissue of lower limb, including hip**

D21.3 **Connective and other soft tissue of thorax**
Axilla
Diaphragm
Great vessels
Excludes: heart (D15.1)
        mediastinum (D15.2)
        thymus (D15.0)

D21.4 **Connective and other soft tissue of abdomen**

D21.5 **Connective and other soft tissue of pelvis**
Excludes: uterine:
        • leiomyoma (D25.–)
        • ligament, any (D28.2)

D21.6 **Connective and other soft tissue of trunk, unspecified**
Back NOS

D21.9 **Connective and other soft tissue, unspecified**

D22   Melanocytic naevi

Includes: morphology codes M872–M879 with behaviour code /0
naevus:
• NOS
• blue
• hairy
• pigmented

D22.0 **Melanocytic naevi of lip**

D22.1 **Melanocytic naevi of eyelid, including canthus**

D22.2 **Melanocytic naevi of ear and external auricular canal**

D22.3 **Melanocytic naevi of other and unspecified parts of face**

D22.4 **Melanocytic naevi of scalp and neck**

D22.5 **Melanocytic naevi of trunk**
Anal:
• margin
• skin
Perianal skin
Skin of breast

D22.6 **Melanocytic naevi of upper limb, including shoulder**

D22.7 **Melanocytic naevi of lower limb, including hip**

D22.9 **Melanocytic naevi, unspecified**

D23   Other benign neoplasms of skin

Includes: benign neoplasm of:
- hair follicles
- sebaceous glands
- sweat glands

Excludes: benign lipomatous neoplasms (D17.0–D17.3)
              melanocytic naevi (D22.–)

D23.0   **Skin of lip**

Excludes: vermilion border of lip (D10.0)

D23.1   **Skin of eyelid, including canthus**

D23.2   **Skin of ear and external auricular canal**

D23.3   **Skin of other and unspecified parts of face**

D23.4   **Skin of scalp and neck**

D23.5   **Skin of trunk**

Anal:
- margin
- skin

Perianal skin
Skin of breast

Excludes: anus NOS (D12.9)
              skin of genital organs (D28–D29)

D23.6   **Skin of upper limb, including shoulder**

D23.7   **Skin of lower limb, including hip**

D23.9   **Skin, unspecified**

D24   Benign neoplasm of breast

Breast:
- connective tissue
- soft parts

Excludes: benign mammary dysplasia (N60.–)
              skin of breast (D22.5, D23.5)

D25   Leiomyoma of uterus

Includes: benign neoplasms of uterus with morphology code
              M889 and behaviour code /0
              fibromyoma of uterus

D25.0   Submucous leiomyoma of uterus

D25.1   Intramural leiomyoma of uterus

D25.2   Subserosal leiomyoma of uterus

D25.9   Leiomyoma of uterus, unspecified

D26 Other benign neoplasms of uterus

D26.0   Cervix uteri

D26.1   Corpus uteri

D26.7   Other parts of uterus

D26.9   Uterus, unspecified

D27 Benign neoplasm of ovary

D28 Benign neoplasm of other and unspecified female genital organs

Includes: adenomatous polyp
skin of female genital organs

D28.0   Vulva

D28.1   Vagina

D28.2   Uterine tubes and ligaments
Fallopian tube
Uterine ligament (broad)(round)

D28.7   Other specified female genital organs

D28.9   Female genital organ, unspecified

D29 Benign neoplasm of male genital organs

Includes: skin of male genital organs

D29.0   Penis

D29.1 **Prostate**

Excludes: hyperplasia of prostate (adenomatous) (N40)
prostatic:
- adenoma (N40)
- enlargement (N40)
- hypertrophy (N40)

D29.2 **Testis**

D29.3 **Epididymis**

D29.4 **Scrotum**
Skin of scrotum

D29.7 **Other male genital organs**
Seminal vesicle
Spermatic cord
Tunica vaginalis

D29.9 **Male genital organ, unspecified**

D30 Benign neoplasm of urinary organs

D30.0 **Kidney**

Excludes: renal:
- calyces (D30.1)
- pelvis (D30.1)

D30.1 **Renal pelvis**

D30.2 **Ureter**

Excludes: ureteric orifice of bladder (D30.3)

D30.3 **Bladder**
Orifice of bladder:
- urethral
- ureteric

D30.4 **Urethra**

Excludes: urethral orifice of bladder (D30.3)

D30.7 **Other urinary organs**
Paraurethral glands

D30.9 **Urinary organ, unspecified**
Urinary system NOS

D31 Benign neoplasm of eye and adnexa

Excludes: connective tissue of eyelid (D21.0)
optic nerve (D33.3)
skin of eyelid (D22.1, D23.1)

D31.0 Conjunctiva

D31.1 Cornea

D31.2 Retina

D31.3 Choroid

D31.4 Ciliary body
Eyeball

D31.5 Lacrimal gland and duct
Lacrimal sac
Nasolacrimal duct

D31.6 Orbit, unspecified
Connective tissue of orbit
Extraocular muscle
Peripheral nerves of orbit
Retrobulbar tissue
Retro-ocular tissue
Excludes: orbital bone (D16.4)

D31.9 Eye, unspecified

D32 Benign neoplasm of meninges

D32.0 Cerebral meninges

D32.1 Spinal meninges

D32.9 Meninges, unspecified
Meningioma NOS

D33 Benign neoplasm of brain and other parts of central nervous system

Excludes: angioma (D18.0)
meninges (D32.–)
peripheral nerves and autonomic nervous system
(D36.1)
retro-ocular tissue (D31.6)

D33.0   **Brain, supratentorial**
Cerebral ventricle
Cerebrum
Frontal ⎫
Occipital ⎬ lobe
Parietal ⎪
Temporal ⎭
Excludes: fourth ventricle (D33.1)

D33.1   **Brain, infratentorial**
Brain stem
Cerebellum
Fourth ventricle

D33.2   **Brain, unspecified**

D33.3   **Cranial nerves**
Olfactory bulb

D33.4   **Spinal cord**

D33.7   **Other specified parts of central nervous system**

D33.9   **Central nervous system, unspecified**
Nervous system (central) NOS

D34   Benign neoplasm of thyroid gland

D35   Benign neoplasm of other and unspecified
endocrine glands
Excludes: endocrine pancreas (D13.7)
ovary (D27)
testis (D29.2)
thymus (D15.0)

D35.0   **Adrenal gland**

D35.1   **Parathyroid gland**

D35.2   **Pituitary gland**

D35.3   **Craniopharyngeal duct**

D35.4   **Pineal gland**

D35.5   **Carotid body**

D35.6   **Aortic body and other paraganglia**

D35.7   Other specified endocrine glands

D35.8   Pluriglandular involvement

D35.9   Endocrine gland, unspecified

D36   Benign neoplasm of other and unspecified sites

D36.0   Lymph nodes

D36.1   Peripheral nerves and autonomic nervous system
Excludes: peripheral nerves of orbit (D31.6)

D36.7   Other specified sites
Nose NOS

D36.9   Benign neoplasm of unspecified site

Neoplasms of uncertain or unknown behaviour (D37–D48)

Note: Categories D37–D48 classify by site neoplasms of uncertain or unknown behaviour, i.e., there is doubt whether the neoplasm is malignant or benign. Such neoplasms are assigned behaviour code /1 in the classification of the morphology of neoplasms.

D37   Neoplasm of uncertain or unknown behaviour of oral cavity and digestive organs

D37.0   Lip, oral cavity and pharynx
Aryepiglottic fold:
• NOS
• hypopharyngeal aspect
• marginal zone
Major and minor salivary glands
Vermilion border of lip
Excludes: aryepiglottic fold, laryngeal aspect (D38.0)
  epiglottis:
  • NOS (D38.0)
  • suprahyoid portion (D38.0)
  skin of lip (D48.5)

D37.1   Stomach

D37.2   **Small intestine**

D37.3   **Appendix**

D37.4   **Colon**

D37.5   **Rectum**
Rectosigmoid junction

D37.6   **Liver, gallbladder and bile ducts**
Ampulla of Vater

D37.7   **Other digestive organs**
Anal:
- canal
- sphincter

Anus NOS
Intestine NOS
Oesophagus
Pancreas
Excludes: anal:
- margin (D48.5)
- skin (D48.5)

perianal skin (D48.5)

D37.9   **Digestive organ, unspecified**

D38   **Neoplasm of uncertain or unknown behaviour of middle ear and respiratory and intrathoracic organs**
Excludes: heart (D48.7)

D38.0   **Larynx**
Aryepiglottic fold, laryngeal aspect
Epiglottis (suprahyoid portion)
Excludes: aryepiglottic fold:
- NOS (D37.0)
- hypopharyngeal aspect (D37.0)
- marginal zone (D37.0)

D38.1   **Trachea, bronchus and lung**

D38.2   **Pleura**

D38.3   **Mediastinum**

D38.4   **Thymus**

D38.5   **Other respiratory organs**
Accessory sinuses
Cartilage of nose
Middle ear
Nasal cavities
Excludes: ear (external)(skin) (D48.5)
nose:
• NOS (D48.7)
• skin (D48.5)

D38.6   **Respiratory organ, unspecified**

D39   Neoplasm of uncertain or unknown behaviour of female genital organs

D39.0   **Uterus**

D39.1   **Ovary**

D39.2   **Placenta**
Chorioadenoma destruens
Hydatidiform mole:
• invasive
• malignant
Excludes: hydatidiform mole NOS (O01.9)

D39.7   **Other female genital organs**
Skin of female genital organs

D39.9   **Female genital organ, unspecified**

D40   Neoplasm of uncertain or unknown behaviour of male genital organs

D40.0   **Prostate**

D40.1   **Testis**

D40.7   **Other male genital organs**
Skin of male genital organs

D40.9   **Male genital organ, unspecified**

D41 Neoplasm of uncertain or unknown behaviour of urinary organs

D41.0 Kidney
Excludes: renal pelvis (D41.1)

D41.1 Renal pelvis

D41.2 Ureter

D41.3 Urethra

D41.4 Bladder

D41.7 Other urinary organs

D41.9 Urinary organ, unspecified

D42 Neoplasm of uncertain or unknown behaviour of meninges

D42.0 Cerebral meninges

D42.1 Spinal meninges

D42.9 Meninges, unspecified

D43 Neoplasm of uncertain or unknown behaviour of brain and central nervous system

Excludes: peripheral nerves and autonomic nervous system (D48.2)

D43.0 Brain, supratentorial
Cerebral ventricle
Cerebrum
Frontal ⎫
Occipital ⎬ lobe
Parietal ⎪
Temporal ⎭
Excludes: fourth ventricle (D43.1)

D43.1 Brain, infratentorial
Brain stem
Cerebellum
Fourth ventricle

D43.2 Brain, unspecified

D43.3   **Cranial nerves**

D43.4   **Spinal cord**

D43.7   **Other parts of central nervous system**

D43.9   **Central nervous system, unspecified**
Nervous system (central) NOS

D44   Neoplasm of uncertain or unknown behaviour of endocrine glands

Excludes: endocrine pancreas (D37.7)
ovary (D39.1)
testis (D40.1)
thymus (D38.4)

D44.0   **Thyroid gland**

D44.1   **Adrenal gland**

D44.2   **Parathyroid gland**

D44.3   **Pituitary gland**

D44.4   **Craniopharyngeal duct**

D44.5   **Pineal gland**

D44.6   **Carotid body**

D44.7   **Aortic body and other paraganglia**

D44.8   **Pluriglandular involvement**
Multiple endocrine adenomatosis

D44.9   **Endocrine gland, unspecified**

D45   Polycythaemia vera
Morphology code M9950 with behaviour code /1

D46   Myelodysplastic syndromes
Includes: morphology code M998 with behaviour code /1

D46.0   **Refractory anaemia without sideroblasts, so stated**

D46.1   **Refractory anaemia with sideroblasts**

D46.2   **Refractory anaemia with excess of blasts**

D46.3 **Refractory anaemia with excess of blasts with transformation**

D46.4 **Refractory anaemia, unspecified**

D46.7 **Other myelodysplastic syndromes**

D46.9 **Myelodysplastic syndrome, unspecified**
Myelodysplasia NOS
Preleukaemia (syndrome) NOS

D47 Other neoplasms of uncertain or unknown behaviour of lymphoid, haematopoietic and related tissue

Includes: morphology codes M974, M976, M996–M997 with behaviour code /1

D47.0 **Histiocytic and mast cell tumours of uncertain and unknown behaviour**
Mast cell tumour NOS
Mastocytoma NOS

Excludes: mastocytosis (cutaneous) (Q82.2)

D47.1 **Chronic myeloproliferative disease**
Myelofibrosis (with myeloid metaplasia)
Myeloproliferative disease, unspecified
Myelosclerosis (megakaryocytic) with myeloid metaplasia

D47.2 **Monoclonal gammopathy**

D47.3 **Essential (haemorrhagic) thrombocythaemia**
Idiopathic haemorrhagic thrombocythaemia

D47.7 **Other specified neoplasms of uncertain or unknown behaviour of lymphoid, haematopoietic and related tissue**

D47.9 **Neoplasm of uncertain or unknown behaviour of lymphoid, haematopoietic and related tissue, unspecified**
Lymphoproliferative disease NOS

D48   Neoplasm of uncertain or unknown behaviour of other and unspecified sites

Excludes: neurofibromatosis (nonmalignant) (Q85.0)

D48.0   **Bone and articular cartilage**

Excludes: cartilage of:
- ear (D48.1)
- larynx (D38.0)
- nose (D38.5)

connective tissue of eyelid (D48.1)

synovia (D48.1)

D48.1   **Connective and other soft tissue**

Connective tissue of:
- ear
- eyelid

Excludes: cartilage (of):
- articular (D48.0)
- larynx (D38.0)
- nose (D38.5)

connective tissue of breast (D48.6)

D48.2   **Peripheral nerves and autonomic nervous system**

Excludes: peripheral nerves of orbit (D48.7)

D48.3   **Retroperitoneum**

D48.4   **Peritoneum**

D48.5   **Skin**

Anal:
- margin
- skin

Perianal skin

Skin of breast

Excludes: anus NOS (D37.7)

        skin of genital organs (D39.7, D40.7)

        vermilion border of lip (D37.0)

D48.6   **Breast**

Connective tissue of breast

Cystosarcoma phyllodes

Excludes: skin of breast (D48.5)

D48.7 **Other specified sites**
Eye
Heart
Peripheral nerves of orbit

Excludes: connective tissue (D48.1)
skin of eyelid (D48.5)

D48.9 **Neoplasm of uncertain or unknown behaviour, unspecified**
"Growth" NOS
Neoplasm NOS
New growth NOS
Tumour NOS

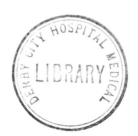

Diseases of the blood and blood-forming organs and certain disorders involving the immune mechanism (D50–D89)

Excludes: autoimmune disease (systemic) NOS (M35.9)

certain conditions originating in the perinatal period (P00–P96)

complications of pregnancy, childbirth and the puerperium (O00–O99)

congenital malformations, deformations and chromosomal abnormalities (Q00–Q99)

endocrine, nutritional and metabolic diseases (E00–E90)

human immunodeficiency virus [HIV] disease (B20–B24)

injury, poisoning and certain other consequences of external causes (S00–T98)

neoplasms (C00–D48)

symptoms, signs and abnormal clinical and laboratory findings, not elsewhere classified (R00–R99)

This chapter contains the following blocks:

D50–D53 Nutritional anaemias
D55–D59 Haemolytic anaemias
D60–D64 Aplastic and other anaemias
D65–D69 Coagulation defects, purpura and other haemorrhagic conditions
D70–D77 Other diseases of blood and blood-forming organs
D80–D89 Certain disorders involving the immune mechanism

Asterisk categories for this chapter are provided as follows:

D63* Anaemia in chronic diseases classified elsewhere
D77* Other disorders of blood and blood-forming organs in diseases classified elsewhere

Nutritional anaemias (D50–D53)

D50 Iron deficiency anaemia

Includes: anaemia:
- asiderotic
- hypochromic

D50.0 Iron deficiency anaemia secondary to blood loss (chronic)
Posthaemorrhagic anaemia (chronic)
Excludes: acute posthaemorrhagic anaemia (D62)
congenital anaemia from fetal blood loss (P61.3)

D50.1 Sideropenic dysphagia
Kelly–Paterson syndrome
Plummer–Vinson syndrome

D50.8 Other iron deficiency anaemias

D50.9 Iron deficiency anaemia, unspecified

D51 Vitamin B_{12} deficiency anaemia

Excludes: vitamin B_{12} deficiency (E53.8)

D51.0 Vitamin B_{12} deficiency anaemia due to intrinsic factor deficiency
Anaemia:
- Addison
- Biermer
- pernicious (congenital)
Congenital intrinsic factor deficiency

D51.1 Vitamin B_{12} deficiency anaemia due to selective vitamin B_{12} malabsorption with proteinuria
Imerslund(–Gräsbeck) syndrome
Megaloblastic hereditary anaemia

D51.2 Transcobalamin II deficiency

D51.3 Other dietary vitamin B_{12} deficiency anaemia
Vegan anaemia

D51.8 Other vitamin B_{12} deficiency anaemias

D51.9 Vitamin B_{12} deficiency anaemia, unspecified

D52 Folate deficiency anaemia

D52.0 **Dietary folate deficiency anaemia**
Nutritional megaloblastic anaemia

D52.1 **Drug-induced folate deficiency anaemia**
Use additional external cause code (Chapter XX), if desired, to identify drug.

D52.8 **Other folate deficiency anaemias**

D52.9 **Folate deficiency anaemia, unspecified**
Folic acid deficiency anaemia NOS

D53 Other nutritional anaemias

Includes: megaloblastic anaemia unresponsive to vitamin B_{12} or folate therapy

D53.0 **Protein deficiency anaemia**
Amino-acid deficiency anaemia
Orotaciduric anaemia
Excludes: Lesch–Nyhan syndrome (E79.1)

D53.1 **Other megaloblastic anaemias, not elsewhere classified**
Megaloblastic anaemia NOS
Excludes: Di Guglielmo's disease (C94.0)

D53.2 **Scorbutic anaemia**
Excludes: scurvy (E54)

D53.8 **Other specified nutritional anaemias**
Anaemia associated with deficiency of:
- copper
- molybdenum
- zinc

Excludes: nutritional deficiencies without mention of anaemia, such as:
- copper deficiency (E61.0)
- molybdenum deficiency (E61.5)
- zinc deficiency (E60)

D53.9 **Nutritional anaemia, unspecified**
Simple chronic anaemia
Excludes: anaemia NOS (D64.9)

Haemolytic anaemias
(D55–D59)

D55 ## Anaemia due to enzyme disorders
Excludes: drug-induced enzyme deficiency anaemia (D59.2)

D55.0 **Anaemia due to glucose-6-phosphate dehydrogenase [G6PD] deficiency**
Favism
G6PD deficiency anaemia

D55.1 **Anaemia due to other disorders of glutathione metabolism**
Anaemia (due to):
• enzyme deficiencies, except G6PD, related to the hexose monophosphate [HMP] shunt pathway
• haemolytic nonspherocytic (hereditary), type I

D55.2 **Anaemia due to disorders of glycolytic enzymes**
Anaemia:
• haemolytic nonspherocytic (hereditary), type II
• hexokinase deficiency
• pyruvate kinase [PK] deficiency
• triose-phosphate isomerase deficiency

D55.3 **Anaemia due to disorders of nucleotide metabolism**

D55.8 **Other anaemias due to enzyme disorders**

D55.9 **Anaemia due to enzyme disorder, unspecified**

D56 ## Thalassaemia

D56.0 **Alpha thalassaemia**
Excludes: hydrops fetalis due to haemolytic disease (P56.–)

D56.1   **Beta thalassaemia**
Cooley's anaemia
Severe beta thalassaemia
Sickle-cell beta thalassaemia
Thalassaemia:
• intermedia
• major

D56.2   **Delta-beta thalassaemia**

D56.3   **Thalassaemia trait**

D56.4   **Hereditary persistence of fetal haemoglobin [HPFH]**

D56.8   **Other thalassaemias**

D56.9   **Thalassaemia, unspecified**
Mediterranean anaemia (with other haemoglobinopathy)
Thalassaemia (minor)(mixed)(with other haemoglobinopathy)

D57   Sickle-cell disorders

Excludes: other haemoglobinopathies (D58.–)
sickle-cell beta thalassaemia (D56.1)

D57.0   **Sickle-cell anaemia with crisis**
Hb-SS disease with crisis

D57.1   **Sickle-cell anaemia without crisis**
Sickle-cell:
• anaemia ⎤
• disease ⎬ NOS
• disorder ⎦

D57.2   **Double heterozygous sickling disorders**
Disease:
• Hb-SC
• Hb-SD
• Hb-SE

D57.3   **Sickle-cell trait**
Hb-S trait
Heterozygous haemoglobin S

D57.8   **Other sickle-cell disorders**

D58 Other hereditary haemolytic anaemias

D58.0 **Hereditary spherocytosis**
Acholuric (familial) jaundice
Congenital (spherocytic) haemolytic icterus
Minkowski–Chauffard syndrome

D58.1 **Hereditary elliptocytosis**
Elliptocytosis (congenital)
Ovalocytosis (congenital)(hereditary)

D58.2 **Other haemoglobinopathies**
Abnormal haemoglobin NOS
Congenital Heinz body anaemia
Disease:
• Hb-C
• Hb-D
• Hb-E
Haemoglobinopathy NOS
Unstable haemoglobin haemolytic disease
Excludes: familial polycythaemia (D75.0)
Hb-M disease (D74.0)
hereditary persistence of fetal haemoglobin [HPFH]
(D56.4)
high-altitude polycythaemia (D75.1)
methaemoglobinaemia (D74.–)

D58.8 **Other specified hereditary haemolytic anaemias**
Stomatocytosis

D58.9 **Hereditary haemolytic anaemia, unspecified**

D59 Acquired haemolytic anaemia

D59.0 **Drug-induced autoimmune haemolytic anaemia**
Use additional external cause code (Chapter XX), if desired, to identify drug.

D59.1 **Other autoimmune haemolytic anaemias**
Autoimmune haemolytic disease (cold type)(warm type)
Chronic cold haemagglutinin disease
Cold agglutinin:
- disease
- haemoglobinuria

Haemolytic anaemia:
- cold type (secondary)(symptomatic)
- warm type (secondary)(symptomatic)

Excludes: Evans' syndrome (D69.3)
     haemolytic disease of fetus and newborn (P55.–)
     paroxysmal cold haemoglobinuria (D59.6)

D59.2 **Drug-induced nonautoimmune haemolytic anaemia**
Drug-induced enzyme deficiency anaemia

Use additional external cause code (Chapter XX), if desired, to identify drug.

D59.3 **Haemolytic-uraemic syndrome**

D59.4 **Other nonautoimmune haemolytic anaemias**
Haemolytic anaemia:
- mechanical
- microangiopathic
- toxic

Use additional external cause code (Chapter XX), if desired, to identify cause.

D59.5 **Paroxysmal nocturnal haemoglobinuria [Marchiafava–Micheli]**
Excludes: haemoglobinuria NOS (R82.3)

D59.6 **Haemoglobinuria due to haemolysis from other external causes**
Haemoglobinuria:
- from exertion
- march
- paroxysmal cold

Use additional external cause code (Chapter XX), if desired, to identify cause.

Excludes: haemoglobinuria NOS (R82.3)

D59.8 **Other acquired haemolytic anaemias**

D59.9 **Acquired haemolytic anaemia, unspecified**
Idiopathic haemolytic anaemia, chronic

Aplastic and other anaemias (D60–D64)

D60 Acquired pure red cell aplasia [erythroblastopenia]
Includes: red cell aplasia (acquired)(adult)(with thymoma)

D60.0 Chronic acquired pure red cell aplasia

D60.1 Transient acquired pure red cell aplasia

D60.8 Other acquired pure red cell aplasias

D60.9 Acquired pure red cell aplasia, unspecified

D61 Other aplastic anaemias
Excludes: agranulocytosis (D70)

D61.0 **Constitutional aplastic anaemia**
Aplasia, (pure) red cell (of):
• congenital
• infants
• primary
Blackfan–Diamond syndrome
Familial hypoplastic anaemia
Fanconi's anaemia
Pancytopenia with malformations

D61.1 **Drug-induced aplastic anaemia**
Use additional external cause code (Chapter XX), if desired, to identify drug.

D61.2 **Aplastic anaemia due to other external agents**
Use additional external cause code (Chapter XX), if desired, to identify cause.

D61.3 Idiopathic aplastic anaemia

D61.8 Other specified aplastic anaemias

D61.9 **Aplastic anaemia, unspecified**
Hypoplastic anaemia NOS
Medullary hypoplasia
Panmyelophthisis

D62 Acute posthaemorrhagic anaemia

Excludes: congenital anaemia from fetal blood loss (P61.3)

D63* Anaemia in chronic diseases classified elsewhere

D63.0* Anaemia in neoplastic disease (C00–D48†)

D63.8* Anaemia in other chronic diseases classified elsewhere

D64 Other anaemias

Excludes: refractory anaemia:
- NOS (D46.4)
- with excess of blasts (D46.2)
  - with transformation (D46.3)
- with sideroblasts (D46.1)
- without sideroblasts (D46.0)

D64.0 Hereditary sideroblastic anaemia
Sex-linked hypochromic sideroblastic anaemia

D64.1 Secondary sideroblastic anaemia due to disease
Use additional code, if desired, to identify disease.

D64.2 Secondary sideroblastic anaemia due to drugs and toxins
Use additional external cause code (Chapter XX), if desired, to identify cause.

D64.3 Other sideroblastic anaemias
Sideroblastic anaemia:
- NOS
- pyridoxine-responsive NEC

D64.4 Congenital dyserythropoietic anaemia
Dyshaematopoietic anaemia (congenital)
Excludes: Blackfan–Diamond syndrome (D61.0)
Di Guglielmo's disease (C94.0)

D64.8 Other specified anaemias
Infantile pseudoleukaemia
Leukoerythroblastic anaemia

D64.9 Anaemia, unspecified

Coagulation defects, purpura and other haemorrhagic conditions
(D65–D69)

D65 Disseminated intravascular coagulation [defibrination syndrome]
Afibrinogenaemia, acquired
Consumption coagulopathy
Diffuse or disseminated intravascular coagulation [DIC]
Fibrinolytic haemorrhage, acquired
Purpura:
• fibrinolytic
• fulminans

Excludes: that (complicating):
• abortion or ectopic or molar pregnancy (O00–O07, O08.1)
• in newborn (P60)
• pregnancy, childbirth and the puerperium (O45.0, O46.0, O67.0, O72.3)

D66 Hereditary factor VIII deficiency
Deficiency factor VIII (with functional defect)
Haemophilia:
• NOS
• A
• classical

Excludes: factor VIII deficiency with vascular defect (D68.0)

D67 Hereditary factor IX deficiency
Christmas disease
Deficiency:
• factor IX (with functional defect)
• plasma thromboplastin component [PTC]
Haemophilia B

D68 Other coagulation defects

Excludes: those complicating:
- abortion or ectopic or molar pregnancy (O00–O07, O08.1)
- pregnancy, childbirth and the puerperium (O45.0, O46.0, O67.0, O72.3)

D68.0 Von Willebrand's disease
Angiohaemophilia
Factor VIII deficiency with vascular defect
Vascular haemophilia

Excludes: capillary fragility (hereditary) (D69.8)
factor VIII deficiency:
- NOS (D66)
- with functional defect (D66)

D68.1 Hereditary factor XI deficiency
Haemophilia C
Plasma thromboplastin antecedent [PTA] deficiency

D68.2 Hereditary deficiency of other clotting factors
Congenital afibrinogenaemia
Deficiency:
- AC globulin
- proaccelerin
Deficiency of factor:
- I [fibrinogen]
- II [prothrombin]
- V [labile]
- VII [stable]
- X [Stuart–Prower]
- XII [Hageman]
- XIII [fibrin-stabilizing]
Dysfibrinogenaemia (congenital)
Hypoproconvertinaemia
Owren's disease

D68.3   **Haemorrhagic disorder due to circulating anticoagulants**
Hyperheparinaemia
Increase in:
• antithrombin
• anti-VIIIa
• anti-IXa
• anti-Xa
• anti-XIa

Use additional external cause code (Chapter XX), if desired, to identify any administered anticoagulant.

D68.4   **Acquired coagulation factor deficiency**
Deficiency of coagulation factor due to:
• liver disease
• vitamin K deficiency
Excludes: vitamin K deficiency of newborn (P53)

D68.8   **Other specified coagulation defects**
Presence of systemic lupus erythematosus [SLE] inhibitor

D68.9   **Coagulation defect, unspecified**

D69   **Purpura and other haemorrhagic conditions**
Excludes: benign hypergammaglobulinaemic purpura (D89.0)
cryoglobulinaemic purpura (D89.1)
essential (haemorrhagic) thrombocythaemia (D47.3)
purpura fulminans (D65)
thrombotic thrombocytopenic purpura (M31.1)

D69.0   **Allergic purpura**
Purpura:
• anaphylactoid
• Henoch(–Schönlein)
• nonthrombocytopenic:
  • haemorrhagic
  • idiopathic
• vascular
Vasculitis, allergic

D69.1 **Qualitative platelet defects**
Bernard–Soulier [giant platelet] syndrome
Glanzmann's disease
Grey platelet syndrome
Thromboasthenia (haemorrhagic)(hereditary)
Thrombocytopathy
Excludes: von Willebrand's disease (D68.0)

D69.2 **Other nonthrombocytopenic purpura**
Purpura:
• NOS
• senile
• simplex

D69.3 **Idiopathic thrombocytopenic purpura**
Evans' syndrome

D69.4 **Other primary thrombocytopenia**
Excludes: thrombocytopenia with absent radius (Q87.2)
transient neonatal thrombocytopenia (P61.0)
Wiskott–Aldrich syndrome (D82.0)

D69.5 **Secondary thrombocytopenia**
Use additional external cause code (Chapter XX), if desired, to
identify cause.

D69.6 **Thrombocytopenia, unspecified**

D69.8 **Other specified haemorrhagic conditions**
Capillary fragility (hereditary)
Vascular pseudohaemophilia

D69.9 **Haemorrhagic condition, unspecified**

Other diseases of blood and blood-forming organs (D70–D77)

D70 Agranulocytosis

Agranulocytic angina
Infantile genetic agranulocytosis
Kostmann's disease
Neutropenia:
- NOS
- congenital
- cyclic
- drug-induced
- periodic
- splenic (primary)
- toxic

Neutropenic splenomegaly

Use additional external cause code (Chapter XX), if desired, to identify drug, if drug-induced.

Excludes: transient neonatal neutropenia (P61.5)

D71 Functional disorders of polymorphonuclear neutrophils

Cell membrane receptor complex [CR3] defect
Chronic (childhood) granulomatous disease
Congenital dysphagocytosis
Progressive septic granulomatosis

D72 Other disorders of white blood cells

Excludes: basophilia (D75.8)
immunity disorders (D80–D89)
neutropenia (D70)
preleukaemia (syndrome) (D46.9)

D72.0   **Genetic anomalies of leukocytes**
Anomaly (granulation)(granulocyte) or syndrome:
- Alder
- May–Hegglin
- Pelger–Huët

Hereditary:
- leukocytic:
  - hypersegmentation
  - hyposegmentation
- leukomelanopathy

Excludes: Chediak(–Steinbrinck)–Higashi syndrome (E70.3)

D72.1   **Eosinophilia**
Eosinophilia:
- allergic
- hereditary

D72.8   **Other specified disorders of white blood cells**
Leukaemoid reaction:
- lymphocytic
- monocytic
- myelocytic

Leukocytosis
Lymphocytosis (symptomatic)
Lymphopenia
Monocytosis (symptomatic)
Plasmacytosis

D72.9   **Disorder of white blood cells, unspecified**

D73   Diseases of spleen

D73.0   **Hyposplenism**
Asplenia, postsurgical
Atrophy of spleen
Excludes: asplenia (congenital) (Q89.0)

D73.1   **Hypersplenism**
Excludes: splenomegaly:
- NOS (R16.1)
- congenital (Q89.0)

D73.2   **Chronic congestive splenomegaly**

D73.3   **Abscess of spleen**

D73.4 **Cyst of spleen**

D73.5 **Infarction of spleen**
Splenic rupture, nontraumatic
Torsion of spleen
Excludes: traumatic rupture of spleen (S36.0)

D73.8 **Other diseases of spleen**
Fibrosis of spleen NOS
Perisplenitis
Splenitis NOS

D73.9 **Disease of spleen, unspecified**

D74 Methaemoglobinaemia

D74.0 **Congenital methaemoglobinaemia**
Congenital NADH-methaemoglobin reductase deficiency
Haemoglobin-M [Hb-M] disease
Methaemoglobinaemia, hereditary

D74.8 **Other methaemoglobinaemias**
Acquired methaemoglobinaemia (with sulfhaemoglobinaemia)
Toxic methaemoglobinaemia

Use additional external cause code (Chapter XX), if desired, to identify cause.

D74.9 **Methaemoglobinaemia, unspecified**

D75 Other diseases of blood and blood-forming organs
Excludes: enlarged lymph nodes (R59.–)
hypergammaglobulinaemia NOS (D89.2)
lymphadenitis:
- NOS (I88.9)
- acute (L04.–)
- chronic (I88.1)
- mesenteric (acute)(chronic) (I88.0)

D75.0 **Familial erythrocytosis**
Polycythaemia:
- benign
- familial
Excludes: hereditary ovalocytosis (D58.1)

264

D75.1 **Secondary polycythaemia**
Polycythaemia:
- acquired
- due to:
  - erythropoietin
  - fall in plasma volume
  - high altitude
  - stress
- emotional
- hypoxaemic
- nephrogenous
- relative

Excludes: polycythaemia:
- neonatorum (P61.1)
- vera (D45)

D75.2 **Essential thrombocytosis**
Excludes: essential (haemorrhagic) thrombocythaemia (D47.3)

D75.8 **Other specified diseases of blood and blood-forming organs**
Basophilia

D75.9 **Disease of blood and blood-forming organs, unspecified**

D76 **Certain diseases involving lymphoreticular tissue and reticulohistiocytic system**
Excludes: Letterer–Siwe disease (C96.0)
malignant histiocytosis (C96.1)
reticuloendotheliosis or reticulosis:
- histiocytic medullary (C96.1)
- leukaemic (C91.4)
- lipomelanotic (I89.8)
- malignant (C85.7)
- nonlipid (C96.0)

D76.0 **Langerhans' cell histiocytosis, not elsewhere classified**
Eosinophilic granuloma
Hand–Schüller–Christian disease
Histiocytosis X (chronic)

D76.1 **Haemophagocytic lymphohistiocytosis**
Familial haemophagocytic reticulosis
Histiocytoses of mononuclear phagocytes other than Langerhans' cells NOS

265

D76.2 **Haemophagocytic syndrome, infection-associated**
Use additional code, if desired, to identify infectious agent or disease.

D76.3 **Other histiocytosis syndromes**
Reticulohistiocytoma (giant-cell)
Sinus histiocytosis with massive lymphadenopathy
Xanthogranuloma

D77* Other disorders of blood and blood-forming organs in diseases classified elsewhere
Fibrosis of spleen in schistosomiasis [bilharziasis] (B65.–†)

Certain disorders involving the immune mechanism (D80–D89)

Includes: defects in the complement system
immunodeficiency disorders, except human immunodeficiency
    virus [HIV] disease
sarcoidosis

Excludes: autoimmune disease (systemic) NOS (M35.9)
functional disorders of polymorphonuclear neutrophils (D71)
human immunodeficiency virus [HIV] disease (B20–B24)

D80 Immunodeficiency with predominantly antibody defects

D80.0 **Hereditary hypogammaglobulinaemia**
Autosomal recessive agammaglobulinaemia (Swiss type)
X-linked agammaglobulinaemia [Bruton] (with growth hormone deficiency)

D80.1 **Nonfamilial hypogammaglobulinaemia**
Agammaglobulinaemia with immunoglobulin-bearing B-lymphocytes
Common variable agammaglobulinaemia [CVAgamma]
Hypogammaglobulinaemia NOS

D80.2 **Selective deficiency of immunoglobulin A [IgA]**

D80.3 **Selective deficiency of immunoglobulin G [IgG] subclasses**

D80.4   **Selective deficiency of immunoglobulin M [IgM]**

D80.5   **Immunodeficiency with increased immunoglobulin M [IgM]**

D80.6   **Antibody deficiency with near-normal immunoglobulins or with hyperimmunoglobulinaemia**

D80.7   **Transient hypogammaglobulinaemia of infancy**

D80.8   **Other immunodeficiencies with predominantly antibody defects**
Kappa light chain deficiency

D80.9   **Immunodeficiency with predominantly antibody defects, unspecified**

D81   Combined immunodeficiencies

Excludes: autosomal recessive agammaglobulinaemia (Swiss type) (D80.0)

D81.0   **Severe combined immunodeficiency [SCID] with reticular dysgenesis**

D81.1   **Severe combined immunodeficiency [SCID] with low T- and B-cell numbers**

D81.2   **Severe combined immunodeficiency [SCID] with low or normal B-cell numbers**

D81.3   **Adenosine deaminase [ADA] deficiency**

D81.4   **Nezelof's syndrome**

D81.5   **Purine nucleoside phosphorylase [PNP] deficiency**

D81.6   **Major histocompatibility complex class I deficiency**
Bare lymphocyte syndrome

D81.7   **Major histocompatibility complex class II deficiency**

D81.8   **Other combined immunodeficiencies**
Biotin-dependent carboxylase deficiency

D81.9   **Combined immunodeficiency, unspecified**
Severe combined immunodeficiency disorder [SCID] NOS

D82   Immunodeficiency associated with other major defects

Excludes: ataxia telangiectasia [Louis-Bar] (G11.3)

D82.0   **Wiskott-Aldrich syndrome**
Immunodeficiency with thrombocytopenia and eczema

D82.1   **Di George's syndrome**
Pharyngeal pouch syndrome
Thymic:
- alymphoplasia
- aplasia or hypoplasia with immunodeficiency

D82.2   **Immunodeficiency with short-limbed stature**

D82.3   **Immunodeficiency following hereditary defective response to Epstein–Barr virus**
X-linked lymphoproliferative disease

D82.4   **Hyperimmunoglobulin E [IgE] syndrome**

D82.8   **Immunodeficiency associated with other specified major defects**

D82.9   **Immunodeficiency associated with major defect, unspecified**

D83   Common variable immunodeficiency

D83.0   **Common variable immunodeficiency with predominant abnormalities of B-cell numbers and function**

D83.1   **Common variable immunodeficiency with predominant immunoregulatory T-cell disorders**

D83.2   **Common variable immunodeficiency with autoantibodies to B- or T-cells**

D83.8   **Other common variable immunodeficiencies**

D83.9   **Common variable immunodeficiency, unspecified**

D84   Other immunodeficiencies

D84.0   **Lymphocyte function antigen-1 [LFA-1] defect**

D84.1   **Defects in the complement system**
C1 esterase inhibitor [C1-INH] deficiency

D84.8   **Other specified immunodeficiencies**

D84.9   **Immunodeficiency, unspecified**

D86   Sarcoidosis

D86.0   Sarcoidosis of lung

D86.1   Sarcoidosis of lymph nodes

D86.2   Sarcoidosis of lung with sarcoidosis of lymph nodes

D86.3   Sarcoidosis of skin

D86.8   Sarcoidosis of other and combined sites
Iridocyclitis in sarcoidosis† (H22.1*)
Multiple cranial nerve palsies in sarcoidosis† (G53.2*)
Sarcoid:
• arthropathy† (M14.8*)
• myocarditis† (I41.8*)
• myositis† (M63.3*)
Uveoparotid fever [Heerfordt]

D86.9   Sarcoidosis, unspecified

D89   Other disorders involving the immune mechanism, not elsewhere classified
Excludes: hyperglobulinaemia NOS (R77.1)
monoclonal gammopathy (D47.2)
transplant failure and rejection (T86.–)

D89.0   Polyclonal hypergammaglobulinaemia
Benign hypergammaglobulinaemic purpura
Polyclonal gammopathy NOS

D89.1   Cryoglobulinaemia
Cryoglobulinaemia:
• essential
• idiopathic
• mixed
• primary
• secondary
Cryoglobulinaemic:
• purpura
• vasculitis

D89.2   Hypergammaglobulinaemia, unspecified

D89.8   Other specified disorders involving the immune mechanism, not elsewhere classified

D89.9   **Disorder involving the immune mechanism, unspecified**
Immune disease NOS

CHAPTER IV

Endocrine, nutritional and metabolic diseases (E00–E90)

Note: All neoplasms, whether functionally active or not, are classified in Chapter II. Appropriate codes in this chapter (i.e. E05.8, E07.0, E16–E31, E34.–) may be used, if desired, as additional codes to indicate either functional activity by neoplasms and ectopic endocrine tissue or hyperfunction and hypofunction of endocrine glands associated with neoplasms and other conditions classified elsewhere.

Excludes: complications of pregnancy, childbirth and the puerperium (O00–O99)
symptoms, signs and abnormal clinical and laboratory findings, not elsewhere classified (R00–R99)
transitory endocrine and metabolic disorders specific to fetus and newborn (P70–P74)

This chapter contains the following blocks:

E00–E07 Disorders of thyroid gland
E10–E14 Diabetes mellitus
E15–E16 Other disorders of glucose regulation and pancreatic internal secretion
E20–E35 Disorders of other endocrine glands
E40–E46 Malnutrition
E50–E64 Other nutritional deficiencies
E65–E68 Obesity and other hyperalimentation
E70–E90 Metabolic disorders

Asterisk categories for this chapter are provided as follows:

E35* Disorders of endocrine glands in diseases classified elsewhere
E90* Nutritional and metabolic disorders in diseases classified elsewhere

Disorders of thyroid gland
(E00–E07)

E00 Congenital iodine-deficiency syndrome

Includes: endemic conditions associated with environmental iodine deficiency either directly or as a consequence of maternal iodine deficiency. Some of the conditions have no current hypothyroidism but are the consequence of inadequate thyroid hormone secretion in the developing fetus. Environmental goitrogens may be associated.

Use additional code (F70–F79), if desired, to identify associated mental retardation.

Excludes: subclinical iodine-deficiency hypothyroidism (E02)

E00.0   **Congenital iodine-deficiency syndrome, neurological type**
Endemic cretinism, neurological type

E00.1   **Congenital iodine-deficiency syndrome, myxoedematous type**
Endemic cretinism:
• hypothyroid
• myxoedematous type

E00.2   **Congenital iodine-deficiency syndrome, mixed type**
Endemic cretinism, mixed type

E00.9   **Congenital iodine-deficiency syndrome, unspecified**
Congenital iodine-deficiency hypothyroidism NOS
Endemic cretinism NOS

E01 Iodine-deficiency-related thyroid disorders and allied conditions

Excludes: congenital iodine-deficiency syndrome (E00.–)
subclinical iodine-deficiency hypothyroidism (E02)

E01.0   **Iodine-deficiency-related diffuse (endemic) goitre**

E01.1   **Iodine-deficiency-related multinodular (endemic) goitre**
Iodine-deficiency-related nodular goitre

E01.2   **Iodine-deficiency-related (endemic) goitre, unspecified**
Endemic goitre NOS

E01.8 **Other iodine-deficiency-related thyroid disorders and allied conditions**
Acquired iodine-deficiency hypothyroidism NOS

E02 Subclinical iodine-deficiency hypothyroidism

E03 Other hypothyroidism
Excludes: iodine-deficiency-related hypothyroidism (E00–E02)
postprocedural hypothyroidism (E89.0)

E03.0 **Congenital hypothyroidism with diffuse goitre**
Goitre (nontoxic) congenital:
- NOS
- parenchymatous

Excludes: transitory congenital goitre with normal function (P72.0)

E03.1 **Congenital hypothyroidism without goitre**
Aplasia of thyroid (with myxoedema)
Congenital:
- atrophy of thyroid
- hypothyroidism NOS

E03.2 **Hypothyroidism due to medicaments and other exogenous substances**
Use additional external cause code (Chapter XX), if desired, to identify cause.

E03.3 **Postinfectious hypothyroidism**

E03.4 **Atrophy of thyroid (acquired)**
Excludes: congenital atrophy of thyroid (E03.1)

E03.5 **Myxoedema coma**

E03.8 **Other specified hypothyroidism**

E03.9 **Hypothyroidism, unspecified**
Myxoedema NOS

E04   Other nontoxic goitre

Excludes: congenital goitre:
- NOS   ⎫
- diffuse   ⎬ (E03.0)
- parenchymatous ⎭

iodine-deficiency-related goitre (E00–E02)

E04.0   **Nontoxic diffuse goitre**
Goitre, nontoxic:
- diffuse (colloid)
- simple

E04.1   **Nontoxic single thyroid nodule**
Colloid nodule (cystic)(thyroid)
Nontoxic uninodular goitre
Thyroid (cystic) nodule NOS

E04.2   **Nontoxic multinodular goitre**
Cystic goitre NOS
Multinodular (cystic) goitre NOS

E04.8   **Other specified nontoxic goitre**

E04.9   **Nontoxic goitre, unspecified**
Goitre NOS
Nodular goitre (nontoxic) NOS

E05   Thyrotoxicosis [hyperthyroidism]

Excludes: chronic thyroiditis with transient thyrotoxicosis
(E06.2)
neonatal thyrotoxicosis (P72.1)

E05.0   **Thyrotoxicosis with diffuse goitre**
Exophthalmic or toxic goitre NOS
Graves' disease
Toxic diffuse goitre

E05.1   **Thyrotoxicosis with toxic single thyroid nodule**
Thyrotoxicosis with toxic uninodular goitre

E05.2   **Thyrotoxicosis with toxic multinodular goitre**
Toxic nodular goitre NOS

E05.3   **Thyrotoxicosis from ectopic thyroid tissue**

E05.4   **Thyrotoxicosis factitia**

E05.5   **Thyroid crisis or storm**

E05.8   **Other thyrotoxicosis**
Overproduction of thyroid-stimulating hormone

Use additional external cause code (Chapter XX), if desired, to identify cause.

E05.9   **Thyrotoxicosis, unspecified**
Hyperthyroidism NOS
Thyrotoxic heart disease† (I43.8*)

E06   Thyroiditis
Excludes: postpartum thyroiditis (O90.5)

E06.0   **Acute thyroiditis**
Abscess of thyroid
Thyroiditis:
- pyogenic
- suppurative

Use additional code (B95–B97), if desired, to identify infectious agent.

E06.1   **Subacute thyroiditis**
Thyroiditis:
- de Quervain
- giant-cell
- granulomatous
- nonsuppurative

Excludes: autoimmune thyroiditis (E06.3)

E06.2   **Chronic thyroiditis with transient thyrotoxicosis**

Excludes: autoimmune thyroiditis (E06.3)

E06.3   **Autoimmune thyroiditis**
Hashimoto's thyroiditis
Hashitoxicosis (transient)
Lymphadenoid goitre
Lymphocytic thyroiditis
Struma lymphomatosa

E06.4   **Drug-induced thyroiditis**
Use additional external cause code (Chapter XX), if desired, to identify drug.

E06.5   Other chronic thyroiditis
Thyroiditis:
- chronic:
  - NOS
  - fibrous
- ligneous
- Riedel

E06.9   Thyroiditis, unspecified

E07   Other disorders of thyroid

E07.0   Hypersecretion of calcitonin
C-cell hyperplasia of thyroid
Hypersecretion of thyrocalcitonin

E07.1   Dyshormogenetic goitre
Familial dyshormogenetic goitre
Pendred's syndrome

Excludes: transitory congenital goitre with normal function
(P72.0)

E07.8   Other specified disorders of thyroid
Abnormality of thyroid-binding globulin
Haemorrhage ⎱
Infarction ⎰ of thyroid
Sick-euthyroid syndrome

E07.9   Disorder of thyroid, unspecified

Diabetes mellitus
(E10–E14)

Use additional external cause code (Chapter XX), if desired, to identify
drug, if drug-induced.

The following fourth-character subdivisions are for use with categories
E10–E14:

.0   With coma
Diabetic:
- coma with or without ketoacidosis
- hyperosmolar coma
- hypoglycaemic coma

Hyperglycaemic coma NOS

.1   With ketoacidosis
Diabetic:
- acidosis } without mention of coma
- ketoacidosis

.2† With renal complications
Diabetic nephropathy (N08.3*)
Intracapillary glomerulonephrosis (N08.3*)
Kimmelstiel–Wilson syndrome (N08.3*)

.3† With ophthalmic complications
Diabetic:
- cataract (H28.0*)
- retinopathy (H36.0*)

.4† With neurological complications
Diabetic:
- amyotrophy (G73.0*)
- autonomic neuropathy (G99.0*)
- mononeuropathy (G59.0*)
- polyneuropathy (G63.2*)
  - autonomic (G99.0*)

.5   With peripheral circulatory complications
Diabetic:
- gangrene
- peripheral angiopathy† (I79.2*)
- ulcer

.6   With other specified complications
Diabetic arthropathy† (M14.2*)
- neuropathic† (M14.6*)

.7   With multiple complications

.8   With unspecified complications

.9   Without complications

E10 Insulin-dependent diabetes mellitus

[See page 277 for subdivisions]

Includes: diabetes (mellitus):
- brittle
- juvenile-onset
- ketosis-prone
- type I

Excludes: diabetes mellitus (in):
- malnutrition-related (E12.–)
- neonatal (P70.2)
- pregnancy, childbirth and the puerperium (O24.–)

glycosuria:
- NOS (R81)
- renal (E74.8)

impaired glucose tolerance (R73.0)

postsurgical hypoinsulinaemia (E89.1)

E11 Non-insulin-dependent diabetes mellitus

[See page 277 for subdivisions]

Includes: diabetes (mellitus)(nonobese)(obese):
- adult-onset
- maturity-onset
- nonketotic
- stable
- type II

non-insulin-dependent diabetes of the young

Excludes: diabetes mellitus (in):
- malnutrition-related (E12.–)
- neonatal (P70.2)
- pregnancy, childbirth and the puerperium (O24.–)

glycosuria:
- NOS (R81)
- renal (E74.8)

impaired glucose tolerance (R73.0)

postsurgical hypoinsulinaemia (E89.1)

E12 Malnutrition-related diabetes mellitus

[See page 277 for subdivisions]

Includes: malnutrition-related diabetes mellitus:
- insulin-dependent
- non-insulin-dependent

Excludes: diabetes mellitus in pregnancy, childbirth and the puerperium (O24.–)

glycosuria:
- NOS (R81)
- renal (E74.8)

impaired glucose tolerance (R73.0)

neonatal diabetes mellitus (P70.2)

postsurgical hypoinsulinaemia (E89.1)

E13 Other specified diabetes mellitus

[See page 277 for subdivisions]

Excludes: diabetes mellitus (in):
- insulin-dependent (E10.–)
- malnutrition-related (E12.–)
- neonatal (P70.2)
- non-insulin-dependent (E11.–)
- pregnancy, childbirth and the puerperium (O24.–)

glycosuria:
- NOS (R81)
- renal (E74.8)

impaired glucose tolerance (R73.0)

postsurgical hypoinsulinaemia (E89.1)

E14 Unspecified diabetes mellitus
[See page 277 for subdivisions]

Includes: diabetes NOS

Excludes: diabetes mellitus (in):
- insulin-dependent (E10.–)
- malnutrition-related (E12.–)
- neonatal (P70.2)
- non-insulin-dependent (E11.–)
- pregnancy, childbirth and the puerperium (O24.–)

glycosuria:
- NOS (R81)
- renal (E74.8)

impaired glucose tolerance (R73.0)

postsurgical hypoinsulinaemia (E89.1)

Other disorders of glucose regulation and pancreatic internal secretion (E15–E16)

E15 Nondiabetic hypoglycaemic coma
Drug-induced insulin coma in nondiabetic

Hyperinsulinism with hypoglycaemic coma

Hypoglycaemic coma NOS

Use additional external cause code (Chapter XX), if desired, to identify drug, if drug-induced.

E16 Other disorders of pancreatic internal secretion

E16.0 Drug-induced hypoglycaemia without coma

Use additional external cause code (Chapter XX), if desired, to identify drug.

E16.1   **Other hypoglycaemia**
Functional nonhyperinsulinaemic hypoglycaemia
Hyperinsulinism:
- NOS
- functional

Hyperplasia of pancreatic islet beta cells NOS
Posthypoglycaemic coma encephalopathy

E16.2   **Hypoglycaemia, unspecified**

E16.3   **Increased secretion of glucagon**
Hyperplasia of pancreatic endocrine cells with glucagon excess

E16.8   **Other specified disorders of pancreatic internal secretion**
Hypergastrinaemia
Increased secretion from endocrine pancreas of:
- growth hormone-releasing hormone
- pancreatic polypeptide
- somatostatin
- vasoactive-intestinal polypeptide

Zollinger–Ellison syndrome

E16.9   **Disorder of pancreatic internal secretion, unspecified**
Islet-cell hyperplasia NOS
Pancreatic endocrine cell hyperplasia NOS

Disorders of other endocrine glands (E20–E35)

Excludes: galactorrhoea (N64.3)
gynaecomastia (N62)

E20   Hypoparathyroidism

Excludes: Di George's syndrome (D82.1)
postprocedural hypoparathyroidism (E89.2)
tetany NOS (R29.0)
transitory neonatal hypoparathyroidism (P71.4)

E20.0   **Idiopathic hypoparathyroidism**

E20.1   **Pseudohypoparathyroidism**

E20.8   **Other hypoparathyroidism**

E20.9   Hypoparathyroidism, unspecified
Parathyroid tetany

E21 Hyperparathyroidism and other disorders of parathyroid gland
Excludes: osteomalacia:
- adult (M83.–)
- infantile and juvenile (E55.0)

E21.0   Primary hyperparathyroidism
Hyperplasia of parathyroid
Osteitis fibrosa cystica generalisata [von Recklinghausen's disease of bone]

E21.1   Secondary hyperparathyroidism, not elsewhere classified
Excludes: secondary hyperparathyroidism of renal origin (N25.8)

E21.2   Other hyperparathyroidism
Excludes: familial hypocalciuric hypercalcaemia (E83.5)

E21.3   Hyperparathyroidism, unspecified

E21.4   Other specified disorders of parathyroid gland

E21.5   Disorder of parathyroid gland, unspecified

E22 Hyperfunction of pituitary gland
Excludes: Cushing's syndrome (E24.–)
Nelson's syndrome (E24.1)
overproduction of:
- ACTH not associated with Cushing's disease (E27.0)
- pituitary ACTH (E24.0)
- thyroid-stimulating hormone (E05.8)

E22.0   Acromegaly and pituitary gigantism
Arthropathy associated with acromegaly† (M14.5*)
Overproduction of growth hormone
Excludes: constitutional:
- gigantism (E34.4)
- tall stature (E34.4)
increased secretion from endocrine pancreas of growth hormone-releasing hormone (E16.8)

E22.1 **Hyperprolactinaemia**
Use additional external cause code (Chapter XX), if desired, to identify drug, if drug-induced.

E22.2 **Syndrome of inappropriate secretion of antidiuretic hormone**

E22.8 **Other hyperfunction of pituitary gland**
Central precocious puberty

E22.9 **Hyperfunction of pituitary gland, unspecified**

E23 Hypofunction and other disorders of pituitary gland

Includes: the listed conditions whether the disorder is in the pituitary or the hypothalamus
Excludes: postprocedural hypopituitarism (E89.3)

E23.0 **Hypopituitarism**
Fertile eunuch syndrome
Hypogonadotropic hypogonadism
Idiopathic growth hormone deficiency
Isolated deficiency of:
• gonadotropin
• growth hormone
• pituitary hormone
Kallmann's syndrome
Lorain–Levi short stature
Necrosis of pituitary gland (postpartum)
Panhypopituitarism
Pituitary:
• cachexia
• insufficiency NOS
• short stature
Sheehan's syndrome
Simmonds' disease

E23.1 **Drug-induced hypopituitarism**
Use additional external cause code (Chapter XX), if desired, to identify drug.

E23.2 **Diabetes insipidus**
Excludes: nephrogenic diabetes insipidus (N25.1)

E23.3 **Hypothalamic dysfunction, not elsewhere classified**
Excludes: Prader–Willi syndrome (Q87.1)
Russell–Silver syndrome (Q87.1)

E23.6 **Other disorders of pituitary gland**
Abscess of pituitary
Adiposogenital dystrophy

E23.7 **Disorder of pituitary gland, unspecified**

E24 Cushing's syndrome

E24.0 **Pituitary-dependent Cushing's disease**
Overproduction of pituitary ACTH
Pituitary-dependent hyperadrenocorticism

E24.1 **Nelson's syndrome**

E24.2 **Drug-induced Cushing's syndrome**
Use additional external cause code (Chapter XX), if desired, to identify drug.

E24.3 **Ectopic ACTH syndrome**

E24.4 **Alcohol-induced pseudo-Cushing's syndrome**

E24.8 **Other Cushing's syndrome**

E24.9 **Cushing's syndrome, unspecified**

E25 Adrenogenital disorders

Includes: adrenogenital syndromes, virilizing or feminizing, whether acquired or due to adrenal hyperplasia consequent on inborn enzyme defects in hormone synthesis
female:
• adrenal pseudohermaphroditism
• heterosexual precocious pseudopuberty
male:
• isosexual precocious pseudopuberty
• macrogenitosomia praecox
• sexual precocity with adrenal hyperplasia
virilization (female)

E25.0 **Congenital adrenogenital disorders associated with enzyme deficiency**
Congenital adrenal hyperplasia
21-Hydroxylase deficiency
Salt-losing congenital adrenal hyperplasia

E25.8 **Other adrenogenital disorders**
Idiopathic adrenogenital disorder

Use additional external cause code (Chapter XX), if desired, to identify drug, if drug-induced.

E25.9 **Adrenogenital disorder, unspecified**
Adrenogenital syndrome NOS

E26 Hyperaldosteronism

E26.0 **Primary hyperaldosteronism**
Conn's syndrome
Primary aldosteronism due to adrenal hyperplasia (bilateral)

E26.1 **Secondary hyperaldosteronism**

E26.8 **Other hyperaldosteronism**
Bartter's syndrome

E26.9 **Hyperaldosteronism, unspecified**

E27 Other disorders of adrenal gland

E27.0 **Other adrenocortical overactivity**
Overproduction of ACTH, not associated with Cushing's disease
Premature adrenarche
Excludes: Cushing's syndrome (E24.–)

E27.1 **Primary adrenocortical insufficiency**
Addison's disease
Autoimmune adrenalitis
Excludes: amyloidosis (E85.–)
tuberculous Addison's disease (A18.7)
Waterhouse–Friderichsen syndrome (A39.1)

E27.2 **Addisonian crisis**
Adrenal crisis
Adrenocortical crisis

E27.3 **Drug-induced adrenocortical insufficiency**
Use additional external cause code (Chapter XX), if desired, to identify drug.

E27.4 **Other and unspecified adrenocortical insufficiency**
Adrenal:
- haemorrhage
- infarction

Adrenocortical insufficiency NOS
Hypoaldosteronism
Excludes: adrenoleukodystrophy [Addison–Schilder] (E71.3)
Waterhouse–Friderichsen syndrome (A39.1)

E27.5 **Adrenomedullary hyperfunction**
Adrenomedullary hyperplasia
Catecholamine hypersecretion

E27.8 **Other specified disorders of adrenal gland**
Abnormality of cortisol-binding globulin

E27.9 **Disorder of adrenal gland, unspecified**

E28 **Ovarian dysfunction**
Excludes: isolated gonadotropin deficiency (E23.0)
postprocedural ovarian failure (E89.4)

E28.0 **Estrogen excess**
Use additional external cause code (Chapter XX), if desired, to identify drug, if drug-induced.

E28.1 **Androgen excess**
Hypersecretion of ovarian androgens

Use additional external cause code (Chapter XX), if desired, to identify drug, if drug-induced.

E28.2 **Polycystic ovarian syndrome**
Sclerocystic ovary syndrome
Stein–Leventhal syndrome

E28.3 **Primary ovarian failure**
Decreased estrogen
Premature menopause NOS
Resistant ovary syndrome
Excludes: menopausal and female climacteric states (N95.1)
pure gonadal dysgenesis (Q99.1)
Turner's syndrome (Q96.–)

E28.8 **Other ovarian dysfunction**
Ovarian hyperfunction NOS

E28.9 **Ovarian dysfunction, unspecified**

E29 Testicular dysfunction

Excludes: androgen resistance syndrome (E34.5)
azoospermia or oligospermia NOS (N46)
isolated gonadotropin deficiency (E23.0)
Klinefelter's syndrome (Q98.0–Q98.2, Q98.4)
postprocedural testicular hypofunction (E89.5)
testicular feminization (syndrome) (E34.5)

E29.0 **Testicular hyperfunction**
Hypersecretion of testicular hormones

E29.1 **Testicular hypofunction**
Defective biosynthesis of testicular androgen NOS
5-α-Reductase deficiency (with male pseudohermaphroditism)
Testicular hypogonadism NOS

Use additional external cause code (Chapter XX), if desired, to
identify drug, if drug-induced.

E29.8 **Other testicular dysfunction**

E29.9 **Testicular dysfunction, unspecified**

E30 Disorders of puberty, not elsewhere classified

E30.0 **Delayed puberty**
Constitutional delay of puberty
Delayed sexual development

E30.1 **Precocious puberty**
Precocious menstruation
Excludes: Albright(–McCune)(–Sternberg) syndrome (Q78.1)
central precocious puberty (E22.8)
congenital adrenal hyperplasia (E25.0)
female heterosexual precocious pseudopuberty (E25.–)
male isosexual precocious pseudopuberty (E25.–)

E30.8 **Other disorders of puberty**
Premature thelarche

E30.9 **Disorder of puberty, unspecified**

E31 Polyglandular dysfunction

Excludes: ataxia telangiectasia [Louis-Bar] (G11.3)
dystrophia myotonica [Steinert] (G71.1)
pseudohypoparathyroidism (E20.1)

E31.0 Autoimmune polyglandular failure
Schmidt's syndrome

E31.1 Polyglandular hyperfunction

Excludes: multiple endocrine adenomatosis (D44.8)

E31.8 Other polyglandular dysfunction

E31.9 Polyglandular dysfunction, unspecified

E32 Diseases of thymus

Excludes: aplasia or hypoplasia with immunodeficiency (D82.1)
myasthenia gravis (G70.0)

E32.0 Persistent hyperplasia of thymus
Hypertrophy of thymus

E32.1 Abscess of thymus

E32.8 Other diseases of thymus

E32.9 Disease of thymus, unspecified

E34 Other endocrine disorders

Excludes: pseudohypoparathyroidism (E20.1)

E34.0 Carcinoid syndrome
Note: May be used as an additional code, if desired, to identify
functional activity associated with a carcinoid tumour.

E34.1 Other hypersecretion of intestinal hormones

E34.2 Ectopic hormone secretion, not elsewhere classified

E34.3   **Short stature, not elsewhere classified**

Short stature:

- NOS
- constitutional
- Laron-type
- psychosocial

Excludes: progeria (E34.8)
         Russell–Silver syndrome (Q87.1)
         short-limbed stature with immunodeficiency (D82.2)
         short stature:
         - achondroplastic (Q77.4)
         - hypochondroplastic (Q77.4)
         - in specific dysmorphic syndromes—code to
          syndrome—see Alphabetical Index
         - nutritional (E45)
         - pituitary (E23.0)
         - renal (N25.0)

E34.4   **Constitutional tall stature**

Constitutional gigantism

E34.5   **Androgen resistance syndrome**

Male pseudohermaphroditism with androgen resistance
Peripheral hormonal receptor disorder
Reifenstein's syndrome
Testicular feminization (syndrome)

E34.8   **Other specified endocrine disorders**

Pineal gland dysfunction
Progeria

E34.9   **Endocrine disorder, unspecified**

Disturbance:

- endocrine NOS
- hormone NOS

E35*   Disorders of endocrine glands in diseases classified elsewhere

E35.0*   **Disorders of thyroid gland in diseases classified elsewhere**

Tuberculosis of thyroid gland (A18.8†)

E35.1*   **Disorders of adrenal glands in diseases classified elsewhere**

Tuberculous Addison's disease (A18.7†)
Waterhouse–Friderichsen syndrome (meningococcal) (A39.1†)

E35.8* **Disorders of other endocrine glands in diseases classified elsewhere**

Malnutrition
(E40–E46)

Note: The degree of malnutrition is usually measured in terms of weight, expressed in standard deviations from the mean of the relevant reference population. When one or more previous measurements are available, lack of weight gain in children, or evidence of weight loss in children or adults, is usually indicative of malnutrition. When only one measurement is available, the diagnosis is based on probabilities and is not definitive without other clinical or laboratory tests. In the exceptional circumstances that no measurement of weight is available, reliance should be placed on clinical evidence.

If an observed weight is below the mean value of the reference population, there is a high probability of severe malnutrition if there is an observed value situated 3 or more standard deviations below the mean value of the reference population; a high probability of moderate malnutrition for an observed value located between 2 and less than 3 standard deviations below this mean; and a high probability of mild malnutrition for an observed value located between 1 and less than 2 standard deviations below this mean.

Excludes: intestinal malabsorption (K90.–)
nutritional anaemias (D50–D53)
sequelae of protein-energy malnutrition (E64.0)
slim disease (B22.2)
starvation (T73.0)

E40 **Kwashiorkor**
Severe malnutrition with nutritional oedema with dyspigmentation of skin and hair.

Excludes: marasmic kwashiorkor (E42)

E41   Nutritional marasmus

Severe malnutrition with marasmus

Excludes: marasmic kwashiorkor (E42)

E42   Marasmic kwashiorkor

Severe protein-energy malnutrition [as in E43]:
• intermediate form
• with signs of both kwashiorkor and marasmus

E43   Unspecified severe protein-energy malnutrition

Severe loss of weight [wasting] in children or adults, or lack of weight gain in children leading to an observed weight that is at least 3 standard deviations below the mean value for the reference population (or a similar loss expressed through other statistical approaches). When only one measurement is available, there is a high probability of severe wasting when the observed weight is 3 or more standard deviations below the mean of the reference population.

Starvation oedema

E44   Protein-energy malnutrition of moderate and mild degree

E44.0   Moderate protein-energy malnutrition

Weight loss in children or adults, or lack of weight gain in children leading to an observed weight that is 2 or more but less than 3 standard deviations below the mean value for the reference population (or a similar loss expressed through other statistical approaches). When only one measurement is available, there is a high probability of moderate protein-energy malnutrition when the observed weight is 2 or more but less than 3 standard deviations below the mean of the reference population.

E44.1   Mild protein-energy malnutrition

Weight loss in children or adults, or lack of weight gain in children leading to an observed weight that is 1 or more but less than 2 standard deviations below the mean value for the reference population (or a similar loss expressed through other statistical approaches). When only one measurement is available, there is a high probability of mild protein-energy malnutrition when the observed weight is 1 or more but less than 2 standard deviations below the mean of the reference population.

E45   Retarded development following protein-energy malnutrition

Nutritional:
- short stature
- stunting

Physical retardation due to malnutrition

E46   Unspecified protein-energy malnutrition

Malnutrition NOS

Protein-energy imbalance NOS

Other nutritional deficiencies (E50–E64)

Excludes: nutritional anaemias (D50–D53)

E50   Vitamin A deficiency

Excludes: sequelae of vitamin A deficiency (E64.1)

E50.0   **Vitamin A deficiency with conjunctival xerosis**

E50.1   **Vitamin A deficiency with Bitot's spot and conjunctival xerosis**

Bitot's spot in the young child

E50.2   **Vitamin A deficiency with corneal xerosis**

E50.3   **Vitamin A deficiency with corneal ulceration and xerosis**

E50.4   **Vitamin A deficiency with keratomalacia**

E50.5   **Vitamin A deficiency with night blindness**

E50.6   **Vitamin A deficiency with xerophthalmic scars of cornea**

E50.7   **Other ocular manifestations of vitamin A deficiency**

Xerophthalmia NOS

E50.8   **Other manifestations of vitamin A deficiency**

Follicular keratosis ⎫
Xeroderma   ⎬ due to vitamin A deficiency† (L86*)
            ⎭

E50.9   **Vitamin A deficiency, unspecified**

Hypovitaminosis A NOS

E51   Thiamine deficiency
Excludes: sequelae of thiamine deficiency (E64.8)

E51.1   **Beriberi**
Beriberi:
- dry
- wet† (I98.8*)

E51.2   **Wernicke's encephalopathy**

E51.8   **Other manifestations of thiamine deficiency**

E51.9   **Thiamine deficiency, unspecified**

E52   Niacin deficiency [pellagra]
Deficiency:
- niacin(-tryptophan)
- nicotinamide

Pellagra (alcoholic)
Excludes: sequelae of niacin deficiency (E64.8)

E53   Deficiency of other B group vitamins
Excludes: sequelae of vitamin B deficiency (E64.8)
          vitamin B_{12} deficiency anaemia (D51.–)

E53.0   **Riboflavin deficiency**
Ariboflavinosis

E53.1   **Pyridoxine deficiency**
Vitamin B_6 deficiency
Excludes: pyridoxine-responsive sideroblastic anaemia (D64.3)

E53.8   **Deficiency of other specified B group vitamins**
Deficiency:
- biotin
- cyanocobalamin
- folate
- folic acid
- pantothenic acid
- vitamin B_{12}

E53.9   **Vitamin B deficiency, unspecified**

E54   Ascorbic acid deficiency

Deficiency of vitamin C
Scurvy

Excludes: scorbutic anaemia (D53.2)
sequelae of vitamin C deficiency (E64.2)

E55   Vitamin D deficiency

Excludes: adult osteomalacia (M83.–)
osteoporosis (M80–M81)
sequelae of rickets (E64.3)

E55.0   **Rickets, active**

Osteomalacia:
• infantile
• juvenile

Excludes: rickets:
• coeliac (K90.0)
• Crohn's (K50.–)
• inactive (E64.3)
• renal (N25.0)
• vitamin-D-resistant (E83.3)

E55.9   **Vitamin D deficiency, unspecified**

Avitaminosis D

E56   Other vitamin deficiencies

Excludes: sequelae of other vitamin deficiencies (E64.8)

E56.0   **Deficiency of vitamin E**

E56.1   **Deficiency of vitamin K**

Excludes: deficiency of coagulation factor due to vitamin K
deficiency (D68.4)
vitamin K deficiency of newborn (P53)

E56.8   **Deficiency of other vitamins**

E56.9   **Vitamin deficiency, unspecified**

E58   Dietary calcium deficiency

Excludes: disorders of calcium metabolism (E83.5)
sequelae of calcium deficiency (E64.8)

E59 Dietary selenium deficiency

Keshan disease

Excludes: sequelae of selenium deficiency (E64.8)

E60 Dietary zinc deficiency

E61 Deficiency of other nutrient elements

Use additional external cause code (Chapter XX), if desired, to identify drug, if drug-induced.

Excludes: disorders of mineral metabolism (E83.–)
iodine-deficiency-related thyroid disorders (E00–E02)
sequelae of malnutrition and other nutritional deficiencies (E64.–)

E61.0 **Copper deficiency**

E61.1 **Iron deficiency**

Excludes: iron deficiency anaemia (D50.–)

E61.2 **Magnesium deficiency**

E61.3 **Manganese deficiency**

E61.4 **Chromium deficiency**

E61.5 **Molybdenum deficiency**

E61.6 **Vanadium deficiency**

E61.7 **Deficiency of multiple nutrient elements**

E61.8 **Deficiency of other specified nutrient elements**

E61.9 **Deficiency of nutrient element, unspecified**

E63 Other nutritional deficiencies

Excludes: dehydration (E86)
failure to thrive (R62.8)
feeding problems in newborn (P92.–)
sequelae of malnutrition and other nutritional deficiencies (E64.–)

E63.0 **Essential fatty acid [EFA] deficiency**

E63.1 **Imbalance of constituents of food intake**

E63.8   Other specified nutritional deficiencies

E63.9   Nutritional deficiency, unspecified
Nutritional cardiomyopathy NOS† (I43.2*)

E64   Sequelae of malnutrition and other nutritional deficiencies

E64.0   Sequelae of protein-energy malnutrition
Excludes: retarded development following protein-energy malnutrition (E45)

E64.1   Sequelae of vitamin A deficiency

E64.2   Sequelae of vitamin C deficiency

E64.3   Sequelae of rickets

E64.8   Sequelae of other nutritional deficiencies

E64.9   Sequelae of unspecified nutritional deficiency

Obesity and other hyperalimentation (E65–E68)

E65   Localized adiposity
Fat pad

E66   Obesity
Excludes: adiposogenital dystrophy (E23.6)
lipomatosis:
• NOS (E88.2)
• dolorosa [Dercum] (E88.2)
Prader–Willi syndrome (Q87.1)

E66.0   Obesity due to excess calories

E66.1   Drug-induced obesity
Use additional external cause code (Chapter XX), if desired, to identify drug.

E66.2   Extreme obesity with alveolar hypoventilation
Pickwickian syndrome

E66.8 **Other obesity**
Morbid obesity

E66.9 **Obesity, unspecified**
Simple obesity NOS

E67 Other hyperalimentation

Excludes: hyperalimentation NOS (R63.2)
sequelae of hyperalimentation (E68)

E67.0 **Hypervitaminosis A**

E67.1 **Hypercarotenaemia**

E67.2 **Megavitamin-B$_6$ syndrome**

E67.3 **Hypervitaminosis D**

E67.8 **Other specified hyperalimentation**

E68 Sequelae of hyperalimentation

Metabolic disorders
(E70–E90)

Excludes: androgen resistance syndrome (E34.5)
congenital adrenal hyperplasia (E25.0)
Ehlers–Danlos syndrome (Q79.6)
haemolytic anaemias due to enzyme disorders (D55.–)
Marfan's syndrome (Q87.4)
5-α-reductase deficiency (E29.1)

E70 Disorders of aromatic amino-acid metabolism

E70.0 **Classical phenylketonuria**

E70.1 **Other hyperphenylalaninaemias**

E70.2 **Disorders of tyrosine metabolism**
Alkaptonuria
Hypertyrosinaemia
Ochronosis
Tyrosinaemia
Tyrosinosis

E70.3 **Albinism**
Albinism:
• ocular
• oculocutaneous
Syndrome:
• Chediak(–Steinbrinck)–Higashi
• Cross
• Hermansky–Pudlak

E70.8 **Other disorders of aromatic amino-acid metabolism**
Disorders of:
• histidine metabolism
• tryptophan metabolism

E70.9 **Disorder of aromatic amino-acid metabolism, unspecified**

E71 **Disorders of branched-chain amino-acid metabolism and fatty-acid metabolism**

E71.0 **Maple-syrup-urine disease**

E71.1 **Other disorders of branched-chain amino-acid metabolism**
Hyperleucine-isoleucinaemia
Hypervalinaemia
Isovaleric acidaemia
Methylmalonic acidaemia
Propionic acidaemia

E71.2 **Disorder of branched-chain amino-acid metabolism, unspecified**

E71.3 **Disorders of fatty-acid metabolism**
Adrenoleukodystrophy [Addison–Schilder]
Muscle carnitine palmityltransferase deficiency
Excludes: Refsum's disease (G60.1)
Schilder's disease (G37.0)
Zellweger's syndrome (Q87.8)

E72 Other disorders of amino-acid metabolism

Excludes: abnormal findings without manifest disease
(R70–R89)
disorders of:
- aromatic amino-acid metabolism (E70.–)
- branched-chain amino-acid metabolism
(E71.0–E71.2)
- fatty-acid metabolism (E71.3)
- purine and pyrimidine metabolism (E79.–)
gout (M10.–)

E72.0 Disorders of amino-acid transport

Cystinosis
Cystinuria
Fanconi(–de Toni)(–Debré) syndrome
Hartnup's disease
Lowe's syndrome

Excludes: disorders of tryptophan metabolism (E70.8)

E72.1 Disorders of sulfur-bearing amino-acid metabolism

Cystathioninuria
Homocystinuria
Methioninaemia
Sulfite oxidase deficiency

Excludes: transcobalamin II deficiency (D51.2)

E72.2 Disorders of urea cycle metabolism

Argininaemia
Argininosuccinic aciduria
Citrullinaemia
Hyperammonaemia

Excludes: disorders of ornithine metabolism (E72.4)

E72.3 Disorders of lysine and hydroxylysine metabolism

Glutaric aciduria
Hydroxylysinaemia
Hyperlysinaemia

E72.4 Disorders of ornithine metabolism

Ornithinaemia (types I, II)

E72.5 Disorders of glycine metabolism

Hyperhydroxyprolinaemia
Hyperprolinaemia (types I, II)
Non-ketotic hyperglycinaemia
Sarcosinaemia

E72.8   Other specified disorders of amino-acid metabolism
Disorders of:
- β-amino-acid metabolism
- γ-glutamyl cycle

E72.9   Disorder of amino-acid metabolism, unspecified

E73   Lactose intolerance

E73.0   Congenital lactase deficiency

E73.1   Secondary lactase deficiency

E73.8   Other lactose intolerance

E73.9   Lactose intolerance, unspecified

E74   Other disorders of carbohydrate metabolism
Excludes: increased secretion of glucagon (E16.3)
diabetes mellitus (E10–E14)
hypoglycaemia NOS (E16.2)
mucopolysaccharidosis (E76.0–E76.3)

E74.0   Glycogen storage disease
Cardiac glycogenosis
Disease:
- Andersen
- Cori
- Forbes
- Hers
- McArdle
- Pompe
- Tauri
- von Gierke
Liver phosphorylase deficiency

E74.1   Disorders of fructose metabolism
Essential fructosuria
Fructose-1,6-diphosphatase deficiency
Hereditary fructose intolerance

E74.2   Disorders of galactose metabolism
Galactokinase deficiency
Galactosaemia

E74.3   **Other disorders of intestinal carbohydrate absorption**
Glucose-galactose malabsorption
Sucrase deficiency
Excludes: lactose intolerance (E73.–)

E74.4   **Disorders of pyruvate metabolism and gluconeogenesis**
Deficiency of:
• phosphoenolpyruvate carboxykinase
• pyruvate:
  • carboxylase
  • dehydrogenase
Excludes: with anaemia (D55.–)

E74.8   **Other specified disorders of carbohydrate metabolism**
Essential pentosuria
Oxalosis
Oxaluria
Renal glycosuria

E74.9   **Disorder of carbohydrate metabolism, unspecified**

E75   Disorders of sphingolipid metabolism and other lipid storage disorders
Excludes: mucolipidosis, types I–III (E77.0–E77.1)
Refsum's disease (G60.1)

E75.0   **GM$_2$ gangliosidosis**
Disease:
• Sandhoff
• Tay–Sachs
GM$_2$ gangliosidosis:
• NOS
• adult
• juvenile

E75.1   **Other gangliosidosis**
Gangliosidosis:
• NOS
• GM$_1$
• GM$_3$
Mucolipidosis IV

E75.2 **Other sphingolipidosis**
Disease:
- Fabry(–Anderson)
- Gaucher
- Krabbe
- Niemann–Pick

Farber's syndrome
Metachromatic leukodystrophy
Sulfatase deficiency
Excludes: adrenoleukodystrophy [Addison–Schilder] (E71.3)

E75.3 **Sphingolipidosis, unspecified**

E75.4 **Neuronal ceroid lipofuscinosis**
Disease:
- Batten
- Bielschowsky–Jansky
- Kufs
- Spielmeyer–Vogt

E75.5 **Other lipid storage disorders**
Cerebrotendinous cholesterosis [van Bogaert–Scherer–Epstein]
Wolman's disease

E75.6 **Lipid storage disorder, unspecified**

E76 Disorders of glycosaminoglycan metabolism

E76.0 **Mucopolysaccharidosis, type I**
Syndrome:
- Hurler
- Hurler–Scheie
- Scheie

E76.1 **Mucopolysaccharidosis, type II**
Hunter's syndrome

E76.2 **Other mucopolysaccharidoses**
β-Glucuronidase deficiency
Mucopolysaccharidosis, types III, IV, VI, VII
Syndrome:
- Maroteaux–Lamy (mild)(severe)
- Morquio(-like)(classic)
- Sanfilippo (type B)(type C)(type D)

E76.3 **Mucopolysaccharidosis, unspecified**

E76.8   Other disorders of glucosaminoglycan metabolism

E76.9   Disorder of glucosaminoglycan metabolism, unspecified

E77   Disorders of glycoprotein metabolism

E77.0   **Defects in post-translational modification of lysosomal enzymes**
Mucolipidosis II [I-cell disease]
Mucolipidosis III [pseudo-Hurler polydystrophy]

E77.1   **Defects in glycoprotein degradation**
Aspartylglucosaminuria
Fucosidosis
Mannosidosis
Sialidosis [mucolipidosis I]

E77.8   Other disorders of glycoprotein metabolism

E77.9   Disorder of glycoprotein metabolism, unspecified

E78   Disorders of lipoprotein metabolism and other lipidaemias

Excludes: sphingolipidosis (E75.0–E75.3)

E78.0   **Pure hypercholesterolaemia**
Familial hypercholesterolaemia
Fredrickson's hyperlipoproteinaemia, type IIa
Hyperbetalipoproteinaemia
Hyperlipidaemia, group A
Low-density-lipoprotein-type [LDL] hyperlipoproteinaemia

E78.1   **Pure hyperglyceridaemia**
Endogenous hyperglyceridaemia
Fredrickson's hyperlipoproteinaemia, type IV
Hyperlipidaemia, group B
Hyperprebetalipoproteinaemia
Very-low-density-lipoprotein-type [VLDL] hyperlipoproteinaemia

E78.2 **Mixed hyperlipidaemia**
Broad- or floating-betalipoproteinaemia
Fredrickson's hyperlipoproteinaemia, type IIb or III
Hyperbetalipoproteinaemia with prebetalipoproteinaemia
Hypercholesterolaemia with endogenous hyperglyceridaemia
Hyperlipidaemia, group C
Tubero-eruptive xanthoma
Xanthoma tuberosum
Excludes: cerebrotendinous cholesterosis [van Bogaert–Scherer–Epstein] (E75.5)

E78.3 **Hyperchylomicronaemia**
Fredrickson's hyperlipoproteinaemia, type I or V
Hyperlipidaemia, group D
Mixed hyperglyceridaemia

E78.4 **Other hyperlipidaemia**
Familial combined hyperlipidaemia

E78.5 **Hyperlipidaemia, unspecified**

E78.6 **Lipoprotein deficiency**
Abetalipoproteinaemia
High-density lipoprotein deficiency
Hypoalphalipoproteinaemia
Hypobetalipoproteinaemia (familial)
Lecithin cholesterol acyltransferase deficiency
Tangier disease

E78.8 **Other disorders of lipoprotein metabolism**

E78.9 **Disorder of lipoprotein metabolism, unspecified**

E79 Disorders of purine and pyrimidine metabolism
Excludes: calculus of kidney (N20.0)
combined immunodeficiency disorders (D81.–)
gout (M10.–)
orotaciduric anaemia (D53.0)
xeroderma pigmentosum (Q82.1)

E79.0 **Hyperuricaemia without signs of inflammatory arthritis and tophaceous disease**
Asymptomatic hyperuricaemia

E79.1 **Lesch–Nyhan syndrome**

E79.8 **Other disorders of purine and pyrimidine metabolism**
Hereditary xanthinuria

E79.9 **Disorder of purine and pyrimidine metabolism, unspecified**

E80 Disorders of porphyrin and bilirubin metabolism
Includes: defects of catalase and peroxidase

E80.0 **Hereditary erythropoietic porphyria**
Congenital erythropoietic porphyria
Erythropoietic protoporphyria

E80.1 **Porphyria cutanea tarda**

E80.2 **Other porphyria**
Hereditary coproporphyria
Porphyria:
• NOS
• acute intermittent (hepatic)

Use additional external cause code (Chapter XX), if desired, to
identify cause.

E80.3 **Defects of catalase and peroxidase**
Acatalasia [Takahara]

E80.4 **Gilbert's syndrome**

E80.5 **Crigler–Najjar syndrome**

E80.6 **Other disorders of bilirubin metabolism**
Dubin–Johnson syndrome
Rotor's syndrome

E80.7 **Disorder of bilirubin metabolism, unspecified**

E83 Disorders of mineral metabolism
Excludes: dietary mineral deficiency (E58–E61)
parathyroid disorders (E20–E21)
vitamin D deficiency (E55.–)

E83.0 **Disorders of copper metabolism**
Menkes' (kinky hair)(steely hair) disease
Wilson's disease

E83.1 **Disorders of iron metabolism**
Haemochromatosis
Excludes: anaemia:
- iron deficiency (D50.–)
- sideroblastic (D64.0–D64.3)

E83.2 **Disorders of zinc metabolism**
Acrodermatitis enteropathica

E83.3 **Disorders of phosphorus metabolism**
Acid phosphatase deficiency
Familial hypophosphataemia
Hypophosphatasia
Vitamin-D-resistant:
- osteomalacia
- rickets
Excludes: adult osteomalacia (M83.–)
osteoporosis (M80–M81)

E83.4 **Disorders of magnesium metabolism**
Hypermagnesaemia
Hypomagnesaemia

E83.5 **Disorders of calcium metabolism**
Familial hypocalciuric hypercalcaemia
Idiopathic hypercalciuria
Excludes: chondrocalcinosis (M11.1–M11.2)
hyperparathyroidism (E21.0–E21.3)

E83.8 **Other disorders of mineral metabolism**

E83.9 **Disorder of mineral metabolism, unspecified**

E84 **Cystic fibrosis**
Includes: mucoviscidosis

E84.0 **Cystic fibrosis with pulmonary manifestations**

E84.1 **Cystic fibrosis with intestinal manifestations**
Meconium ileus† (P75*)

E84.8 **Cystic fibrosis with other manifestations**
Cystic fibrosis with combined manifestations

E84.9 **Cystic fibrosis, unspecified**

E85 Amyloidosis

Excludes: Alzheimer's disease (G30.–)

E85.0 Non-neuropathic heredofamilial amyloidosis
Familial Mediterranean fever
Hereditary amyloid nephropathy

E85.1 Neuropathic heredofamilial amyloidosis
Amyloid polyneuropathy (Portuguese)

E85.2 Heredofamilial amyloidosis, unspecified

E85.3 Secondary systemic amyloidosis
Haemodialysis-associated amyloidosis

E85.4 Organ-limited amyloidosis
Localized amyloidosis

E85.8 Other amyloidosis

E85.9 Amyloidosis, unspecified

E86 Volume depletion

Dehydration
Depletion of volume of plasma or extracellular fluid
Hypovolaemia

Excludes: dehydration of newborn (P74.1)
hypovolaemic shock:
• NOS (R57.1)
• postoperative (T81.1)
• traumatic (T79.4)

E87 Other disorders of fluid, electrolyte and acid–base balance

E87.0 Hyperosmolality and hypernatraemia
Sodium [Na] excess
Sodium [Na] overload

E87.1 Hypo-osmolality and hyponatraemia
Sodium [Na] deficiency

Excludes: syndrome of inappropriate secretion of antidiuretic hormone (E22.2)

E87.2   Acidosis
Acidosis:
- NOS
- lactic
- metabolic
- respiratory

Excludes: diabetic acidosis (E10–E14 with common fourth
              character .1)

E87.3   Alkalosis
Alkalosis:
- NOS
- metabolic
- respiratory

E87.4   Mixed disorder of acid-base balance

E87.5   Hyperkalaemia
Potassium [K] excess
Potassium [K] overload

E87.6   Hypokalaemia
Potassium [K] deficiency

E87.7   Fluid overload
Excludes: oedema (R60.–)

**E87.8   Other disorders of electrolyte and fluid balance, not
           elsewhere classified**
Electrolyte imbalance NOS
Hyperchloraemia
Hypochloraemia

E88   Other metabolic disorders
Excludes: histiocytosis X (chronic) (D76.0)

Use additional external cause code (Chapter XX), if desired, to
identify drug, if drug-induced.

**E88.0   Disorders of plasma-protein metabolism, not elsewhere
           classified**
α-1-Antitrypsin deficiency
Bisalbuminaemia

Excludes: disorder of lipoprotein metabolism (E78.–)
              monoclonal gammopathy (D47.2)
              polyclonal hypergammaglobulinaemia (D89.0)
              Waldenström's macroglobulinaemia (C88.0)

E88.1 **Lipodystrophy, not elsewhere classified**
Lipodystrophy NOS
Excludes: Whipple's disease (K90.8)

E88.2 **Lipomatosis, not elsewhere classified**
Lipomatosis:
• NOS
• dolorosa [Dercum]

E88.8 **Other specified metabolic disorders**
Launois–Bensaude adenolipomatosis
Trimethylaminuria

E88.9 **Metabolic disorder, unspecified**

E89 **Postprocedural endocrine and metabolic disorders, not elsewhere classified**

E89.0 **Postprocedural hypothyroidism**
Postirradiation hypothyroidism
Postsurgical hypothyroidism

E89.1 **Postprocedural hypoinsulinaemia**
Postpancreatectomy hyperglycaemia
Postsurgical hypoinsulinaemia

E89.2 **Postprocedural hypoparathyroidism**
Parathyroprival tetany

E89.3 **Postprocedural hypopituitarism**
Postirradiation hypopituitarism

E89.4 **Postprocedural ovarian failure**

E89.5 **Postprocedural testicular hypofunction**

E89.6 **Postprocedural adrenocortical(-medullary) hypofunction**

E89.8 **Other postprocedural endocrine and metabolic disorders**

E89.9 **Postprocedural endocrine and metabolic disorder, unspecified**

E90* **Nutritional and metabolic disorders in diseases classified elsewhere**

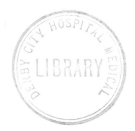

CHAPTER V

Mental and behavioural disorders (F00–F99)

Includes: disorders of psychological development

Excludes: symptoms, signs and abnormal clinical and laboratory findings, not elsewhere classified (R00–R99)

This chapter contains the following blocks:

F00–F09 Organic, including symptomatic, mental disorders
F10–F19 Mental and behavioural disorders due to psychoactive substance use
F20–F29 Schizophrenia, schizotypal and delusional disorders
F30–F39 Mood [affective] disorders
F40–F48 Neurotic, stress-related and somatoform disorders
F50–F59 Behavioural syndromes associated with physiological disturbances and physical factors
F60–F69 Disorders of adult personality and behaviour
F70–F79 Mental retardation
F80–F89 Disorders of psychological development
F90–F98 Behavioural and emotional disorders with onset usually occurring in childhood and adolescence
F99 Unspecified mental disorder

Asterisk categories for this chapter are provided as follows:

F00* Dementia in Alzheimer's disease
F02* Dementia in other diseases classified elsewhere

Organic, including symptomatic, mental disorders (F00–F09)

This block comprises a range of mental disorders grouped together on the basis of their having in common a demonstrable etiology in cerebral disease, brain injury, or other insult leading to cerebral dysfunction. The dysfunction may be primary, as in diseases, injuries, and insults that affect the brain directly and selectively; or secondary, as in systemic diseases and disorders that attack the brain only as one of the multiple organs or systems of the body that are involved.

Dementia (F00–F03) is a syndrome due to disease of the brain, usually of a chronic or progressive nature, in which there is disturbance of multiple higher cortical functions, including memory, thinking, orientation, comprehension, calculation, learning capacity, language, and judgement. Consciousness is not clouded. The impairments of cognitive function are commonly accompanied, and occasionally preceded, by deterioration in emotional control, social behaviour, or motivation. This syndrome occurs in Alzheimer's disease, in cerebrovascular disease, and in other conditions primarily or secondarily affecting the brain.

Use additional code, if desired, to identify the underlying disease.

F00* Dementia in Alzheimer's disease (G30.–†)
Alzheimer's disease is a primary degenerative cerebral disease of unknown etiology with characteristic neuropathological and neurochemical features. The disorder is usually insidious in onset and develops slowly but steadily over a period of several years.

F00.0* Dementia in Alzheimer's disease with early onset (G30.0†)
Dementia in Alzheimer's disease with onset before the age of 65, with a relatively rapid deteriorating course and with marked multiple disorders of the higher cortical functions.

Alzheimer's disease, type 2
Presenile dementia, Alzheimer's type
Primary degenerative dementia of the Alzheimer's type, presenile onset

F00.1*   **Dementia in Alzheimer's disease with late onset (G30.1†)**

Dementia in Alzheimer's disease with onset after the age of 65, usually in the late 70s or thereafter, with a slow progression, and with memory impairment as the principal feature.

Alzheimer's disease, type 1

Primary degenerative dementia of the Alzheimer's type, senile onset

Senile dementia, Alzheimer's type

F00.2*   **Dementia in Alzheimer's disease, atypical or mixed type (G30.8†)**

Atypical dementia, Alzheimer's type

F00.9*   **Dementia in Alzheimer's disease, unspecified (G30.9†)**

F01 Vascular dementia

Vascular dementia is the result of infarction of the brain due to vascular disease, including hypertensive cerebrovascular disease. The infarcts are usually small but cumulative in their effect. Onset is usually in later life.

Includes: arteriosclerotic dementia

F01.0   **Vascular dementia of acute onset**

Usually develops rapidly after a succession of strokes from cerebrovascular thrombosis, embolism or haemorrhage. In rare cases, a single large infarction may be the cause.

F01.1   **Multi-infarct dementia**

Gradual in onset, following a number of transient ischaemic episodes which produce an accumulation of infarcts in the cerebral parenchyma.

Predominantly cortical dementia

F01.2   **Subcortical vascular dementia**

Includes cases with a history of hypertension and foci of ischaemic destruction in the deep white matter of the cerebral hemispheres. The cerebral cortex is usually preserved and this contrasts with the clinical picture which may closely resemble that of dementia in Alzheimer's disease.

F01.3   **Mixed cortical and subcortical vascular dementia**

F01.8   **Other vascular dementia**

F01.9   **Vascular dementia, unspecified**

F02* Dementia in other diseases classified elsewhere

Cases of dementia due, or presumed to be due, to causes other than Alzheimer's disease or cerebrovascular disease. Onset may be at any time in life, though rarely in old age.

F02.0* Dementia in Pick's disease (G31.0†)

A progressive dementia, commencing in middle age, characterized by early, slowly progressing changes of character and social deterioration, followed by impairment of intellect, memory, and language functions, with apathy, euphoria and, occasionally, extrapyramidal phenomena.

F02.1* Dementia in Creutzfeldt-Jakob disease (A81.0†)

A progressive dementia with extensive neurological signs, due to specific neuropathological changes that are presumed to be caused by a transmissible agent. Onset is usually in middle or later life, but may be at any adult age. The course is subacute, leading to death within one to two years.

F02.2* Dementia in Huntington's disease (G10†)

A dementia occurring as part of a widespread degeneration of the brain. The disorder is transmitted by a single autosomal dominant gene. Symptoms typically emerge in the third and fourth decade. Progression is slow, leading to death usually within 10 to 15 years.

Dementia in Huntington's chorea

F02.3* Dementia in Parkinson's disease (G20†)

A dementia developing in the course of established Parkinson's disease. No particular distinguishing clinical features have yet been demonstrated.

Dementia in:
- paralysis agitans
- parkinsonism

F02.4* Dementia in human immunodeficiency virus [HIV] disease (B22.0†)

Dementia developing in the course of HIV disease, in the absence of a concurrent illness or condition other than HIV infection that could explain the clinical features.

F02.8* Dementia in other specified diseases classified elsewhere

Dementia in:
- cerebral lipidosis (E75.–†)
- epilepsy (G40.–†)
- hepatolenticular degeneration (E83.0†)
- hypercalcaemia (E83.5†)
- hypothyroidism, acquired (E01, E03.–†)
- intoxications (T36–T65†)
- multiple sclerosis (G35†)
- neurosyphilis (A52.1†)
- niacin deficiency [pellagra] (E52†)
- polyarteritis nodosa (M30.0†)
- systemic lupus erythematosus (M32.–†)
- trypanosomiasis (B56.–†, B57.–†)
- vitamin B_{12} deficiency (E53.8†)

F03 Unspecified dementia

Presenile:

- dementia NOS
- psychosis NOS

Primary degenerative dementia NOS

Senile:

- dementia:
  - NOS
  - depressed or paranoid type
- psychosis NOS

Excludes: senile dementia with delirium or acute confusional
state (F05.1)
senility NOS (R54)

F04 Organic amnesic syndrome, not induced by alcohol and other psychoactive substances

A syndrome of prominent impairment of recent and remote memory
while immediate recall is preserved, with reduced ability to learn new
material and disorientation in time. Confabulation may be a marked
feature, but perception and other cognitive functions, including the
intellect, are usually intact. The prognosis depends on the course of the
underlying lesion.

Korsakov's psychosis or syndrome, nonalcoholic

Excludes: amnesia:

- NOS (R41.3)
- anterograde (R41.1)
- dissociative (F44.0)
- retrograde (R41.2)

Korsakov's syndrome:

- alcohol-induced or unspecified (F10.6)
- induced by other psychoactive substances (F11–
  F19 with common fourth character .6)

F05 Delirium, not induced by alcohol and other psychoactive substances

An etiologically nonspecific organic cerebral syndrome characterized by concurrent disturbances of consciousness and attention, perception, thinking, memory, psychomotor behaviour, emotion, and the sleep–wake schedule. The duration is variable and the degree of severity ranges from mild to very severe.

Includes: acute or subacute:
- brain syndrome
- confusional state (nonalcoholic)
- infective psychosis
- organic reaction
- psycho-organic syndrome

Excludes: delirium tremens, alcohol-induced or unspecified (F10.4)

F05.0 **Delirium not superimposed on dementia, so described**

F05.1 **Delirium superimposed on dementia**
Conditions meeting the above criteria but developing in the course of a dementia (F00–F03).

F05.8 **Other delirium**
Delirium of mixed origin

F05.9 **Delirium, unspecified**

F06 Other mental disorders due to brain damage and dysfunction and to physical disease

Includes miscellaneous conditions causally related to brain disorder due to primary cerebral disease, to systemic disease affecting the brain secondarily, to exogenous toxic substances or hormones, to endocrine disorders, or to other somatic illnesses.

Excludes: associated with:
- delirium (F05.–)
- dementia as classified in F00–F03

resulting from use of alcohol and other psychoactive substances (F10–F19)

F06.0 **Organic hallucinosis**

A disorder of persistent or recurrent hallucinations, usually visual or auditory, that occur in clear consciousness and may or may not be recognized by the subject as such. Delusional elaboration of the hallucinations may occur, but delusions do not dominate the clinical picture; insight may be preserved.

Organic hallucinatory state (nonalcoholic)

Excludes: alcoholic hallucinosis (F10.5)

schizophrenia (F20.–)

F06.1 **Organic catatonic disorder**

A disorder of diminished (stupor) or increased (excitement) psychomotor activity associated with catatonic symptoms. The extremes of psychomotor disturbance may alternate.

Excludes: catatonic schizophrenia (F20.2)

stupor:

• NOS (R40.1)

• dissociative (F44.2)

F06.2 **Organic delusional [schizophrenia-like] disorder**

A disorder in which persistent or recurrent delusions dominate the clinical picture. The delusions may be accompanied by hallucinations. Some features suggestive of schizophrenia, such as bizarre hallucinations or thought disorder, may be present.

Paranoid and paranoid-hallucinatory organic states
Schizophrenia-like psychosis in epilepsy

Excludes: disorder:

• acute and transient psychotic (F23.–)

• persistent delusional (F22.–)

• psychotic drug-induced (F11–F19 with common fourth character .5)

schizophrenia (F20.–)

F06.3 **Organic mood [affective] disorders**

Disorders characterized by a change in mood or affect, usually accompanied by a change in the overall level of activity, depressive, hypomanic, manic or bipolar (see F30–F32), but arising as a consequence of an organic disorder.

Excludes: mood disorders, nonorganic or unspecified (F30–F39)

F06.4 **Organic anxiety disorder**

A disorder characterized by the essential descriptive features of a generalized anxiety disorder (F41.1), a panic disorder (F41.0), or a combination of both, but arising as a consequence of an organic disorder.

Excludes: anxiety disorders, nonorganic or unspecified (F41.–)

F06.5   Organic dissociative disorder

A disorder characterized by a partial or complete loss of the normal integration between memories of the past, awareness of identity and immediate sensations, and control of bodily movements (see F44.–), but arising as a consequence of an organic disorder.

Excludes: dissociative [conversion] disorders, nonorganic or unspecified (F44.–)

F06.6   Organic emotionally labile [asthenic] disorder

A disorder characterized by emotional incontinence or lability, fatigability, and a variety of unpleasant physical sensations (e.g. dizziness) and pains, but arising as a consequence of an organic disorder.

Excludes: somatoform disorders, nonorganic or unspecified (F45.–)

F06.7   Mild cognitive disorder

A disorder characterized by impairment of memory, learning difficulties, and reduced ability to concentrate on a task for more than brief periods. There is often a marked feeling of mental fatigue when mental tasks are attempted, and new learning is found to be subjectively difficult even when objectively successful. None of these symptoms is so severe that a diagnosis of either dementia (F00–F03) or delirium (F05.–) can be made. This diagnosis should be made only in association with a specified physical disorder, and should not be made in the presence of any of the mental or behavioural disorders classified to F10–F99. The disorder may precede, accompany, or follow a wide variety of infections and physical disorders, both cerebral and systemic, but direct evidence of cerebral involvement is not necessarily present. It can be differentiated from postencephalitic syndrome (F07.1) and postconcussional syndrome (F07.2) by its different etiology, more restricted range of generally milder symptoms, and usually shorter duration.

F06.8   Other specified mental disorders due to brain damage and dysfunction and to physical disease

Epileptic psychosis NOS

F06.9   Unspecified mental disorder due to brain damage and dysfunction and to physical disease

Organic:
• brain syndrome NOS
• mental disorder NOS

F07   Personality and behavioural disorders due to brain disease, damage and dysfunction

Alteration of personality and behaviour can be a residual or concomitant disorder of brain disease, damage or dysfunction.

F07.0   Organic personality disorder

A disorder characterized by a significant alteration of the habitual patterns of behaviour displayed by the subject premorbidly, involving the expression of emotions, needs and impulses. Impairment of cognitive and thought functions, and altered sexuality may also be part of the clinical picture.

Organic:

- pseudopsychopathic personality
- pseudoretarded personality

Syndrome:

- frontal lobe
- limbic epilepsy personality
- lobotomy
- postleucotomy

Excludes: enduring personality change after:
- catastrophic experience (F62.0)
- psychiatric illness (F62.1)
postconcussional syndrome (F07.2)
postencephalitic syndrome (F07.1)
specific personality disorder (F60.–)

F07.1   Postencephalitic syndrome

Residual nonspecific and variable behavioural change following recovery from either viral or bacterial encephalitis. The principal difference between this disorder and the organic personality disorders is that it is reversible.

Excludes: organic personality disorder (F07.0)

F07.2   Postconcussional syndrome

A syndrome that occurs following head trauma (usually sufficiently severe to result in loss of consciousness) and includes a number of disparate symptoms such as headache, dizziness, fatigue, irritability, difficulty in concentration and performing mental tasks, impairment of memory, insomnia, and reduced tolerance to stress, emotional excitement, or alcohol.

Postcontusional syndrome (encephalopathy)
Post-traumatic brain syndrome, nonpsychotic

F07.8   Other organic personality and behavioural disorders due to brain disease, damage and dysfunction

Right hemispheric organic affective disorder

F07.9   Unspecified organic personality and behavioural disorder due to brain disease, damage and dysfunction

Organic psychosyndrome

F09 Unspecified organic or symptomatic mental disorder

Psychosis:
- organic NOS
- symptomatic NOS

Excludes: psychosis NOS (F29)

Mental and behavioural disorders due to psychoactive substance use
(F10–F19)

This block contains a wide variety of disorders that differ in severity and clinical form but that are all attributable to the use of one or more psychoactive substances, which may or may not have been medically prescribed. The third character of the code identifies the substance involved, and the fourth character specifies the clinical state. The codes should be used, as required, for each substance specified, but it should be noted that not all fourth-character codes are applicable to all substances.

Identification of the psychoactive substance should be based on as many sources of information as possible. These include self-report data, analysis of blood and other body fluids, characteristic physical and psychological symptoms, clinical signs and behaviour, and other evidence such as a drug being in the patient's possession or reports from informed third parties. Many drug users take more than one type of psychoactive substance. The main diagnosis should be classified, whenever possible, according to the substance or class of substances that has caused or contributed most to the presenting clinical syndrome. Other diagnoses should be coded when other psychoactive substances have been taken in intoxicating amounts (common fourth character .0) or to the extent of causing harm (common fourth character .1), dependence (common fourth character .2) or other disorders (common fourth character .3–.9).

Only in cases in which patterns of psychoactive substance-taking are chaotic and indiscriminate, or in which the contributions of different psychoactive substances are inextricably mixed, should the diagnosis of disorders resulting from multiple drug use (F19.–) be used.

Excludes: abuse of non-dependence-producing substances (F55)

The following fourth-character subdivisions are for use with categories F10–F19:

.0 Acute intoxication

A condition that follows the administration of a psychoactive substance resulting in disturbances in level of consciousness, cognition, perception, affect or behaviour, or other psychophysiological functions and responses. The disturbances are directly related to the acute pharmacological effects of the substance and resolve with time, with complete recovery, except where tissue damage or other complications have arisen. Complications may include trauma, inhalation of vomitus, delirium, coma, convulsions, and other medical complications. The nature of these complications depends on the pharmacological class of substance and mode of administration.

Acute drunkenness in alcoholism

"Bad trips" (drugs)

Drunkenness NOS

Pathological intoxication

Trance and possession disorders in psychoactive substance intoxication

.1 Harmful use

A pattern of psychoactive substance use that is causing damage to health. The damage may be physical (as in cases of hepatitis from the self-administration of injected psychoactive substances) or mental (e.g. episodes of depressive disorder secondary to heavy consumption of alcohol).

Psychoactive substance abuse

.2 Dependence syndrome

A cluster of behavioural, cognitive, and physiological phenomena that develop after repeated substance use and that typically include a strong desire to take the drug, difficulties in controlling its use, persisting in its use despite harmful consequences, a higher priority given to drug use than to other activities and obligations, increased tolerance, and sometimes a physical withdrawal state.

The dependence syndrome may be present for a specific psychoactive substance (e.g. tobacco, alcohol, or diazepam), for a class of substances (e.g. opioid drugs), or for a wider range of pharmacologically different psychoactive substances.

Chronic alcoholism

Dipsomania

Drug addiction

.3 Withdrawal state

A group of symptoms of variable clustering and severity occurring on absolute or relative withdrawal of a psychoactive substance after persistent use of that substance. The onset and course of the withdrawal state are time-limited and are related to the type of psychoactive substance and dose being used immediately before cessation or reduction of use. The withdrawal state may be complicated by convulsions.

.4 Withdrawal state with delirium

A condition where the withdrawal state as defined in the common fourth character .3 is complicated by delirium as defined in F05.–. Convulsions may also occur. When organic factors are also considered to play a role in the etiology, the condition should be classified to F05.8.

Delirium tremens (alcohol-induced)

.5 Psychotic disorder

A cluster of psychotic phenomena that occur during or following psychoactive substance use but that are not explained on the basis of acute intoxication alone and do not form part of a withdrawal state. The disorder is characterized by hallucinations (typically auditory, but often in more than one sensory modality), perceptual distortions, delusions (often of a paranoid or persecutory nature), psychomotor disturbances (excitement or stupor), and an abnormal affect, which may range from intense fear to ecstasy. The sensorium is usually clear but some degree of clouding of consciousness, though not severe confusion, may be present.

Alcoholic:
- hallucinosis
- jealousy
- paranoia
- psychosis NOS

Excludes: alcohol- or other psychoactive substance-induced residual and late-onset psychotic disorder (F10–F19 with common fourth character .7)

.6 Amnesic syndrome

A syndrome associated with chronic prominent impairment of recent and remote memory. Immediate recall is usually preserved and recent memory is characteristically more disturbed than remote memory. Disturbances of time sense and ordering of events are usually evident, as are difficulties in learning new material. Confabulation may be marked but is not invariably present. Other cognitive functions are usually relatively well preserved and amnesic defects are out of proportion to other disturbances.

Amnestic disorder, alcohol- or drug-induced

Korsakov's psychosis or syndrome, alcohol- or other psychoactive substance-induced or unspecified

Excludes: nonalcoholic Korsakov's psychosis or syndrome (F04)

.7 Residual and late-onset psychotic disorder

A disorder in which alcohol- or psychoactive substance-induced changes of cognition, affect, personality, or behaviour persist beyond the period during which a direct psychoactive substance-related effect might reasonably be assumed to be operating. Onset of the disorder should be directly related to the use of the psychoactive substance. Cases in which initial onset of the state occurs later than episode(s) of such substance use should be coded here only where clear and strong evidence is available to attribute the state to the residual effect of the psychoactive substance. Flashbacks may be distinguished from psychotic state partly by their episodic nature, frequently of very short duration, and by their duplication of previous alcohol- or other psychoactive substance-related experiences.

Alcoholic dementia NOS

Chronic alcoholic brain syndrome

Dementia and other milder forms of persisting impairment of cognitive functions

Flashbacks

Late-onset psychoactive substance-induced psychotic disorder

Posthallucinogen perception disorder

Residual:

- affective disorder
- disorder of personality and behaviour

Excludes: alcohol- or psychoactive substance-induced:

- Korsakov's syndrome (F10–F19 with common fourth character .6)
- psychotic state (F10–F19 with common fourth character .5)

.8 Other mental and behavioural disorders

.9 Unspecified mental and behavioural disorder

F10.– Mental and behavioural disorders due to use of alcohol
[See pages 321–323 for subdivisions]

F11.– Mental and behavioural disorders due to use of opioids
[See pages 321–323 for subdivisions]

F12.– Mental and behavioural disorders due to use of cannabinoids
[See pages 321–323 for subdivisions]

F13.– Mental and behavioural disorders due to use of sedatives or hypnotics
[See pages 321–323 for subdivisions]

F14.– **Mental and behavioural disorders due to use of cocaine**

[See pages 321–323 for subdivisions]

F15.– **Mental and behavioural disorders due to use of other stimulants, including caffeine**

[See pages 321–323 for subdivisions]

F16.– **Mental and behavioural disorders due to use of hallucinogens**

[See pages 321–323 for subdivisions]

F17.– **Mental and behavioural disorders due to use of tobacco**

[See pages 321–323 for subdivisions]

F18.– **Mental and behavioural disorders due to use of volatile solvents**

[See pages 321–323 for subdivisions]

F19.– **Mental and behavioural disorders due to multiple drug use and use of other psychoactive substances**

[See pages 321–323 for subdivisions]

This category should be used when two or more psychoactive substances are known to be involved, but it is impossible to assess which substance is contributing most to the disorders. It should also be used when the exact identity of some or even all the psychoactive substances being used is uncertain or unknown, since many multiple drug users themselves often do not know the details of what they are taking.

Includes: misuse of drugs NOS

Schizophrenia, schizotypal and delusional disorders (F20–F29)

This block brings together schizophrenia, as the most important member of the group, schizotypal disorder, persistent delusional disorders, and a larger group of acute and transient psychotic disorders. Schizoaffective disorders have been retained here in spite of their controversial nature.

F20 Schizophrenia

The schizophrenic disorders are characterized in general by fundamental and characteristic distortions of thinking and perception, and affects that are inappropriate or blunted. Clear consciousness and intellectual capacity are usually maintained although certain cognitive deficits may evolve in the course of time. The most important psychopathological phenomena include thought echo; thought insertion or withdrawal; thought broadcasting; delusional perception and delusions of control; influence or passivity; hallucinatory voices commenting or discussing the patient in the third person; thought disorders and negative symptoms.

The course of schizophrenic disorders can be either continuous, or episodic with progressive or stable deficit, or there can be one or more episodes with complete or incomplete remission. The diagnosis of schizophrenia should not be made in the presence of extensive depressive or manic symptoms unless it is clear that schizophrenic symptoms antedate the affective disturbance. Nor should schizophrenia be diagnosed in the presence of overt brain disease or during states of drug intoxication or withdrawal. Similar disorders developing in the presence of epilepsy or other brain disease should be classified under F06.2, and those induced by psychoactive substances under F10–F19 with common fourth character .5.

Excludes: schizophrenia:
- acute (undifferentiated) (F23.2)
- cyclic (F25.2)
schizophrenic reaction (F23.2)
schizotypal disorder (F21)

F20.0 Paranoid schizophrenia

Paranoid schizophrenia is dominated by relatively stable, often paranoid delusions, usually accompanied by hallucinations, particularly of the auditory variety, and perceptual disturbances. Disturbances of affect, volition and speech, and catatonic symptoms, are either absent or relatively inconspicuous.

Paraphrenic schizophrenia

Excludes: involutional paranoid state (F22.8)
paranoia (F22.0)

F20.1   Hebephrenic schizophrenia

A form of schizophrenia in which affective changes are prominent, delusions and hallucinations fleeting and fragmentary, behaviour irresponsible and unpredictable, and mannerisms common. The mood is shallow and inappropriate, thought is disorganized, and speech is incoherent. There is a tendency to social isolation. Usually the prognosis is poor because of the rapid development of "negative" symptoms, particularly flattening of affect and loss of volition. Hebephrenia should normally be diagnosed only in adolescents or young adults.

Disorganized schizophrenia
Hebephrenia

F20.2   Catatonic schizophrenia

Catatonic schizophrenia is dominated by prominent psychomotor disturbances that may alternate between extremes such as hyperkinesis and stupor, or automatic obedience and negativism. Constrained attitudes and postures may be maintained for long periods. Episodes of violent excitement may be a striking feature of the condition. The catatonic phenomena may be combined with a dream-like (oneiroid) state with vivid scenic hallucinations.

Catatonic stupor
Schizophrenic:
- catalepsy
- catatonia
- flexibilitas cerea

F20.3   Undifferentiated schizophrenia

Psychotic conditions meeting the general diagnostic criteria for schizophrenia but not conforming to any of the subtypes in F20.0–F20.2, or exhibiting the features of more than one of them without a clear predominance of a particular set of diagnostic characteristics.

Atypical schizophrenia

Excludes: acute schizophrenia-like psychotic disorder (F23.2)
chronic undifferentiated schizophrenia (F20.5)
post-schizophrenic depression (F20.4)

F20.4   Post-schizophrenic depression

A depressive episode, which may be prolonged, arising in the aftermath of a schizophrenic illness. Some schizophrenic symptoms, either "positive" or "negative", must still be present but they no longer dominate the clinical picture. These depressive states are associated with an increased risk of suicide. If the patient no longer has any schizophrenic symptoms, a depressive episode should be diagnosed (F32.–). If schizophrenic symptoms are still florid and prominent, the diagnosis should remain that of the appropriate schizophrenic subtype (F20.0–F20.3).

F20.5   Residual schizophrenia

A chronic stage in the development of a schizophrenic illness in which there has been a clear progression from an early stage to a later stage characterized by long-term, though not necessarily irreversible, "negative" symptoms, e.g. psychomotor slowing; underactivity; blunting of affect; passivity and lack of initiative; poverty of quantity or content of speech; poor nonverbal communication by facial expression, eye contact, voice modulation and posture; poor self-care and social performance.

Chronic undifferentiated schizophrenia

Restzustand (schizophrenic)

Schizophrenic residual state

F20.6   Simple schizophrenia

A disorder in which there is an insidious but progressive development of oddities of conduct, inability to meet the demands of society, and decline in total performance. The characteristic negative features of residual schizophrenia (e.g. blunting of affect and loss of volition) develop without being preceded by any overt psychotic symptoms.

F20.8   Other schizophrenia

Cenesthopathic schizophrenia

Schizophreniform:

- disorder NOS
- psychosis NOS

Excludes: brief schizophreniform disorders (F23.2)

F20.9   Schizophrenia, unspecified

F21   Schizotypal disorder

A disorder characterized by eccentric behaviour and anomalies of thinking and affect which resemble those seen in schizophrenia, though no definite and characteristic schizophrenic anomalies occur at any stage. The symptoms may include a cold or inappropriate affect; anhedonia; odd or eccentric behaviour; a tendency to social withdrawal; paranoid or bizarre ideas not amounting to true delusions; obsessive ruminations; thought disorder and perceptual disturbances; occasional transient quasi-psychotic episodes with intense illusions, auditory or other hallucinations, and delusion-like ideas, usually occurring without external provocation. There is no definite onset and evolution and course are usually those of a personality disorder.

Latent schizophrenic reaction
Schizophrenia:
- borderline
- latent
- prepsychotic
- prodromal
- pseudoneurotic
- pseudopsychopathic
Schizotypal personality disorder

Excludes: Asperger's syndrome (F84.5)
schizoid personality disorder (F60.1)

F22   Persistent delusional disorders

Includes a variety of disorders in which long-standing delusions constitute the only, or the most conspicuous, clinical characteristic and which cannot be classified as organic, schizophrenic or affective. Delusional disorders that have lasted for less than a few months should be classified, at least temporarily, under F23.–.

F22.0   Delusional disorder

A disorder characterized by the development either of a single delusion or of a set of related delusions that are usually persistent and sometimes lifelong. The content of the delusion or delusions is very variable. Clear and persistent auditory hallucinations (voices), schizophrenic symptoms such as delusions of control and marked blunting of affect, and definite evidence of brain disease are all incompatible with this diagnosis. However, the presence of occasional or transitory auditory hallucinations, particularly in elderly patients, does not rule out this diagnosis, provided that they are not typically schizophrenic and form only a small part of the overall clinical picture.

Paranoia

Paranoid:

- psychosis
- state

Paraphrenia (late)

Sensitiver Beziehungswahn

Excludes: paranoid:
- personality disorder (F60.0)
- psychosis, psychogenic (F23.3)
- reaction (F23.3)
- schizophrenia (F20.0)

F22.8   Other persistent delusional disorders

Disorders in which the delusion or delusions are accompanied by persistent hallucinatory voices or by schizophrenic symptoms that do not justify a diagnosis of schizophrenia (F20.–).

Delusional dysmorphophobia

Involutional paranoid state

Paranoia querulans

F22.9   Persistent delusional disorder, unspecified

F23   Acute and transient psychotic disorders

A heterogeneous group of disorders characterized by the acute onset of psychotic symptoms such as delusions, hallucinations, and perceptual disturbances, and by the severe disruption of ordinary behaviour. Acute onset is defined as a crescendo development of a clearly abnormal clinical picture in about two weeks or less. For these disorders there is no evidence of organic causation. Perplexity and puzzlement are often present but disorientation for time, place and person is not persistent or severe enough to justify a diagnosis of organically caused delirium (F05.–). Complete recovery usually occurs within a few months, often within a few weeks or even days. If the disorder persists, a change in classification will be necessary. The disorder may or may not be associated with acute stress, defined as usually stressful events preceding the onset by one to two weeks.

F23.0 **Acute polymorphic psychotic disorder without symptoms of schizophrenia**

An acute psychotic disorder in which hallucinations, delusions or perceptual disturbances are obvious but markedly variable, changing from day to day or even from hour to hour. Emotional turmoil with intense transient feelings of happiness or ecstasy, or anxiety and irritability, is also frequently present. The polymorphism and instability are characteristic for the overall clinical picture and the psychotic features do not justify a diagnosis of schizophrenia (F20.–). These disorders often have an abrupt onset, developing rapidly within a few days, and they frequently show a rapid resolution of symptoms with no recurrence. If the symptoms persist the diagnosis should be changed to persistent delusional disorder (F22.–).

Bouffée délirante without symptoms of schizophrenia or unspecified

Cycloid psychosis without symptoms of schizophrenia or unspecified

F23.1 **Acute polymorphic psychotic disorder with symptoms of schizophrenia**

An acute psychotic disorder in which the polymorphic and unstable clinical picture is present, as described in F23.0; despite this instability, however, some symptoms typical of schizophrenia are also in evidence for the majority of the time. If the schizophrenic symptoms persist the diagnosis should be changed to schizophrenia (F20.–).

Bouffée délirante with symptoms of schizophrenia

Cycloid psychosis with symptoms of schizophrenia

F23.2 **Acute schizophrenia-like psychotic disorder**

An acute psychotic disorder in which the psychotic symptoms are comparatively stable and justify a diagnosis of schizophrenia, but have lasted for less than about one month; the polymorphic unstable features, as described in F23.0, are absent. If the schizophrenic symptoms persist the diagnosis should be changed to schizophrenia (F20.–).

Acute (undifferentiated) schizophrenia

Brief schizophreniform:

• disorder

• psychosis

Oneirophrenia

Schizophrenic reaction

Excludes: organic delusional [schizophrenia-like] disorder (F06.2)
schizophreniform disorder NOS (F20.8)

F23.3 **Other acute predominantly delusional psychotic disorders**

Acute psychotic disorders in which comparatively stable delusions or hallucinations are the main clinical features, but do not justify a diagnosis of schizophrenia (F20.–). If the delusions persist the diagnosis should be changed to persistent delusional disorder (F22.–).

Paranoid reaction

Psychogenic paranoid psychosis

F23.8 **Other acute and transient psychotic disorders**

Any other specified acute psychotic disorders for which there is no evidence of organic causation and which do not justify classification to F23.0–F23.3.

F23.9 **Acute and transient psychotic disorder, unspecified**

Brief reactive psychosis NOS

Reactive psychosis

F24 **Induced delusional disorder**

A delusional disorder shared by two or more people with close emotional links. Only one of the people suffers from a genuine psychotic disorder; the delusions are induced in the other(s) and usually disappear when the people are separated.

Folie à deux

Induced:

• paranoid disorder
• psychotic disorder

F25 **Schizoaffective disorders**

Episodic disorders in which both affective and schizophrenic symptoms are prominent but which do not justify a diagnosis of either schizophrenia or depressive or manic episodes. Other conditions in which affective symptoms are superimposed on a pre-existing schizophrenic illness, or co-exist or alternate with persistent delusional disorders of other kinds, are classified under F20–F29. Mood-incongruent psychotic symptoms in affective disorders do not justify a diagnosis of schizoaffective disorder.

F25.0 **Schizoaffective disorder, manic type**

A disorder in which both schizophrenic and manic symptoms are prominent so that the episode of illness does not justify a diagnosis of either schizophrenia or a manic episode. This category should be used for both a single episode and a recurrent disorder in which the majority of episodes are schizoaffective, manic type.

Schizoaffective psychosis, manic type

Schizophreniform psychosis, manic type

F25.1   Schizoaffective disorder, depressive type

A disorder in which both schizophrenic and depressive symptoms are prominent so that the episode of illness does not justify a diagnosis of either schizophrenia or a depressive episode. This category should be used for both a single episode and a recurrent disorder in which the majority of episodes are schizoaffective, depressive type.

Schizoaffective psychosis, depressive type
Schizophreniform psychosis, depressive type

F25.2   Schizoaffective disorder, mixed type

Cyclic schizophrenia
Mixed schizophrenic and affective psychosis

F25.8   Other schizoaffective disorders

F25.9   Schizoaffective disorder, unspecified

Schizoaffective psychosis NOS

F28   Other nonorganic psychotic disorders

Delusional or hallucinatory disorders that do not justify a diagnosis of schizophrenia (F20.–), persistent delusional disorders (F22.–), acute and transient psychotic disorders (F23.–), psychotic types of manic episode (F30.2), or severe depressive episode (F32.3).

Chronic hallucinatory psychosis

F29   Unspecified nonorganic psychosis

Psychosis NOS

Excludes: mental disorder NOS (F99)
           organic or symptomatic psychosis NOS (F09)

Mood [affective] disorders (F30–F39)

This block contains disorders in which the fundamental disturbance is a change in affect or mood to depression (with or without associated anxiety) or to elation. The mood change is usually accompanied by a change in the overall level of activity; most of the other symptoms are either secondary to, or easily understood in the context of, the change in mood and activity. Most of these disorders tend to be recurrent and the onset of individual episodes can often be related to stressful events or situations.

F30 Manic episode

All the subdivisions of this category should be used only for a single episode. Hypomanic or manic episodes in individuals who have had one or more previous affective episodes (depressive, hypomanic, manic, or mixed) should be coded as bipolar affective disorder (F31.–).

Includes: bipolar disorder, single manic episode

F30.0 Hypomania

A disorder characterized by a persistent mild elevation of mood, increased energy and activity, and usually marked feelings of well-being and both physical and mental efficiency. Increased sociability, talkativeness, over-familiarity, increased sexual energy, and a decreased need for sleep are often present but not to the extent that they lead to severe disruption of work or result in social rejection. Irritability, conceit, and boorish behaviour may take the place of the more usual euphoric sociability. The disturbances of mood and behaviour are not accompanied by hallucinations or delusions.

F30.1 Mania without psychotic symptoms

Mood is elevated out of keeping with the patient's circumstances and may vary from carefree joviality to almost uncontrollable excitement. Elation is accompanied by increased energy, resulting in overactivity, pressure of speech, and a decreased need for sleep. Attention cannot be sustained, and there is often marked distractibility. Self-esteem is often inflated with grandiose ideas and overconfidence. Loss of normal social inhibitions may result in behaviour that is reckless, foolhardy, or inappropriate to the circumstances, and out of character.

F30.2 Mania with psychotic symptoms

In addition to the clinical picture described in F30.1, delusions (usually grandiose) or hallucinations (usually of voices speaking directly to the patient) are present, or the excitement, excessive motor activity, and flight of ideas are so extreme that the subject is incomprehensible or inaccessible to ordinary communication.

Mania with:
• mood-congruent psychotic symptoms
• mood-incongruent psychotic symptoms
Manic stupor

F30.8 Other manic episodes

F30.9 Manic episode, unspecified

Mania NOS

F31 Bipolar affective disorder

A disorder characterized by two or more episodes in which the patient's mood and activity levels are significantly disturbed, this disturbance consisting on some occasions of an elevation of mood and increased energy and activity (hypomania or mania) and on others of a lowering of mood and decreased energy and activity (depression). Repeated episodes of hypomania or mania only are classified as bipolar (F31.8).

Includes: manic–depressive:
- illness
- psychosis
- reaction

Excludes: bipolar disorder, single manic episode (F30.–)
cyclothymia (F34.0)

F31.0 **Bipolar affective disorder, current episode hypomanic**
The patient is currently hypomanic, and has had at least one other affective episode (hypomanic, manic, depressive, or mixed) in the past.

F31.1 **Bipolar affective disorder, current episode manic without psychotic symptoms**
The patient is currently manic, without psychotic symptoms (as in F30.1), and has had at least one other affective episode (hypomanic, manic, depressive, or mixed) in the past.

F31.2 **Bipolar affective disorder, current episode manic with psychotic symptoms**
The patient is currently manic, with psychotic symptoms (as in F30.2), and has had at least one other affective episode (hypomanic, manic, depressive, or mixed) in the past.

F31.3 **Bipolar affective disorder, current episode mild or moderate depression**
The patient is currently depressed, as in a depressive episode of either mild or moderate severity (F32.0 or F32.1), and has had at least one authenticated hypomanic, manic, or mixed affective episode in the past.

F31.4 **Bipolar affective disorder, current episode severe depression without psychotic symptoms**
The patient is currently depressed, as in severe depressive episode without psychotic symptoms (F32.2), and has had at least one authenticated hypomanic, manic, or mixed affective episode in the past.

F31.5 **Bipolar affective disorder, current episode severe depression with psychotic symptoms**
The patient is currently depressed, as in severe depressive episode with psychotic symptoms (F32.3), and has had at least one authenticated hypomanic, manic, or mixed affective episode in the past.

F31.6 **Bipolar affective disorder, current episode mixed**

The patient has had at least one authenticated hypomanic, manic, depressive, or mixed affective episode in the past, and currently exhibits either a mixture or a rapid alteration of manic and depressive symptoms.

Excludes: single mixed affective episode (F38.0)

F31.7 **Bipolar affective disorder, currently in remission**

The patient has had at least one authenticated hypomanic, manic, or mixed affective episode in the past, and at least one other affective episode (hypomanic, manic, depressive, or mixed) in addition, but is not currently suffering from any significant mood disturbance, and has not done so for several months. Periods of remission during prophylactic treatment should be coded here.

F31.8 **Other bipolar affective disorders**

Bipolar II disorder
Recurrent manic episodes

F31.9 **Bipolar affective disorder, unspecified**

F32 **Depressive episode**

In typical mild, moderate, or severe depressive episodes, the patient suffers from lowering of mood, reduction of energy, and decrease in activity. Capacity for enjoyment, interest, and concentration is reduced, and marked tiredness after even minimum effort is common. Sleep is usually disturbed and appetite diminished. Self-esteem and self-confidence are almost always reduced and, even in the mild form, some ideas of guilt or worthlessness are often present. The lowered mood varies little from day to day, is unresponsive to circumstances and may be accompanied by so-called "somatic" symptoms, such as loss of interest and pleasurable feelings, waking in the morning several hours before the usual time, depression worst in the morning, marked psychomotor retardation, agitation, loss of appetite, weight loss, and loss of libido. Depending upon the number and severity of the symptoms, a depressive episode may be specified as mild, moderate or severe.

Includes: single episodes of:
- depressive reaction
- psychogenic depression
- reactive depression

Excludes: adjustment disorder (F43.2)
recurrent depressive disorder (F33.–)
when associated with conduct disorders in F91.–
(F92.0)

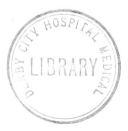

F32.0   Mild depressive episode

Two or three of the above symptoms are usually present. The patient is usually distressed by these but will probably be able to continue with most activities.

F32.1   Moderate depressive episode

Four or more of the above symptoms are usually present and the patient is likely to have great difficulty in continuing with ordinary activities.

F32.2   Severe depressive episode without psychotic symptoms

An episode of depression in which several of the above symptoms are marked and distressing, typically loss of self-esteem and ideas of worthlessness or guilt. Suicidal thoughts and acts are common and a number of "somatic" symptoms are usually present.

Agitated depression
Major depression   } single episode without psychotic symptoms
Vital depression

F32.3   Severe depressive episode with psychotic symptoms

An episode of depression as described in F32.2, but with the presence of hallucinations, delusions, psychomotor retardation, or stupor so severe that ordinary social activities are impossible; there may be danger to life from suicide, dehydration, or starvation. The hallucinations and delusions may or may not be mood-congruent.

Single episodes of:
- major depression with psychotic symptoms
- psychogenic depressive psychosis
- psychotic depression
- reactive depressive psychosis

F32.8   Other depressive episodes

Atypical depression
Single episodes of "masked" depression NOS

F32.9   Depressive episode, unspecified

Depression NOS
Depressive disorder NOS

F33   Recurrent depressive disorder

A disorder characterized by repeated episodes of depression as described for depressive episode (F32.–), without any history of independent episodes of mood elevation and increased energy (mania). There may, however, be brief episodes of mild mood elevation and overactivity (hypomania) immediately after a depressive episode, sometimes precipitated by antidepressant treatment. The more severe forms of recurrent depressive disorder (F33.2 and F33.3) have much in common with earlier concepts such as manic-depressive depression, melancholia, vital depression and endogenous depression. The first episode may occur at any age from childhood to old age, the onset may be either acute or insidious, and the duration varies from a few weeks to many months. The risk that a patient with recurrent depressive disorder will have an episode of mania never disappears completely, however many depressive episodes have been experienced. If such an episode does occur, the diagnosis should be changed to bipolar affective disorder (F31.–).

Includes: recurrent episodes of:
- depressive reaction
- psychogenic depression
- reactive depression

seasonal depressive disorder

Excludes: recurrent brief depressive episodes (F38.1)

F33.0 Recurrent depressive disorder, current episode mild

A disorder characterized by repeated episodes of depression, the current episode being mild, as in F32.0, and without any history of mania.

F33.1 Recurrent depressive disorder, current episode moderate

A disorder characterized by repeated episodes of depression, the current episode being of moderate severity, as in F32.1, and without any history of mania.

F33.2 Recurrent depressive disorder, current episode severe without psychotic symptoms

A disorder characterized by repeated episodes of depression, the current episode being severe without psychotic symptoms, as in F32.2, and without any history of mania.

Endogenous depression without psychotic symptoms

Major depression, recurrent without psychotic symptoms

Manic–depressive psychosis, depressed type without psychotic symptoms

Vital depression, recurrent without psychotic symptoms

F33.3 Recurrent depressive disorder, current episode severe with psychotic symptoms

A disorder characterized by repeated episodes of depression, the current episode being severe with psychotic symptoms, as in F32.3, and with no previous episodes of mania.

Endogenous depression with psychotic symptoms

Manic–depressive psychosis, depressed type with psychotic symptoms

Recurrent severe episodes of:
- major depression with psychotic symptoms
- psychogenic depressive psychosis
- psychotic depression
- reactive depressive psychosis

F33.4   Recurrent depressive disorder, currently in remission

The patient has had two or more depressive episodes as described in F33.0–F33.3, in the past, but has been free from depressive symptoms for several months.

F33.8   Other recurrent depressive disorders

F33.9   Recurrent depressive disorder, unspecified

Monopolar depression NOS

F34   Persistent mood [affective] disorders

Persistent and usually fluctuating disorders of mood in which the majority of the individual episodes are not sufficiently severe to warrant being described as hypomanic or mild depressive episodes. Because they last for many years, and sometimes for the greater part of the patient's adult life, they involve considerable distress and disability. In some instances, recurrent or single manic or depressive episodes may become superimposed on a persistent affective disorder.

F34.0   Cyclothymia

A persistent instability of mood involving numerous periods of depression and mild elation, none of which is sufficiently severe or prolonged to justify a diagnosis of bipolar affective disorder (F31.–) or recurrent depressive disorder (F33.–). This disorder is frequently found in the relatives of patients with bipolar affective disorder. Some patients with cyclothymia eventually develop bipolar affective disorder.

Affective personality disorder
Cycloid personality
Cyclothymic personality

F34.1   Dysthymia

A chronic depression of mood, lasting at least several years, which is not sufficiently severe, or in which individual episodes are not sufficiently prolonged, to justify a diagnosis of severe, moderate, or mild recurrent depressive disorder (F33.–).

Depressive:
• neurosis
• personality disorder
Neurotic depression
Persistent anxiety depression

Excludes: anxiety depression (mild or not persistent) (F41.2)

F34.8   Other persistent mood [affective] disorders

F34.9   Persistent mood [affective] disorder, unspecified

F38 Other mood [affective] disorders

Any other mood disorders that do not justify classification to F30–F34, because they are not of sufficient severity or duration.

F38.0 Other single mood [affective] disorders

Mixed affective episode

F38.1 Other recurrent mood [affective] disorders

Recurrent brief depressive episodes

F38.8 Other specified mood [affective] disorders

F39 Unspecified mood [affective] disorder

Affective psychosis NOS

Neurotic, stress-related and somatoform disorders (F40–F48)

Excludes: when associated with conduct disorders in F91.– (F92.8)

F40 Phobic anxiety disorders

A group of disorders in which anxiety is evoked only, or predominantly, in certain well-defined situations that are not currently dangerous. As a result these situations are characteristically avoided or endured with dread. The patient's concern may be focused on individual symptoms like palpitations or feeling faint and is often associated with secondary fears of dying, losing control, or going mad. Contemplating entry to the phobic situation usually generates anticipatory anxiety. Phobic anxiety and depression often coexist. Whether two diagnoses, phobic anxiety and depressive episode, are needed, or only one, is determined by the time course of the two conditions and by therapeutic considerations at the time of consultation.

F40.0 Agoraphobia

A fairly well-defined cluster of phobias embracing fears of leaving home, entering shops, crowds and public places, or travelling alone in trains, buses or planes. Panic disorder is a frequent feature of both present and past episodes. Depressive and obsessional symptoms and social phobias are also commonly present as subsidiary features. Avoidance of the phobic situation is often prominent, and some agoraphobics experience little anxiety because they are able to avoid their phobic situations.

Agoraphobia without history of panic disorder
Panic disorder with agoraphobia

F40.1   **Social phobias**

Fear of scrutiny by other people leading to avoidance of social situations. More pervasive social phobias are usually associated with low self-esteem and fear of criticism. They may present as a complaint of blushing, hand tremor, nausea, or urgency of micturition, the patient sometimes being convinced that one of these secondary manifestations of their anxiety is the primary problem. Symptoms may progress to panic attacks.

Anthropophobia

Social neurosis

F40.2   **Specific (isolated) phobias**

Phobias restricted to highly specific situations such as proximity to particular animals, heights, thunder, darkness, flying, closed spaces, urinating or defecating in public toilets, eating certain foods, dentistry, or the sight of blood or injury. Though the triggering situation is discrete, contact with it can evoke panic as in agoraphobia or social phobia.

Acrophobia

Animal phobias

Claustrophobia

Simple phobia

Excludes: dysmorphophobia (nondelusional) (F45.2)
nosophobia (F45.2)

F40.8   **Other phobic anxiety disorders**

F40.9   **Phobic anxiety disorder, unspecified**

Phobia NOS

Phobic state NOS

F41   **Other anxiety disorders**

Disorders in which manifestation of anxiety is the major symptom and is not restricted to any particular environmental situation. Depressive and obsessional symptoms, and even some elements of phobic anxiety, may also be present, provided that they are clearly secondary or less severe.

F41.0 **Panic disorder [episodic paroxysmal anxiety]**

The essential feature is recurrent attacks of severe anxiety (panic), which are not restricted to any particular situation or set of circumstances and are therefore unpredictable. As with other anxiety disorders, the dominant symptoms include sudden onset of palpitations, chest pain, choking sensations, dizziness, and feelings of unreality (depersonalization or derealization). There is often also a secondary fear of dying, losing control, or going mad. Panic disorder should not be given as the main diagnosis if the patient has a depressive disorder at the time the attacks start; in these circumstances the panic attacks are probably secondary to depression.

Panic:

- attack
- state

Excludes: panic disorder with agoraphobia (F40.0)

F41.1 **Generalized anxiety disorder**

Anxiety that is generalized and persistent but not restricted to, or even strongly predominating in, any particular environmental circumstances (i.e. it is "free-floating"). The dominant symptoms are variable but include complaints of persistent nervousness, trembling, muscular tensions, sweating, lightheadedness, palpitations, dizziness, and epigastric discomfort. Fears that the patient or a relative will shortly become ill or have an accident are often expressed.

Anxiety:

- neurosis
- reaction
- state

Excludes: neurasthenia (F48.0)

F41.2 **Mixed anxiety and depressive disorder**

This category should be used when symptoms of anxiety and depression are both present, but neither is clearly predominant, and neither type of symptom is present to the extent that justifies a diagnosis if considered separately. When both anxiety and depressive symptoms are present and severe enough to justify individual diagnoses, both diagnoses should be recorded and this category should not be used.

Anxiety depression (mild or not persistent)

F41.3 **Other mixed anxiety disorders**

Symptoms of anxiety mixed with features of other disorders in F42–F48. Neither type of symptom is severe enough to justify a diagnosis if considered separately.

F41.8 **Other specified anxiety disorders**

Anxiety hysteria

F41.9 **Anxiety disorder, unspecified**

Anxiety NOS

F42 Obsessive–compulsive disorder

The essential feature is recurrent obsessional thoughts or compulsive acts. Obsessional thoughts are ideas, images, or impulses that enter the patient's mind again and again in a stereotyped form. They are almost invariably distressing and the patient often tries, unsuccessfully, to resist them. They are, however, recognized as his or her own thoughts, even though they are involuntary and often repugnant. Compulsive acts or rituals are stereotyped behaviours that are repeated again and again. They are not inherently enjoyable, nor do they result in the completion of inherently useful tasks. Their function is to prevent some objectively unlikely event, often involving harm to or caused by the patient, which he or she fears might otherwise occur. Usually, this behaviour is recognized by the patient as pointless or ineffectual and repeated attempts are made to resist. Anxiety is almost invariably present. If compulsive acts are resisted the anxiety gets worse.

Includes: anankastic neurosis
obsessive–compulsive neurosis

Excludes: obsessive–compulsive personality (disorder) (F60.5)

F42.0 Predominantly obsessional thoughts or ruminations

These may take the form of ideas, mental images, or impulses to act, which are nearly always distressing to the subject. Sometimes the ideas are an indecisive, endless consideration of alternatives, associated with an inability to make trivial but necessary decisions in day-to-day living. The relationship between obsessional ruminations and depression is particularly close and a diagnosis of obsessive–compulsive disorder should be preferred only if ruminations arise or persist in the absence of a depressive episode.

F42.1 Predominantly compulsive acts [obsessional rituals]

The majority of compulsive acts are concerned with cleaning (particularly handwashing), repeated checking to ensure that a potentially dangerous situation has not been allowed to develop, or orderliness and tidiness. Underlying the overt behaviour is a fear, usually of danger either to or caused by the patient, and the ritual is an ineffectual or symbolic attempt to avert that danger.

F42.2 Mixed obsessional thoughts and acts

F42.8 Other obsessive–compulsive disorders

F42.9 Obsessive–compulsive disorder, unspecified

F43 Reaction to severe stress, and adjustment disorders

This category differs from others in that it includes disorders identifiable on the basis of not only symptoms and course but also the existence of one or other of two causative influences: an exceptionally stressful life event producing an acute stress reaction, or a significant life change leading to continued unpleasant circumstances that result in an adjustment disorder. Although less severe psychosocial stress ("life events") may precipitate the onset or contribute to the presentation of a very wide range of disorders classified elsewhere in this chapter, its etiological importance is not always clear and in each case will be found to depend on individual, often idiosyncratic, vulnerability, i.e. the life events are neither necessary nor sufficient to explain the occurrence and form of the disorder. In contrast, the disorders brought together here are thought to arise always as a direct consequence of acute severe stress or continued trauma. The stressful events or the continuing unpleasant circumstances are the primary and overriding causal factor and the disorder would not have occurred without their impact. The disorders in this section can thus be regarded as maladaptive responses to severe or continued stress, in that they interfere with successful coping mechanisms and therefore lead to problems of social functioning.

F43.0 Acute stress reaction

A transient disorder that develops in an individual without any other apparent mental disorder in response to exceptional physical and mental stress and that usually subsides within hours or days. Individual vulnerability and coping capacity play a role in the occurrence and severity of acute stress reactions. The symptoms show a typically mixed and changing picture and include an initial state of "daze" with some constriction of the field of consciousness and narrowing of attention, inability to comprehend stimuli, and disorientation. This state may be followed either by further withdrawal from the surrounding situation (to the extent of a dissociative stupor—F44.2), or by agitation and over-activity (flight reaction or fugue). Autonomic signs of panic anxiety (tachycardia, sweating, flushing) are commonly present. The symptoms usually appear within minutes of the impact of the stressful stimulus or event, and disappear within two to three days (often within hours). Partial or complete amnesia (F44.0) for the episode may be present. If the symptoms persist, a change in diagnosis should be considered.

Acute:
- crisis reaction
- reaction to stress

Combat fatigue
Crisis state
Psychic shock

F43.1   Post-traumatic stress disorder

Arises as a delayed or protracted response to a stressful event or situation (of either brief or long duration) of an exceptionally threatening or catastrophic nature, which is likely to cause pervasive distress in almost anyone. Predisposing factors, such as personality traits (e.g. compulsive, asthenic) or previous history of neurotic illness, may lower the threshold for the development of the syndrome or aggravate its course, but they are neither necessary nor sufficient to explain its occurrence. Typical features include episodes of repeated reliving of the trauma in intrusive memories ("flashbacks"), dreams or nightmares, occurring against the persisting background of a sense of "numbness" and emotional blunting, detachment from other people, unresponsiveness to surroundings, anhedonia, and avoidance of activities and situations reminiscent of the trauma. There is usually a state of autonomic hyperarousal with hypervigilance, an enhanced startle reaction, and insomnia. Anxiety and depression are commonly associated with the above symptoms and signs, and suicidal ideation is not infrequent. The onset follows the trauma with a latency period that may range from a few weeks to months. The course is fluctuating but recovery can be expected in the majority of cases. In a small proportion of cases the condition may follow a chronic course over many years, with eventual transition to an enduring personality change (F62.0).

Traumatic neurosis

F43.2   Adjustment disorders

States of subjective distress and emotional disturbance, usually interfering with social functioning and performance, arising in the period of adaptation to a significant life change or a stressful life event. The stressor may have affected the integrity of an individual's social network (bereavement, separation experiences) or the wider system of social supports and values (migration, refugee status), or represented a major developmental transition or crisis (going to school, becoming a parent, failure to attain a cherished personal goal, retirement). Individual predisposition or vulnerability plays an important role in the risk of occurrence and the shaping of the manifestations of adjustment disorders, but it is nevertheless assumed that the condition would not have arisen without the stressor. The manifestations vary and include depressed mood, anxiety or worry (or mixture of these), a feeling of inability to cope, plan ahead, or continue in the present situation, as well as some degree of disability in the performance of daily routine. Conduct disorders may be an associated feature, particularly in adolescents. The predominant feature may be a brief or prolonged depressive reaction, or a disturbance of other emotions and conduct.

Culture shock

Grief reaction

Hospitalism in children

Excludes: separation anxiety disorder of childhood (F93.0)

F43.8   Other reactions to severe stress

F43.9   Reaction to severe stress, unspecified

F44 Dissociative [conversion] disorders

The common themes that are shared by dissociative or conversion disorders are a partial or complete loss of the normal integration between memories of the past, awareness of identity and immediate sensations, and control of bodily movements. All types of dissociative disorders tend to remit after a few weeks or months, particularly if their onset is associated with a traumatic life event. More chronic disorders, particularly paralyses and anaesthesias, may develop if the onset is associated with insoluble problems or interpersonal difficulties. These disorders have previously been classified as various types of "conversion hysteria". They are presumed to be psychogenic in origin, being associated closely in time with traumatic events, insoluble and intolerable problems, or disturbed relationships. The symptoms often represent the patient's concept of how a physical illness would be manifest. Medical examination and investigation do not reveal the presence of any known physical or neurological disorder. In addition, there is evidence that the loss of function is an expression of emotional conflicts or needs. The symptoms may develop in close relationship to psychological stress, and often appear suddenly. Only disorders of physical functions normally under voluntary control and loss of sensations are included here. Disorders involving pain and other complex physical sensations mediated by the autonomic nervous system are classified under somatization disorder (F45.0). The possibility of the later appearance of serious physical or psychiatric disorders should always be kept in mind.

Includes: conversion:
- hysteria
- reaction

hysteria

hysterical psychosis

Excludes: malingering [conscious simulation] (Z76.5)

F44.0 **Dissociative amnesia**

The main feature is loss of memory, usually of important recent events, that is not due to organic mental disorder, and is too great to be explained by ordinary forgetfulness or fatigue. The amnesia is usually centred on traumatic events, such as accidents or unexpected bereavements, and is usually partial and selective. Complete and generalized amnesia is rare, and is usually part of a fugue (F44.1). If this is the case, the disorder should be classified as such. The diagnosis should not be made in the presence of organic brain disorders, intoxication, or excessive fatigue.

Excludes: alcohol- or other psychoactive substance-induced
amnesic disorder (F10–F19 with common fourth
character .6)
amnesia:
- NOS (R41.3)
- anterograde (R41.1)
- retrograde (R41.2)
nonalcoholic organic amnesic syndrome (F04)
postictal amnesia in epilepsy (G40.–)

F44.1 **Dissociative fugue**

Dissociative fugue has all the features of dissociative amnesia, plus purposeful travel beyond the usual everyday range. Although there is amnesia for the period of the fugue, the patient's behaviour during this time may appear completely normal to independent observers.

Excludes: postictal fugue in epilepsy (G40.–)

F44.2 **Dissociative stupor**

Dissociative stupor is diagnosed on the basis of a profound diminution or absence of voluntary movement and normal responsiveness to external stimuli such as light, noise, and touch, but examination and investigation reveal no evidence of a physical cause. In addition, there is positive evidence of psychogenic causation in the form of recent stressful events or problems.

Excludes: organic catatonic disorder (F06.1)
stupor:
- NOS (R40.1)
- catatonic (F20.2)
- depressive (F31–F33)
- manic (F30.2)

F44.3   **Trance and possession disorders**

Disorders in which there is a temporary loss of the sense of personal identity and full awareness of the surroundings. Include here only trance states that are involuntary or unwanted, occurring outside religious or culturally accepted situations.

Excludes: states associated with:
- acute and transient psychotic disorders (F23.–)
- organic personality disorder (F07.0)
- postconcussional syndrome (F07.2)
- psychoactive substance intoxication (F10–F19 with common fourth character .0)
- schizophrenia (F20.–)

F44.4   **Dissociative motor disorders**

In the commonest varieties there is loss of ability to move the whole or a part of a limb or limbs. There may be close resemblance to almost any variety of ataxia, apraxia, akinesia, aphonia, dysarthria, dyskinesia, seizures, or paralysis.

Psychogenic:
- aphonia
- dysphonia

F44.5   **Dissociative convulsions**

Dissociative convulsions may mimic epileptic seizures very closely in terms of movements, but tongue-biting, bruising due to falling, and incontinence of urine are rare, and consciousness is maintained or replaced by a state of stupor or trance.

F44.6   **Dissociative anaesthesia and sensory loss**

Anaesthetic areas of skin often have boundaries that make it clear that they are associated with the patient's ideas about bodily functions, rather than medical knowledge. There may be differential loss between the sensory modalities which cannot be due to a neurological lesion. Sensory loss may be accompanied by complaints of paraesthesia. Loss of vision and hearing are rarely total in dissociative disorders.

Psychogenic deafness

F44.7   **Mixed dissociative [conversion] disorders**

Combination of disorders specified in F44.0–F44.6

F44.8   **Other dissociative [conversion] disorders**

Ganser's syndrome
Multiple personality
Psychogenic:
- confusion
- twilight state

F44.9   **Dissociative [conversion] disorder, unspecified**

347

F45 Somatoform disorders

The main feature is repeated presentation of physical symptoms together with persistent requests for medical investigations, in spite of repeated negative findings and reassurances by doctors that the symptoms have no physical basis. If any physical disorders are present, they do not explain the nature and extent of the symptoms or the distress and preoccupation of the patient.

Excludes: dissociative disorders (F44.–)
    hair-plucking (F98.4)
    lalling (F80.0)
    lisping (F80.8)
    nail-biting (F98.8)
    psychological or behavioural factors associated with
        disorders or diseases classified elsewhere (F54)
    sexual dysfunction, not caused by organic disorder or
        disease (F52.–)
    thumb-sucking (F98.8)
    tic disorders (in childhood and adolescence) (F95.–)
    Tourette's syndrome (F95.2)
    trichotillomania (F63.3)

F45.0 Somatization disorder

The main features are multiple, recurrent and frequently changing physical symptoms of at least two years' duration. Most patients have a long and complicated history of contact with both primary and specialist medical care services, during which many negative investigations or fruitless exploratory operations may have been carried out. Symptoms may be referred to any part or system of the body. The course of the disorder is chronic and fluctuating, and is often associated with disruption of social, interpersonal, and family behaviour. Short-lived (less than two years) and less striking symptom patterns should be classified under undifferentiated somatoform disorder (F45.1).

Multiple psychosomatic disorder

Excludes: malingering [conscious simulation] (Z76.5)

F45.1 Undifferentiated somatoform disorder

When somatoform complaints are multiple, varying and persistent, but the complete and typical clinical picture of somatization disorder is not fulfilled, the diagnosis of undifferentiated somatoform disorder should be considered.

Undifferentiated psychosomatic disorder

F45.2 Hypochondriacal disorder

The essential feature is a persistent preoccupation with the possibility of having one or more serious and progressive physical disorders. Patients manifest persistent somatic complaints or a persistent preoccupation with their physical appearance. Normal or commonplace sensations and appearances are often interpreted by patients as abnormal and distressing, and attention is usually focused upon only one or two organs or systems of the body. Marked depression and anxiety are often present, and may justify additional diagnoses.

Body dysmorphic disorder
Dysmorphophobia (nondelusional)
Hypochondriacal neurosis
Hypochondriasis
Nosophobia

Excludes: delusional dysmorphophobia (F22.8)
        fixed delusions about bodily functions or shape (F22.–)

F45.3   Somatoform autonomic dysfunction

Symptoms are presented by the patient as if they were due to a physical disorder of a system or organ that is largely or completely under autonomic innervation and control, i.e. the cardiovascular, gastrointestinal, respiratory and urogenital systems. The symptoms are usually of two types, neither of which indicates a physical disorder of the organ or system concerned. First, there are complaints based upon objective signs of autonomic arousal, such as palpitations, sweating, flushing, tremor, and expression of fear and distress about the possibility of a physical disorder. Second, there are subjective complaints of a nonspecific or changing nature such as fleeting aches and pains, sensations of burning, heaviness, tightness, and feelings of being bloated or distended, which are referred by the patient to a specific organ or system.

Cardiac neurosis
Da Costa's syndrome
Gastric neurosis
Neurocirculatory asthenia
Psychogenic forms of:
• aerophagy
• cough
• diarrhoea
• dyspepsia
• dysuria
• flatulence
• hiccough
• hyperventilation
• increased frequency of micturition
• irritable bowel syndrome
• pylorospasm

Excludes: psychological and behavioural factors associated with disorders or diseases classified elsewhere (F54)

F45.4　　**Persistent somatoform pain disorder**

The predominant complaint is of persistent, severe, and distressing pain, which cannot be explained fully by a physiological process or a physical disorder, and which occurs in association with emotional conflict or psychosocial problems that are sufficient to allow the conclusion that they are the main causative influences. The result is usually a marked increase in support and attention, either personal or medical. Pain presumed to be of psychogenic origin occurring during the course of depressive disorders or schizophrenia should not be included here.

Psychalgia
Psychogenic:
- backache
- headache
Somatoform pain disorder

Excludes:　backache NOS (M54.9)
　　　　　　pain:
　　　　　　- NOS (R52.9)
　　　　　　- acute (R52.0)
　　　　　　- chronic (R52.2)
　　　　　　- intractable (R52.1)
　　　　　　tension headache (G44.2)

F45.8　　**Other somatoform disorders**

Any other disorders of sensation, function and behaviour, not due to physical disorders, which are not mediated through the autonomic nervous system, which are limited to specific systems or parts of the body, and which are closely associated in time with stressful events or problems.

Psychogenic:
- dysmenorrhoea
- dysphagia, including "globus hystericus"
- pruritus
- torticollis
Teeth-grinding

F45.9　　**Somatoform disorder, unspecified**

Psychosomatic disorder NOS

F48　Other neurotic disorders

F48.0   Neurasthenia

Considerable cultural variations occur in the presentation of this disorder, and two main types occur, with substantial overlap. In one type, the main feature is a complaint of increased fatigue after mental effort, often associated with some decrease in occupational performance or coping efficiency in daily tasks. The mental fatiguability is typically described as an unpleasant intrusion of distracting associations or recollections, difficulty in concentrating, and generally inefficient thinking. In the other type, the emphasis is on feelings of bodily or physical weakness and exhaustion after only minimal effort, accompanied by a feeling of muscular aches and pains and inability to relax. In both types a variety of other unpleasant physical feelings is common, such as dizziness, tension headaches, and feelings of general instability. Worry about decreasing mental and bodily well-being, irritability, anhedonia, and varying minor degrees of both depression and anxiety are all common. Sleep is often disturbed in its initial and middle phases but hypersomnia may also be prominent.

Fatigue syndrome

Use additional code, if desired, to identify previous physical illness.

Excludes: asthenia NOS (R53)
burn-out (Z73.0)
malaise and fatigue (R53)
postviral fatigue syndrome (G93.3)
psychasthenia (F48.8)

F48.1   Depersonalization–derealization syndrome

A rare disorder in which the patient complains spontaneously that his or her mental activity, body, and surroundings are changed in their quality, so as to be unreal, remote, or automatized. Among the varied phenomena of the syndrome, patients complain most frequently of loss of emotions and feelings of estrangement or detachment from their thinking, their body, or the real world. In spite of the dramatic nature of the experience, the patient is aware of the unreality of the change. The sensorium is normal and the capacity for emotional expression intact. Depersonalization–derealization symptoms may occur as part of a diagnosable schizophrenic, depressive, phobic, or obsessive–compulsive disorder. In such cases the diagnosis should be that of the main disorder.

F48.8   Other specified neurotic disorders

Briquet's disorder
Dhat syndrome
Occupational neurosis, including writer's cramp
Psychasthenia
Psychasthenic neurosis
Psychogenic syncope

F48.9   Neurotic disorder, unspecified

Neurosis NOS

351

Behavioural syndromes associated with physiological disturbances and physical factors (F50–F59)

F50 Eating disorders

Excludes: anorexia NOS (R63.0)
feeding:
• difficulties and mismanagement (R63.3)
• disorder of infancy or childhood (F98.2)
polyphagia (R63.2)

F50.0 Anorexia nervosa

A disorder characterized by deliberate weight loss, induced and sustained by the patient. It occurs most commonly in adolescent girls and young women, but adolescent boys and young men may also be affected, as may children approaching puberty and older women up to the menopause. The disorder is associated with a specific psychopathology whereby a dread of fatness and flabbiness of body contour persists as an intrusive overvalued idea, and the patients impose a low weight threshold on themselves. There is usually undernutrition of varying severity with secondary endocrine and metabolic changes and disturbances of bodily function. The symptoms include restricted dietary choice, excessive exercise, induced vomiting and purgation, and use of appetite suppressants and diuretics.

Excludes: loss of appetite (R63.0)
• psychogenic (F50.8)

F50.1 Atypical anorexia nervosa

Disorders that fulfil some of the features of anorexia nervosa but in which the overall clinical picture does not justify that diagnosis. For instance, one of the key symptoms, such as amenorrhoea or marked dread of being fat, may be absent in the presence of marked weight loss and weight-reducing behaviour. This diagnosis should not be made in the presence of known physical disorders associated with weight loss.

F50.2 Bulimia nervosa

A syndrome characterized by repeated bouts of overeating and an excessive preoccupation with the control of body weight, leading to a pattern of overeating followed by vomiting or use of purgatives. This disorder shares many psychological features with anorexia nervosa, including an overconcern with body shape and weight. Repeated vomiting is likely to give rise to disturbances of body electrolytes and physical complications. There is often, but not always, a history of an earlier episode of anorexia nervosa, the interval ranging from a few months to several years.

Bulimia NOS
Hyperorexia nervosa

F50.3   **Atypical bulimia nervosa**
Disorders that fulfil some of the features of bulimia nervosa, but in which the overall clinical picture does not justify that diagnosis. For instance, there may be recurrent bouts of overeating and overuse of purgatives without significant weight change, or the typical overconcern about body shape and weight may be absent.

F50.4   **Overeating associated with other psychological disturbances**
Overeating due to stressful events, such as bereavement, accident, childbirth, etc.

Psychogenic overeating

Excludes: obesity (E66.–)

F50.5   **Vomiting associated with other psychological disturbances**
Repeated vomiting that occurs in dissociative disorders (F44.–) and hypochondriacal disorder (F45.2), and that is not solely due to conditions classified outside this chapter. This subcategory may also be used in addition to O21.– (excessive vomiting in pregnancy) when emotional factors are predominant in the causation of recurrent nausea and vomiting in pregnancy.

Psychogenic vomiting

Excludes: nausea (R11)
vomiting NOS (R11)

F50.8   **Other eating disorders**
Pica in adults
Psychogenic loss of appetite

Excludes: pica of infancy and childhood (F98.3)

F50.9   **Eating disorder, unspecified**

F51   Nonorganic sleep disorders
In many cases, a disturbance of sleep is one of the symptoms of another disorder, either mental or physical. Whether a sleep disorder in a given patient is an independent condition or simply one of the features of another disorder classified elsewhere, either in this chapter or in others, should be determined on the basis of its clinical presentation and course as well as on the therapeutic considerations and priorities at the time of the consultation. Generally, if the sleep disorder is one of the major complaints and is perceived as a condition in itself, the present code should be used along with other pertinent diagnoses describing the psychopathology and pathophysiology involved in a given case. This category includes only those sleep disorders in which emotional causes are considered to be a primary factor, and which are not due to identifiable physical disorders classified elsewhere.

Excludes: sleep disorders (organic) (G47.–)

F51.0   Nonorganic insomnia

A condition of unsatisfactory quantity and/or quality of sleep, which persists for a considerable period of time, including difficulty falling asleep, difficulty staying asleep, or early final wakening. Insomnia is a common symptom of many mental and physical disorders, and should be classified here in addition to the basic disorder only if it dominates the clinical picture.

Excludes: insomnia (organic) (G47.0)

F51.1   Nonorganic hypersomnia

Hypersomnia is defined as a condition of either excessive daytime sleepiness and sleep attacks (not accounted for by an inadequate amount of sleep) or prolonged transition to the fully aroused state upon awakening. In the absence of an organic factor for the occurrence of hypersomnia, this condition is usually associated with mental disorders.

Excludes: hypersomnia (organic) (G47.1)
            narcolepsy (G47.4)

F51.2   Nonorganic disorder of the sleep–wake schedule

A lack of synchrony between the sleep–wake schedule and the desired sleep–wake schedule for the individual's environment, resulting in a complaint of either insomnia or hypersomnia.

Psychogenic inversion of:
- circadian ⎫
- nyctohemeral ⎬ rhythm
- sleep ⎭

Excludes: disorders of the sleep–wake schedule (organic) (G47.2)

F51.3   Sleepwalking [somnambulism]

A state of altered consciousness in which phenomena of sleep and wakefulness are combined. During a sleepwalking episode the individual arises from bed, usually during the first third of nocturnal sleep, and walks about, exhibiting low levels of awareness, reactivity, and motor skill. Upon awakening, there is usually no recall of the event.

F51.4   Sleep terrors [night terrors]

Nocturnal episodes of extreme terror and panic associated with intense vocalization, motility, and high levels of autonomic discharge. The individual sits up or gets up, usually during the first third of nocturnal sleep, with a panicky scream. Quite often he or she rushes to the door as if trying to escape, although very seldom leaves the room. Recall of the event, if any, is very limited (usually to one or two fragmentary mental images).

F51.5   Nightmares

Dream experiences loaded with anxiety or fear. There is very detailed recall of the dream content. The dream experience is very vivid and usually includes themes involving threats to survival, security, or self-esteem. Quite often there is a recurrence of the same or similar frightening nightmare themes. During a typical episode there is a degree of autonomic discharge but no appreciable vocalization or body motility. Upon awakening the individual rapidly becomes alert and oriented.

Dream anxiety disorder

F51.8   Other nonorganic sleep disorders

F51.9   Nonorganic sleep disorder, unspecified

Emotional sleep disorder NOS

F52   Sexual dysfunction, not caused by organic disorder or disease

Sexual dysfunction covers the various ways in which an individual is unable to participate in a sexual relationship as he or she would wish. Sexual response is a psychosomatic process and both psychological and somatic processes are usually involved in the causation of sexual dysfunction.

Excludes: Dhat syndrome (F48.8)

F52.0   Lack or loss of sexual desire

Loss of sexual desire is the principal problem and is not secondary to other sexual difficulties, such as erectile failure or dyspareunia.

Frigidity

Hypoactive sexual desire disorder

F52.1   Sexual aversion and lack of sexual enjoyment

Either the prospect of sexual interaction produces sufficient fear or anxiety that sexual activity is avoided (sexual aversion) or sexual responses occur normally and orgasm is experienced but there is a lack of appropriate pleasure (lack of sexual enjoyment).

Anhedonia (sexual)

F52.2   Failure of genital response

The principal problem in men is erectile dysfunction (difficulty in developing or maintaining an erection suitable for satisfactory intercourse). In women, the principal problem is vaginal dryness or failure of lubrication.

Female sexual arousal disorder

Male erectile disorder

Psychogenic impotence

Excludes: impotence of organic origin (N48.4)

F52.3   Orgasmic dysfunction

Orgasm either does not occur or is markedly delayed.

Inhibited orgasm (male)(female)

Psychogenic anorgasmy

F52.4   Premature ejaculation

The inability to control ejaculation sufficiently for both partners to enjoy sexual interaction.

F52.5   Nonorganic vaginismus

Spasm of the pelvic floor muscles that surround the vagina, causing occlusion of the vaginal opening. Penile entry is either impossible or painful.

Psychogenic vaginismus

Excludes: vaginismus (organic) (N94.2)

F52.6   Nonorganic dyspareunia

Dyspareunia (or pain during sexual intercourse) occurs in both women and men. It can often be attributed to local pathology and should then properly be categorized under the pathological condition. This category is to be used only if there is no primary nonorganic sexual dysfunction (e.g. vaginismus or vaginal dryness).

Psychogenic dyspareunia

Excludes: dyspareunia (organic) (N94.1)

F52.7   Excessive sexual drive

Nymphomania

Satyriasis

F52.8   Other sexual dysfunction, not caused by organic disorder or disease

F52.9   Unspecified sexual dysfunction, not caused by organic disorder or disease

F53 Mental and behavioural disorders associated with the puerperium, not elsewhere classified

This category includes only mental disorders associated with the puerperium (commencing within six weeks of delivery) that do not meet the criteria for disorders classified elsewhere in this chapter, either because insufficient information is available, or because it is considered that special additional clinical features are present that make their classification elsewhere inappropriate.

F53.0   Mild mental and behavioural disorders associated with the puerperium, not elsewhere classified

Depression:
- postnatal NOS
- postpartum NOS

F53.1   Severe mental and behavioural disorders associated with the puerperium, not elsewhere classified

Puerperal psychosis NOS

F53.8   Other mental and behavioural disorders associated with the puerperium, not elsewhere classified

F53.9   Puerperal mental disorder, unspecified

F54 Psychological and behavioural factors associated with disorders or diseases classified elsewhere

This category should be used to record the presence of psychological or behavioural influences thought to have played a major part in the etiology of physical disorders which can be classified to other chapters. Any resulting mental disturbances are usually mild, and often prolonged (such as worry, emotional conflict, apprehension) and do not of themselves justify the use of any of the categories in this chapter.

Psychological factors affecting physical conditions

Examples of the use of this category are:
- asthma F54 and J45.−
- dermatitis F54 and L23–L25
- gastric ulcer F54 and K25.−
- mucous colitis F54 and K58.−
- ulcerative colitis F54 and K51.−
- urticaria F54 and L50.−

Use additional code, if desired, to identify the associated physical disorder.

Excludes: tension-type headache (G44.2)

F55 Abuse of non-dependence-producing substances

A wide variety of medicaments and folk remedies may be involved, but the particularly important groups are: (a) psychotropic drugs that do not produce dependence, such as antidepressants, (b) laxatives, and (c) analgesics that may be purchased without medical prescription, such as aspirin and paracetamol.

Persistent use of these substances often involves unnecessary contacts with medical professionals or supporting staff, and is sometimes accompanied by harmful physical effects of the substances. Attempts to dissuade or forbid the use of the substance are often met with resistance; for laxatives and analgesics this may be in spite of warnings about (or even the development of) physical harm such as renal dysfunction or electrolyte disturbances. Although it is usually clear that the patient has a strong motivation to take the substance, dependence or withdrawal symptoms do not develop as in the case of the psychoactive substances specified in F10–F19.

Abuse of:
- antacids
- herbal or folk remedies
- steroids or hormones
- vitamins

Laxative habit

Excludes: abuse of psychoactive substances (F10–F19)

F59 Unspecified behavioural syndromes associated with physiological disturbances and physical factors

Psychogenic physiological dysfunction NOS

Disorders of adult personality and behaviour (F60–F69)

This block includes a variety of conditions and behaviour patterns of clinical significance which tend to be persistent and appear to be the expression of the individual's characteristic lifestyle and mode of relating to himself or herself and others. Some of these conditions and patterns of behaviour emerge early in the course of individual development, as a result of both constitutional factors and social experience, while others are acquired later in life. Specific personality disorders (F60.–), mixed and other personality disorders (F61.–), and enduring personality changes (F62.–) are deeply ingrained and enduring behaviour patterns, manifesting as inflexible responses to a broad range of personal and social situations. They represent extreme or significant deviations from the way in which the average individual in a given culture perceives, thinks, feels and, particularly, relates to others. Such behaviour patterns tend to be stable and to encompass multiple domains of behaviour and psychological functioning. They are frequently, but not always, associated with various degrees of subjective distress and problems of social performance.

F60 Specific personality disorders

These are severe disturbances in the personality and behavioural tendencies of the individual; not directly resulting from disease, damage, or other insult to the brain, or from another psychiatric disorder; usually involving several areas of the personality; nearly always associated with considerable personal distress and social disruption; and usually manifest since childhood or adolescence and continuing throughout adulthood.

F60.0 Paranoid personality disorder

Personality disorder characterized by excessive sensitivity to setbacks, unforgiveness of insults; suspiciousness and a tendency to distort experience by misconstruing the neutral or friendly actions of others as hostile or contemptuous; recurrent suspicions, without justification, regarding the sexual fidelity of the spouse or sexual partner; and a combative and tenacious sense of personal rights. There may be excessive self-importance, and there is often excessive self-reference.

Personality (disorder):
• expansive paranoid
• fanatic
• querulant
• paranoid
• sensitive paranoid

Excludes: paranoia (F22.0)
            • querulans (F22.8)
           paranoid:
            • psychosis (F22.0)
            • schizophrenia (F20.0)
            • state (F22.0)

F60.1 **Schizoid personality disorder**

Personality disorder characterized by withdrawal from affectional, social and other contacts with preference for fantasy, solitary activities, and introspection. There is a limited capacity to express feelings and to experience pleasure.

Excludes: Asperger's syndrome (F84.5)

delusional disorder (F22.0)

schizoid disorder of childhood (F84.5)

schizophrenia (F20.–)

schizotypal disorder (F21)

F60.2 **Dissocial personality disorder**

Personality disorder characterized by disregard for social obligations, and callous unconcern for the feelings of others. There is gross disparity between behaviour and the prevailing social norms. Behaviour is not readily modifiable by adverse experience, including punishment. There is a low tolerance to frustration and a low threshold for discharge of aggression, including violence; there is a tendency to blame others, or to offer plausible rationalizations for the behaviour bringing the patient into conflict with society.

Personality (disorder):

• amoral

• antisocial

• asocial

• psychopathic

• sociopathic

Excludes: conduct disorders (F91.–)

emotionally unstable personality disorder (F60.3)

F60.3 **Emotionally unstable personality disorder**

Personality disorder characterized by a definite tendency to act impulsively and without consideration of the consequences; the mood is unpredictable and capricious. There is a liability to outbursts of emotion and an incapacity to control the behavioural explosions. There is a tendency to quarrelsome behaviour and to conflicts with others, especially when impulsive acts are thwarted or censored. Two types may be distinguished: the impulsive type, characterized predominantly by emotional instability and lack of impulse control, and the borderline type, characterized in addition by disturbances in self-image, aims, and internal preferences, by chronic feelings of emptiness, by intense and unstable interpersonal relationships, and by a tendency to self-destructive behaviour, including suicide gestures and attempts.

Personality (disorder):

• aggressive

• borderline

• explosive

Excludes: dissocial personality disorder (F60.2)

F60.4   Histrionic personality disorder

Personality disorder characterized by shallow and labile affectivity, self-dramatization, theatricality, exaggerated expression of emotions, suggestibility, egocentricity, self-indulgence, lack of consideration for others, easily hurt feelings, and continuous seeking for appreciation, excitement and attention.

Personality (disorder):

- hysterical
- psychoinfantile

F60.5   Anankastic personality disorder

Personality disorder characterized by feelings of doubt, perfectionism, excessive conscientiousness, checking and preoccupation with details, stubbornness, caution, and rigidity. There may be insistent and unwelcome thoughts or impulses that do not attain the severity of an obsessive–compulsive disorder.

Personality (disorder):

- compulsive
- obsessional
- obsessive–compulsive

Excludes: obsessive–compulsive disorder (F42.–)

F60.6   Anxious [avoidant] personality disorder

Personality disorder characterized by feelings of tension and apprehension, insecurity and inferiority. There is a continuous yearning to be liked and accepted, a hypersensitivity to rejection and criticism with restricted personal attachments, and a tendency to avoid certain activities by habitual exaggeration of the potential dangers or risks in everyday situations.

F60.7   Dependent personality disorder

Personality disorder characterized by pervasive passive reliance on other people to make one's major and minor life decisions, great fear of abandonment, feelings of helplessness and incompetence, passive compliance with the wishes of elders and others, and a weak response to the demands of daily life. Lack of vigour may show itself in the intellectual or emotional spheres; there is often a tendency to transfer responsibility to others.

Personality (disorder):

- asthenic
- inadequate
- passive
- self-defeating

F60.8   **Other specific personality disorders**
Personality (disorder):
- eccentric
- "haltlose" type
- immature
- narcissistic
- passive–aggressive
- psychoneurotic

F60.9   **Personality disorder, unspecified**
Character neurosis NOS
Pathological personality NOS

F61   Mixed and other personality disorders

This category is intended for personality disorders that are often troublesome but do not demonstrate the specific pattern of symptoms that characterize the disorders described in F60.–. As a result they are often more difficult to diagnose than the disorders in F60.–.

Examples include:
- mixed personality disorders with features of several of the disorders in F60.– but without a predominant set of symptoms that would allow a more specific diagnosis
- troublesome personality changes, not classifiable to F60.– or F62.–, and regarded as secondary to a main diagnosis of a coexisting affective or anxiety disorder.

Excludes: accentuated personality traits (Z73.1)

F62   Enduring personality changes, not attributable to brain damage and disease

Disorders of adult personality and behaviour that have developed in persons with no previous personality disorder following exposure to catastrophic or excessive prolonged stress, or following a severe psychiatric illness. These diagnoses should be made only when there is evidence of a definite and enduring change in a person's pattern of perceiving, relating to, or thinking about the environment and himself or herself. The personality change should be significant and be associated with inflexible and maladaptive behaviour not present before the pathogenic experience. The change should not be a direct manifestation of another mental disorder or a residual symptom of any antecedent mental disorder.

Excludes: personality and behavioural disorder due to brain disease, damage and dysfunction (F07.–)

F62.0 **Enduring personality change after catastrophic experience**
Enduring personality change, present for at least two years, following exposure to catastrophic stress. The stress must be so extreme that it is not necessary to consider personal vulnerability in order to explain its profound effect on the personality. The disorder is characterized by a hostile or distrustful attitude towards the world, social withdrawal, feelings of emptiness or hopelessness, a chronic feeling of "being on edge" as if constantly threatened, and estrangement. Post-traumatic stress disorder (F43.1) may precede this type of personality change.

Personality change after:
- concentration camp experiences
- disasters
- prolonged:
  - captivity with an imminent possibility of being killed
  - exposure to life-threatening situations such as being a victim of terrorism
- torture

Excludes: post-traumatic stress disorder (F43.1)

F62.1 **Enduring personality change after psychiatric illness**
Personality change, persisting for at least two years, attributable to the traumatic experience of suffering from a severe psychiatric illness. The change cannot be explained by a previous personality disorder and should be differentiated from residual schizophrenia and other states of incomplete recovery from an antecedent mental disorder. This disorder is characterized by an excessive dependence on and a demanding attitude towards others; conviction of being changed or stigmatized by the illness, leading to an inability to form and maintain close and confiding personal relationships and to social isolation; passivity, reduced interests, and diminished involvement in leisure activities; persistent complaints of being ill, which may be associated with hypochondriacal claims and illness behaviour; dysphoric or labile mood, not due to the presence of a current mental disorder or antecedent mental disorder with residual affective symptoms; and longstanding problems in social and occupational functioning.

F62.8 **Other enduring personality changes**
Chronic pain personality syndrome

F62.9 **Enduring personality change, unspecified**

F63 Habit and impulse disorders

This category includes certain disorders of behaviour that are not classifiable under other categories. They are characterized by repeated acts that have no clear rational motivation, cannot be controlled, and generally harm the patient's own interests and those of other people. The patient reports that the behaviour is associated with impulses to action. The cause of these disorders is not understood and they are grouped together because of broad descriptive similarities, not because they are known to share any other important features.

Excludes: habitual excessive use of alcohol or psychoactive substances (F10–F19)
impulse and habit disorders involving sexual behaviour (F65.–)

F63.0 Pathological gambling

The disorder consists of frequent, repeated episodes of gambling that dominate the patient's life to the detriment of social, occupational, material, and family values and commitments.

Compulsive gambling

Excludes: excessive gambling by manic patients (F30.–)
gambling and betting NOS (Z72.6)
gambling in dissocial personality disorder (F60.2)

F63.1 Pathological fire-setting [pyromania]

Disorder characterized by multiple acts of, or attempts at, setting fire to property or other objects, without apparent motive, and by a persistent preoccupation with subjects related to fire and burning. This behaviour is often associated with feelings of increasing tension before the act, and intense excitement immediately afterwards.

Excludes: fire-setting (by)(in):
- adult with dissocial personality disorder (F60.2)
- alcohol or psychoactive substance intoxication (F10–F19, with common fourth character .0)
- as the reason for observation for suspected mental disorder (Z03.2)
- conduct disorders (F91.–)
- organic mental disorders (F00–F09)
- schizophrenia (F20.–)

F63.2 **Pathological stealing [kleptomania]**

Disorder characterized by repeated failure to resist impulses to steal objects that are not acquired for personal use or monetary gain. The objects may instead be discarded, given away, or hoarded. This behaviour is usually accompanied by an increasing sense of tension before, and a sense of gratification during and immediately after, the act.

Excludes: depressive disorder with stealing (F31–F33)

organic mental disorders (F00–F09)

shoplifting as the reason for observation for suspected mental disorder (Z03.2)

F63.3 **Trichotillomania**

A disorder characterized by noticeable hair-loss due to a recurrent failure to resist impulses to pull out hairs. The hair-pulling is usually preceded by mounting tension and is followed by a sense of relief or gratification. This diagnosis should not be made if there is a pre-existing inflammation of the skin, or if the hair-pulling is in response to a delusion or a hallucination.

Excludes: stereotyped movement disorder with hair-plucking (F98.4)

F63.8 **Other habit and impulse disorders**

Other kinds of persistently repeated maladaptive behaviour that are not secondary to a recognized psychiatric syndrome, and in which it appears that the patient is repeatedly failing to resist impulses to carry out the behaviour. There is a prodromal period of tension with a feeling of release at the time of the act.

Intermittent explosive disorder

F63.9 **Habit and impulse disorder, unspecified**

F64 Gender identity disorders

F64.0 **Transsexualism**

A desire to live and be accepted as a member of the opposite sex, usually accompanied by a sense of discomfort with, or inappropriateness of, one's anatomic sex, and a wish to have surgery and hormonal treatment to make one's body as congruent as possible with one's preferred sex.

F64.1 **Dual-role transvestism**

The wearing of clothes of the opposite sex for part of the individual's existence in order to enjoy the temporary experience of membership of the opposite sex, but without any desire for a more permanent sex change or associated surgical reassignment, and without sexual excitement accompanying the cross-dressing.

Gender identity disorder of adolescence or adulthood, nontranssexual type

Excludes: fetishistic transvestism (F65.1)

F64.2 **Gender identity disorder of childhood**

A disorder, usually first manifest during early childhood (and always well before puberty), characterized by a persistent and intense distress about assigned sex, together with a desire to be (or insistence that one is) of the other sex. There is a persistent preoccupation with the dress and activities of the opposite sex and repudiation of the individual's own sex. The diagnosis requires a profound disturbance of the normal gender identity; mere tomboyishness in girls or girlish behaviour in boys is not sufficient. Gender identity disorders in individuals who have reached or are entering puberty should not be classified here but in F66.–.

Excludes: egodystonic sexual orientation (F66.1)
sexual maturation disorder (F66.0)

F64.8 **Other gender identity disorders**

F64.9 **Gender identity disorder, unspecified**

Gender-role disorder NOS

F65 Disorders of sexual preference

Includes: paraphilias

F65.0 **Fetishism**

Reliance on some non-living object as a stimulus for sexual arousal and sexual gratification. Many fetishes are extensions of the human body, such as articles of clothing or footwear. Other common examples are characterized by some particular texture such as rubber, plastic or leather. Fetish objects vary in their importance to the individual. In some cases they simply serve to enhance sexual excitement achieved in ordinary ways (e.g. having the partner wear a particular garment).

F65.1 **Fetishistic transvestism**

The wearing of clothes of the opposite sex principally to obtain sexual excitement and to create the appearance of a person of the opposite sex. Fetishistic transvestism is distinguished from transsexual transvestism by its clear association with sexual arousal and the strong desire to remove the clothing once orgasm occurs and sexual arousal declines. It can occur as an earlier phase in the development of transsexualism.

Transvestic fetishism

F65.2 **Exhibitionism**

A recurrent or persistent tendency to expose the genitalia to strangers (usually of the opposite sex) or to people in public places, without inviting or intending closer contact. There is usually, but not invariably, sexual excitement at the time of the exposure and the act is commonly followed by masturbation.

F65.3   **Voyeurism**

A recurrent or persistent tendency to look at people engaging in sexual or intimate behaviour such as undressing. This is carried out without the observed people being aware, and usually leads to sexual excitement and masturbation.

F65.4   **Paedophilia**

A sexual preference for children, boys or girls or both, usually of prepubertal or early pubertal age.

F65.5   **Sadomasochism**

A preference for sexual activity which involves the infliction of pain or humiliation, or bondage. If the subject prefers to be the recipient of such stimulation this is called masochism; if the provider, sadism. Often an individual obtains sexual excitement from both sadistic and masochistic activities.

Masochism
Sadism

F65.6   **Multiple disorders of sexual preference**

Sometimes more than one abnormal sexual preference occurs in one person and there is none of first rank. The most common combination is fetishism, transvestism and sadomasochism.

F65.8   **Other disorders of sexual preference**

A variety of other patterns of sexual preference and activity, including making obscene telephone calls, rubbing up against people for sexual stimulation in crowded public places, sexual activity with animals, and use of strangulation or anoxia for intensifying sexual excitement.

Frotteurism
Necrophilia

F65.9   **Disorder of sexual preference, unspecified**

Sexual deviation NOS

F66   Psychological and behavioural disorders associated with sexual development and orientation

Note: Sexual orientation by itself is not to be regarded as a disorder.

F66.0   **Sexual maturation disorder**

The patient suffers from uncertainty about his or her gender identity or sexual orientation, which causes anxiety or depression. Most commonly this occurs in adolescents who are not certain whether they are homosexual, heterosexual or bisexual in orientation, or in individuals who, after a period of apparently stable sexual orientation (often within a longstanding relationship), find that their sexual orientation is changing.

367

F66.1   Egodystonic sexual orientation

The gender identity or sexual preference (heterosexual, homosexual, bisexual, or prepubertal) is not in doubt, but the individual wishes it were different because of associated psychological and behavioural disorders, and may seek treatment in order to change it.

F66.2   Sexual relationship disorder

The gender identity or sexual orientation (heterosexual, homosexual, or bisexual) is responsible for difficulties in forming or maintaining a relationship with a sexual partner.

F66.8   Other psychosexual development disorders

F66.9   Psychosexual development disorder, unspecified

F68   Other disorders of adult personality and behaviour

F68.0   Elaboration of physical symptoms for psychological reasons

Physical symptoms compatible with and originally due to a confirmed physical disorder, disease or disability become exaggerated or prolonged due to the psychological state of the patient. The patient is commonly distressed by this pain or disability, and is often preoccupied with worries, which may be justified, of the possibility of prolonged or progressive disability or pain.

Compensation neurosis

F68.1   Intentional production or feigning of symptoms or disabilities, either physical or psychological [factitious disorder]

The patient feigns symptoms repeatedly for no obvious reason and may even inflict self-harm in order to produce symptoms or signs. The motivation is obscure and presumably internal with the aim of adopting the sick role. The disorder is often combined with marked disorders of personality and relationships.

Hospital hopper syndrome
Münchhausen's syndrome
Peregrinating patient

Excludes: factitial dermatitis (L98.1)
           person feigning illness (with obvious motivation)
           (Z76.5)

F68.8   Other specified disorders of adult personality and behaviour

Character disorder NOS
Relationship disorder NOS

F69 **Unspecified disorder of adult personality and behaviour**

Mental retardation
(F70–F79)

A condition of arrested or incomplete development of the mind, which is especially characterized by impairment of skills manifested during the developmental period, skills which contribute to the overall level of intelligence, i.e. cognitive, language, motor, and social abilities. Retardation can occur with or without any other mental or physical condition.

Degrees of mental retardation are conventionally estimated by standardized intelligence tests. These can be supplemented by scales assessing social adaptation in a given environment. These measures provide an approximate indication of the degree of mental retardation. The diagnosis will also depend on the overall assessment of intellectual functioning by a skilled diagnostician.

Intellectual abilities and social adaptation may change over time, and, however poor, may improve as a result of training and rehabilitation. Diagnosis should be based on the current levels of functioning.

The following fourth-character subdivisions are for use with categories F70–F79 to identify the extent of impairment of behaviour:

.0 With the statement of no, or minimal, impairment of behaviour

.1 Significant impairment of behaviour requiring attention or treatment

.8 Other impairments of behaviour

.9 Without mention of impairment of behaviour

Use additional code, if desired, to identify associated conditions such as autism, other developmental disorders, epilepsy, conduct disorders, or severe physical handicap.

F70 **Mild mental retardation**

Approximate IQ range of 50 to 69 (in adults, mental age from 9 to under 12 years). Likely to result in some learning difficulties in school. Many adults will be able to work and maintain good social relationships and contribute to society.

Includes: feeble-mindedness
mild mental subnormality

369

F71 Moderate mental retardation

Approximate IQ range of 35 to 49 (in adults, mental age from 6 to under 9 years). Likely to result in marked developmental delays in childhood but most can learn to develop some degree of independence in self-care and acquire adequate communication and academic skills. Adults will need varying degrees of support to live and work in the community.

Includes: moderate mental subnormality

F72 Severe mental retardation

Approximate IQ range of 20 to 34 (in adults, mental age from 3 to under 6 years). Likely to result in continuous need of support.

Includes: severe mental subnormality

F73 Profound mental retardation

IQ under 20 (in adults, mental age below 3 years). Results in severe limitation in self-care, continence, communication and mobility.

Includes: profound mental subnormality

F78 Other mental retardation

F79 Unspecified mental retardation

Includes: mental:
- deficiency NOS
- subnormality NOS

Disorders of psychological development (F80–F89)

The disorders included in this block have in common: (a) onset invariably during infancy or childhood; (b) impairment or delay in development of functions that are strongly related to biological maturation of the central nervous system; and (c) a steady course without remissions and relapses. In most cases, the functions affected include language, visuo-spatial skills, and motor coordination. Usually, the delay or impairment has been present from as early as it could be detected reliably and will diminish progressively as the child grows older, although milder deficits often remain in adult life.

F80 Specific developmental disorders of speech and language

Disorders in which normal patterns of language acquisition are disturbed from the early stages of development. The conditions are not directly attributable to neurological or speech mechanism abnormalities, sensory impairments, mental retardation, or environmental factors. Specific developmental disorders of speech and language are often followed by associated problems, such as difficulties in reading and spelling, abnormalities in interpersonal relationships, and emotional and behavioural disorders.

F80.0 Specific speech articulation disorder

A specific developmental disorder in which the child's use of speech sounds is below the appropriate level for its mental age, but in which there is a normal level of language skills.

Developmental:
• phonological disorder
• speech articulation disorder
Dyslalia
Functional speech articulation disorder
Lalling

Excludes: speech articulation impairment (due to):
• aphasia NOS (R47.0)
• apraxia (R48.2)
• hearing loss (H90–H91)
• mental retardation (F70–F79)
• with language developmental disorder:
 • expressive (F80.1)
 • receptive (F80.2)

371

F80.1   Expressive language disorder

A specific developmental disorder in which the child's ability to use expressive spoken language is markedly below the appropriate level for its mental age, but in which language comprehension is within normal limits. There may or may not be abnormalities in articulation.

Developmental dysphasia or aphasia, expressive type

Excludes: acquired aphasia with epilepsy [Landau–Kleffner] (F80.3)

developmental dysphasia or aphasia, receptive type (F80.2)

dysphasia and aphasia NOS (R47.0)

elective mutism (F94.0)

mental retardation (F70–F79)

pervasive developmental disorders (F84.–)

F80.2   Receptive language disorder

A specific developmental disorder in which the child's understanding of language is below the appropriate level for its mental age. In virtually all cases expressive language will also be markedly affected and abnormalities in word-sound production are common.

Congenital auditory imperception
Developmental:
• dysphasia or aphasia, receptive type
• Wernicke's aphasia
Word deafness

Excludes: acquired aphasia with epilepsy [Landau–Kleffner] (F80.3)

autism (F84.0–F84.1)

dysphasia and aphasia:
• NOS (R47.0)
• expressive type (F80.1)
elective mutism (F94.0)

language delay due to deafness (H90–H91)

mental retardation (F70–F79)

F80.3   Acquired aphasia with epilepsy [Landau–Kleffner]

A disorder in which the child, having previously made normal progress in language development, loses both receptive and expressive language skills but retains general intelligence; the onset of the disorder is accompanied by paroxysmal abnormalities on the EEG, and in the majority of cases also by epileptic seizures. Usually the onset is between the ages of three and seven years, with skills being lost over days or weeks. The temporal association between the onset of seizures and loss of language is variable, with one preceding the other (either way round) by a few months to two years. An inflammatory encephalitic process has been suggested as a possible cause of this disorder. About two-thirds of patients are left with a more or less severe receptive language deficit.

Excludes: aphasia (due to):
- NOS (R47.0)
- autism (F84.0–F84.1)
- disintegrative disorders of childhood (F84.2–F84.3)

F80.8   Other developmental disorders of speech and language
Lisping

F80.9   Developmental disorder of speech and language, unspecified
Language disorder NOS

F81   Specific developmental disorders of scholastic skills

Disorders in which the normal patterns of skill acquisition are disturbed from the early stages of development. This is not simply a consequence of a lack of opportunity to learn, it is not solely a result of mental retardation, and it is not due to any form of acquired brain trauma or disease.

F81.0   Specific reading disorder
The main feature is a specific and significant impairment in the development of reading skills that is not solely accounted for by mental age, visual acuity problems, or inadequate schooling. Reading comprehension skill, reading word recognition, oral reading skill, and performance of tasks requiring reading may all be affected. Spelling difficulties are frequently associated with specific reading disorder and often remain into adolescence even after some progress in reading has been made. Specific developmental disorders of reading are commonly preceded by a history of disorders in speech or language development. Associated emotional and behavioural disturbances are common during the school age period.

"Backward reading"
Developmental dyslexia
Specific reading retardation

Excludes: alexia NOS (R48.0)
dyslexia NOS (R48.0)
reading difficulties secondary to emotional disorders (F93.–)

F81.1   Specific spelling disorder

The main feature is a specific and significant impairment in the development of spelling skills in the absence of a history of specific reading disorder, which is not solely accounted for by low mental age, visual acuity problems, or inadequate schooling. The ability to spell orally and to write out words correctly are both affected.

Specific spelling retardation (without reading disorder)

Excludes: agraphia NOS (R48.8)

spelling difficulties:

- associated with a reading disorder (F81.0)
- due to inadequate teaching (Z55.8)

F81.2   Specific disorder of arithmetical skills

Involves a specific impairment in arithmetical skills that is not solely explicable on the basis of general mental retardation or of inadequate schooling. The deficit concerns mastery of basic computational skills of addition, subtraction, multiplication, and division rather than of the more abstract mathematical skills involved in algebra, trigonometry, geometry, or calculus.

Developmental:

- acalculia
- arithmetical disorder
- Gerstmann's syndrome

Excludes: acalculia NOS (R48.8)

arithmetical difficulties:

- associated with a reading or spelling disorder (F81.3)
- due to inadequate teaching (Z55.8)

F81.3   Mixed disorder of scholastic skills

An ill-defined residual category of disorders in which both arithmetical and reading or spelling skills are significantly impaired, but in which the disorder is not solely explicable in terms of general mental retardation or of inadequate schooling. It should be used for disorders meeting the criteria for both F81.2 and either F81.0 or F81.1.

Excludes: specific:

- disorder of arithmetical skills (F81.2)
- reading disorder (F81.0)
- spelling disorder (F81.1)

F81.8   Other developmental disorders of scholastic skills

Developmental expressive writing disorder

F81.9   Developmental disorder of scholastic skills, unspecified

Knowledge acquisition disability NOS
Learning:

- disability NOS
- disorder NOS

F82 Specific developmental disorder of motor function

A disorder in which the main feature is a serious impairment in the development of motor coordination that is not solely explicable in terms of general intellectual retardation or of any specific congenital or acquired neurological disorder. Nevertheless, in most cases a careful clinical examination shows marked neurodevelopmental immaturities such as choreiform movements of unsupported limbs or mirror movements and other associated motor features, as well as signs of impaired fine and gross motor coordination.

Clumsy child syndrome
Developmental:
• coordination disorder
• dyspraxia

Excludes: abnormalities of gait and mobility (R26.–)
lack of coordination (R27.–)
• secondary to mental retardation (F70–F79)

F83 Mixed specific developmental disorders

A residual category for disorders in which there is some admixture of specific developmental disorders of speech and language, of scholastic skills, and of motor function, but in which none predominates sufficiently to constitute the prime diagnosis. This mixed category should be used only when there is a major overlap between each of these specific developmental disorders. The disorders are usually, but not always, associated with some degree of general impairment of cognitive functions. Thus, the category should be used when there are dysfunctions meeting the criteria for two or more of F80.–, F81.– and F82.

F84 Pervasive developmental disorders

A group of disorders characterized by qualitative abnormalities in reciprocal social interactions and in patterns of communication, and by a restricted, stereotyped, repetitive repertoire of interests and activities. These qualitative abnormalities are a pervasive feature of the individual's functioning in all situations.

Use additional code, if desired, to identify any associated medical condition and mental retardation.

F84.0   Childhood autism

A type of pervasive developmental disorder that is defined by: (a) the presence of abnormal or impaired development that is manifest before the age of three years, and (b) the characteristic type of abnormal functioning in all the three areas of psychopathology: reciprocal social interaction, communication, and restricted, stereotyped, repetitive behaviour. In addition to these specific diagnostic features, a range of other nonspecific problems are common, such as phobias, sleeping and eating disturbances, temper tantrums, and (self-directed) aggression.

Autistic disorder
Infantile:
- autism
- psychosis
Kanner's syndrome

Excludes: autistic psychopathy (F84.5)

F84.1   Atypical autism

A type of pervasive developmental disorder that differs from childhood autism either in age of onset or in failing to fulfil all three sets of diagnostic criteria. This subcategory should be used when there is abnormal and impaired development that is present only after age three years, and a lack of sufficient demonstrable abnormalities in one or two of the three areas of psychopathology required for the diagnosis of autism (namely, reciprocal social interactions, communication, and restricted, stereotyped, repetitive behaviour) in spite of characteristic abnormalities in the other area(s). Atypical autism arises most often in profoundly retarded individuals and in individuals with a severe specific developmental disorder of receptive language.

Atypical childhood psychosis
Mental retardation with autistic features

Use additional code (F70–F79), if desired, to identify mental retardation.

F84.2   Rett's syndrome

A condition, so far found only in girls, in which apparently normal early development is followed by partial or complete loss of speech and of skills in locomotion and use of hands, together with deceleration in head growth, usually with an onset between seven and 24 months of age. Loss of purposive hand movements, hand-wringing stereotypies, and hyperventilation are characteristic. Social and play development are arrested but social interest tends to be maintained. Trunk ataxia and apraxia start to develop by age four years and choreoathetoid movements frequently follow. Severe mental retardation almost invariably results.

F84.3   **Other childhood disintegrative disorder**

A type of pervasive developmental disorder that is defined by a period of entirely normal development before the onset of the disorder, followed by a definite loss of previously acquired skills in several areas of development over the course of a few months. Typically, this is accompanied by a general loss of interest in the environment, by stereotyped, repetitive motor mannerisms, and by autistic-like abnormalities in social interaction and communication. In some cases the disorder can be shown to be due to some associated encephalopathy but the diagnosis should be made on the behavioural features.

Dementia infantilis

Disintegrative psychosis

Heller's syndrome

Symbiotic psychosis

Use additional code, if desired, to identify any associated neurological condition.

Excludes: Rett's syndrome (F84.2)

F84.4   **Overactive disorder associated with mental retardation and stereotyped movements**

An ill-defined disorder of uncertain nosological validity. The category is designed to include a group of children with severe mental retardation (IQ below 50) who show major problems in hyperactivity and in attention, as well as stereotyped behaviours. They tend not to benefit from stimulant drugs (unlike those with an IQ in the normal range) and may exhibit a severe dysphoric reaction (sometimes with psychomotor retardation) when given stimulants. In adolescence, the overactivity tends to be replaced by underactivity (a pattern that is not usual in hyperkinetic children with normal intelligence). This syndrome is also often associated with a variety of developmental delays, either specific or global. The extent to which the behavioural pattern is a function of low IQ or of organic brain damage is not known.

F84.5   **Asperger's syndrome**

A disorder of uncertain nosological validity, characterized by the same type of qualitative abnormalities of reciprocal social interaction that typify autism, together with a restricted, stereotyped, repetitive repertoire of interests and activities. It differs from autism primarily in the fact that there is no general delay or retardation in language or in cognitive development. This disorder is often associated with marked clumsiness. There is a strong tendency for the abnormalities to persist into adolescence and adult life. Psychotic episodes occasionally occur in early adult life.

Autistic psychopathy

Schizoid disorder of childhood

F84.8   **Other pervasive developmental disorders**

F84.9   **Pervasive developmental disorder, unspecified**

F88 **Other disorders of psychological development**
Developmental agnosia

F89 **Unspecified disorder of psychological development**
Developmental disorder NOS

Behavioural and emotional disorders with onset usually occurring in childhood and adolescence (F90–F98)

F90 **Hyperkinetic disorders**

A group of disorders characterized by an early onset (usually in the first five years of life), lack of persistence in activities that require cognitive involvement, and a tendency to move from one activity to another without completing any one, together with disorganized, ill-regulated, and excessive activity. Several other abnormalities may be associated. Hyperkinetic children are often reckless and impulsive, prone to accidents, and find themselves in disciplinary trouble because of unthinking breaches of rules rather than deliberate defiance. Their relationships with adults are often socially disinhibited, with a lack of normal caution and reserve. They are unpopular with other children and may become isolated. Impairment of cognitive functions is common, and specific delays in motor and language development are disproportionately frequent. Secondary complications include dissocial behaviour and low self-esteem.

Excludes: anxiety disorders (F41.–)
mood [affective] disorders (F30–F39)
pervasive developmental disorders (F84.–)
schizophrenia (F20.–)

F90.0 **Disturbance of activity and attention**
Attention deficit:
- disorder with hyperactivity
- hyperactivity disorder
- syndrome with hyperactivity

Excludes: hyperkinetic disorder associated with conduct disorder (F90.1)

F90.1 **Hyperkinetic conduct disorder**
Hyperkinetic disorder associated with conduct disorder

F90.8   Other hyperkinetic disorders

F90.9   Hyperkinetic disorder, unspecified
Hyperkinetic reaction of childhood or adolescence NOS
Hyperkinetic syndrome NOS

F91 Conduct disorders

Disorders characterized by a repetitive and persistent pattern of dissocial, aggressive, or defiant conduct. Such behaviour should amount to major violations of age-appropriate social expectations; it should therefore be more severe than ordinary childish mischief or adolescent rebelliousness and should imply an enduring pattern of behaviour (six months or longer). Features of conduct disorder can also be symptomatic of other psychiatric conditions, in which case the underlying diagnosis should be preferred.

Examples of the behaviours on which the diagnosis is based include excessive levels of fighting or bullying, cruelty to other people or animals, severe destructiveness to property, fire-setting, stealing, repeated lying, truancy from school and running away from home, unusually frequent and severe temper tantrums, and disobedience. Any one of these behaviours, if marked, is sufficient for the diagnosis, but isolated dissocial acts are not.

Excludes: mood [affective] disorders (F30–F39)
             pervasive developmental disorders (F84.–)
             schizophrenia (F20.–)
             when associated with:
             • emotional disorders (F92.–)
             • hyperkinetic disorders (F90.1)

F91.0   Conduct disorder confined to the family context
Conduct disorder involving dissocial or aggressive behaviour (and not merely oppositional, defiant, disruptive behaviour), in which the abnormal behaviour is entirely, or almost entirely, confined to the home and to interactions with members of the nuclear family or immediate household. The disorder requires that the overall criteria for F91.– be met; even severely disturbed parent–child relationships are not of themselves sufficient for diagnosis.

F91.1   Unsocialized conduct disorder
Disorder characterized by the combination of persistent dissocial or aggressive behaviour (meeting the overall criteria for F91.– and not merely comprising oppositional, defiant, disruptive behaviour) with significant pervasive abnormalities in the individual's relationships with other children.

Conduct disorder, solitary aggressive type
Unsocialized aggressive disorder

F91.2   Socialized conduct disorder

Disorder involving persistent dissocial or aggressive behaviour (meeting the overall criteria for F91.– and not merely comprising oppositional, defiant, disruptive behaviour) occurring in individuals who are generally well integrated into their peer group.

Conduct disorder, group type

Group delinquency

Offences in the context of gang membership

Stealing in company with others

Truancy from school

F91.3   Oppositional defiant disorder

Conduct disorder, usually occurring in younger children, primarily characterized by markedly defiant, disobedient, disruptive behaviour that does not include delinquent acts or the more extreme forms of aggressive or dissocial behaviour. The disorder requires that the overall criteria for F91.– be met; even severely mischievous or naughty behaviour is not in itself sufficient for diagnosis. Caution should be employed before using this category, especially with older children, because clinically significant conduct disorder will usually be accompanied by dissocial or aggressive behaviour that goes beyond mere defiance, disobedience, or disruptiveness.

F91.8   Other conduct disorders

F91.9   Conduct disorder, unspecified

Childhood:

- behavioural disorder NOS
- conduct disorder NOS

F92   Mixed disorders of conduct and emotions

A group of disorders characterized by the combination of persistently aggressive, dissocial or defiant behaviour with overt and marked symptoms of depression, anxiety or other emotional upsets. The criteria for both conduct disorders of childhood (F91.–) and emotional disorders of childhood (F93.–) or an adult-type neurotic diagnosis (F40–F48) or a mood disorder (F30–F39) must be met.

F92.0   Depressive conduct disorder

This category requires the combination of conduct disorder (F91.–) with persistent and marked depression of mood (F32.–), as demonstrated by symptoms such as excessive misery, loss of interest and pleasure in usual activities, self-blame, and hopelessness; disturbances of sleep or appetite may also be present.

Conduct disorder in F91.– associated with depressive disorder in F32.–

F92.8   **Other mixed disorders of conduct and emotions**

This category requires the combination of conduct disorder (F91.–) with persistent and marked emotional symptoms such as anxiety, obsessions or compulsions, depersonalization or derealization, phobias, or hypochondriasis.

Conduct disorder in F91.– associated with:

- emotional disorder in F93.–
- neurotic disorder in F40–F48

F92.9   **Mixed disorder of conduct and emotions, unspecified**

F93   Emotional disorders with onset specific to childhood

Mainly exaggerations of normal developmental trends rather than phenomena that are qualitatively abnormal in themselves. Developmental appropriateness is used as the key diagnostic feature in defining the difference between these emotional disorders, with onset specific to childhood, and the neurotic disorders (F40–F48).

Excludes: when associated with conduct disorder (F92.–)

F93.0   **Separation anxiety disorder of childhood**

Should be diagnosed when fear of separation constitutes the focus of the anxiety and when such anxiety first arose during the early years of childhood. It is differentiated from normal separation anxiety when it is of a degree (severity) that is statistically unusual (including an abnormal persistence beyond the usual age period), and when it is associated with significant problems in social functioning.

Excludes: mood [affective] disorders (F30–F39)
neurotic disorders (F40–F48)
phobic anxiety disorder of childhood (F93.l)
social anxiety disorder of childhood (F93.2)

F93.1   **Phobic anxiety disorder of childhood**

Fears in childhood that show a marked developmental phase specificity and arise (to some extent) in a majority of children, but that are abnormal in degree. Other fears that arise in childhood but that are not a normal part of psychosocial development (for example agoraphobia) should be coded under the appropriate category in section F40–F48.

Excludes: generalized anxiety disorder (F41.1)

F93.2   **Social anxiety disorder of childhood**

In this disorder there is a wariness of strangers and social apprehension or anxiety when encountering new, strange, or socially threatening situations. This category should be used only where such fears arise during the early years, and are both unusual in degree and accompanied by problems in social functioning.

Avoidant disorder of childhood or adolescence

381

F93.3   Sibling rivalry disorder

Some degree of emotional disturbance usually following the birth of an immediately younger sibling is shown by a majority of young children. A sibling rivalry disorder should be diagnosed only if the degree or persistence of the disturbance is both statistically unusual and associated with abnormalities of social interaction.

Sibling jealousy

F93.8   Other childhood emotional disorders

Identity disorder

Overanxious disorder

Excludes: gender identity disorder of childhood (F64.2)

F93.9   Childhood emotional disorder, unspecified

F94   Disorders of social functioning with onset specific to childhood and adolescence

A somewhat heterogeneous group of disorders that have in common abnormalities in social functioning which begin during the developmental period, but which (unlike the pervasive developmental disorders) are not primarily characterized by an apparently constitutional social incapacity or deficit that pervades all areas of functioning. In many instances, serious environmental distortions or privations probably play a crucial role in etiology.

F94.0   Elective mutism

Characterized by a marked, emotionally determined selectivity in speaking, such that the child demonstrates a language competence in some situations but fails to speak in other (definable) situations. The disorder is usually associated with marked personality features involving social anxiety, withdrawal, sensitivity, or resistance.

Selective mutism

Excludes: pervasive developmental disorders (F84.–)

schizophrenia (F20.–)

specific developmental disorders of speech and
    language (F80.–)

transient mutism as part of separation anxiety in
    young children (F93.0)

F94.1   **Reactive attachment disorder of childhood**

Starts in the first five years of life and is characterized by persistent abnormalities in the child's pattern of social relationships that are associated with emotional disturbance and are reactive to changes in environmental circumstances (e.g. fearfulness and hypervigilance, poor social interaction with peers, aggression towards self and others, misery, and growth failure in some cases). The syndrome probably occurs as a direct result of severe parental neglect, abuse, or serious mishandling.

Use additional code, if desired, to identify any associated failure to thrive or growth retardation.

Excludes: Asperger's syndrome (F84.5)
disinhibited attachment disorder of childhood (F94.2)
maltreatment syndromes (T74.–)
normal variation in pattern of selective attachment
sexual or physical abuse in childhood, resulting in
psychosocial problems (Z61.4–Z61.6)

F94.2   **Disinhibited attachment disorder of childhood**

A particular pattern of abnormal social functioning that arises during the first five years of life and that tends to persist despite marked changes in environmental circumstances, e.g. diffuse, nonselectively focused attachment behaviour, attention-seeking and indiscriminately friendly behaviour, poorly modulated peer interactions; depending on circumstances there may also be associated emotional or behavioural disturbance.

Affectionless psychopathy
Institutional syndrome

Excludes: Asperger's syndrome (F84.5)
hospitalism in children (F43.2)
hyperkinetic disorders (F90.–)
reactive attachment disorder of childhood (F94.l)

F94.8   **Other childhood disorders of social functioning**

F94.9   **Childhood disorder of social functioning, unspecified**

F95 Tic disorders

Syndromes in which the predominant manifestation is some form of tic. A tic is an involuntary, rapid, recurrent, nonrhythmic motor movement (usually involving circumscribed muscle groups) or vocal production that is of sudden onset and that serves no apparent purpose. Tics tend to be experienced as irresistible but usually they can be suppressed for varying periods of time, are exacerbated by stress, and disappear during sleep. Common simple motor tics include only eye-blinking, neck-jerking, shoulder-shrugging, and facial grimacing. Common simple vocal tics include throat-clearing, barking, sniffing, and hissing. Common complex tics include hitting oneself, jumping, and hopping. Common complex vocal tics include the repetition of particular words, and sometimes the use of socially unacceptable (often obscene) words (coprolalia), and the repetition of one's own sounds or words (palilalia).

F95.0 Transient tic disorder

Meets the general criteria for a tic disorder but the tics do not persist longer than 12 months. The tics usually take the form of eye-blinking, facial grimacing, or head-jerking.

F95.1 Chronic motor or vocal tic disorder

Meets the general criteria for a tic disorder, in which there are motor or vocal tics (but not both), that may be either single or multiple (but usually multiple), and last for more than a year.

F95.2 Combined vocal and multiple motor tic disorder [de la Tourette]

A form of tic disorder in which there are, or have been, multiple motor tics and one or more vocal tics, although these need not have occurred concurrently. The disorder usually worsens during adolescence and tends to persist into adult life. The vocal tics are often multiple with explosive repetitive vocalizations, throat-clearing, and grunting, and there may be the use of obscene words or phrases. Sometimes there is associated gestural echopraxia which may also be of an obscene nature (copropraxia).

F95.8 Other tic disorders

F95.9 Tic disorder, unspecified

Tic NOS

F98 Other behavioural and emotional disorders with onset usually occurring in childhood and adolescence

A heterogeneous group of disorders that share the characteristic of an onset in childhood but otherwise differ in many respects. Some of the conditions represent well-defined syndromes but others are no more than symptom complexes that need inclusion because of their frequency and association with psychosocial problems, and because they cannot be incorporated into other syndromes.

Excludes: breath-holding spells (R06.8)
gender identity disorder of childhood (F64.2)
Kleine–Levin syndrome (G47.8)
obsessive–compulsive disorder (F42.–)
sleep disorders due to emotional causes (F51.–)

F98.0 Nonorganic enuresis

A disorder characterized by involuntary voiding of urine, by day and by night, which is abnormal in relation to the individual's mental age, and which is not a consequence of a lack of bladder control due to any neurological disorder, to epileptic attacks, or to any structural abnormality of the urinary tract. The enuresis may have been present from birth or it may have arisen following a period of acquired bladder control. The enuresis may or may not be associated with a more widespread emotional or behavioural disorder.

Enuresis (primary)(secondary) of nonorganic origin
Functional enuresis
Psychogenic enuresis
Urinary incontinence of nonorganic origin

Excludes: enuresis NOS (R32)

F98.1 Nonorganic encopresis

Repeated, voluntary or involuntary passage of faeces, usually of normal or near-normal consistency, in places not appropriate for that purpose in the individual's own sociocultural setting. The condition may represent an abnormal continuation of normal infantile incontinence, it may involve a loss of continence following the acquisition of bowel control, or it may involve the deliberate deposition of faeces in inappropriate places in spite of normal physiological bowel control. The condition may occur as a monosymptomatic disorder, or it may form part of a wider disorder, especially an emotional disorder (F93.–) or a conduct disorder (F91.–).

Functional encopresis
Incontinence of faeces of nonorganic origin
Psychogenic encopresis

Use additional code, if desired, to identify the cause of any coexisting constipation.

Excludes: encopresis NOS (R15)

385

F98.2   **Feeding disorder of infancy and childhood**

A feeding disorder of varying manifestations usually specific to infancy and early childhood. It generally involves food refusal and extreme faddiness in the presence of an adequate food supply, a reasonably competent caregiver, and the absence of organic disease. There may or may not be associated rumination (repeated regurgitation without nausea or gastrointestinal illness).

Rumination disorder of infancy

Excludes: anorexia nervosa and other eating disorders (F50.–)
feeding:
- difficulties and mismanagement (R63.3)
- problems of newborn (P92.–)
pica of infancy or childhood (F98.3)

F98.3   **Pica of infancy and childhood**

Persistent eating of non-nutritive substances (such as soil, paint chippings, etc.). It may occur as one of many symptoms that are part of a more widespread psychiatric disorder (such as autism), or as a relatively isolated psychopathological behaviour; only the latter is classified here. The phenomenon is most common in mentally retarded children and, if mental retardation is also present, F70–F79 should be selected as the main diagnosis.

F98.4   **Stereotyped movement disorders**

Voluntary, repetitive, stereotyped, nonfunctional (and often rhythmic) movements that do not form part of any recognized psychiatric or neurological condition. When such movements occur as symptoms of some other disorder, only the overall disorder should be recorded. The movements that are of a non self-injurious variety include: body-rocking, head-rocking, hair-plucking, hair-twisting, finger-flicking mannerisms, and hand-flapping. Stereotyped self-injurious behaviour includes repetitive head-banging, face-slapping, eye-poking, and biting of hands, lips or other body parts. All the stereotyped movement disorders occur most frequently in association with mental retardation (when this is the case, both should be recorded). If eye-poking occurs in a child with visual impairment, both should be coded: eye-poking under this category and the visual condition under the appropriate somatic disorder code.

Stereotype/habit disorder

Excludes: abnormal involuntary movements (R25.–)
movement disorders of organic origin (G20–G25)
nail-biting (F98.8)
nose-picking (F98.8)
stereotypies that are part of a broader psychiatric condition (F00–F95)
thumb-sucking (F98.8)
tic disorders (F95.–)
trichotillomania (F63.3)

F98.5 **Stuttering [stammering]**
Speech that is characterized by frequent repetition or prolongation of sounds or syllables or words, or by frequent hesitations or pauses that disrupt the rhythmic flow of speech. It should be classified as a disorder only if its severity is such as to markedly disturb the fluency of speech.

Excludes: tic disorders (F95.–)
cluttering (F98.6)

F98.6 **Cluttering**
A rapid rate of speech with breakdown in fluency, but no repetitions or hesitations, of a severity to give rise to diminished speech intelligibility. Speech is erratic and dysrhythmic, with rapid jerky spurts that usually involve faulty phrasing patterns.

Excludes: stuttering (F98.5)
tic disorders (F95.–)

F98.8 **Other specified behavioural and emotional disorders with onset usually occurring in childhood and adolescence**
Attention deficit disorder without hyperactivity
Excessive masturbation
Nail-biting
Nose-picking
Thumb-sucking

F98.9 **Unspecified behavioural and emotional disorders with onset usually occurring in childhood and adolescence**

Unspecified mental disorder (F99)

F99 **Mental disorder, not otherwise specified**
Mental illness NOS

Excludes: organic mental disorder NOS (F06.9)

CHAPTER VI

Diseases of the nervous system (G00–G99)

Excludes: certain conditions originating in the perinatal period (P00–P96)

certain infectious and parasitic diseases (A00–B99)

complications of pregnancy, childbirth and the puerperium (O00–O99)

congenital malformations, deformations and chromosomal abnormalities (Q00–Q99)

endocrine, nutritional and metabolic diseases (E00–E90)

injury, poisoning and certain other consequences of external causes (S00–T98)

neoplasms (C00–D48)

symptoms, signs and abnormal clinical and laboratory findings, not elsewhere classified (R00–R99)

This chapter contains the following blocks:

G00–G09 Inflammatory diseases of the central nervous system

G10–G13 Systemic atrophies primarily affecting the central nervous system

G20–G26 Extrapyramidal and movement disorders

G30–G32 Other degenerative diseases of the nervous system

G35–G37 Demyelinating diseases of the central nervous system

G40–G47 Episodic and paroxysmal disorders

G50–G59 Nerve, nerve root and plexus disorders

G60–G64 Polyneuropathies and other disorders of the peripheral nervous system

G70–G73 Diseases of myoneural junction and muscle

G80–G83 Cerebral palsy and other paralytic syndromes

G90–G99 Other disorders of the nervous system

Asterisk categories for this chapter are provided as follows:

G01* Meningitis in bacterial diseases classified elsewhere

G02* Meningitis in other infectious and parasitic diseases classified elsewhere

G05* Encephalitis, myelitis and encephalomyelitis in diseases classified elsewhere

G07* Intracranial and intraspinal abscess and granuloma in diseases classified elsewhere

G13*   Systemic atrophies primarily affecting central nervous system in diseases classified elsewhere
G22*   Parkinsonism in diseases classified elsewhere
G26*   Extrapyramidal and movement disorders in diseases classified elsewhere
G32*   Other degenerative disorders of nervous system in diseases classified elsewhere
G46*   Vascular syndromes of brain in cerebrovascular diseases
G53*   Cranial nerve disorders in diseases classified elsewhere
G55*   Nerve root and plexus compressions in diseases classified elsewhere
G59*   Mononeuropathy in diseases classified elsewhere
G63*   Polyneuropathy in diseases classified elsewhere
G73*   Disorders of myoneural junction and muscle in diseases classified elsewhere
G94*   Other disorders of brain in diseases classified elsewhere
G99*   Other disorders of nervous system in diseases classified elsewhere

Inflammatory diseases of the central nervous system (G00–G09)

G00 Bacterial meningitis, not elsewhere classified

Includes: arachnoiditis
leptomeningitis
meningitis   } bacterial
pachymeningitis

Excludes: bacterial:
• meningoencephalitis (G04.2)
• meningomyelitis (G04.2)

G00.0   Haemophilus meningitis
Meningitis due to *Haemophilus influenzae*

G00.1   Pneumococcal meningitis

G00.2   Streptococcal meningitis

G00.3   Staphylococcal meningitis

G00.8 **Other bacterial meningitis**
Meningitis due to:
- *Escherichia coli*
- Friedländer bacillus
- *Klebsiella*

G00.9 **Bacterial meningitis, unspecified**
Meningitis:
- purulent NOS
- pyogenic NOS
- suppurative NOS

G01* Meningitis in bacterial diseases classified elsewhere
Meningitis (in):
- anthrax (A22.8†)
- gonococcal (A54.8†)
- leptospirosis (A27.–†)
- listerial (A32.1†)
- Lyme disease (A69.2†)
- meningococcal (A39.0†)
- neurosyphilis (A52.1†)
- salmonella infection (A02.2†)
- syphilis:
  - congenital (A50.4†)
  - secondary (A51.4†)
- tuberculous (A17.0†)
- typhoid fever (A01.0†)

Excludes: meningoencephalitis and meningomyelitis in bacterial
diseases classified elsewhere (G05.0*)

G02* Meningitis in other infectious and parasitic diseases classified elsewhere
Excludes: meningoencephalitis and meningomyelitis in other
infectious and parasitic diseases classified
elsewhere (G05.1–G05.2*)

G02.0* **Meningitis in viral diseases classified elsewhere**
Meningitis (due to):
- adenoviral (A87.1†)
- enteroviral (A87.0†)
- herpesviral [herpes simplex] (B00.3†)
- infectious mononucleosis (B27.–†)
- measles (B05.1†)
- mumps (B26.1†)
- rubella (B06.0†)
- varicella [chickenpox] (B01.0†)
- zoster (B02.1†)

G02.1* **Meningitis in mycoses**
Meningitis (in):
- candidal (B37.5†)
- coccidioidomycosis (B38.4†)
- cryptococcal (B45.1†)

G02.8* **Meningitis in other specified infectious and parasitic diseases classified elsewhere**
Meningitis due to:
- African trypanosomiasis (B56.–†)
- Chagas' disease (chronic) (B57.4†)

G03 Meningitis due to other and unspecified causes

Includes: arachnoiditis
leptomeningitis
meningitis   due to other and unspecified
pachymeningitis   causes

Excludes: meningoencephalitis (G04.–)
meningomyelitis (G04.–)

G03.0 **Nonpyogenic meningitis**
Nonbacterial meningitis

G03.1 **Chronic meningitis**

G03.2 **Benign recurrent meningitis [Mollaret]**

G03.8 **Meningitis due to other specified causes**

G03.9 **Meningitis, unspecified**
Arachnoiditis (spinal) NOS

G04 — Encephalitis, myelitis and encephalomyelitis

Includes: acute ascending myelitis
meningoencephalitis
meningomyelitis

Excludes: benign myalgic encephalomyelitis (G93.3)
encephalopathy:
- NOS (G93.4)
- alcoholic (G31.2)
- toxic (G92)
multiple sclerosis (G35)
myelitis:
- acute transverse (G37.3)
- subacute necrotizing (G37.4)

G04.0 Acute disseminated encephalitis
Encephalitis ⎱
Encephalomyelitis ⎰ postimmunization

Use additional external cause code (Chapter XX), if desired, to identify vaccine.

G04.1 Tropical spastic paraplegia

G04.2 Bacterial meningoencephalitis and meningomyelitis, not elsewhere classified

G04.8 Other encephalitis, myelitis and encephalomyelitis
Postinfectious encephalitis and encephalomyelitis NOS

G04.9 Encephalitis, myelitis and encephalomyelitis, unspecified
Ventriculitis (cerebral) NOS

G05* Encephalitis, myelitis and encephalomyelitis in diseases classified elsewhere

Includes: meningoencephalitis and meningomyelitis in diseases classified elsewhere

G05.0* Encephalitis, myelitis and encephalomyelitis in bacterial diseases classified elsewhere

Encephalitis, myelitis or encephalomyelitis (in):
- listerial (A32.1†)
- meningococcal (A39.8†)
- syphilis:
  - congenital (A50.4†)
  - late (A52.1†)
- tuberculous (A17.8†)

G05.1* Encephalitis, myelitis and encephalomyelitis in viral diseases classified elsewhere

Encephalitis, myelitis or encephalomyelitis (in):
- adenoviral (A85.1†)
- cytomegaloviral (B25.8†)
- enteroviral (A85.0†)
- herpesviral [herpes simplex] (B00.4†)
- influenza (J10.8†, J11.8†)
- measles (B05.0†)
- mumps (B26.2†)
- postchickenpox (B01.1†)
- rubella (B06.0†)
- zoster (B02.0†)

G05.2* Encephalitis, myelitis and encephalomyelitis in other infectious and parasitic diseases classified elsewhere

Encephalitis, myclitis or encephalomyelitis in:
- African trypanosomiasis (B56.–†)
- Chagas' disease (chronic) (B57.4†)
- naegleriasis (B60.2†)
- toxoplasmosis (B58.2†)

Eosinophilic meningoencephalitis (B83.2†)

G05.8* Encephalitis, myelitis and encephalomyelitis in other diseases classified elsewhere

Encephalitis in systemic lupus erythematosus (M32.1†)

G06 Intracranial and intraspinal abscess and granuloma

Use additional code (B95–B97), if desired, to identify infectious agent.

G06.0 Intracranial abscess and granuloma

Abscess (embolic)(of):
- brain [any part]
- cerebellar
- cerebral
- otogenic

Intracranial abscess or granuloma:
- epidural
- extradural
- subdural

G06.1 Intraspinal abscess and granuloma

Abscess (embolic) of spinal cord [any part]
Intraspinal abscess or granuloma:
- epidural
- extradural
- subdural

G06.2 Extradural and subdural abscess, unspecified

G07* Intracranial and intraspinal abscess and granuloma in diseases classified elsewhere

Abscess of brain:
- amoebic (A06.6†)
- gonococcal (A54.8†)
- tuberculous (A17.8†)

Schistosomiasis granuloma of brain (B65.–†)
Tuberculoma of:
- brain (A17.8†)
- meninges (A17.1†)

G08 Intracranial and intraspinal phlebitis and thrombophlebitis

Septic:
- embolism
- endophlebitis
- phlebitis
- thrombophlebitis
- thrombosis

of intracranial or intraspinal venous sinuses and veins

Excludes: intracranial phlebitis and thrombophlebitis:
- complicating:
  - abortion or ectopic or molar pregnancy (O00–O07, O08.7)
  - pregnancy, childbirth and the puerperium (O22.5, O87.3)
- of nonpyogenic origin (I67.6)
- nonpyogenic intraspinal phlebitis and thrombophlebitis (G95.1)

G09 Sequelae of inflammatory diseases of central nervous system

Note: This category is to be used to indicate conditions whose primary classification is to G00–G08 (i.e. excluding those marked with an asterisk (*)) as the cause of sequelae, themselves classifiable elsewhere. The "sequelae" include conditions specified as such or as late effects, or those present one year or more after onset of the causal condition. For use of this category reference should be made to the relevant morbidity and mortality coding rules and guidelines in Volume 2.

Systemic atrophies primarily affecting the central nervous system (G10–G13)

G10 Huntington's disease
Huntington's chorea

G11 Hereditary ataxia
Excludes: hereditary and idiopathic neuropathy (G60.–)
infantile cerebral palsy (G80.–)
metabolic disorders (E70–E90)

G11.0 **Congenital nonprogressive ataxia**

G11.1 **Early-onset cerebellar ataxia**

Note: Onset usually before the age of 20

Early-onset cerebellar ataxia with:
• essential tremor
• myoclonus [Hunt's ataxia]
• retained tendon reflexes
Friedreich's ataxia (autosomal recessive)
X-linked recessive spinocerebellar ataxia

G11.2 **Late-onset cerebellar ataxia**

Note: Onset usually after the age of 20

G11.3 **Cerebellar ataxia with defective DNA repair**
Ataxia telangiectasia [Louis–Bar]
Excludes: Cockayne's syndrome (Q87.1)
xeroderma pigmentosum (Q82.1)

G11.4 **Hereditary spastic paraplegia**

G11.8 **Other hereditary ataxias**

G11.9 **Hereditary ataxia, unspecified**
Hereditary cerebellar:
• ataxia NOS
• degeneration
• disease
• syndrome

G12   Spinal muscular atrophy and related syndromes

G12.0   **Infantile spinal muscular atrophy, type I [Werdnig–Hoffman]**

G12.1   **Other inherited spinal muscular atrophy**
Progressive bulbar palsy of childhood [Fazio–Londe]
Spinal muscular atrophy:
- adult form
- childhood form, type II
- distal
- juvenile form, type III [Kugelberg–Welander]
- scapuloperoneal form

G12.2   **Motor neuron disease**
Familial motor neuron disease
Lateral sclerosis:
- amyotrophic
- primary
Progressive:
- bulbar palsy
- spinal muscular atrophy

G12.8   **Other spinal muscular atrophies and related syndromes**

G12.9   **Spinal muscular atrophy, unspecified**

G13*   Systemic atrophies primarily affecting central nervous system in diseases classified elsewhere

G13.0*   **Paraneoplastic neuromyopathy and neuropathy**
Carcinomatous neuromyopathy (C00–C97†)
Sensorial paraneoplastic neuropathy [Denny Brown] (C00–D48†)

G13.1*   **Other systemic atrophy primarily affecting central nervous system in neoplastic disease**
Paraneoplastic limbic encephalopathy (C00–D48†)

G13.2*   **Systemic atrophy primarily affecting central nervous system in myxoedema (E00.1†, E03.–†)**

G13.8*   **Systemic atrophy primarily affecting central nervous system in other diseases classified elsewhere**

Extrapyramidal and movement disorders (G20–G26)

G20 Parkinson's disease

Hemiparkinsonism
Paralysis agitans
Parkinsonism or Parkinson's disease:
- NOS
- idiopathic
- primary

G21 Secondary parkinsonism

G21.0 Malignant neuroleptic syndrome
Use additional external cause code (Chapter XX), if desired, to identify drug.

G21.1 Other drug-induced secondary parkinsonism
Use additional external cause code (Chapter XX), if desired, to identify drug.

G21.2 Secondary parkinsonism due to other external agents
Use additional external cause code (Chapter XX), if desired, to identify external agent.

G21.3 Postencephalitic parkinsonism

G21.8 Other secondary parkinsonism

G21.9 Secondary parkinsonism, unspecified

G22* Parkinsonism in diseases classified elsewhere

Syphilitic parkinsonism (A52.1†)

G23 Other degenerative diseases of basal ganglia

Excludes: multi-system degeneration (G90.3)

G23.0 Hallervorden–Spatz disease
Pigmentary pallidal degeneration

G23.1 Progressive supranuclear ophthalmoplegia [Steele–Richardson–Olszewski]

G23.2 **Striatonigral degeneration**

G23.8 **Other specified degenerative diseases of basal ganglia**
Calcification of basal ganglia

G23.9 **Degenerative disease of basal ganglia, unspecified**

G24 Dystonia
Includes: dyskinesia
Excludes: athetoid cerebral palsy (G80.3)

G24.0 **Drug-induced dystonia**
Use additional external cause code (Chapter XX), if desired, to
identify drug.

G24.1 **Idiopathic familial dystonia**
Idiopathic dystonia NOS

G24.2 **Idiopathic nonfamilial dystonia**

G24.3 **Spasmodic torticollis**
Excludes: torticollis NOS (M43.6)

G24.4 **Idiopathic orofacial dystonia**
Orofacial dyskinesia

G24.5 **Blepharospasm**

G24.8 **Other dystonia**

G24.9 **Dystonia, unspecified**
Dyskinesia NOS

G25 Other extrapyramidal and movement disorders

G25.0 **Essential tremor**
Familial tremor
Excludes: tremor NOS (R25.1)

G25.1 **Drug-induced tremor**
Use additional external cause code (Chapter XX), if desired, to
identify drug.

G25.2 **Other specified forms of tremor**
Intention tremor

G25.3 **Myoclonus**
Drug-induced myoclonus

Use additional external cause code (Chapter XX), if desired, to identify drug, if drug-induced.

Excludes: facial myokymia (G51.4)
myoclonic epilepsy (G40.–)

G25.4 **Drug-induced chorea**
Use additional external cause code (Chapter XX), if desired, to identify drug.

G25.5 **Other chorea**
Chorea NOS

Excludes: chorea NOS with heart involvement (I02.0)
Huntington's chorea (G10)
rheumatic chorea (I02.–)
Sydenham's chorea (I02.–)

G25.6 **Drug-induced tics and other tics of organic origin**
Use additional external cause code (Chapter XX), if desired, to identify drug, if drug-induced.

Excludes: de la Tourette's syndrome (F95.2)
tic NOS (F95.9)

G25.8 **Other specified extrapyramidal and movement disorders**
Restless legs syndrome
Stiff-man syndrome

G25.9 **Extrapyramidal and movement disorder, unspecified**

G26* **Extrapyramidal and movement disorders in diseases classified elsewhere**

Other degenerative diseases of the nervous system (G30–G32)

G30 Alzheimer's disease

Includes: senile and presenile forms
Excludes: senile:
- degeneration of brain NEC (G31.1)
- dementia NOS (F03)
senility NOS (R54)

G30.0 Alzheimer's disease with early onset

Note: Onset usually before the age of 65

G30.1 Alzheimer's disease with late onset

Note: Onset usually after the age of 65

G30.8 Other Alzheimer's disease

G30.9 Alzheimer's disease, unspecified

G31 Other degenerative diseases of nervous system, not elsewhere classified

Excludes: Reye's syndrome (G93.7)

G31.0 Circumscribed brain atrophy
Pick's disease
Progressive isolated aphasia

G31.1 Senile degeneration of brain, not elsewhere classified
Excludes: Alzheimer's disease (G30.–)
senility NOS (R54)

G31.2 Degeneration of nervous system due to alcohol
Alcoholic:
- cerebellar:
  - ataxia
  - degeneration
- cerebral degeneration
- encephalopathy
Dysfunction of autonomic nervous system due to alcohol

G31.8 Other specified degenerative diseases of nervous system
Grey-matter degeneration [Alpers]
Subacute necrotizing encephalopathy [Leigh]

G31.9   **Degenerative disease of nervous system, unspecified**

G32* Other degenerative disorders of nervous system in diseases classified elsewhere

G32.0*   **Subacute combined degeneration of spinal cord in diseases classified elsewhere**
Subacute combined degeneration of spinal cord in vitamin B_{12} deficiency (E53.8†)

G32.8*   **Other specified degenerative disorders of nervous system in diseases classified elsewhere**

Demyelinating diseases of the central nervous system (G35–G37)

G35 Multiple sclerosis
Multiple sclerosis (of):
- NOS
- brain stem
- cord
- disseminated
- generalized

G36 Other acute disseminated demyelination
Excludes: postinfectious encephalitis and encephalomyelitis NOS (G04.8)

G36.0   **Neuromyelitis optica [Devic]**
Demyelination in optic neuritis
Excludes: optic neuritis NOS (H46)

G36.1   **Acute and subacute haemorrhagic leukoencephalitis [Hurst]**

G36.8   **Other specified acute disseminated demyelination**

G36.9   **Acute disseminated demyelination, unspecified**

G37 Other demyelinating diseases of central nervous system

G37.0 Diffuse sclerosis
Periaxial encephalitis
Schilder's disease
Excludes: adrenoleukodystrophy [Addison–Schilder] (E71.3)

G37.1 Central demyelination of corpus callosum

G37.2 Central pontine myelinolysis

G37.3 Acute transverse myelitis in demyelinating disease of central nervous system
Acute transverse myelitis NOS
Excludes: multiple sclerosis (G35)
neuromyelitis optica [Devic] (G36.0)

G37.4 Subacute necrotizing myelitis

G37.5 Concentric sclerosis [Baló]

G37.8 Other specified demyelinating diseases of central nervous system

G37.9 Demyelinating disease of central nervous system, unspecified

Episodic and paroxysmal disorders (G40–G47)

G40 Epilepsy
Excludes: Landau–Kleffner syndrome (F80.3)
seizure (convulsive) NOS (R56.8)
status epilepticus (G41.–)
Todd's paralysis (G83.8)

G40.0 Localization-related (focal)(partial) idiopathic epilepsy and epileptic syndromes with seizures of localized onset
Benign childhood epilepsy with centrotemporal EEG spikes
Childhood epilepsy with occipital EEG paroxysms

G40.1   **Localization-related (focal)(partial) symptomatic epilepsy and epileptic syndromes with simple partial seizures**
Attacks without alteration of consciousness
Simple partial seizures developing into secondarily generalized seizures

G40.2   **Localization-related (focal)(partial) symptomatic epilepsy and epileptic syndromes with complex partial seizures**
Attacks with alteration of consciousness, often with automatisms
Complex partial seizures developing into secondarily generalized seizures

G40.3   **Generalized idiopathic epilepsy and epileptic syndromes**
Benign:
• myoclonic epilepsy in infancy
• neonatal convulsions (familial)
Childhood absence epilepsy [pyknolepsy]
Epilepsy with grand mal seizures on awakening
Juvenile:
• absence epilepsy
• myoclonic epilepsy [impulsive petit mal]
Nonspecific epileptic seizures:
• atonic
• clonic
• myoclonic
• tonic
• tonic-clonic

G40.4   **Other generalized epilepsy and epileptic syndromes**
Epilepsy with:
• myoclonic absences
• myoclonic-astatic seizures
Infantile spasms
Lennox–Gastaut syndrome
Salaam attacks
Symptomatic early myoclonic encephalopathy
West's syndrome

G40.5   Special epileptic syndromes
Epilepsia partialis continua [Kozhevnikof]
Epileptic seizures related to:
- alcohol
- drugs
- hormonal changes
- sleep deprivation
- stress

Use additional external cause code (Chapter XX), if desired, to identify drug, if drug-induced.

G40.6   Grand mal seizures, unspecified (with or without petit mal)

G40.7   Petit mal, unspecified, without grand mal seizures

G40.8   Other epilepsy
Epilepsies and epileptic syndromes undetermined as to whether they are focal or generalized

G40.9   Epilepsy, unspecified
Epileptic:
- convulsions NOS
- fits NOS
- seizures NOS

G41 Status epilepticus

G41.0   Grand mal status epilepticus
Tonic-clonic status epilepticus
Excludes: epilepsia partialis continua [Kozhevnikof] (G40.5)

G41.1   Petit mal status epilepticus
Epileptic absence status

G41.2   Complex partial status epilepticus

G41.8   Other status epilepticus

G41.9   Status epilepticus, unspecified

G43 Migraine
Use additional external cause code (Chapter XX), if desired, to identify drug, if drug-induced.
Excludes: headache NOS (R51)

G43.0   Migraine without aura [common migraine]

G43.1 **Migraine with aura [classical migraine]**
Migraine:
- aura without headache
- basilar
- equivalents
- familial hemiplegic
- with:
  - acute-onset aura
  - prolonged aura
  - typical aura

G43.2 **Status migrainosus**

G43.3 **Complicated migraine**

G43.8 **Other migraine**
Ophthalmoplegic migraine
Retinal migraine

G43.9 **Migraine, unspecified**

G44 Other headache syndromes

Excludes: atypical facial pain (G50.1)
headache NOS (R51)
trigeminal neuralgia (G50.0)

G44.0 **Cluster headache syndrome**
Chronic paroxysmal hemicrania
Cluster headache:
- chronic
- episodic

G44.1 **Vascular headache, not elsewhere classified**
Vascular headache NOS

G44.2 **Tension-type headache**
Chronic tension-type headache
Episodic tension headache
Tension headache NOS

G44.3 **Chronic post-traumatic headache**

G44.4 **Drug-induced headache, not elsewhere classified**
Use additional external cause code (Chapter XX), if desired, to identify drug.

G44.8 **Other specified headache syndromes**

G45 Transient cerebral ischaemic attacks and related syndromes

Excludes: neonatal cerebral ischaemia (P91.0)

G45.0 **Vertebro-basilar artery syndrome**

G45.1 **Carotid artery syndrome (hemispheric)**

G45.2 **Multiple and bilateral precerebral artery syndromes**

G45.3 **Amaurosis fugax**

G45.4 **Transient global amnesia**

Excludes: amnesia NOS (R41.3)

G45.8 **Other transient cerebral ischaemic attacks and related syndromes**

G45.9 **Transient cerebral ischaemic attack, unspecified**

Spasm of cerebral artery

Transient cerebral ischaemia NOS

G46* Vascular syndromes of brain in cerebrovascular diseases (I60–I67†)

G46.0* **Middle cerebral artery syndrome (I66.0†)**

G46.1* **Anterior cerebral artery syndrome (I66.1†)**

G46.2* **Posterior cerebral artery syndrome (I66.2†)**

G46.3* **Brain stem stroke syndrome (I60–I67†)**

Syndrome:

- Benedikt
- Claude
- Foville
- Millard–Gubler
- Wallenberg
- Weber

G46.4* **Cerebellar stroke syndrome (I60–I67†)**

G46.5* **Pure motor lacunar syndrome (I60–I67†)**

G46.6* **Pure sensory lacunar syndrome (I60–I67†)**

G46.7* **Other lacunar syndromes (I60–I67†)**

G46.8* **Other vascular syndromes of brain in cerebrovascular diseases (I60–I67†)**

G47 Sleep disorders

Excludes: nightmares (F51.5)
nonorganic sleep disorders (F51.–)
sleep terrors (F51.4)
sleepwalking (F51.3)

G47.0 Disorders of initiating and maintaining sleep [insomnias]

G47.1 Disorders of excessive somnolence [hypersomnias]

G47.2 Disorders of the sleep–wake schedule
Delayed sleep phase syndrome
Irregular sleep–wake pattern

G47.3 Sleep apnoea
Sleep apnoea:
• central
• obstructive

Excludes: pickwickian syndrome (E66.2)
sleep apnoea of newborn (P28.3)

G47.4 Narcolepsy and cataplexy

G47.8 Other sleep disorders
Kleine–Levin syndrome

G47.9 Sleep disorder, unspecified

Nerve, nerve root and plexus disorders (G50–G59)

Excludes: current traumatic nerve, nerve root and plexus disorders—see
nerve injury by body region
neuralgia ⎫
neuritis ⎬ NOS (M79.2)
peripheral neuritis in pregnancy (O26.8)
radiculitis NOS (M54.1)

G50 Disorders of trigeminal nerve

Includes: disorders of 5th cranial nerve

G50.0 Trigeminal neuralgia
Syndrome of paroxysmal facial pain
Tic douloureux

G50.1 Atypical facial pain

G50.8 Other disorders of trigeminal nerve

G50.9 Disorder of trigeminal nerve, unspecified

G51 Facial nerve disorders

Includes: disorders of 7th cranial nerve

G51.0 Bell's palsy
Facial palsy

G51.1 Geniculate ganglionitis
Excludes: postherpetic geniculate ganglionitis (B02.2)

G51.2 Melkersson's syndrome
Melkersson–Rosenthal syndrome

G51.3 Clonic hemifacial spasm

G51.4 Facial myokymia

G51.8 Other disorders of facial nerve

G51.9 Disorder of facial nerve, unspecified

G52 Disorders of other cranial nerves

Excludes: disorders of:
- acoustic [8th] nerve (H93.3)
- optic [2nd] nerve (H46, H47.0)
paralytic strabismus due to nerve palsy
(H49.0–H49.2)

G52.0 Disorders of olfactory nerve
Disorder of 1st cranial nerve

G52.1 Disorders of glossopharyngeal nerve
Disorder of 9th cranial nerve
Glossopharyngeal neuralgia

G52.2 **Disorders of vagus nerve**
Disorder of pneumogastric [10th] nerve

G52.3 **Disorders of hypoglossal nerve**
Disorder of 12th cranial nerve

G52.7 **Disorders of multiple cranial nerves**
Polyneuritis cranialis

G52.8 **Disorders of other specified cranial nerves**

G52.9 **Cranial nerve disorder, unspecified**

G53* Cranial nerve disorders in diseases classified elsewhere

G53.0* **Postzoster neuralgia (B02.2†)**
Postherpetic:
• geniculate ganglionitis
• trigeminal neuralgia

G53.1* **Multiple cranial nerve palsies in infectious and parasitic diseases classified elsewhere (A00–B99†)**

G53.2* **Multiple cranial nerve palsies in sarcoidosis (D86.8†)**

G53.3* **Multiple cranial nerve palsies in neoplastic disease (C00–D48†)**

G53.8* **Other cranial nerve disorders in other diseases classified elsewhere**

G54 Nerve root and plexus disorders

Excludes: current traumatic nerve root and plexus disorders—
see nerve injury by body region
intervertebral disc disorders (M50–M51)
neuralgia or neuritis NOS (M79.2)
neuritis or radiculitis:
• brachial NOS
• lumbar NOS
• lumbosacral NOS ⎫ (M54.1)
• thoracic NOS ⎬
radiculitis NOS ⎭
radiculopathy NOS
spondylosis (M47.–)

G54.0 **Brachial plexus disorders**
Thoracic outlet syndrome

G54.1 **Lumbosacral plexus disorders**

G54.2 **Cervical root disorders, not elsewhere classified**

G54.3 **Thoracic root disorders, not elsewhere classified**

G54.4 **Lumbosacral root disorders, not elsewhere classified**

G54.5 **Neuralgic amyotrophy**
Parsonage–Aldren–Turner syndrome
Shoulder-girdle neuritis

G54.6 **Phantom limb syndrome with pain**

G54.7 **Phantom limb syndrome without pain**
Phantom limb syndrome NOS

G54.8 **Other nerve root and plexus disorders**

G54.9 **Nerve root and plexus disorder, unspecified**

G55* Nerve root and plexus compressions in diseases classified elsewhere

G55.0* **Nerve root and plexus compressions in neoplastic disease (C00–D48†)**

G55.1* **Nerve root and plexus compressions in intervertebral disc disorders (M50–M51†)**

G55.2* **Nerve root and plexus compressions in spondylosis (M47.–†)**

G55.3* **Nerve root and plexus compressions in other dorsopathies (M45–M46†, M48.–†, M53–M54†)**

G55.8* **Nerve root and plexus compressions in other diseases classified elsewhere**

G56 Mononeuropathies of upper limb

Excludes: current traumatic nerve disorder—see nerve injury by body region

G56.0 **Carpal tunnel syndrome**

G56.1 **Other lesions of median nerve**

G56.2 **Lesion of ulnar nerve**
Tardy ulnar nerve palsy

G56.3 **Lesion of radial nerve**

G56.4 **Causalgia**

G56.8 **Other mononeuropathies of upper limb**
Interdigital neuroma of upper limb

G56.9 **Mononeuropathy of upper limb, unspecified**

G57 Mononeuropathies of lower limb

Excludes: current traumatic nerve disorder—see nerve injury by body region

G57.0 **Lesion of sciatic nerve**
Excludes: sciatica:
• NOS (M54.3)
• attributed to intervertebral disc disorder (M51.1)

G57.1 **Meralgia paraesthetica**
Lateral cutaneous nerve of thigh syndrome

G57.2 **Lesion of femoral nerve**

G57.3 **Lesion of lateral popliteal nerve**
Peroneal nerve palsy

G57.4 **Lesion of medial popliteal nerve**

G57.5 **Tarsal tunnel syndrome**

G57.6 **Lesion of plantar nerve**
Morton's metatarsalgia

G57.8   **Other mononeuropathies of lower limb**
Interdigital neuroma of lower limb

G57.9   **Mononeuropathy of lower limb, unspecified**

G58   Other mononeuropathies

G58.0   **Intercostal neuropathy**

G58.7   **Mononeuritis multiplex**

G58.8   **Other specified mononeuropathies**

G58.9   **Mononeuropathy, unspecified**

G59*   Mononeuropathy in diseases classified elsewhere

G59.0*   **Diabetic mononeuropathy (E10–E14† with common fourth character .4)**

G59.8*   **Other mononeuropathies in diseases classified elsewhere**

Polyneuropathies and other disorders of the peripheral nervous system (G60–G64)

Excludes: neuralgia NOS (M79.2)
neuritis NOS (M79.2)
peripheral neuritis in pregnancy (O26.8)
radiculitis NOS (M54.1)

G60   Hereditary and idiopathic neuropathy

G60.0   **Hereditary motor and sensory neuropathy**
Disease:
• Charcot–Marie–Tooth
• Déjerine–Sottas
Hereditary motor and sensory neuropathy, types I–IV
Hypertrophic neuropathy of infancy
Peroneal muscular atrophy (axonal type)(hypertrophic type)
Roussy–Lévy syndrome

G60.1   **Refsum's disease**

G60.2   **Neuropathy in association with hereditary ataxia**

G60.3   **Idiopathic progressive neuropathy**

G60.8   **Other hereditary and idiopathic neuropathies**
Morvan's disease
Nelaton's syndrome
Sensory neuropathy:
- dominantly inherited
- recessively inherited

G60.9   **Hereditary and idiopathic neuropathy, unspecified**

G61   Inflammatory polyneuropathy

G61.0   **Guillain–Barré syndrome**
Acute (post-)infective polyneuritis

G61.1   **Serum neuropathy**
Use additional external cause code (Chapter XX), if desired, to identify cause.

G61.8   **Other inflammatory polyneuropathies**

G61.9   **Inflammatory polyneuropathy, unspecified**

G62   Other polyneuropathies

G62.0   **Drug-induced polyneuropathy**
Use additional external cause code (Chapter XX), if desired, to identify drug.

G62.1   **Alcoholic polyneuropathy**

G62.2   **Polyneuropathy due to other toxic agents**
Use additional external cause code (Chapter XX), if desired, to identify toxic agent.

G62.8   **Other specified polyneuropathies**
Radiation-induced polyneuropathy

Use additional external cause code (Chapter XX), if desired, to identify cause.

G62.9   **Polyneuropathy, unspecified**
Neuropathy NOS

G63* Polyneuropathy in diseases classified elsewhere

G63.0* **Polyneuropathy in infectious and parasitic diseases classified elsewhere**
Polyneuropathy (in):
- diphtheria (A36.8†)
- infectious mononucleosis (B27.–†)
- leprosy (A30.–†)
- Lyme disease (A69.2†)
- mumps (B26.8†)
- postherpetic (B02.2†)
- syphilis, late (A52.1†)
  - congenital (A50.4†)
- tuberculous (A17.8†)

G63.1* **Polyneuropathy in neoplastic disease (C00–D48†)**

G63.2* **Diabetic polyneuropathy (E10–E14† with common fourth character .4)**

G63.3* **Polyneuropathy in other endocrine and metabolic diseases (E00–E07†, E15–E16†, E20–E34†, E70–E89†)**

G63.4* **Polyneuropathy in nutritional deficiency (E40–E64†)**

G63.5* **Polyneuropathy in systemic connective tissue disorders (M30–M35†)**

G63.6* **Polyneuropathy in other musculoskeletal disorders (M00–M25†, M40–M96†)**

G63.8* **Polyneuropathy in other diseases classified elsewhere**
Uraemic neuropathy (N18.8†)

G64 Other disorders of peripheral nervous system
Disorder of peripheral nervous system NOS

Diseases of myoneural junction and muscle (G70–G73)

G70 Myasthenia gravis and other myoneural disorders

Excludes: botulism (A05.1)
transient neonatal myasthenia gravis (P94.0)

G70.0 Myasthenia gravis
Use additional external cause code (Chapter XX), if desired, to identify drug, if drug-induced.

G70.1 Toxic myoneural disorders
Use additional external cause code (Chapter XX), if desired, to identify toxic agent.

G70.2 Congenital and developmental myasthenia

G70.8 Other specified myoneural disorders

G70.9 Myoneural disorder, unspecified

G71 Primary disorders of muscles

Excludes: arthrogryposis multiplex congenita (Q74.3)
metabolic disorders (E70–E90)
myositis (M60.–)

G71.0 Muscular dystrophy
Muscular dystrophy:
- autosomal recessive, childhood type, resembling Duchenne or Becker
- benign [Becker]
- benign scapuloperoneal with early contractures [Emery–Dreifuss]
- distal
- facioscapulohumeral
- limb-girdle
- ocular
- oculopharyngeal
- scapuloperoneal
- severe [Duchenne]

Excludes: congenital muscular dystrophy:
  - NOS (G71.2)
  - with specific morphological abnormalities of the muscle fibre (G71.2)

417

G71.1 **Myotonic disorders**
Dystrophia myotonica [Steinert]
Myotonia:
- chondrodystrophic
- drug-induced
- symptomatic

Myotonia congenita:
- NOS
- dominant [Thomsen]
- recessive [Becker]

Neuromyotonia [Isaacs]
Paramyotonia congenita
Pseudomyotonia

Use additional external cause code (Chapter XX), if desired, to identify drug, if drug-induced.

G71.2 **Congenital myopathies**
Congenital muscular dystrophy:
- NOS
- with specific morphological abnormalities of the muscle fibre

Disease:
- central core
- minicore
- multicore

Fibre-type disproportion
Myopathy:
- myotubular (centronuclear)
- nemaline

G71.3 **Mitochondrial myopathy, not elsewhere classified**

G71.8 **Other primary disorders of muscles**

G71.9 **Primary disorder of muscle, unspecified**
Hereditary myopathy NOS

G72 Other myopathies

Excludes: arthrogryposis multiplex congenita (Q74.3)
dermatopolymyositis (M33.–)
ischaemic infarction of muscle (M62.2)
myositis (M60.–)
polymyositis (M33.2)

G72.0 **Drug-induced myopathy**
Use additional external cause code (Chapter XX), if desired, to identify drug.

G72.1 **Alcoholic myopathy**

G72.2 **Myopathy due to other toxic agents**
Use additional external cause code (Chapter XX), if desired, to identify toxic agent.

G72.3 **Periodic paralysis**
Periodic paralysis (familial):
• hyperkalaemic
• hypokalaemic
• myotonic
• normokalaemic

G72.4 **Inflammatory myopathy, not elsewhere classified**

G72.8 **Other specified myopathies**

G72.9 **Myopathy, unspecified**

G73* Disorders of myoneural junction and muscle in diseases classified elsewhere

G73.0* **Myasthenic syndromes in endocrine diseases**
Myasthenic syndromes in:
• diabetic amyotrophy (E10–E14† with common fourth character .4)
• thyrotoxicosis [hyperthyroidism] (E05.–†)

G73.1* **Eaton–Lambert syndrome (C80†)**

G73.2* **Other myasthenic syndromes in neoplastic disease (C00–D48†)**

G73.3* **Myasthenic syndromes in other diseases classified elsewhere**

G73.4* **Myopathy in infectious and parasitic diseases classified elsewhere**

G73.5* **Myopathy in endocrine diseases**
Myopathy in:
• hyperparathyroidism (E21.0–E21.3†)
• hypoparathyroidism (E20.–†)
Thyrotoxic myopathy (E05.–†)

G73.6* **Myopathy in metabolic diseases**
Myopathy in:
- glycogen storage disease (E74.0†)
- lipid storage disorders (E75.–†)

G73.7* **Myopathy in other diseases classified elsewhere**
Myopathy in:
- rheumatoid arthritis (M05–M06†)
- scleroderma (M34.8†)
- sicca syndrome [Sjögren] (M35.0†)
- systemic lupus erythematosus (M32.1†)

Cerebral palsy and other paralytic syndromes (G80–G83)

G80 **Infantile cerebral palsy**
Includes: Little's disease
Excludes: hereditary spastic paraplegia (G11.4)

G80.0 **Spastic cerebral palsy**
Congenital spastic paralysis (cerebral)

G80.1 **Spastic diplegia**

G80.2 **Infantile hemiplegia**

G80.3 **Dyskinetic cerebral palsy**
Athetoid cerebral palsy

G80.4 **Ataxic cerebral palsy**

G80.8 **Other infantile cerebral palsy**
Mixed cerebral palsy syndromes

G80.9 **Infantile cerebral palsy, unspecified**
Cerebral palsy NOS

G81 Hemiplegia

Note: For primary coding, this category is to be used only when hemiplegia (complete)(incomplete) is reported without further specification, or is stated to be old or longstanding but of unspecified cause. The category is also for use in multiple coding to identify these types of hemiplegia resulting from any cause.

Excludes: congenital and infantile cerebral palsy (G80.–)

G81.0   **Flaccid hemiplegia**

G81.1   **Spastic hemiplegia**

G81.9   **Hemiplegia, unspecified**

G82 Paraplegia and tetraplegia

Note: For primary coding, this category is to be used only when the listed conditions are reported without further specification, or are stated to be old or longstanding but of unspecified cause. The category is also for use in multiple coding to identify these conditions resulting from any cause.

Excludes: congenital and infantile cerebral palsy (G80.–)

G82.0   **Flaccid paraplegia**

G82.1   **Spastic paraplegia**

G82.2   **Paraplegia, unspecified**
Paralysis of both lower limbs NOS
Paraplegia (lower) NOS

G82.3   **Flaccid tetraplegia**

G82.4   **Spastic tetraplegia**

G82.5   **Tetraplegia, unspecified**
Quadriplegia NOS

G83 Other paralytic syndromes

Note: For primary coding, this category is to be used only when the listed conditions are reported without further specification, or are stated to be old or longstanding but of unspecified cause. The category is also for use in multiple coding to identify these conditions resulting from any cause.

Includes: paralysis (complete)(incomplete), except as in G80–G82

G83.0 Diplegia of upper limbs
Diplegia (upper)
Paralysis of both upper limbs

G83.1 Monoplegia of lower limb
Paralysis of lower limb

G83.2 Monoplegia of upper limb
Paralysis of upper limb

G83.3 Monoplegia, unspecified

G83.4 Cauda equina syndrome
Neurogenic bladder due to cauda equina syndrome
Excludes: cord bladder NOS (G95.8)

G83.8 Other specified paralytic syndromes
Todd's paralysis (postepileptic)

G83.9 Paralytic syndrome, unspecified

Other disorders of the nervous system (G90–G99)

G90 Disorders of autonomic nervous system

Excludes: dysfunction of autonomic nervous system due to alcohol (G31.2)

G90.0 Idiopathic peripheral autonomic neuropathy
Carotid sinus syncope

G90.1 Familial dysautonomia [Riley–Day]

G90.2 **Horner's syndrome**
Bernard(–Horner) syndrome

G90.3 **Multi-system degeneration**
Neurogenic orthostatic hypotension [Shy–Drager]
Excludes: orthostatic hypotension NOS (I95.1)

G90.8 **Other disorders of autonomic nervous system**

G90.9 **Disorder of autonomic nervous system, unspecified**

G91 Hydrocephalus

Includes: acquired hydrocephalus
Excludes: hydrocephalus:
- congenital (Q03.–)
- due to congenital toxoplasmosis (P37.1)

G91.0 **Communicating hydrocephalus**

G91.1 **Obstructive hydrocephalus**

G91.2 **Normal-pressure hydrocephalus**

G91.3 **Post-traumatic hydrocephalus, unspecified**

G91.8 **Other hydrocephalus**

G91.9 **Hydrocephalus, unspecified**

G92 Toxic encephalopathy

Use additional external cause code (Chapter XX), if desired, to identify toxic agent.

G93 Other disorders of brain

G93.0 **Cerebral cysts**
Arachnoid cyst
Porencephalic cyst, acquired
Excludes: acquired periventricular cysts of newborn (P91.1)
congenital cerebral cysts (Q04.6)

G93.1   Anoxic brain damage, not elsewhere classified

Excludes: complicating:
- abortion or ectopic or molar pregnancy (O00–O07, O08.8)
- pregnancy, labour or delivery (O29.2, O74.3, O89.2)
- surgical and medical care (T80–T88)

neonatal anoxia (P21.9)

G93.2   Benign intracranial hypertension

Excludes: hypertensive encephalopathy (I67.4)

G93.3   Postviral fatigue syndrome

Benign myalgic encephalomyelitis

G93.4   Encephalopathy, unspecified

Excludes: encephalopathy:
- alcoholic (G31.2)
- toxic (G92)

G93.5   Compression of brain

Compression ⎫
Herniation ⎬ of brain (stem)

Excludes: traumatic compression of brain (diffuse) (S06.2)
- focal (S06.3)

G93.6   Cerebral oedema

Excludes: cerebral oedema:
- due to birth injury (P11.0)
- traumatic (S06.1)

G93.7   Reye's syndrome

Use additional external cause code (Chapter XX), if desired, to identify cause.

G93.8   Other specified disorders of brain

Postradiation encephalopathy

Use additional external cause code (Chapter XX), if desired, to identify cause.

G93.9   Disorder of brain, unspecified

G94* Other disorders of brain in diseases classified elsewhere

G94.0* **Hydrocephalus in infectious and parasitic diseases classified elsewhere (A00–B99†)**

G94.1* **Hydrocephalus in neoplastic disease (C00–D48†)**

G94.2* **Hydrocephalus in other diseases classified elsewhere**

G94.8* **Other specified disorders of brain in diseases classified elsewhere**

G95 Other diseases of spinal cord
Excludes: myelitis (G04.–)

G95.0 **Syringomyelia and syringobulbia**

G95.1 **Vascular myelopathies**
Acute infarction of spinal cord (embolic)(nonembolic)
Arterial thrombosis of spinal cord
Haematomyelia
Nonpyogenic intraspinal phlebitis and thrombophlebitis
Oedema of spinal cord
Subacute necrotic myelopathy
Excludes: intraspinal phlebitis and thrombophlebitis, except non-pyogenic (G08)

G95.2 **Cord compression, unspecified**

G95.8 **Other specified diseases of spinal cord**
Cord bladder NOS
Myelopathy:
• drug-induced
• radiation-induced

Use additional external cause code (Chapter XX), if desired, to identify external agent.
Excludes: neurogenic bladder:
• NOS (N31.9)
• due to cauda equina syndrome (G83.4)
neuromuscular dysfunction of bladder without mention of spinal cord lesion (N31.–)

G95.9 **Disease of spinal cord, unspecified**
Myelopathy NOS

G96 Other disorders of central nervous system

G96.0 **Cerebrospinal fluid leak**
Excludes: from spinal puncture (G97.0)

G96.1 **Disorders of meninges, not elsewhere classified**
Meningeal adhesions (cerebral)(spinal)

G96.8 **Other specified disorders of central nervous system**

G96.9 **Disorder of central nervous system, unspecified**

G97 Postprocedural disorders of nervous system, not elsewhere classified

G97.0 **Cerebrospinal fluid leak from spinal puncture**

G97.1 **Other reaction to spinal and lumbar puncture**

G97.2 **Intracranial hypotension following ventricular shunting**

G97.8 **Other postprocedural disorders of nervous system**

G97.9 **Postprocedural disorder of nervous system, unspecified**

G98 Other disorders of nervous system, not elsewhere classified
Nervous system disorder NOS

G99* Other disorders of nervous system in diseases classified elsewhere

G99.0* **Autonomic neuropathy in endocrine and metabolic diseases**
Amyloid autonomic neuropathy (E85.–†)
Diabetic autonomic neuropathy (E10–E14† with common fourth
character .4)

G99.1* **Other disorders of autonomic nervous system in other diseases classified elsewhere**

426

G99.2* **Myelopathy in diseases classified elsewhere**

Anterior spinal and vertebral artery compression syndromes (M47.0†)

Myelopathy in:

- intervertebral disc disorders (M50.0†, M51.0†)
- neoplastic disease (C00–D48†)
- spondylosis (M47.–†)

G99.8* **Other specified disorders of nervous system in diseases classified elsewhere**

CHAPTER VII

Diseases of the eye and adnexa (H00–H59)

Excludes: certain conditions originating in the perinatal period (P00–P96)

certain infectious and parasitic diseases (A00–B99)

complications of pregnancy, childbirth and the puerperium (O00–O99)

congenital malformations, deformations and chromosomal abnormalities (Q00–Q99)

endocrine, nutritional and metabolic diseases (E00–E90)

injury, poisoning and certain other consequences of external causes (S00–T98)

neoplasms (C00–D48)

symptoms, signs and abnormal clinical and laboratory findings, not elsewhere classified (R00–R99)

This chapter contains the following blocks:

H00–H06 Disorders of eyelid, lacrimal system and orbit

H10–H13 Disorders of conjunctiva

H15–H22 Disorders of sclera, cornea, iris and ciliary body

H25–H28 Disorders of lens

H30–H36 Disorders of choroid and retina

H40–H42 Glaucoma

H43–H45 Disorders of vitreous body and globe

H46–H48 Disorders of optic nerve and visual pathways

H49–H52 Disorders of ocular muscles, binocular movement, accommodation and refraction

H53–H54 Visual disturbances and blindness

H55–H59 Other disorders of eye and adnexa

Asterisk categories for this chapter are provided as follows:

H03* Disorders of eyelid in diseases classified elsewhere

H06* Disorders of lacrimal system and orbit in diseases classified elsewhere

H13* Disorders of conjunctiva in diseases classified elsewhere

H19* Disorders of sclera and cornea in diseases classified elsewhere

H22* Disorders of iris and ciliary body in diseases classified elsewhere

H28* Cataract and other disorders of lens in diseases classified elsewhere

H32*	Chorioretinal disorders in diseases classified elsewhere
H36*	Retinal disorders in diseases classified elsewhere
H42*	Glaucoma in diseases classified elsewhere
H45*	Disorders of vitreous body and globe in diseases classified elsewhere
H48*	Disorders of optic nerve and visual pathways in diseases classified elsewhere
H58*	Other disorders of eye and adnexa in diseases classified elsewhere

Disorders of eyelid, lacrimal system and orbit (H00–H06)

H00 Hordeolum and chalazion

H00.0 **Hordeolum and other deep inflammation of eyelid**
Abscess ⎫
Furuncle ⎬ of eyelid
Stye ⎭

H00.1 **Chalazion**

H01 Other inflammation of eyelid

H01.0 **Blepharitis**
Excludes: blepharoconjunctivitis (H10.5)

H01.1 **Noninfectious dermatoses of eyelid**
Dermatitis:
• allergic ⎫
• contact ⎪
• eczematous ⎬ of eyelid
Discoid lupus erythematosus ⎪
Xeroderma ⎭

H01.8 **Other specified inflammation of eyelid**

H01.9 **Inflammation of eyelid, unspecified**

H02   Other disorders of eyelid

Excludes: congenital malformations of eyelid (Q10.0–Q10.3)

H02.0   **Entropion and trichiasis of eyelid**

H02.1   **Ectropion of eyelid**

H02.2   **Lagophthalmos**

H02.3   **Blepharochalasis**

H02.4   **Ptosis of eyelid**

H02.5   **Other disorders affecting eyelid function**
Ankyloblepharon
Blepharophimosis
Lid retraction
Excludes: blepharospasm (G24.5)
        tic (psychogenic) (F95.–)
        • organic (G25.6)

H02.6   **Xanthelasma of eyelid**

H02.7   **Other degenerative disorders of eyelid and periocular area**
Chloasma ⎫
Madarosis ⎬ of eyelid
Vitiligo ⎭

H02.8   **Other specified disorders of eyelid**
Hypertrichosis of eyelid
Retained foreign body in eyelid

H02.9   **Disorder of eyelid, unspecified**

H03*   Disorders of eyelid in diseases classified elsewhere

H03.0*   **Parasitic infestation of eyelid in diseases classified elsewhere**
Dermatitis of eyelid due to *Demodex* species (B88.0†)
Parasitic infestation of eyelid in:
• leishmaniasis (B55.–†)
• loiasis (B74.3†)
• onchocerciasis (B73†)
• phthiriasis (B85.3†)

H03.1* **Involvement of eyelid in other infectious diseases classified elsewhere**
Involvement of eyelid in:
- herpesviral [herpes simplex] infection (B00.5†)
- leprosy (A30.–†)
- molluscum contagiosum (B08.1†)
- tuberculosis (A18.4†)
- yaws (A66.–†)
- zoster (B02.3†)

H03.8* **Involvement of eyelid in other diseases classified elsewhere**
Involvement of eyelid in impetigo (L01.0†)

H04 Disorders of lacrimal system
Excludes: congenital malformations of lacrimal system
(Q10.4–Q10.6)

H04.0 **Dacryoadenitis**
Chronic enlargement of lacrimal gland

H04.1 **Other disorders of lacrimal gland**
Dacryops
Dry eye syndrome
Lacrimal:
- cyst
- gland atrophy

H04.2 **Epiphora**

H04.3 **Acute and unspecified inflammation of lacrimal passages**
Dacryocystitis (phlegmonous) ⎫
Dacryopericystitis ⎬ acute, subacute or
Lacrimal canaliculitis ⎭ unspecified
Excludes: neonatal dacryocystitis (P39.1)

H04.4 **Chronic inflammation of lacrimal passages**
Dacryocystitis ⎫
Lacrimal: ⎬ chronic
- canaliculitis ⎭
- mucocele

H04.5 **Stenosis and insufficiency of lacrimal passages**
Dacryolith
Eversion of lacrimal punctum
Stenosis of lacrimal:
- canaliculi
- duct
- sac

H04.6 **Other changes in lacrimal passages**
Lacrimal fistula

H04.8 **Other disorders of lacrimal system**

H04.9 **Disorder of lacrimal system, unspecified**

H05 Disorders of orbit

Excludes: congenital malformation of orbit (Q10.7)

H05.0 **Acute inflammation of orbit**
Abscess
Cellulitis
Osteomyelitis } of orbit
Periostitis
Tenonitis

H05.1 **Chronic inflammatory disorders of orbit**
Granuloma of orbit

H05.2 **Exophthalmic conditions**
Displacement of globe (lateral) NOS
Haemorrhage } of orbit
Oedema

H05.3 **Deformity of orbit**
Atrophy } of orbit
Exostosis

H05.4 **Enophthalmos**

H05.5 **Retained (old) foreign body following penetrating wound of orbit**
Retrobulbar foreign body

H05.8 **Other disorders of orbit**
Cyst of orbit

H05.9 **Disorder of orbit, unspecified**

H06* Disorders of lacrimal system and orbit in diseases classified elsewhere

H06.0* **Disorders of lacrimal system in diseases classified elsewhere**

H06.1* **Parasitic infestation of orbit in diseases classified elsewhere**
Echinococcus infection of orbit (B67.–†)
Myiasis of orbit (B87.2†)

H06.2* **Dysthyroid exophthalmos (E05.–†)**

H06.3* **Other disorders of orbit in diseases classified elsewhere**

Disorders of conjunctiva (H10–H13)

H10 Conjunctivitis
Excludes: keratoconjunctivitis (H16.2)

H10.0 **Mucopurulent conjunctivitis**

H10.1 **Acute atopic conjunctivitis**

H10.2 **Other acute conjunctivitis**

H10.3 **Acute conjunctivitis, unspecified**
Excludes: ophthalmia neonatorum NOS (P39.1)

H10.4 **Chronic conjunctivitis**

H10.5 **Blepharoconjunctivitis**

H10.8 **Other conjunctivitis**

H10.9 **Conjunctivitis, unspecified**

H11 Other disorders of conjunctiva
Excludes: keratoconjunctivitis (H16.2)

H11.0 **Pterygium**
Excludes: pseudopterygium (H11.8)

H11.1 **Conjunctival degenerations and deposits**
Conjunctival:
• argyrosis [argyria]
• concretions
• pigmentation
• xerosis NOS

H11.2 **Conjunctival scars**
Symblepharon

H11.3 **Conjunctival haemorrhage**
Subconjunctival haemorrhage

H11.4 **Other conjunctival vascular disorders and cysts**
Conjunctival:
• aneurysm
• hyperaemia
• oedema

H11.8 **Other specified disorders of conjunctiva**
Pseudopterygium

H11.9 **Disorder of conjunctiva, unspecified**

H13* Disorders of conjunctiva in diseases classified elsewhere

H13.0* **Filarial infection of conjunctiva (B74.–†)**

H13.1* **Conjunctivitis in infectious and parasitic diseases classified elsewhere**
Conjunctivitis (due to):
• *Acanthamoeba* (B60.1†)
• adenoviral follicular (acute) (B30.1†)
• chlamydial (A74.0†)
• diphtheritic (A36.8†)
• gonococcal (A54.3†)
• haemorrhagic (acute)(epidemic) (B30.3†)
• herpesviral [herpes simplex] (B00.5†)
• meningococcal (A39.8†)
• Newcastle (B30.8†)
• zoster (B02.3†)

H13.2* **Conjunctivitis in other diseases classified elsewhere**

H13.3* **Ocular pemphigoid (L12.–†)**

H13.8* **Other disorders of conjunctiva in diseases classified elsewhere**

Disorders of sclera, cornea, iris and ciliary body (H15–H22)

H15 Disorders of sclera

H15.0 **Scleritis**

H15.1 **Episcleritis**

H15.8 **Other disorders of sclera**
Equatorial staphyloma
Scleral ectasia
Excludes: degenerative myopia (H44.2)

H15.9 **Disorder of sclera, unspecified**

H16 Keratitis

H16.0 **Corneal ulcer**
Ulcer:
- corneal:
  - NOS
  - central
  - marginal
  - perforated
  - ring
  - with hypopyon
- Mooren

H16.1 **Other superficial keratitis without conjunctivitis**
Keratitis:
- areolar
- filamentary
- nummular
- stellate
- striate
- superficial punctate
Photokeratitis
Snow blindness

H16.2 **Keratoconjunctivitis**
Keratoconjunctivitis:
- NOS
- exposure
- neurotrophic
- phlyctenular

Ophthalmia nodosa
Superficial keratitis with conjunctivitis

H16.3 **Interstitial and deep keratitis**

H16.4 **Corneal neovascularization**
Ghost vessels (corneal)
Pannus (corneal)

H16.8 **Other keratitis**

H16.9 **Keratitis, unspecified**

H17 Corneal scars and opacities

H17.0 **Adherent leukoma**

H17.1 **Other central corneal opacity**

H17.8 **Other corneal scars and opacities**

H17.9 **Corneal scar and opacity, unspecified**

H18 Other disorders of cornea

H18.0 **Corneal pigmentations and deposits**
Haematocornea
Kayser–Fleischer ring
Krukenberg's spindle
Staehli's line

Use additional external cause code (Chapter XX), if desired, to identify drug, if drug-induced.

H18.1 **Bullous keratopathy**

H18.2 **Other corneal oedema**

H18.3 **Changes in corneal membranes**
Fold ⎫
Rupture ⎬ in Descemet's membrane

H18.4   **Corneal degeneration**
Arcus senilis
Band keratopathy
Excludes: Mooren's ulcer (H16.0)

H18.5   **Hereditary corneal dystrophies**
Dystrophy:
- corneal:
  - epithelial
  - granular
  - lattice
  - macular
- Fuchs

H18.6   **Keratoconus**

H18.7   **Other corneal deformities**
Corneal:
- ectasia
- staphyloma
Descemetocele
Excludes: congenital malformations of cornea (Q13.3–Q13.4)

H18.8   **Other specified disorders of cornea**
Anaesthesia
Hypaesthesia   } of cornea
Recurrent erosion

H18.9   **Disorder of cornea, unspecified**

H19* **Disorders of sclera and cornea in diseases classified elsewhere**

H19.0*   **Scleritis and episcleritis in diseases classified elsewhere**
Syphilitic episcleritis (A52.7†)
Tuberculous episcleritis (A18.5†)
Zoster scleritis (B02.3†)

H19.1*   **Herpesviral keratitis and keratoconjunctivitis (B00.5†)**
Dendritic and disciform keratitis

H19.2* **Keratitis and keratoconjunctivitis in other infectious and parasitic diseases classified elsewhere**
Epidemic keratoconjunctivitis (B30.0†)
Keratitis and keratoconjunctivitis (interstitial) in:
- acanthamoebiasis (B60.1†)
- measles (B05.8†)
- syphilis (A50.3†)
- tuberculosis (A18.5†)
- zoster (B02.3†)

H19.3* **Keratitis and keratoconjunctivitis in other diseases classified elsewhere**
Keratoconjunctivitis sicca (M35.0†)

H19.8* **Other disorders of sclera and cornea in diseases classified elsewhere**
Keratoconus in Down's syndrome (Q90.–†)

H20 Iridocyclitis

H20.0 **Acute and subacute iridocyclitis**
Anterior uveitis ⎫
Cyclitis ⎬ acute, recurrent or subacute
Iritis ⎭

H20.1 **Chronic iridocyclitis**

H20.2 **Lens-induced iridocyclitis**

H20.8 **Other iridocyclitis**

H20.9 **Iridocyclitis, unspecified**

H21 Other disorders of iris and ciliary body
Excludes: sympathetic uveitis (H44.1)

H21.0 **Hyphaema**
Excludes: traumatic hyphaema (S05.1)

H21.1 **Other vascular disorders of iris and ciliary body**
Neovascularization of iris or ciliary body
Rubeosis of iris

H21.2   Degeneration of iris and ciliary body
Degeneration of:
- iris (pigmentary)
- pupillary margin

Iridoschisis
Iris atrophy (essential)(progressive)
Miotic pupillary cyst
Translucency of iris

H21.3   Cyst of iris, ciliary body and anterior chamber
Cyst of iris, ciliary body or anterior chamber:
- NOS
- exudative
- implantation
- parasitic

Excludes: miotic pupillary cyst (H21.2)

H21.4   Pupillary membranes
Iris bombé
Pupillary:
- occlusion
- seclusion

H21.5   Other adhesions and disruptions of iris and ciliary body
Goniosynechiae
Iridodialysis
Recession, chamber angle
Synechiae (iris):
- NOS
- anterior
- posterior

Excludes: corectopia (Q13.2)

H21.8   Other specified disorders of iris and ciliary body

H21.9   Disorder of iris and ciliary body, unspecified

H22* Disorders of iris and ciliary body in diseases classified elsewhere

H22.0* **Iridocyclitis in infectious and parasitic diseases classified elsewhere**
Iridocyclitis in:
- gonococcal infection (A54.3†)
- herpesviral [herpes simplex] infection (B00.5†)
- syphilis (secondary) (A51.4†)
- tuberculosis (A18.5†)
- zoster (B02.3†)

H22.1* **Iridocyclitis in other diseases classified elsewhere**
Iridocyclitis in:
- ankylosing spondylitis (M45†)
- sarcoidosis (D86.8†)

H22.8* **Other disorders of iris and ciliary body in diseases classified elsewhere**

Disorders of lens
(H25–H28)

H25 Senile cataract
Excludes: capsular glaucoma with pseudoexfoliation of lens
(H40.1)

H25.0 **Senile incipient cataract**
Senile cataract:
- coronary
- cortical
- punctate
Subcapsular polar senile cataract (anterior)(posterior)
Water clefts

H25.1 **Senile nuclear cataract**
Cataracta brunescens
Nuclear sclerosis cataract

H25.2 **Senile cataract, morgagnian type**
Senile hypermature cataract

H25.8 **Other senile cataract**
Combined forms of senile cataract

H25.9 **Senile cataract, unspecified**

H26 Other cataract

Excludes: congenital cataract (Q12.0)

H26.0 **Infantile, juvenile and presenile cataract**

H26.1 **Traumatic cataract**
Use additional external cause code (Chapter XX), if desired, to identify cause.

H26.2 **Complicated cataract**
Cataract in chronic iridocyclitis
Cataract secondary to ocular disorders
Glaucomatous flecks (subcapsular)

H26.3 **Drug-induced cataract**
Use additional external cause code (Chapter XX), if desired, to identify drug.

H26.4 **After-cataract**
Secondary cataract
Soemmerring's ring

H26.8 **Other specified cataract**

H26.9 **Cataract, unspecified**

H27 Other disorders of lens

Excludes: congenital lens malformations (Q12.–)
mechanical complications of intraocular lens (T85.2)
pseudophakia (Z96.1)

H27.0 **Aphakia**

H27.1 **Dislocation of lens**

H27.8 **Other specified disorders of lens**

H27.9 **Disorder of lens, unspecified**

H28* Cataract and other disorders of lens in diseases classified elsewhere

H28.0* **Diabetic cataract (E10–E14† with common fourth character .3)**

H28.1* **Cataract in other endocrine, nutritional and metabolic diseases**
Cataract in hypoparathyroidism (E20.–†)
Malnutrition-dehydration cataract (E40–E46†)

H28.2* **Cataract in other diseases classified elsewhere**
Myotonic cataract (G71.1†)

H28.8* **Other disorders of lens in diseases classified elsewhere**

Disorders of choroid and retina (H30–H36)

H30 Chorioretinal inflammation

H30.0 **Focal chorioretinal inflammation**
Focal:
- chorioretinitis
- choroiditis
- retinitis
- retinochoroiditis

H30.1 **Disseminated chorioretinal inflammation**
Disseminated:
- chorioretinitis
- choroiditis
- retinitis
- retinochoroiditis

Excludes: exudative retinopathy (H35.0)

H30.2 **Posterior cyclitis**
Pars planitis

H30.8 **Other chorioretinal inflammations**
Harada's disease

443

H30.9　　**Chorioretinal inflammation, unspecified**
Chorioretinitis
Choroiditis
Retinitis ⎬ NOS
Retinochoroiditis

H31　Other disorders of choroid

H31.0　　**Chorioretinal scars**
Macula scars of posterior pole (postinflammatory)(post-traumatic)
Solar retinopathy

H31.1　　**Choroidal degeneration**
Atrophy ⎫
Sclerosis ⎬ of choroid
Excludes: angioid streaks (H35.3)

H31.2　　**Hereditary choroidal dystrophy**
Choroideremia
Dystrophy, choroidal (central areolar)(generalized)(peripapillary)
Gyrate atrophy, choroid
Excludes: ornithinaemia (E72.4)

H31.3　　**Choroidal haemorrhage and rupture**
Choroidal haemorrhage:
• NOS
• expulsive

H31.4　　**Choroidal detachment**

H31.8　　**Other specified disorders of choroid**

H31.9　　**Disorder of choroid, unspecified**

H32*　Chorioretinal disorders in diseases classified elsewhere

H32.0*　　**Chorioretinal inflammation in infectious and parasitic diseases classified elsewhere**
Chorioretinitis:
• syphilitic, late (A52.7†)
• toxoplasma (B58.0†)
• tuberculous (A18.5†)

H32.8*　　**Other chorioretinal disorders in diseases classified elsewhere**

H33 Retinal detachments and breaks

Excludes: detachment of retinal pigment epithelium (H35.7)

H33.0 Retinal detachment with retinal break
Rhegmatogenous retinal detachment

H33.1 Retinoschisis and retinal cysts
Cyst of ora serrata
Parasitic cyst of retina NOS
Pseudocyst of retina
Excludes: congenital retinoschisis (Q14.1)
microcystoid degeneration of retina (H35.4)

H33.2 Serous retinal detachment
Retinal detachment:
• NOS
• without retinal break
Excludes: central serous chorioretinopathy (H35.7)

H33.3 Retinal breaks without detachment
Horseshoe tear ⎫
Round hole ⎬ of retina, without detachment
Operculum ⎭
Retinal break NOS
Excludes: chorioretinal scars after surgery for detachment
(H59.8)
peripheral retinal degeneration without break (H35.4)

H33.4 Traction detachment of retina
Proliferative vitreo-retinopathy with retinal detachment

H33.5 Other retinal detachments

H34 Retinal vascular occlusions

Excludes: amaurosis fugax (G45.3)

H34.0 Transient retinal artery occlusion

H34.1 Central retinal artery occlusion

H34.2 **Other retinal artery occlusions**
Hollenhorst's plaque
Retinal:
- artery occlusion:
  - branch
  - partial
- microembolism

H34.8 **Other retinal vascular occlusions**
Retinal vein occlusion:
- central
- incipient
- partial
- tributary

H34.9 **Retinal vascular occlusion, unspecified**

H35 Other retinal disorders

H35.0 **Background retinopathy and retinal vascular changes**
Changes in retinal vascular appearance
Retinal:
- micro-aneurysms
- neovascularization
- perivasculitis
- varices
- vascular sheathing
- vasculitis
Retinopathy:
- NOS
- background NOS
- Coats
- exudative
- hypertensive

H35.1 **Retinopathy of prematurity**
Retrolental fibroplasia

H35.2 **Other proliferative retinopathy**
Proliferative vitreo-retinopathy
Excludes: proliferative vitreo-retinopathy with retinal
detachment (H33.4)

H35.3 **Degeneration of macula and posterior pole**

Angioid streaks
Cyst
Drusen (degenerative) } of macula
Hole
Puckering
Kuhnt–Junius degeneration
Senile macular degeneration (atrophic)(exudative)
Toxic maculopathy

Use additional external cause code (Chapter XX), if desired, to identify drug, if drug-induced.

H35.4 **Peripheral retinal degeneration**

Degeneration, retina:
- NOS
- lattice
- microcystoid
- palisade
- paving stone
- reticular

Excludes: with retinal break (H33.3)

H35.5 **Hereditary retinal dystrophy**

Dystrophy:
- retinal (albipunctate)(pigmentary)(vitelliform)
- tapetoretinal
- vitreoretinal
Retinitis pigmentosa
Stargardt's disease

H35.6 **Retinal haemorrhage**

H35.7 **Separation of retinal layers**

Central serous chorioretinopathy
Detachment of retinal pigment epithelium

H35.8 **Other specified retinal disorders**

H35.9 **Retinal disorder, unspecified**

H36* Retinal disorders in diseases classified elsewhere

H36.0* **Diabetic retinopathy (E10–E14† with common fourth character .3)**

H36.8* **Other retinal disorders in diseases classified elsewhere**
Atherosclerotic retinopathy (I70.8†)
Proliferative sickle-cell retinopathy (D57.–†)
Retinal dystrophy in lipid storage disorders (E75.–†)

Glaucoma
(H40–H42)

H40 **Glaucoma**
Excludes: absolute glaucoma (H44.5)
congenital glaucoma (Q15.0)
traumatic glaucoma due to birth injury (P15.3)

H40.0 **Glaucoma suspect**
Ocular hypertension

H40.1 **Primary open-angle glaucoma**
Glaucoma (primary)(residual stage):
• capsular with pseudoexfoliation of lens
• chronic simple
• low-tension
• pigmentary

H40.2 **Primary angle-closure glaucoma**
Angle-closure glaucoma (primary)(residual stage):
• acute
• chronic
• intermittent

H40.3 **Glaucoma secondary to eye trauma**
Use additional code, if desired, to identify cause.

H40.4 **Glaucoma secondary to eye inflammation**
Use additional code, if desired, to identify cause.

H40.5 **Glaucoma secondary to other eye disorders**
Use additional code, if desired, to identify cause.

H40.6 **Glaucoma secondary to drugs**
Use additional external cause code (Chapter XX), if desired, to
identify drug.

H40.8 **Other glaucoma**

H40.9 **Glaucoma, unspecified**

H42* Glaucoma in diseases classified elsewhere

H42.0* **Glaucoma in endocrine, nutritional and metabolic diseases**
Glaucoma in:
- amyloidosis (E85.–†)
- Lowe's syndrome (E72.0†)

H42.8* **Glaucoma in other diseases classified elsewhere**
Glaucoma in onchocerciasis (B73†)

Disorders of vitreous body and globe (H43–H45)

H43 Disorders of vitreous body

H43.0 **Vitreous prolapse**
Excludes: vitreous syndrome following cataract surgery (H59.0)

H43.1 **Vitreous haemorrhage**

H43.2 **Crystalline deposits in vitreous body**

H43.3 **Other vitreous opacities**
Vitreous membranes and strands

H43.8 **Other disorders of vitreous body**
Vitreous:
- degeneration
- detachment
Excludes: proliferative vitreo-retinopathy with retinal detachment (H33.4)

H43.9 **Disorder of vitreous body, unspecified**

H44 Disorders of globe
Includes: disorders affecting multiple structures of eye

H44.0 **Purulent endophthalmitis**
Panophthalmitis
Vitreous abscess

H44.1   **Other endophthalmitis**
Parasitic endophthalmitis NOS
Sympathetic uveitis

H44.2   **Degenerative myopia**

H44.3   **Other degenerative disorders of globe**
Chalcosis
Siderosis of eye

H44.4   **Hypotony of eye**

H44.5   **Degenerated conditions of globe**
Absolute glaucoma
Atrophy of globe
Phthisis bulbi

H44.6   **Retained (old) intraocular foreign body, magnetic**
Retained (old) magnetic foreign body (in):
• anterior chamber
• ciliary body
• iris
• lens
• posterior wall of globe
• vitreous body

H44.7   **Retained (old) intraocular foreign body, nonmagnetic**
Retained (nonmagnetic)(old) foreign body (in):
• anterior chamber
• ciliary body
• iris
• lens
• posterior wall of globe
• vitreous body

H44.8   **Other disorders of globe**
Haemophthalmos
Luxation of globe

H44.9   **Disorder of globe, unspecified**

H45*   **Disorders of vitreous body and globe in diseases classified elsewhere**

H45.0*   **Vitreous haemorrhage in diseases classified elsewhere**

H45.1* **Endophthalmitis in diseases classified elsewhere**
Endophthalmitis in:
- cysticercosis (B69.1†)
- onchocerciasis (B73†)
- toxocariasis (B83.0†)

H45.8* **Other disorders of vitreous body and globe in diseases classified elsewhere**

Disorders of optic nerve and visual pathways (H46–H48)

H46 Optic neuritis
Optic
- neuropathy, except ischaemic
- papillitis

Retrobulbar neuritis NOS

Excludes: ischaemic optic neuropathy (H47.0)
neuromyelitis optica [Devic] (G36.0)

H47 Other disorders of optic [2nd] nerve and visual pathways

H47.0 **Disorders of optic nerve, not elsewhere classified**
Compression of optic nerve
Haemorrhage in optic nerve sheath
Ischaemic optic neuropathy

H47.1 **Papilloedema, unspecified**

H47.2 **Optic atrophy**
Temporal pallor of optic disc

H47.3 **Other disorders of optic disc**
Drusen of optic disc
Pseudopapilloedema

H47.4 **Disorders of optic chiasm**

H47.5 **Disorders of other visual pathways**
Disorders of optic tracts, geniculate nuclei and optic radiations

H47.6 **Disorders of visual cortex**

H47.7   Disorder of visual pathways, unspecified

H48*   Disorders of optic [2nd] nerve and visual pathways in diseases classified elsewhere

H48.0*   Optic atrophy in diseases classified elsewhere
Optic atrophy in late syphilis (A52.1†)

H48.1*   Retrobulbar neuritis in diseases classified elsewhere
Retrobulbar neuritis in:
- late syphilis (A52.1†)
- meningococcal infection (A39.8†)
- multiple sclerosis (G35†)

H48.8*   Other disorders of optic nerve and visual pathways in diseases classified elsewhere

Disorders of ocular muscles, binocular movement, accommodation and refraction (H49–H52)

Excludes: nystagmus and other irregular eye movements (H55)

H49   Paralytic strabismus
Excludes: ophthalmoplegia:
- internal (H52.5)
- internuclear (H51.2)
- progressive supranuclear (G23.1)

H49.0   Third [oculomotor] nerve palsy

H49.1   Fourth [trochlear] nerve palsy

H49.2   Sixth [abducent] nerve palsy

H49.3   Total (external) ophthalmoplegia

H49.4   Progressive external ophthalmoplegia

H49.8   Other paralytic strabismus
External ophthalmoplegia NOS
Kearns–Sayre syndrome

H49.9   Paralytic strabismus, unspecified

H50 Other strabismus

H50.0 **Convergent concomitant strabismus**
Esotropia (alternating)(monocular), except intermittent

H50.1 **Divergent concomitant strabismus**
Exotropia (alternating)(monocular), except intermittent

H50.2 **Vertical strabismus**

H50.3 **Intermittent heterotropia**
Intermittent:
- esotropia ⎱
- exotropia ⎰ (alternating)(monocular)

H50.4 **Other and unspecified heterotropia**
Concomitant strabismus NOS
Cyclotropia
Hypertropia
Hypotropia
Microtropia
Monofixation syndrome

H50.5 **Heterophoria**
Alternating hyperphoria
Esophoria
Exophoria

H50.6 **Mechanical strabismus**
Brown's sheath syndrome
Strabismus due to adhesions
Traumatic limitation of duction of eye muscle

H50.8 **Other specified strabismus**
Duane's syndrome

H50.9 **Strabismus, unspecified**

H51 Other disorders of binocular movement

H51.0 **Palsy of conjugate gaze**

H51.1 **Convergence insufficiency and excess**

H51.2 **Internuclear ophthalmoplegia**

H51.8 **Other specified disorders of binocular movement**

H51.9 **Disorder of binocular movement, unspecified**

H52   Disorders of refraction and accommodation

H52.0   **Hypermetropia**

H52.1   **Myopia**
Excludes: degenerative myopia (H44.2)

H52.2   **Astigmatism**

H52.3   **Anisometropia and aniseikonia**

H52.4   **Presbyopia**

H52.5   **Disorders of accommodation**
Internal ophthalmoplegia (complete)(total)
Paresis ⎫
Spasm ⎬ of accommodation

H52.6   **Other disorders of refraction**

H52.7   **Disorder of refraction, unspecified**

Visual disturbances and blindness (H53–H54)

H53   Visual disturbances

H53.0   **Amblyopia ex anopsia**
Amblyopia:
• anisometropic
• deprivation
• strabismic

H53.1   **Subjective visual disturbances**
Asthenopia
Day blindness
Hemeralopia
Metamorphopsia
Photophobia
Scintillating scotoma
Sudden visual loss
Visual halos
Excludes: visual hallucinations (R44.1)

H53.2 **Diplopia**
Double vision

H53.3 **Other disorders of binocular vision**
Abnormal retinal correspondence
Fusion with defective stereopsis
Simultaneous visual perception without fusion
Suppression of binocular vision

H53.4 **Visual field defects**
Enlarged blind spot
Generalized contraction of visual field
Hemianop(s)ia (heteronymous)(homonymous)
Quadrant anop(s)ia
Scotoma:
• arcuate
• Bjerrum
• central
• ring

H53.5 **Colour vision deficiencies**
Achromatopsia
Acquired colour vision deficiency
Colour blindness
Deuteranomaly
Deuteranopia
Protanomaly
Protanopia
Tritanomaly
Tritanopia
Excludes: day blindness (H53.1)

H53.6 **Night blindness**
Excludes: due to vitamin A deficiency (E50.5)

H53.8 **Other visual disturbances**

H53.9 **Visual disturbance, unspecified**

H54 Blindness and low vision

Note: For definition of visual impairment categories see
table opposite.

Excludes: amaurosis fugax (G45.3)

H54.0 **Blindness, both eyes**
Visual impairment categories 3, 4, 5 in both eyes.

H54.1 **Blindness, one eye, low vision other eye**
Visual impairment categories 3, 4, 5 in one eye, with categories
1 or 2 in the other eye.

H54.2 **Low vision, both eyes**
Visual impairment categories 1 or 2 in both eyes.

H54.3 **Unqualified visual loss, both eyes**
Visual impairment category 9 in both eyes.

H54.4 **Blindness, one eye**
Visual impairment categories 3, 4, 5 in one eye [normal vision
in other eye].

H54.5 **Low vision, one eye**
Visual impairment categories 1 or 2 in one eye [normal vision in
other eye].

H54.6 **Unqualified visual loss, one eye**
Visual impairment category 9 in one eye [normal vision in other
eye].

H54.7 **Unspecified visual loss**
Visual impairment category 9 NOS.

Note: The table opposite gives a classification of severity of visual
impairment recommended by a WIIO Study Group on the Prevention
of Blindness, Geneva, 6–10 November 1972.[1]

The term "low vision" in category H54 comprises categories 1 and 2
of the table, the term "blindness" categories 3, 4 and 5, and the term
"unqualified visual loss" category 9.

If the extent of the visual field is taken into account, patients with a
field no greater than 10° but greater than 5° around central fixation
should be placed in category 3 and patients with a field no greater
than 5° around central fixation should be placed in category 4, even
if the central acuity is not impaired.

[1] WHO Technical Report Series, No. 518, 1973.

456

Category of visual impairment	Visual acuity with best possible correction	
	Maximum less than:	Minimum equal to or better than:
1	6/18 3/10 (0.3) 20/70	6/60 1/10 (0.1) 20/200
2	6/60 1/10 (0.1) 20/200	3/60 1/20 (0.5) 20/400
3	3/60 1/20 (0.05) 20/400	1/60 (finger counting at 1 metre) 1/50 (0.02) 5/300 (20/1200)
4	1/60 (finger counting at 1 metre) 1/50 (0.02) 5/300	Light perception
5	No light perception	
9	Undetermined or unspecified	

Other disorders of eye and adnexa (H55–H59)

H55 Nystagmus and other irregular eye movements

Nystagmus:
- NOS
- congenital
- deprivation
- dissociated
- latent

H57 Other disorders of eye and adnexa

H57.0 Anomalies of pupillary function

H57.1 Ocular pain

H57.8 Other specified disorders of eye and adnexa

H57.9 Disorder of eye and adnexa, unspecified

H58* Other disorders of eye and adnexa in diseases classified elsewhere

H58.0* Anomalies of pupillary function in diseases classified elsewhere
Argyll Robertson phenomenon or pupil, syphilitic (A52.1†)

H58.1* Visual disturbances in diseases classified elsewhere

H58.8* Other specified disorders of eye and adnexa in diseases classified elsewhere
Syphilitic oculopathy NEC:
- congenital:
  - early (A50.0†)
  - late (A50.3†)
- early (secondary) (A51.4†)
- late (A52.7†)

H59 Postprocedural disorders of eye and adnexa, not elsewhere classified

Excludes: mechanical complication of:
- intraocular lens (T85.2)
- other ocular prosthetic devices, implants and grafts (T85.3)
pseudophakia (Z96.1)

H59.0 Vitreous syndrome following cataract surgery

H59.8 Other postprocedural disorders of eye and adnexa
Chorioretinal scars after surgery for detachment

H59.9 Postprocedural disorder of eye and adnexa, unspecified

CHAPTER VIII

Diseases of the ear and mastoid process (H60–H95)

Excludes: certain conditions originating in the perinatal period (P00–P96)

certain infectious and parasitic diseases (A00–B99)

complications of pregnancy, childbirth and the puerperium (O00–O99)

congenital malformations, deformations and chromosomal abnormalities (Q00–Q99)

endocrine, nutritional and metabolic diseases (E00–E90)

injury, poisoning and certain other consequences of external causes (S00–T98)

neoplasms (C00–D48)

symptoms, signs and abnormal clinical and laboratory findings, not elsewhere classified (R00–R99)

This chapter contains the following blocks:

H60–H62 Diseases of external ear

H65–H75 Diseases of middle ear and mastoid

H80–H83 Diseases of inner ear

H90–H95 Other disorders of ear

Asterisk categories for this chapter are provided as follows:

H62* Disorders of external ear in diseases classified elsewhere

H67* Otitis media in diseases classified elsewhere

H75* Other disorders of middle ear and mastoid in diseases classified elsewhere

H82* Vertiginous syndromes in diseases classified elsewhere

H94* Other disorders of ear in diseases classified elsewhere

Diseases of external ear
(H60–H62)

H60 Otitis externa

H60.0 Abscess of external ear
Boil ⎤
Carbuncle ⎬ of auricle or external auditory canal
Furuncle ⎦

H60.1 Cellulitis of external ear
Cellulitis of:
• auricle
• external auditory canal

H60.2 Malignant otitis externa

H60.3 Other infective otitis externa
Otitis externa:
• diffuse
• haemorrhagic
Swimmer's ear

H60.4 Cholesteatoma of external ear
Keratosis obturans of external ear (canal)

H60.5 Acute otitis externa, noninfective
Acute otitis externa:
• NOS
• actinic
• chemical
• contact
• eczematoid
• reactive

H60.8 Other otitis externa
Chronic otitis externa NOS

H60.9 Otitis externa, unspecified

H61 Other disorders of external ear

H61.0 Perichondritis of external ear
Chondrodermatitis nodularis chronica helicis
Perichondritis of:
- auricle
- pinna

H61.1 Noninfective disorders of pinna
Acquired deformity of:
- auricle
- pinna

Excludes: cauliflower ear (M95.1)

H61.2 Impacted cerumen
Wax in ear

H61.3 Acquired stenosis of external ear canal
Collapse of external ear canal

H61.8 Other specified disorders of external ear
Exostosis of external canal

H61.9 Disorder of external ear, unspecified

H62* Disorders of external ear in diseases classified elsewhere

H62.0* Otitis externa in bacterial diseases classified elsewhere
Otitis externa in erysipelas (A46†)

H62.1* Otitis externa in viral diseases classified elsewhere
Otitis externa in:
- herpesviral [herpes simplex] infection (B00.1†)
- zoster (B02.8†)

H62.2* Otitis externa in mycoses
Otitis externa in:
- aspergillosis (B44.8†)
- candidiasis (B37.2†)
Otomycosis NOS (B36.9†)

H62.3* Otitis externa in other infectious and parasitic diseases classified elsewhere

H62.4* Otitis externa in other diseases classified elsewhere
Otitis externa in impetigo (L01.–†)

H62.8* **Other disorders of external ear in diseases classified elsewhere**

Diseases of middle ear and mastoid (H65–H75)

H65 Nonsuppurative otitis media

Includes: with myringitis

H65.0 **Acute serous otitis media**
Acute and subacute secretory otitis media

H65.1 **Other acute nonsuppurative otitis media**
Otitis media, acute and subacute:
- allergic (mucoid)(sanguinous)(serous)
- mucoid
- nonsuppurative NOS
- sanguinous
- seromucinous

Excludes: otitic barotrauma (T70.0)
otitis media (acute) NOS (H66.9)

H65.2 **Chronic serous otitis media**
Chronic tubotympanal catarrh

H65.3 **Chronic mucoid otitis media**
Glue ear
Otitis media, chronic:
- mucinous
- secretory
- transudative

Excludes: adhesive middle ear disease (H74.1)

H65.4 **Other chronic nonsuppurative otitis media**
Otitis media, chronic:
- allergic
- exudative
- nonsuppurative NOS
- seromucinous
- with effusion (nonpurulent)

H65.9 **Nonsuppurative otitis media, unspecified**
Otitis media:
- allergic
- catarrhal
- exudative
- mucoid
- secretory
- seromucinous
- serous
- transudative
- with effusion (nonpurulent)

H66 Suppurative and unspecified otitis media
Includes: with myringitis

H66.0 **Acute suppurative otitis media**

H66.1 **Chronic tubotympanic suppurative otitis media**
Benign chronic suppurative otitis media
Chronic tubotympanic disease

H66.2 **Chronic atticoantral suppurative otitis media**
Chronic atticoantral disease

H66.3 **Other chronic suppurative otitis media**
Chronic suppurative otitis media NOS

H66.4 **Suppurative otitis media, unspecified**
Purulent otitis media NOS

H66.9 **Otitis media, unspecified**
Otitis media:
- NOS
- acute NOS
- chronic NOS

H67* Otitis media in diseases classified elsewhere

H67.0* **Otitis media in bacterial diseases classified elsewhere**
Otitis media in:
- scarlet fever (A38†)
- tuberculosis (A18.6†)

H67.1* **Otitis media in viral diseases classified elsewhere**
Otitis media in:
- influenza (J10–J11†)
- measles (B05.3†)

H67.8* **Otitis media in other diseases classified elsewhere**

H68 Eustachian salpingitis and obstruction

H68.0 **Eustachian salpingitis**

H68.1 **Obstruction of Eustachian tube**
Compression ⎫
Stenosis ⎬ of Eustachian tube
Stricture ⎭

H69 Other disorders of Eustachian tube

H69.0 **Patulous Eustachian tube**

H69.8 **Other specified disorders of Eustachian tube**

H69.9 **Eustachian tube disorder, unspecified**

H70 Mastoiditis and related conditions

H70.0 **Acute mastoiditis**
Abscess ⎫
Empyema ⎬ of mastoid

H70.1 **Chronic mastoiditis**
Caries ⎫
Fistula ⎬ of mastoid

H70.2 **Petrositis**
Inflammation of petrous bone (acute)(chronic)

H70.8 **Other mastoiditis and related conditions**

H70.9 **Mastoiditis, unspecified**

H71 Cholesteatoma of middle ear

Cholesteatoma tympani

Excludes: cholesteatoma of external ear (H60.4)
recurrent cholesteatoma of postmastoidectomy cavity
(H95.0)

H72 Perforation of tympanic membrane

Includes: perforation of ear drum:
• persistent post-traumatic
• postinflammatory
Excludes: traumatic rupture of ear drum (S09.2)

H72.0 **Central perforation of tympanic membrane**

H72.1 **Attic perforation of tympanic membrane**
Perforation of pars flaccida

H72.2 **Other marginal perforations of tympanic membrane**

H72.8 **Other perforations of tympanic membrane**
Perforation(s):
• multiple ⎫
            ⎬ of tympanic membrane
• total ⎭

H72.9 **Perforation of tympanic membrane, unspecified**

H73 Other disorders of tympanic membrane

H73.0 **Acute myringitis**
Acute tympanitis
Bullous myringitis
Excludes: with otitis media (H65–H66)

H73.1 **Chronic myringitis**
Chronic tympanitis
Excludes: with otitis media (H65–H66)

H73.8 **Other specified disorders of tympanic membrane**

H73.9 **Disorder of tympanic membrane, unspecified**

H74 Other disorders of middle ear and mastoid

H74.0 Tympanosclerosis

H74.1 Adhesive middle ear disease
Adhesive otitis
Excludes: glue ear (H65.3)

H74.2 Discontinuity and dislocation of ear ossicles

H74.3 Other acquired abnormalities of ear ossicles
Ankylosis
Partial loss } of ear ossicles

H74.4 Polyp of middle ear

H74.8 Other specified disorders of middle ear and mastoid

H74.9 Disorder of middle ear and mastoid, unspecified

H75* Other disorders of middle ear and mastoid in diseases classified elsewhere

H75.0* Mastoiditis in infectious and parasitic diseases classified elsewhere
Tuberculous mastoiditis (A18.0†)

H75.8* Other specified disorders of middle ear and mastoid in diseases classified elsewhere

Diseases of inner ear (H80–H83)

H80 Otosclerosis
Includes: otospongiosis

H80.0 Otosclerosis involving oval window, nonobliterative

H80.1 Otosclerosis involving oval window, obliterative

H80.2 Cochlear otosclerosis
Otosclerosis involving:
• otic capsule
• round window

H80.8   **Other otosclerosis**

H80.9   **Otosclerosis, unspecified**

H81   Disorders of vestibular function

Excludes: vertigo:
- NOS (R42)
- epidemic (A88.1)

H81.0   **Ménière's disease**
Labyrinthine hydrops
Ménière's syndrome or vertigo

H81.1   **Benign paroxysmal vertigo**

H81.2   **Vestibular neuronitis**

H81.3   **Other peripheral vertigo**
Lermoyez' syndrome
Vertigo:
- aural
- otogenic
- peripheral NOS

H81.4   **Vertigo of central origin**
Central positional nystagmus

H81.8   **Other disorders of vestibular function**

H81.9   **Disorder of vestibular function, unspecified**
Vertiginous syndrome NOS

H82*   Vertiginous syndromes in diseases classified elsewhere

H83   Other diseases of inner ear

H83.0   **Labyrinthitis**

H83.1   **Labyrinthine fistula**

H83.2   **Labyrinthine dysfunction**
Hypersensitivity ⎫
Hypofunction   ⎬ of labyrinth
Loss of function ⎭

H83.3 **Noise effects on inner ear**
Acoustic trauma
Noise-induced hearing loss

H83.8 **Other specified diseases of inner ear**

H83.9 **Disease of inner ear, unspecified**

Other disorders of ear
(H90–H95)

H90 Conductive and sensorineural hearing loss
Includes: congenital deafness
Excludes: deaf mutism NEC (H91.3)
deafness NOS (H91.9)
hearing loss:
• NOS (H91.9)
• noise-induced (H83.3)
• ototoxic (H91.0)
• sudden (idiopathic) (H91.2)

H90.0 **Conductive hearing loss, bilateral**

H90.1 **Conductive hearing loss, unilateral with unrestricted hearing on the contralateral side**

H90.2 **Conductive hearing loss, unspecified**
Conductive deafness NOS

H90.3 **Sensorineural hearing loss, bilateral**

H90.4 **Sensorlneural hearing loss, unilateral with unrestricted hearing on the contralateral side**

H90.5 **Sensorineural hearing loss, unspecified**
Congenital deafness NOS
Hearing loss:
• central ⎫
• neural ⎬ NOS
• perceptive ⎪
• sensory ⎭
Sensorineural deafness NOS

H90.6 **Mixed conductive and sensorineural hearing loss, bilateral**

H90.7 **Mixed conductive and sensorineural hearing loss, unilateral with unrestricted hearing on the contralateral side**

H90.8 **Mixed conductive and sensorineural hearing loss, unspecified**

H91 Other hearing loss

Excludes: abnormal auditory perception (H93.2)
hearing loss as classified in H90.–
impacted cerumen (H61.2)
noise-induced hearing loss (H83.3)
psychogenic deafness (F44.6)
transient ischaemic deafness (H93.0)

H91.0 **Ototoxic hearing loss**
Use additional external cause code (Chapter XX), if desired, to identify toxic agent.

H91.1 **Presbycusis**
Presbyacusia

H91.2 **Sudden idiopathic hearing loss**
Sudden hearing loss NOS

H91.3 **Deaf mutism, not elsewhere classified**

H91.8 **Other specified hearing loss**

H91.9 **Hearing loss, unspecified**
Deafness:
• NOS
• high frequency
• low frequency

H92 Otalgia and effusion of ear

H92.0 **Otalgia**

H92.1 **Otorrhoea**
Excludes: leakage of cerebrospinal fluid through ear (G96.0)

H92.2 **Otorrhagia**
Excludes: traumatic otorrhagia—code by type of injury

H93 Other disorders of ear, not elsewhere classified

H93.0 **Degenerative and vascular disorders of ear**
Transient ischaemic deafness
Excludes: presbycusis (H91.1)

H93.1 **Tinnitus**

H93.2 **Other abnormal auditory perceptions**
Auditory recruitment
Diplacusis
Hyperacusis
Temporary auditory threshold shift
Excludes: auditory hallucinations (R44.0)

H93.3 **Disorders of acoustic nerve**
Disorder of 8th cranial nerve

H93.8 **Other specified disorders of ear**

H93.9 **Disorder of ear, unspecified**

H94* Other disorders of ear in diseases classified elsewhere

H94.0* **Acoustic neuritis in infectious and parasitic diseases classified elsewhere**
Acoustic neuritis in syphilis (A52.1†)

H94.8* **Other specified disorders of ear in diseases classified elsewhere**

H95 Postprocedural disorders of ear and mastoid process, not elsewhere classified

H95.0 **Recurrent cholesteatoma of postmastoidectomy cavity**

H95.1 **Other disorders following mastoidectomy**
Chronic inflammation ⎫
Granulation   ⎬ of postmastoidectomy cavity
Mucosal cyst   ⎭

H95.8 **Other postprocedural disorders of ear and mastoid process**

H95.9 **Postprocedural disorder of ear and mastoid process, unspecified**

CHAPTER IX

Diseases of the circulatory system (I00–I99)

Excludes: certain conditions originating in the perinatal period (P00–P96)
certain infectious and parasitic diseases (A00–B99)
complications of pregnancy, childbirth and the puerperium
(O00–O99)
congenital malformations, deformations and chromosomal
abnormalities (Q00–Q99)
endocrine, nutritional and metabolic diseases (E00–E90)
injury, poisoning and certain other consequences of external
causes (S00–T98)
neoplasms (C00–D48)
symptoms, signs and abnormal clinical and laboratory findings,
not elsewhere classified (R00–R99)
systemic connective tissue disorders (M30–M36)
transient cerebral ischaemic attacks and related syndromes
(G45.–)

This chapter contains the following blocks:

I00–I02	Acute rheumatic fever
I05–I09	Chronic rheumatic heart diseases
I10–I15	Hypertensive diseases
I20–I25	Ischaemic heart diseases
I26–I28	Pulmonary heart disease and diseases of pulmonary circulation
I30–I52	Other forms of heart disease
I60–I69	Cerebrovascular diseases
I70–I79	Diseases of arteries, arterioles and capillaries
I80–I89	Diseases of veins, lymphatic vessels and lymph nodes, not elsewhere classified
I95–I99	Other and unspecified disorders of the circulatory system

Asterisk categories for this chapter are provided as follows:

I32*	Pericarditis in diseases classified elsewhere
I39*	Endocarditis and heart valve disorders in diseases classified elsewhere
I41*	Myocarditis in diseases classified elsewhere
I43*	Cardiomyopathy in diseases classified elsewhere
I52*	Other heart disorders in diseases classified elsewhere

I68*   Cerebrovascular disorders in diseases classified elsewhere

I79*   Disorders of arteries, arterioles and capillaries in diseases
          classified elsewhere

I98*   Other disorders of circulatory system in diseases classified
          elsewhere

Acute rheumatic fever (I00–I02)

I00   Rheumatic fever without mention of heart involvement

Arthritis, rheumatic, acute or subacute

I01   Rheumatic fever with heart involvement

Excludes: chronic diseases of rheumatic origin (I05–I09) unless
rheumatic fever is also present or there is evidence
of recrudescence or activity of the rheumatic
process. In cases where there is doubt as to
rheumatic activity at the time of death refer to
the mortality coding rules and guidelines in
Volume 2.

I01.0   Acute rheumatic pericarditis

Any condition in I00 with pericarditis
Rheumatic pericarditis (acute)

Excludes: when not specified as rheumatic (I30.–)

I01.1   Acute rheumatic endocarditis

Any condition in I00 with endocarditis or valvulitis
Acute rheumatic valvulitis

I01.2   Acute rheumatic myocarditis

Any condition in I00 with myocarditis

I01.8   Other acute rheumatic heart disease

Any condition in I00 with other or multiple types of heart
involvement
Acute rheumatic pancarditis

I01.9   **Acute rheumatic heart disease, unspecified**
Any condition in I00 with unspecified type of heart involvement
Rheumatic:
• carditis, acute
• heart disease, active or acute

I02   Rheumatic chorea

Includes: Sydenham's chorea
Excludes: chorea:
• NOS (G25.5)
• Huntington (G10)

I02.0   **Rheumatic chorea with heart involvement**
Chorea NOS with heart involvement
Rheumatic chorea with heart involvement of any type classifiable
under I01.–

I02.9   **Rheumatic chorea without heart involvement**
Rheumatic chorea NOS

Chronic rheumatic heart diseases (I05–I09)

I05   Rheumatic mitral valve diseases

Includes: conditions classifiable to I05.0 and I05.2–I05.9,
whether specified as rheumatic or not
Excludes: when specified as nonrheumatic (I34.–)

I05.0   **Mitral stenosis**
Mitral (valve) obstruction (rheumatic)

I05.1   **Rheumatic mitral insufficiency**
Rheumatic mitral:
• incompetence
• regurgitation

I05.2   **Mitral stenosis with insufficiency**
Mitral stenosis with incompetence or regurgitation

I05.8   **Other mitral valve diseases**
Mitral (valve) failure

473

I05.9   Mitral valve disease, unspecified
Mitral (valve) disorder (chronic) NOS

I06   Rheumatic aortic valve diseases

Excludes: when not specified as rheumatic (I35.–)

I06.0   Rheumatic aortic stenosis
Rheumatic aortic (valve) obstruction

I06.1   Rheumatic aortic insufficiency
Rheumatic aortic:
• incompetence
• regurgitation

I06.2   Rheumatic aortic stenosis with insufficiency
Rheumatic aortic stenosis with incompetence or regurgitation

I06.8   Other rheumatic aortic valve diseases

I06.9   Rheumatic aortic valve disease, unspecified
Rheumatic aortic (valve) disease NOS

I07   Rheumatic tricuspid valve diseases

Includes: whether specified as rheumatic or not
Excludes: when specified as nonrheumatic (I36.–)

I07.0   Tricuspid stenosis
Tricuspid (valve) stenosis (rheumatic)

I07.1   Tricuspid insufficiency
Tricuspid (valve) insufficiency (rheumatic)

I07.2   Tricuspid stenosis with insufficiency

I07.8   Other tricuspid valve diseases

I07.9   Tricuspid valve disease, unspecified
Tricuspid valve disorder NOS

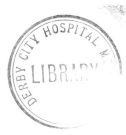

I08 Multiple valve diseases

Includes: whether specified as rheumatic or not

Excludes: endocarditis, valve unspecified (I38)
rheumatic diseases of endocardium, valve unspecified (I09.1)

I08.0 Disorders of both mitral and aortic valves
Involvement of both mitral and aortic valves whether specified as rheumatic or not

I08.1 Disorders of both mitral and tricuspid valves

I08.2 Disorders of both aortic and tricuspid valves

I08.3 Combined disorders of mitral, aortic and tricuspid valves

I08.8 Other multiple valve diseases

I08.9 Multiple valve disease, unspecified

I09 Other rheumatic heart diseases

I09.0 Rheumatic myocarditis
Excludes: myocarditis not specified as rheumatic (I51.4)

I09.1 Rheumatic diseases of endocardium, valve unspecified
Rheumatic:
• endocarditis (chronic)
• valvulitis (chronic)
Excludes: endocarditis, valve unspecified (I38)

I09.2 Chronic rheumatic pericarditis
Adherent pericardium, rheumatic
Chronic rheumatic:
• mediastinopericarditis
• myopericarditis
Excludes: when not specified as rheumatic (I31.–)

I09.8 Other specified rheumatic heart diseases
Rheumatic disease of pulmonary valve

I09.9 Rheumatic heart disease, unspecified
Rheumatic:
• carditis
• heart failure
Excludes: rheumatoid carditis (M05.3)

Hypertensive diseases
(I10–I15)

Excludes: complicating pregnancy, childbirth and the puerperium
(O10–O11, O13–O16)
involving coronary vessels (I20–I25)
neonatal hypertension (P29.2)
pulmonary hypertension (I27.0)

I10 Essential (primary) hypertension
High blood pressure
Hypertension (arterial)(benign)(essential)(malignant)(primary)
(systemic)
Excludes: involving vessels of:
- brain (I60–I69)
- eye (H35.0)

I11 Hypertensive heart disease
Includes: any condition in I50.–, I51.4–I51.9 due to
hypertension

I11.0 **Hypertensive heart disease with (congestive) heart failure**
Hypertensive heart failure

I11.9 **Hypertensive heart disease without (congestive) heart failure**
Hypertensive heart disease NOS

I12 Hypertensive renal disease
Includes: any condition in N18.–, N19.– or N26.– with any
condition in I10
arteriosclerosis of kidney
arteriosclerotic nephritis (chronic)(interstitial)
hypertensive nephropathy
nephrosclerosis
Excludes: secondary hypertension (I15.–)

I12.0 **Hypertensive renal disease with renal failure**
Hypertensive renal failure

I12.9 **Hypertensive renal disease without renal failure**
Hypertensive renal disease NOS

I13 Hypertensive heart and renal disease

Includes: any condition in I11.– with any condition in I12.– disease:
- cardiorenal
- cardiovascular renal

I13.0 **Hypertensive heart and renal disease with (congestive) heart failure**

I13.1 **Hypertensive heart and renal disease with renal failure**

I13.2 **Hypertensive heart and renal disease with both (congestive) heart failure and renal failure**

I13.9 **Hypertensive heart and renal disease, unspecified**

I15 Secondary hypertension

Excludes: involving vessels of:
- brain (I60–I69)
- eye (H35.0)

I15.0 **Renovascular hypertension**

I15.1 **Hypertension secondary to other renal disorders**

I15.2 **Hypertension secondary to endocrine disorders**

I15.8 **Other secondary hypertension**

I15.9 **Secondary hypertension, unspecified**

Ischaemic heart diseases
(I20–I25)

Note: For morbidity, duration as used in categories I21–I25 refers to the interval elapsing between onset of the ischaemic episode and admission to care. For mortality, duration refers to the interval elapsing between onset and death.

Includes: with mention of hypertension (I10–I15)

Use additional code, if desired, to identify presence of hypertension.

I20   Angina pectoris

I20.0   **Unstable angina**
Angina:
- crescendo
- de novo effort
- worsening effort

Intermediate coronary syndrome
Preinfarction syndrome

I20.1   **Angina pectoris with documented spasm**
Angina:
- angiospastic
- Prinzmetal
- spasm-induced
- variant

I20.8   **Other forms of angina pectoris**
Angina of effort
Stenocardia

I20.9   **Angina pectoris, unspecified**
Angina:
- NOS
- cardiac

Anginal syndrome
Ischaemic chest pain

I21   Acute myocardial infarction

Includes: myocardial infarction specified as acute or with a stated duration of 4 weeks (28 days) or less from onset

Excludes: certain current complications following acute myocardial infarction (I23.–)
myocardial infarction:
- old (I25.2)
- specified as chronic or with a stated duration of more than 4 weeks (more than 28 days) from onset (I25.8)
- subsequent (I22.–)

postmyocardial infarction syndrome (I24.1)

I21.0 **Acute transmural myocardial infarction of anterior wall**
Transmural infarction (acute)(of):
- anterior (wall) NOS
- anteroapical
- anterolateral
- anteroseptal

I21.1 **Acute transmural myocardial infarction of inferior wall**
Transmural infarction (acute)(of):
- diaphragmatic wall
- inferior (wall) NOS
- inferolateral
- inferoposterior

I21.2 **Acute transmural myocardial infarction of other sites**
Transmural infarction (acute)(of):
- apical-lateral
- basal-lateral
- high lateral
- lateral (wall) NOS
- posterior (true)
- posterobasal
- posterolateral
- posteroseptal
- septal NOS

I21.3 **Acute transmural myocardial infarction of unspecified site**
Transmural myocardial infarction NOS

I21.4 **Acute subendocardial myocardial infarction**
Nontransmural myocardial infarction NOS

I21.9 **Acute myocardial infarction, unspecified**
Myocardial infarction (acute) NOS

I22 Subsequent myocardial infarction

Includes: recurrent myocardial infarction

Excludes: specified as chronic or with a stated duration of more than 4 weeks (more than 28 days) from onset (I25.8)

I22.0   **Subsequent myocardial infarction of anterior wall**
Subsequent infarction (acute)(of):
- anterior (wall) NOS
- anteroapical
- anterolateral
- anteroseptal

I22.1   **Subsequent myocardial infarction of inferior wall**
Subsequent infarction (acute)(of):
- diaphragmatic wall
- inferior (wall) NOS
- inferolateral
- inferoposterior

I22.8   **Subsequent myocardial infarction of other sites**
Subsequent myocardial infarction (acute)(of):
- apical-lateral
- basal-lateral
- high lateral
- lateral (wall) NOS
- posterior (true)
- posterobasal
- posterolateral
- posteroseptal
- septal NOS

I22.9   **Subsequent myocardial infarction of unspecified site**

I23   Certain current complications following acute myocardial infarction

Excludes: the listed conditions, when:
- concurrent with acute myocardial infarction (I21–I22)
- not specified as current complications following acute myocardial infarction (I31.–, I51.–)

I23.0   **Haemopericardium as current complication following acute myocardial infarction**

I23.1   **Atrial septal defect as current complication following acute myocardial infarction**

I23.2   **Ventricular septal defect as current complication following acute myocardial infarction**

I23.3 **Rupture of cardiac wall without haemopericardium as current complication following acute myocardial infarction**
Excludes: with haemopericardium (I23.0)

I23.4 **Rupture of chordae tendineae as current complication following acute myocardial infarction**

I23.5 **Rupture of papillary muscle as current complication following acute myocardial infarction**

I23.6 **Thrombosis of atrium, auricular appendage, and ventricle as current complications following acute myocardial infarction**

I23.8 **Other current complications following acute myocardial infarction**

I24 Other acute ischaemic heart diseases

Excludes: angina pectoris (I20.–)
transient myocardial ischaemia of newborn (P29.4)

I24.0 **Coronary thrombosis not resulting in myocardial infarction**
Coronary (artery)(vein):
- embolism
- occlusion ⎫ not resulting in myocardial infarction
- thromboembolism ⎭
Excludes: specified as chronic or with a stated duration of more than 4 weeks (more than 28 days) from onset (I25.8)

I24.1 **Dressler's syndrome**
Postmyocardial infarction syndrome

I24.8 **Other forms of acute ischaemic heart disease**
Coronary:
- failure
- insufficiency

I24.9 **Acute ischaemic heart disease, unspecified**
Excludes: ischaemic heart disease (chronic) NOS (I25.9)

I25 Chronic ischaemic heart disease

Excludes: cardiovascular disease NOS (I51.6)

I25.0 Atherosclerotic cardiovascular disease, so described

I25.1 Atherosclerotic heart disease
Coronary (artery):
• atheroma
• atherosclerosis
• disease
• sclerosis

I25.2 Old myocardial infarction
Healed myocardial infarction
Past myocardial infarction diagnosed by ECG or other special
    investigation, but currently presenting no symptoms

I25.3 Aneurysm of heart
Aneurysm:
• mural
• ventricular

I25.4 Coronary artery aneurysm
Coronary arteriovenous fistula, acquired

Excludes: congenital coronary (artery) aneurysm (Q24.5)

I25.5 Ischaemic cardiomyopathy

I25.6 Silent myocardial ischaemia

I25.8 Other forms of chronic ischaemic heart disease
Any condition in I21–I22 and I24.– specified as chronic or with
    a stated duration of more than 4 weeks (more than 28 days)
    from onset

I25.9 Chronic ischaemic heart disease, unspecified
Ischaemic heart disease (chronic) NOS

Pulmonary heart disease and diseases of pulmonary circulation (I26–I28)

I26 Pulmonary embolism

Includes: pulmonary (artery)(vein):
- infarction
- thromboembolism
- thrombosis

Excludes: complicating:
- abortion or ectopic or molar pregnancy (O00–O07, O08.2)
- pregnancy, childbirth and the puerperium (O88.–)

I26.0 Pulmonary embolism with mention of acute cor pulmonale
Acute cor pulmonale NOS

I26.9 Pulmonary embolism without mention of acute cor pulmonale
Pulmonary embolism NOS

I27 Other pulmonary heart diseases

I27.0 Primary pulmonary hypertension
Pulmonary (artery) hypertension (idiopathic)(primary)

I27.1 Kyphoscoliotic heart disease

I27.8 Other specified pulmonary heart diseases

I27.9 Pulmonary heart disease, unspecified
Chronic cardiopulmonary disease
Cor pulmonale (chronic) NOS

I28 Other diseases of pulmonary vessels

I28.0 Arteriovenous fistula of pulmonary vessels

I28.1 Aneurysm of pulmonary artery

I28.8   Other specified diseases of pulmonary vessels

Rupture ⎫
Stenosis ⎬ of pulmonary vessel
Stricture ⎭

I28.9   Disease of pulmonary vessels, unspecified

Other forms of heart disease
(I30–I52)

I30   Acute pericarditis

Includes: acute pericardial effusion
Excludes: rheumatic pericarditis (acute) (I01.0)

I30.0   Acute nonspecific idiopathic pericarditis

I30.1   Infective pericarditis

Pericarditis:
• pneumococcal
• purulent
• staphylococcal
• streptococcal
• viral

Pyopericarditis

Use additional code (B95–B97), if desired, to identify infectious agent.

I30.8   Other forms of acute pericarditis

I30.9   Acute pericarditis, unspecified

I31   Other diseases of pericardium

Excludes: current complications following acute myocardial
              infarction (I23.–)
              postcardiotomy syndrome (I97.0)
              trauma (S26.–)
              when specified as rheumatic (I09.2)

I31.0   **Chronic adhesive pericarditis**
Accretio cordis
Adherent pericardium
Adhesive mediastinopericarditis

I31.1   **Chronic constrictive pericarditis**
Concretio cordis
Pericardial calcification

I31.2   **Haemopericardium, not elsewhere classified**

I31.3   **Pericardial effusion (noninflammatory)**
Chylopericardium

I31.8   **Other specified diseases of pericardium**
Epicardial plaques
Focal pericardial adhesions

I31.9   **Disease of pericardium, unspecified**
Cardiac tamponade
Pericarditis (chronic) NOS

32* Pericarditis in diseases classified elsewhere

I32.0*   **Pericarditis in bacterial diseases classified elsewhere**
Pericarditis:
- gonococcal (A54.8†)
- meningococcal (A39.5†)
- syphilitic (A52.0†)
- tuberculous (A18.8†)

I32.1*   **Pericarditis in other infectious and parasitic diseases
classified elsewhere**

I32.8*   **Pericarditis in other diseases classified elsewhere**
Pericarditis (in):
- rheumatoid (M05.3†)
- systemic lupus erythematosus (M32.1†)
- uraemic (N18.8†)

33 Acute and subacute endocarditis

Excludes: acute rheumatic endocarditis (I01.1)
endocarditis NOS (I38)

485

I33.0 **Acute and subacute infective endocarditis**
Endocarditis (acute)(subacute):
- bacterial
- infective NOS
- lenta
- malignant
- septic
- ulcerative

Use additional code (B95–B97), if desired, to identify infectious agent.

I33.9 **Acute endocarditis, unspecified**
Endocarditis ⎫
Myoendocarditis ⎬ acute or subacute
Periendocarditis ⎭

I34 Nonrheumatic mitral valve disorders

Excludes: mitral (valve):
- disease (I05.9)
- failure (I05.8)
- stenosis (I05.0)
when of unspecified cause but with mention of:
- diseases of aortic valve (I08.0)
- mitral stenosis or obstruction (I05.0)
when specified as rheumatic (I05.–)

I34.0 **Mitral (valve) insufficiency**
Mitral (valve):
- incompetence ⎫
- regurgitation ⎬ NOS or of specified cause, except rheumatic

I34.1 **Mitral (valve) prolapse**
Floppy mitral valve syndrome
Excludes: Marfan's syndrome (Q87.4)

I34.2 **Nonrheumatic mitral (valve) stenosis**

I34.8 **Other nonrheumatic mitral valve disorders**

I34.9 **Nonrheumatic mitral valve disorder, unspecified**

I35 Nonrheumatic aortic valve disorders

Excludes: hypertrophic subaortic stenosis (I42.1)
when of unspecified cause but with mention of
diseases of mitral valve (I08.0)
when specified as rheumatic (I06.–)

I35.0 Aortic (valve) stenosis

I35.1 Aortic (valve) insufficiency
Aortic (valve):
- incompetence
- regurgitation
} NOS or of specified cause, except rheumatic

I35.2 Aortic (valve) stenosis with insufficiency

I35.8 Other aortic valve disorders

I35.9 Aortic valve disorder, unspecified

I36 Nonrheumatic tricuspid valve disorders

Excludes: when of unspecified cause (I07.–)
when specified as rheumatic (I07.–)

I36.0 Nonrheumatic tricuspid (valve) stenosis

I36.1 Nonrheumatic tricuspid (valve) insufficiency
Tricuspid (valve):
- incompetence
- regurgitation
} of specified cause, except rheumatic

I36.2 Nonrheumatic tricuspid (valve) stenosis with insufficiency

I36.8 Other nonrheumatic tricuspid valve disorders

I36.9 Nonrheumatic tricuspid valve disorder, unspecified

I37 Pulmonary valve disorders

Excludes: when specified as rheumatic (I09.8)

I37.0 Pulmonary valve stenosis

I37.1 Pulmonary valve insufficiency
Pulmonary valve:
- incompetence
- regurgitation
} NOS or of specified cause, except rheumatic

487

I37.2   **Pulmonary valve stenosis with insufficiency**

I37.8   **Other pulmonary valve disorders**

I37.9   **Pulmonary valve disorder, unspecified**

I38   Endocarditis, valve unspecified

Endocarditis (chronic) NOS
Valvular:
- incompetence
- insufficiency
- regurgitation
- stenosis
Valvulitis
  (chronic)

of unspecified valve

NOS or of specified cause, except rheumatic

Excludes: endocardial fibroelastosis (I42.4)
             when specified as rheumatic (I09.1)

I39*   Endocarditis and heart valve disorders in diseases classified elsewhere

Includes: endocardial involvement in:
- candidal infection (B37.6†)
- gonococcal infection (A54.8†)
- Libman–Sacks disease (M32.1†)
- meningococcal infection (A39.5†)
- rheumatoid arthritis (M05.3†)
- syphilis (A52.0†)
- tuberculosis (A18.8†)
- typhoid fever (A01.0†)

I39.0*   **Mitral valve disorders in diseases classified elsewhere**

I39.1*   **Aortic valve disorders in diseases classified elsewhere**

I39.2*   **Tricuspid valve disorders in diseases classified elsewhere**

I39.3*   **Pulmonary valve disorders in diseases classified elsewhere**

I39.4*   **Multiple valve disorders in diseases classified elsewhere**

I39.8*   **Endocarditis, valve unspecified, in diseases classified elsewhere**

I40　Acute myocarditis

I40.0　Infective myocarditis
Septic myocarditis

Use additional code (B95–B97), if desired, to identify infectious agent.

I40.1　Isolated myocarditis

I40.8　Other acute myocarditis

I40.9　Acute myocarditis, unspecified

I41*　Myocarditis in diseases classified elsewhere

I41.0*　Myocarditis in bacterial diseases classified elsewhere
Myocarditis:
- diphtheritic (A36.8†)
- gonococcal (A54.8†)
- meningococcal (A39.5†)
- syphilitic (A52.0†)
- tuberculous (A18.8†)

I41.1*　Myocarditis in viral diseases classified elsewhere
Influenzal myocarditis (acute):
- virus identified (J10.8†)
- virus not identified (J11.8†)
Mumps myocarditis (B26.8†)

I41.2*　Myocarditis in other infectious and parasitic diseases classified elsewhere
Myocarditis in:
- Chagas' disease (chronic) (B57.2†)
  - acute (B57.0†)
- toxoplasmosis (B58.8†)

I41.8*　Myocarditis in other diseases classified elsewhere
Rheumatoid myocarditis (M05.3†)
Sarcoid myocarditis (D86.8†)

I42   Cardiomyopathy

Excludes: cardiomyopathy complicating:
- pregnancy (O99.4)
- puerperium (O90.3)

ischaemic cardiomyopathy (I25.5)

I42.0   **Dilated cardiomyopathy**

I42.1   **Obstructive hypertrophic cardiomyopathy**
Hypertrophic subaortic stenosis

I42.2   **Other hypertrophic cardiomyopathy**
Nonobstructive hypertrophic cardiomyopathy

I42.3   **Endomyocardial (eosinophilic) disease**
Endomyocardial (tropical) fibrosis
Löffler's endocarditis

I42.4   **Endocardial fibroelastosis**
Congenital cardiomyopathy

I42.5   **Other restrictive cardiomyopathy**

I42.6   **Alcoholic cardiomyopathy**

I42.7   **Cardiomyopathy due to drugs and other external agents**
Use additional external cause code (Chapter XX), if desired, to identify cause.

I42.8   **Other cardiomyopathies**

I42.9   **Cardiomyopathy, unspecified**
Cardiomyopathy (primary)(secondary) NOS

I43*   Cardiomyopathy in diseases classified elsewhere

I43.0*   **Cardiomyopathy in infectious and parasitic diseases classified elsewhere**
Cardiomyopathy in diphtheria (A36.8†)

I43.1*   **Cardiomyopathy in metabolic diseases**
Cardiac amyloidosis (E85.–†)

I43.2*   **Cardiomyopathy in nutritional diseases**
Nutritional cardiomyopathy NOS (E63.9†)

I43.8*   **Cardiomyopathy in other diseases classified elsewhere**
Gouty tophi of heart (M10.0†)
Thyrotoxic heart disease (E05.9†)

I44   Atrioventricular and left bundle-branch block

I44.0   **Atrioventricular block, first degree**

I44.1   **Atrioventricular block, second degree**
Atrioventricular block, type I and II
Möbitz block, type I and II
Second-degree block, type I and II
Wenckebach's block

I44.2   **Atrioventricular block, complete**
Complete heart block NOS
Third-degree block

I44.3   **Other and unspecified atrioventricular block**
Atrioventricular block NOS

I44.4   **Left anterior fascicular block**

I44.5   **Left posterior fascicular block**

I44.6   **Other and unspecified fascicular block**
Left bundle-branch hemiblock NOS

I44.7   **Left bundle-branch block, unspecified**

I45   Other conduction disorders

I45.0   **Right fascicular block**

I45.1   **Other and unspecified right bundle-branch block**
Right bundle-branch block NOS

I45.2   **Bifascicular block**

I45.3   **Trifascicular block**

I45.4   **Nonspecific intraventricular block**
Bundle-branch block NOS

I45.5   **Other specified heart block**
Sinoatrial block
Sinoauricular block
Excludes: heart block NOS (I45.9)

I45.6 **Pre-excitation syndrome**
Anomalous atrioventricular excitation
Atrioventricular conduction:
- accelerated
- accessory
- pre-excitation
Lown–Ganong–Levine syndrome
Wolff–Parkinson–White syndrome

I45.8 **Other specified conduction disorders**
Atrioventricular [AV] dissociation
Interference dissociation

I45.9 **Conduction disorder, unspecified**
Heart block NOS
Stokes–Adams syndrome

I46 Cardiac arrest

Excludes: cardiogenic shock (R57.0)
complicating:
- abortion or ectopic or molar pregnancy (O00–O07, O08.8)
- obstetric surgery and procedures (O75.4)

I46.0 **Cardiac arrest with successful resuscitation**

I46.1 **Sudden cardiac death, so described**
Excludes: sudden death:
- NOS (R96.–)
- with:
  - conduction disorder (I44–I45)
  - myocardial infarction (I21–I22)

I46.9 **Cardiac arrest, unspecified**

I47 Paroxysmal tachycardia

Excludes: complicating:
- abortion or ectopic or molar pregnancy (O00–O07, O08.8)
- obstetric surgery and procedures (O75.4)
tachycardia NOS (R00.0)

I47.0 **Re-entry ventricular arrhythmia**

I47.1   **Supraventricular tachycardia**
Paroxysmal tachycardia:
- atrial
- atrioventricular [AV]
- junctional
- nodal

I47.2   **Ventricular tachycardia**

I47.9   **Paroxysmal tachycardia, unspecified**
Bouveret(–Hoffmann) syndrome

I48   Atrial fibrillation and flutter

I49   Other cardiac arrhythmias

Excludes: bradycardia NOS (R00.1)
complicating:
- abortion or ectopic or molar pregnancy (O00–O07, O08.8)
- obstetric surgery and procedures (O75.4)
neonatal cardiac dysrhythmia (P29.1)

I49.0   **Ventricular fibrillation and flutter**

I49.1   **Atrial premature depolarization**
Atrial premature beats

I49.2   **Junctional premature depolarization**

I49.3   **Ventricular premature depolarization**

I49.4   **Other and unspecified premature depolarization**
Ectopic beats
Extrasystoles
Extrasystolic arrhythmias
Premature:
- beats NOS
- contractions

I49.5   **Sick sinus syndrome**
Tachycardia-bradycardia syndrome

I49.8   **Other specified cardiac arrhythmias**
Rhythm disorder:
- coronary sinus
- ectopic
- nodal

I49.9   **Cardiac arrhythmia, unspecified**
Arrhythmia (cardiac) NOS

I50   Heart failure

Excludes: complicating:
- abortion or ectopic or molar pregnancy (O00–O07, O08.8)
- obstetric surgery and procedures (O75.4)
due to hypertension (I11.0)
- with renal disease (I13.–)
following cardiac surgery or due to presence of cardiac prosthesis (I97.1)
neonatal cardiac failure (P29.0)

I50.0   **Congestive heart failure**
Congestive heart disease
Right ventricular failure (secondary to left heart failure)

I50.1   **Left ventricular failure**
Acute oedema of lung ⎫ with mention of heart disease
Acute pulmonary oedema ⎭ NOS or heart failure
Cardiac asthma
Left heart failure

I50.9   **Heart failure, unspecified**
Biventricular failure
Cardiac, heart or myocardial failure NOS

I51   Complications and ill-defined descriptions of heart disease

Excludes: any condition in I51.4–I51.9 due to hypertension (I11.–)
- with renal disease (I13.–)
complications following acute myocardial infarction (I23.–)
when specified as rheumatic (I00–I09)

I51.0   **Cardiac septal defect, acquired**
Acquired septal defect (old):
- atrial
- auricular
- ventricular

I51.1   Rupture of chordae tendineae, not elsewhere classified

I51.2   Rupture of papillary muscle, not elsewhere classified

I51.3   Intracardiac thrombosis, not elsewhere classified
Thrombosis (old):
- apical
- atrial
- auricular
- ventricular

I51.4   Myocarditis, unspecified
Myocardial fibrosis
Myocarditis:
- NOS
- chronic (interstitial)

I51.5   Myocardial degeneration
Degeneration of heart or myocardium:
- fatty
- senile
Myocardial disease

I51.6   Cardiovascular disease, unspecified
Cardiovascular accident NOS

Excludes: atherosclerotic cardiovascular disease, so described
(I25.0)

I51.7   Cardiomegaly
Cardiac:
- dilatation
- hypertrophy
Ventricular dilatation

I51.8   Other ill-defined heart diseases
Carditis (acute)(chronic)
Pancarditis (acute)(chronic)

I51.9   Heart disease, unspecified

I52* Other heart disorders in diseases classified elsewhere

Excludes: cardiovascular disorders NOS in diseases classified
elsewhere (I98.–*)

I52.0* **Other heart disorders in bacterial diseases classified
elsewhere**
Meningococcal carditis NEC (A39.5†)

I52.1* **Other heart disorders in other infectious and parasitic
diseases classified elsewhere**
Pulmonary heart disease in schistosomiasis (B65.–†)

I52.8* **Other heart disorders in other diseases classified elsewhere**
Rheumatoid carditis (M05.3†)

Cerebrovascular diseases
(I60–I69)

Includes: with mention of hypertension (conditions in I10 and I15.–)

Use additional code, if desired, to identify presence of hypertension.

Excludes: transient cerebral ischaemic attacks and related syndromes
(G45.–)
traumatic intracranial haemorrhage (S06.–)
vascular dementia (F01.–)

I60 Subarachnoid haemorrhage

Includes: ruptured cerebral aneurysm
Excludes: sequelae of subarachnoid haemorrhage (I69.0)

I60.0 **Subarachnoid haemorrhage from carotid siphon and
bifurcation**

I60.1 **Subarachnoid haemorrhage from middle cerebral artery**

I60.2 **Subarachnoid haemorrhage from anterior communicating
artery**

I60.3 **Subarachnoid haemorrhage from posterior communicating
artery**

I60.4 **Subarachnoid haemorrhage from basilar artery**

I60.5 **Subarachnoid haemorrhage from vertebral artery**

I60.6 **Subarachnoid haemorrhage from other intracranial arteries**
Multiple involvement of intracranial arteries

I60.7 **Subarachnoid haemorrhage from intracranial artery, unspecified**
Ruptured (congenital) berry aneurysm NOS
Subarachnoid haemorrhage from:
- cerebral ⎫
- communicating ⎬ artery NOS
⎭

I60.8 **Other subarachnoid haemorrhage**
Meningeal haemorrhage
Rupture of cerebral arteriovenous malformation

I60.9 **Subarachnoid haemorrhage, unspecified**
Ruptured (congenital) cerebral aneurysm NOS

I61   Intracerebral haemorrhage

Excludes: sequelae of intracerebral haemorrhage (I69.1)

I61.0 **Intracerebral haemorrhage in hemisphere, subcortical**
Deep intracerebral haemorrhage

I61.1 **Intracerebral haemorrhage in hemisphere, cortical**
Cerebral lobe haemorrhage
Superficial intracerebral haemorrhage

I61.2 **Intracerebral haemorrhage in hemisphere, unspecified**

I61.3 **Intracerebral haemorrhage in brain stem**

I61.4 **Intracerebral haemorrhage in cerebellum**

I61.5 **Intracerebral haemorrhage, intraventricular**

I61.6 **Intracerebral haemorrhage, multiple localized**

I61.8 **Other intracerebral haemorrhage**

I61.9 **Intracerebral haemorrhage, unspecified**

I62   Other nontraumatic intracranial haemorrhage

Excludes: sequelae of intracranial haemorrhage (I69.2)

I62.0 **Subdural haemorrhage (acute)(nontraumatic)**

I62.1 **Nontraumatic extradural haemorrhage**
Nontraumatic epidural haemorrhage

I62.9 **Intracranial haemorrhage (nontraumatic), unspecified**

I63   Cerebral infarction

Includes: occlusion and stenosis of cerebral and precerebral
arteries, resulting in cerebral infarction

Excludes: sequelae of cerebral infarction (I69.3)

I63.0	**Cerebral infarction due to thrombosis of precerebral arteries**
I63.1	**Cerebral infarction due to embolism of precerebral arteries**
I63.2	**Cerebral infarction due to unspecified occlusion or stenosis of precerebral arteries**
I63.3	**Cerebral infarction due to thrombosis of cerebral arteries**
I63.4	**Cerebral infarction due to embolism of cerebral arteries**
I63.5	**Cerebral infarction due to unspecified occlusion or stenosis of cerebral arteries**
I63.6	**Cerebral infarction due to cerebral venous thrombosis, nonpyogenic**
I63.8	**Other cerebral infarction**
I63.9	**Cerebral infarction, unspecified**

I64   Stroke, not specified as haemorrhage or infarction

Cerebrovascular accident NOS

Excludes: sequelae of stroke (I69.4)

I65   Occlusion and stenosis of precerebral arteries, not resulting in cerebral infarction

Includes: embolism
narrowing
obstruction (complete)
(partial)
thrombosis
of basilar, carotid or vertebral arteries, not resulting in cerebral infarction

Excludes: when causing cerebral infarction (I63.–)

I65.0	**Occlusion and stenosis of vertebral artery**
I65.1	**Occlusion and stenosis of basilar artery**
I65.2	**Occlusion and stenosis of carotid artery**

I65.3   **Occlusion and stenosis of multiple and bilateral precerebral arteries**

I65.8   **Occlusion and stenosis of other precerebral artery**

I65.9   **Occlusion and stenosis of unspecified precerebral artery**
Precerebral artery NOS

I66   Occlusion and stenosis of cerebral arteries, not resulting in cerebral infarction

Includes: embolism   of middle, anterior and
          narrowing   posterior cerebral
          obstruction (complete)   arteries, and cerebellar
              (partial)   arteries, not resulting
          thrombosis   in cerebral infarction

Excludes: when causing cerebral infarction (I63.–)

I66.0   **Occlusion and stenosis of middle cerebral artery**

I66.1   **Occlusion and stenosis of anterior cerebral artery**

I66.2   **Occlusion and stenosis of posterior cerebral artery**

I66.3   **Occlusion and stenosis of cerebellar arteries**

I66.4   **Occlusion and stenosis of multiple and bilateral cerebral arteries**

I66.8   **Occlusion and stenosis of other cerebral artery**
Occlusion and stenosis of perforating arteries

I66.9   **Occlusion and stenosis of unspecified cerebral artery**

I67   Other cerebrovascular diseases

Excludes: sequelae of the listed conditions (I69.8)

I67.0   **Dissection of cerebral arteries, nonruptured**
Excludes: ruptured cerebral arteries (I60.7)

I67.1   **Cerebral aneurysm, nonruptured**
Cerebral:
- aneurysm NOS
- arteriovenous fistula, acquired

Excludes: congenital cerebral aneurysm, nonruptured (Q28.–)
          ruptured cerebral aneurysm (I60.9)

I67.2 **Cerebral atherosclerosis**
Atheroma of cerebral arteries

I67.3 **Progressive vascular leukoencephalopathy**
Binswanger's disease
Excludes: subcortical vascular dementia (F01.2)

I67.4 **Hypertensive encephalopathy**

I67.5 **Moyamoya disease**

I67.6 **Nonpyogenic thrombosis of intracranial venous system**
Nonpyogenic thrombosis of:
• cerebral vein
• intracranial venous sinus
Excludes: when causing infarction (I63.6)

I67.7 **Cerebral arteritis, not elsewhere classified**

I67.8 **Other specified cerebrovascular diseases**
Acute cerebrovascular insufficiency NOS
Cerebral ischaemia (chronic)

I67.9 **Cerebrovascular disease, unspecified**

I68* Cerebrovascular disorders in diseases classified elsewhere

I68.0* **Cerebral amyloid angiopathy (E85.–†)**

I68.1* **Cerebral arteritis in infectious and parasitic diseases classified elsewhere**
Cerebral arteritis:
• listerial (A32.8†)
• syphilitic (A52.0†)
• tuberculous (A18.8†)

I68.2* **Cerebral arteritis in other diseases classified elsewhere**
Cerebral arteritis in systemic lupus erythematosus (M32.1†)

I68.8* **Other cerebrovascular disorders in diseases classified elsewhere**

I69   Sequelae of cerebrovascular disease

Note: This category is to be used to indicate conditions in I60–I67 as the cause of sequelae, themselves classified elsewhere. The "sequelae" include conditions specified as such or as late effects, or those present one year or more after onset of the causal condition.

I69.0   **Sequelae of subarachnoid haemorrhage**

I69.1   **Sequelae of intracerebral haemorrhage**

I69.2   **Sequelae of other nontraumatic intracranial haemorrhage**

I69.3   **Sequelae of cerebral infarction**

I69.4   **Sequelae of stroke, not specified as haemorrhage or infarction**

I69.8   **Sequelae of other and unspecified cerebrovascular diseases**

Diseases of arteries, arterioles and capillaries (I70–I79)

I70   Atherosclerosis

Includes: arteriolosclerosis
           arteriosclerosis
           arteriosclerotic vascular disease
           atheroma
           degeneration:
           • arterial
           • arteriovascular
           • vascular
           endarteritis deformans or obliterans
           senile:
           • arteritis
           • endarteritis

Excludes: cerebral (I67.2)
           coronary (I25.1)
           mesenteric (K55.1)
           pulmonary (I27.0)

I70.0   **Atherosclerosis of aorta**

I70.1   **Atherosclerosis of renal artery**
Goldblatt's kidney
Excludes: atherosclerosis of renal arterioles (I12.–)

I70.2   **Atherosclerosis of arteries of extremities**
Atherosclerotic gangrene
Mönckeberg's (medial) sclerosis

I70.8   **Atherosclerosis of other arteries**

I70.9   **Generalized and unspecified atherosclerosis**

I71   Aortic aneurysm and dissection

I71.0   **Dissection of aorta [any part]**
Dissecting aneurysm of aorta (ruptured) [any part]

I71.1   **Thoracic aortic aneurysm, ruptured**

I71.2   **Thoracic aortic aneurysm, without mention of rupture**

I71.3   **Abdominal aortic aneurysm, ruptured**

I71.4   **Abdominal aortic aneurysm, without mention of rupture**

I71.5   **Thoracoabdominal aortic aneurysm, ruptured**

I71.6   **Thoracoabdominal aortic aneurysm, without mention of rupture**

I71.8   **Aortic aneurysm of unspecified site, ruptured**
Rupture of aorta NOS

I71.9   **Aortic aneurysm of unspecified site, without mention of rupture**
Aneurysm ⎤
Dilatation ⎬ of aorta
Hyaline necrosis ⎦

I72   Other aneurysm

Includes: aneurysm (cirsoid)(false)(ruptured)

Excludes: aneurysm (of):
- aorta (I71.–)
- arteriovenous NOS (Q27.3)
  - acquired (I77.0)
- cerebral (nonruptured) (I67.1)
  - ruptured (I60.–)
- coronary (I25.4)
- heart (I25.3)
- pulmonary artery (I28.1)
- retinal (H35.0)
- varicose (I77.0)

I72.0   **Aneurysm of carotid artery**

I72.1   **Aneurysm of artery of upper extremity**

I72.2   **Aneurysm of renal artery**

I72.3   **Aneurysm of iliac artery**

I72.4   **Aneurysm of artery of lower extremity**

I72.8   **Aneurysm of other specified arteries**

I72.9   **Aneurysm of unspecified site**

I73   Other peripheral vascular diseases

Excludes: chilblains (T69.1)
         frostbite (T33–T35)
         immersion hand or foot (T69.0)
         spasm of cerebral artery (G45.9)

I73.0   **Raynaud's syndrome**
Raynaud's:
- disease
- gangrene
- phenomenon (secondary)

I73.1   **Thromboangiitis obliterans [Buerger]**

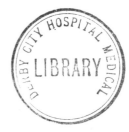

I73.8 **Other specified peripheral vascular diseases**
Acrocyanosis
Acroparaesthesia:
- simple [Schultze's type]
- vasomotor [Nothnagel's type]
Erythrocyanosis
Erythromelalgia

I73.9 **Peripheral vascular disease, unspecified**
Intermittent claudication
Spasm of artery

I74 Arterial embolism and thrombosis

Includes: infarction:
- embolic
- thrombotic
occlusion:
- embolic
- thrombotic

Excludes: embolism and thrombosis:
- basilar (I63.0–I63.2, I65.1)
- carotid (I63.0–I63.2, I65.2)
- cerebral (I63.3–I63.5, I66.9)
- complicating:
  - abortion or ectopic or molar pregnancy (O00–O07, O08.2)
  - pregnancy, childbirth and the puerperium (O88.–)
- coronary (I21–I25)
- mesenteric (K55.0)
- precerebral (I63.0–I63.2, I65.9)
- pulmonary (I26.–)
- renal (N28.0)
- retinal (H34.–)
- vertebral (I63.0–I63.2, I65.0)

I74.0 **Embolism and thrombosis of abdominal aorta**
Aortic bifurcation syndrome
Leriche's syndrome

I74.1 **Embolism and thrombosis of other and unspecified parts of aorta**

I74.2 **Embolism and thrombosis of arteries of upper extremities**

I74.3   **Embolism and thrombosis of arteries of lower extremities**

I74.4   **Embolism and thrombosis of arteries of extremities, unspecified**
Peripheral arterial embolism

I74.5   **Embolism and thrombosis of iliac artery**

I74.8   **Embolism and thrombosis of other arteries**

I74.9   **Embolism and thrombosis of unspecified artery**

I77   Other disorders of arteries and arterioles

Excludes: collagen (vascular) diseases (M30–M36)
hypersensitivity angiitis (M31.0)
pulmonary artery (I28.–)

I77.0   **Arteriovenous fistula, acquired**
Aneurysmal varix
Arteriovenous aneurysm, acquired
Excludes: arteriovenous aneurysm NOS (Q27.3)
cerebral (I67.1)
coronary (I25.4)
traumatic—see injury of blood vessel by body region

I77.1   **Stricture of artery**

I77.2   **Rupture of artery**
Erosion ⎫
Fistula ⎬ of artery
Ulcer ⎭
Excludes: traumatic rupture of artery—see injury of blood
vessel by body region

I77.3   **Arterial fibromuscular dysplasia**

I77.4   **Coeliac artery compression syndrome**

I77.5   **Necrosis of artery**

I77.6   **Arteritis, unspecified**
Aortitis NOS
Endarteritis NOS
Excludes: arteritis or endarteritis:
- aortic arch [Takayasu] (M31.4)
- cerebral NEC (I67.7)
- coronary (I25.8)
- deformans (I70.–)
- giant cell (M31.5–M31.6)
- obliterans (I70.–)
- senile (I70.–)

I77.8   **Other specified disorders of arteries and arterioles**

I77.9   **Disorder of arteries and arterioles, unspecified**

I78   Diseases of capillaries

I78.0   **Hereditary haemorrhagic telangiectasia**
Rendu–Osler–Weber disease

I78.1   **Naevus, non-neoplastic**
Naevus:
- araneus
- spider
- stellar

Excludes: naevus:
- NOS (D22.–)
- blue (D22.–)
- flammeus (Q82.5)
- hairy (D22.–)
- melanocytic (D22.–)
- pigmented (D22.–)
- portwine (Q82.5)
- sanguineous (Q82.5)
- strawberry (Q82.5)
- vascular NOS (Q82.5)
- verrucous (Q82.5)

I78.8   **Other diseases of capillaries**

I78.9   **Disease of capillaries, unspecified**

I79* Disorders of arteries, arterioles and capillaries in diseases classified elsewhere

I79.0* **Aneurysm of aorta in diseases classified elsewhere**
Syphilitic aneurysm of aorta (A52.0†)

I79.1* **Aortitis in diseases classified elsewhere**
Syphilitic aortitis (A52.0†)

I79.2* **Peripheral angiopathy in diseases classified elsewhere**
Diabetic peripheral angiopathy (E10–E14† with common fourth character .5)

I79.8* **Other disorders of arteries, arterioles and capillaries in diseases classified elsewhere**

Diseases of veins, lymphatic vessels and lymph nodes, not elsewhere classified (I80–I89)

I80 Phlebitis and thrombophlebitis

Includes: endophlebitis
inflammation, vein
periphlebitis
suppurative phlebitis

Excludes: phlebitis and thrombophlebitis (of):
• complicating:
  • abortion or ectopic or molar pregnancy (O00–O07, O08.7)
  • pregnancy, childbirth and the puerperium (O22.–, O87.–)
• intracranial and intraspinal, septic or NOS (G08)
• intracranial, nonpyogenic (I67.6)
• intraspinal, nonpyogenic (G95.1)
• portal (vein) (K75.1)
postphlebitic syndrome (I87.0)
thrombophlebitis migrans (I82.1)

Use additional external cause code (Chapter XX), if desired, to identify drug, if drug-induced.

I80.0   **Phlebitis and thrombophlebitis of superficial vessels of lower extremities**

I80.1   **Phlebitis and thrombophlebitis of femoral vein**

I80.2   **Phlebitis and thrombophlebitis of other deep vessels of lower extremities**
Deep vein thrombosis NOS

I80.3   **Phlebitis and thrombophlebitis of lower extremities, unspecified**
Embolism or thrombosis of lower extremity NOS

I80.8   **Phlebitis and thrombophlebitis of other sites**

I80.9   **Phlebitis and thrombophlebitis of unspecified site**

I81   Portal vein thrombosis
Portal (vein) obstruction
Excludes: phlebitis of portal vein (K75.1)

I82   Other venous embolism and thrombosis
Excludes: venous embolism and thrombosis (of):
- cerebral (I63.6, I67.6)
- complicating:
  - abortion or ectopic or molar pregnancy (O00–O07, O08.7)
  - pregnancy, childbirth and the puerperium (O22.–, O87.–)
- coronary (I21–I25)
- intracranial and intraspinal, septic or NOS (G08)
- intracranial, nonpyogenic (I67.6)
- intraspinal, nonpyogenic (G95.1)
- lower extremities (I80.–)
- mesenteric (K55.0)
- portal (I81)
- pulmonary (I26.–)

I82.0   **Budd–Chiari syndrome**

I82.1   **Thrombophlebitis migrans**

I82.2   **Embolism and thrombosis of vena cava**

I82.3   **Embolism and thrombosis of renal vein**

I82.8   **Embolism and thrombosis of other specified veins**

I82.9   **Embolism and thrombosis of unspecified vein**
Embolism of vein NOS
Thrombosis (vein) NOS

I83   Varicose veins of lower extremities

Excludes: complicating:
- pregnancy (O22.0)
- puerperium (O87.8)

I83.0   **Varicose veins of lower extremities with ulcer**
Any condition in I83.9 with ulcer or specified as ulcerated
Varicose ulcer (lower extremity, any part)

I83.1   **Varicose veins of lower extremities with inflammation**
Any condition in I83.9 with inflammation or specified as inflamed
Stasis dermatitis NOS

I83.2   **Varicose veins of lower extremities with both ulcer and inflammation**
Any condition in I83.9 with both ulcer and inflammation

I83.9   **Varicose veins of lower extremities without ulcer or inflammation**
Phlebectasia
Varicose veins   of lower extremity [any part] or of
Varix   unspecified site

I84   Haemorrhoids

Includes: piles
varicose veins of anus and rectum
Excludes: complicating:
- childbirth and the puerperium (O87.2)
- pregnancy (O22.4)

I84.0   **Internal thrombosed haemorrhoids**

I84.1   **Internal haemorrhoids with other complications**
Internal haemorrhoids:
- bleeding
- prolapsed
- strangulated
- ulcerated

I84.2 **Internal haemorrhoids without complication**
Internal haemorrhoids NOS

I84.3 **External thrombosed haemorrhoids**

I84.4 **External haemorrhoids with other complications**
External haemorrhoids:
- bleeding
- prolapsed
- strangulated
- ulcerated

I84.5 **External haemorrhoids without complication**
External haemorrhoids NOS

I84.6 **Residual haemorrhoidal skin tags**
Skin tags of anus or rectum

I84.7 **Unspecified thrombosed haemorrhoids**
Thrombosed haemorrhoids, unspecified whether internal or
external

I84.8 **Unspecified haemorrhoids with other complications**
Haemorrhoids, unspecified whether internal or external:
- bleeding
- prolapsed
- strangulated
- ulcerated

I84.9 **Unspecified haemorrhoids without complication**
Haemorrhoids NOS

I85   Oesophageal varices

I85.0 **Oesophageal varices with bleeding**

I85.9 **Oesophageal varices without bleeding**
Oesophageal varices NOS

I86   Varicose veins of other sites

Excludes: retinal varices (H35.0)
varicose veins of unspecified site (I83.9)

I86.0 **Sublingual varices**

I86.1 **Scrotal varices**
Varicocele

I86.2   **Pelvic varices**

I86.3   **Vulval varices**
Excludes: complicating:
- childbirth and the puerperium (O87.8)
- pregnancy (O22.1)

I86.4   **Gastric varices**

I86.8   **Varicose veins of other specified sites**
Varicose ulcer of nasal septum

I87   Other disorders of veins

I87.0   **Postphlebitic syndrome**

I87.1   **Compression of vein**
Stricture of vein
Vena cava syndrome (inferior)(superior)
Excludes: pulmonary (I28.8)

I87.2   **Venous insufficiency (chronic)(peripheral)**

I87.8   **Other specified disorders of veins**

I87.9   **Disorder of vein, unspecified**

I88   Nonspecific lymphadenitis

Excludes: acute lymphadenitis, except mesenteric (L04.–)
enlarged lymph nodes NOS (R59.–)
human immunodeficiency virus [HIV] disease
resulting in generalized lymphadenopathy (B23.1)

I88.0   **Nonspecific mesenteric lymphadenitis**
Mesenteric lymphadenitis (acute)(chronic)

I88.1   **Chronic lymphadenitis, except mesenteric**
Adenitis ⎫
Lymphadenitis ⎬ chronic, any lymph node except mesenteric

I88.8   **Other nonspecific lymphadenitis**

I88.9   **Nonspecific lymphadenitis, unspecified**
Lymphadenitis NOS

I89   Other noninfective disorders of lymphatic vessels and lymph nodes

Excludes: chylocele:
- filarial (B74.–)
- tunica vaginalis (nonfilarial) NOS (N50.8)

enlarged lymph nodes NOS (R59.–)
hereditary lymphoedema (Q82.0)
postmastectomy lymphoedema (I97.2)

I89.0   Lymphoedema, not elsewhere classified
Lymphangiectasis

I89.1   Lymphangitis
Lymphangitis:
- NOS
- chronic
- subacute

Excludes: acute lymphangitis (L03.–)

I89.8   Other specified noninfective disorders of lymphatic vessels and lymph nodes
Chylocele (nonfilarial)
Lipomelanotic reticulosis

I89.9   Noninfective disorder of lymphatic vessels and lymph nodes, unspecified
Disease of lymphatic vessels NOS

Other and unspecified disorders of the circulatory system (I95–I99)

I95   Hypotension

Excludes: cardiovascular collapse (R57.9)
maternal hypotension syndrome (O26.5)
nonspecific low blood pressure reading NOS (R03.1)

I95.0   Idiopathic hypotension

I95.1 **Orthostatic hypotension**
Hypotension, postural
Excludes: neurogenic orthostatic hypotension [Shy–Drager]
(G90.3)

I95.2 **Hypotension due to drugs**
Use additional external cause code (Chapter XX), if desired, to
identify drug.

I95.8 **Other hypotension**
Chronic hypotension

I95.9 **Hypotension, unspecified**

I97 Postprocedural disorders of circulatory system, not elsewhere classified

Excludes: postoperative shock (T81.1)

I97.0 **Postcardiotomy syndrome**

I97.1 **Other functional disturbances following cardiac surgery**
Cardiac insufficiency ⎱ following cardiac surgery or due to
Heart failure ⎰ presence of cardiac prosthesis

I97.2 **Postmastectomy lymphoedema syndrome**
Elephantiasis ⎱ due to mastectomy
Obliteration of lymphatic vessels ⎰

I97.8 **Other postprocedural disorders of circulatory system, not elsewhere classified**

I97.9 **Postprocedural disorder of circulatory system, unspecified**

I98* Other disorders of circulatory system in diseases classified elsewhere

Excludes: disorders classified to other asterisk categories within
this chapter

I98.0* **Cardiovascular syphilis**
Cardiovascular syphilis:
• NOS (A52.0†)
• congenital, late (A50.5†)

I98.1* **Cardiovascular disorders in other infectious and parasitic diseases classified elsewhere**
Cardiovascular:
- involvement NEC, in Chagas' disease (chronic) (B57.2†)
- lesions of pinta [carate] (A67.2†)

I98.2* **Oesophageal varices in diseases classified elsewhere**
Oesophageal varices in:
- liver disorders (K70–K71†, K74.–†)
- schistosomiasis (B65.–†)

I98.8* **Other specified disorders of circulatory system in diseases classified elsewhere**

I99 **Other and unspecified disorders of circulatory system**

CHAPTER X

Diseases of the respiratory system (J00–J99)

Note: When a respiratory condition is described as occurring in more than one site and is not specifically indexed, it should be classified to the lower anatomic site (e.g., tracheobronchitis to bronchitis in J40).

Excludes: certain conditions originating in the perinatal period (P00–P96)

certain infectious and parasitic diseases (A00–B99)

complications of pregnancy, childbirth and the puerperium (O00–O99)

congenital malformations, deformations and chromosomal abnormalities (Q00–Q99)

endocrine, nutritional and metabolic diseases (E00–E90)

injury, poisoning and certain other consequences of external causes (S00–T98)

neoplasms (C00–D48)

symptoms, signs and abnormal clinical and laboratory findings, not elsewhere classified (R00–R99)

This chapter contains the following blocks:

J00–J06	Acute upper respiratory infections
J10–J18	Influenza and pneumonia
J20–J22	Other acute lower respiratory infections
J30–J39	Other diseases of upper respiratory tract
J40–J47	Chronic lower respiratory diseases
J60–J70	Lung diseases due to external agents
J80–J84	Other respiratory diseases principally affecting the interstitium
J85–J86	Suppurative and necrotic conditions of lower respiratory tract
J90–J94	Other diseases of pleura
J95–J99	Other diseases of the respiratory system

Asterisk categories for this chapter are provided as follows:

J17*	Pneumonia in diseases classified elsewhere
J91*	Pleural effusion in conditions classified elsewhere
J99*	Respiratory disorders in diseases classified elsewhere

Acute upper respiratory infections (J00–J06)

Excludes: chronic obstructive pulmonary disease with acute exacerbation NOS (J44.1)

J00 Acute nasopharyngitis [common cold]

Coryza (acute)
Nasal catarrh, acute
Nasopharyngitis:
- NOS
- infective NOS
Rhinitis:
- acute
- infective

Excludes: nasopharyngitis, chronic (J31.1)
pharyngitis:
- NOS (J02.9)
- acute (J02.–)
- chronic (J31.2)
rhinitis:
- NOS (J31.0)
- allergic (J30.1–J30.4)
- chronic (J31.0)
- vasomotor (J30.0)
sore throat:
- NOS (J02.9)
- acute (J02.–)
- chronic (J31.2)

J01 Acute sinusitis

Includes: abscess
empyema
infection } acute, of sinus (accessory)(nasal)
inflammation
suppuration

Use additional code (B95–B97), if desired, to identify infectious agent.

Excludes: sinusitis, chronic or NOS (J32.–)

J01.0   **Acute maxillary sinusitis**
Acute antritis

J01.1   **Acute frontal sinusitis**

J01.2   **Acute ethmoidal sinusitis**

J01.3   **Acute sphenoidal sinusitis**

J01.4   **Acute pansinusitis**

J01.8   **Other acute sinusitis**
Acute sinusitis involving more than one sinus but not pansinusitis

J01.9   **Acute sinusitis, unspecified**

J02   Acute pharyngitis

Includes: acute sore throat
Excludes: abscess:
- peritonsillar (J36)
- pharyngeal (J39.1)
- retropharyngeal (J39.0)
acute laryngopharyngitis (J06.0)
chronic pharyngitis (J31.2)

J02.0   **Streptococcal pharyngitis**
Streptococcal sore throat
Excludes: scarlet fever (A38)

J02.8   **Acute pharyngitis due to other specified organisms**
Use additional code (B95–B97), if desired, to identify infectious agent.
Excludes: due to:
- infectious mononucleosis (B27.–)
- influenza virus:
  - identified (J10.1)
  - not identified (J11.1)
pharyngitis:
- enteroviral vesicular (B08.5)
- herpesviral [herpes simplex] (B00.2)

J02.9   **Acute pharyngitis, unspecified**
Pharyngitis (acute):
- NOS
- gangrenous
- infective NOS
- suppurative
- ulcerative

Sore throat (acute) NOS

J03   Acute tonsillitis

Excludes: peritonsillar abscess (J36)
sore throat:
- NOS (J02.9)
- acute (J02.–)
- streptococcal (J02.0)

J03.0   **Streptococcal tonsillitis**

J03.8   **Acute tonsillitis due to other specified organisms**
Use additional code (B95–B97), if desired, to identify infectious
agent.

Excludes: herpesviral [herpes simplex] pharyngotonsillitis
(B00.2)

J03.9   **Acute tonsillitis, unspecified**
Tonsillitis (acute):
- NOS
- follicular
- gangrenous
- infective
- ulcerative

J04   Acute laryngitis and tracheitis

Use additional code (B95–B97), if desired, to identify infectious
agent.

Excludes: acute obstructive laryngitis [croup] and epiglottitis
(J05.–)
laryngismus (stridulus) (J38.5)

J04.0   **Acute laryngitis**
Laryngitis (acute):
- NOS
- oedematous
- subglottic
- suppurative
- ulcerative

Excludes: chronic laryngitis (J37.0)
influenzal laryngitis, influenza virus:
- identified (J10.1)
- not identified (J11.1)

J04.1   **Acute tracheitis**
Tracheitis (acute):
- NOS
- catarrhal

Excludes: chronic tracheitis (J42)

J04.2   **Acute laryngotracheitis**
Laryngotracheitis NOS
Tracheitis (acute) with laryngitis (acute)

Excludes: chronic laryngotracheitis (J37.1)

J05   **Acute obstructive laryngitis [croup] and epiglottitis**
Use additional code (B95–B97), if desired, to identify infectious agent.

J05.0   **Acute obstructive laryngitis [croup]**
Obstructive laryngitis NOS

J05.1   **Acute epiglottitis**
Epiglottitis NOS

J06   **Acute upper respiratory infections of multiple and unspecified sites**

Excludes: acute respiratory infection NOS (J22)
influenza virus:
- identified (J10.1)
- not identified (J11.1)

J06.0   **Acute laryngopharyngitis**

J06.8 **Other acute upper respiratory infections of multiple sites**

J06.9 **Acute upper respiratory infection, unspecified**
Upper respiratory:
- disease, acute
- infection NOS

Influenza and pneumonia
(J10–J18)

J10 Influenza due to identified influenza virus
Excludes: *Haemophilus influenzae* [*H. influenzae*]:
- infection NOS (A49.2)
- meningitis (G00.0)
- pneumonia (J14)

J10.0 **Influenza with pneumonia, influenza virus identified**
Influenzal (broncho)pneumonia, influenza virus identified

J10.1 **Influenza with other respiratory manifestations, influenza virus identified**
Influenza
Influenzal:
- acute upper respiratory infection } influenza virus
- laryngitis } identified
- pharyngitis
- pleural effusion

J10.8 **Influenza with other manifestations, influenza virus identified**
Encephalopathy due to influenza
Influenzal: } influenza virus identified
- gastroenteritis
- myocarditis (acute)

520

J11 Influenza, virus not identified

Includes: influenza ⎫ specific virus not stated to have
viral influenza ⎭ been identified

Excludes: *Haemophilus influenzae* [*H. influenzae*]:
- infection NOS (A49.2)
- meningitis (G00.0)
- pneumonia (J14)

J11.0 Influenza with pneumonia, virus not identified
Influenzal (broncho)pneumonia, unspecified or specific virus not
identified

J11.1 Influenza with other respiratory manifestations, virus not identified
Influenza NOS
Influenzal:
- acute upper respiratory infection ⎫
- laryngitis ⎬ unspecified or specific
- pharyngitis virus not identified
- pleural effusion ⎭

J11.8 Influenza with other manifestations, virus not identified
Encephalopathy due to influenza ⎫
Influenzal: ⎪ unspecified or specific
- gastroenteritis ⎬ virus not identified
- myocarditis (acute) ⎭

J12 Viral pneumonia, not elsewhere classified

Includes: bronchopneumonia due to viruses other than influenza viruses

Excludes: congenital rubella pneumonitis (P35.0)
pneumonia:
- aspiration (due to):
  - NOS (J69.0)
  - anaesthesia during:
    - labour and delivery (O74.0)
    - pregnancy (O29.0)
    - puerperium (O89.0)
  - neonatal (P24.9)
  - solids and liquids (J69.–)
- congenital (P23.0)
- in influenza (J10.0, J11.0)
- interstitial NOS (J84.9)
- lipid (J69.1)

J12.0 **Adenoviral pneumonia**

J12.1 **Respiratory syncytial virus pneumonia**

J12.2 **Parainfluenza virus pneumonia**

J12.8 **Other viral pneumonia**

J12.9 **Viral pneumonia, unspecified**

J13 Pneumonia due to *Streptococcus pneumoniae*

Bronchopneumonia due to *S. pneumoniae*

Excludes: congenital pneumonia due to *S. pneumoniae* (P23.6)
pneumonia due to other streptococci (J15.3–J15.4)

J14 Pneumonia due to *Haemophilus influenzae*

Bronchopneumonia due to *H. influenzae*

Excludes: congenital pneumonia due to *H. influenzae* (P23.6)

J15 Bacterial pneumonia, not elsewhere classified

Includes: bronchopneumonia due to bacteria other than
S. pneumoniae and H. influenzae

Excludes: chlamydial pneumonia (J16.0)
congenital pneumonia (P23.–)
Legionnaires' disease (A48.1)

J15.0 Pneumonia due to *Klebsiella pneumoniae*

J15.1 Pneumonia due to *Pseudomonas*

J15.2 Pneumonia due to staphylococcus

J15.3 Pneumonia due to streptococcus, group B

J15.4 Pneumonia due to other streptococci

Excludes: pneumonia due to:
- streptococcus, group B (J15.3)
- *Streptococcus pneumoniae* (J13)

J15.5 Pneumonia due to *Escherichia coli*

J15.6 Pneumonia due to other aerobic Gram-negative bacteria
Pneumonia due to *Serratia marcescens*

J15.7 Pneumonia due to *Mycoplasma pneumoniae*

J15.8 Other bacterial pneumonia

J15.9 Bacterial pneumonia, unspecified

J16 Pneumonia due to other infectious organisms, not elsewhere classified

Excludes: ornithosis (A70)
pneumocystosis (B59)
pneumonia:
- NOS (J18.9)
- congenital (P23.–)

J16.0 Chlamydial pneumonia

J16.8 Pneumonia due to other specified infectious organisms

J17* Pneumonia in diseases classified elsewhere

J17.0* **Pneumonia in bacterial diseases classified elsewhere**
Pneumonia (due to)(in):
- actinomycosis (A42.0†)
- anthrax (A22.1†)
- gonorrhoea (A54.8†)
- nocardiosis (A43.0†)
- salmonella infection (A02.2†)
- tularaemia (A21.2†)
- typhoid fever (A01.0†)
- whooping cough (A37.–†)

J17.1* **Pneumonia in viral diseases classified elsewhere**
Pneumonia in:
- cytomegalovirus disease (B25.0†)
- measles (B05.2†)
- rubella (B06.8†)
- varicella (B01.2†)

J17.2* **Pneumonia in mycoses**
Pneumonia in:
- aspergillosis (B44.0–B44.1†)
- candidiasis (B37.1†)
- coccidioidomycosis (B38.0–B38.2†)
- histoplasmosis (B39.–†)

J17.3* **Pneumonia in parasitic diseases**
Pneumonia in:
- ascariasis (B77.8†)
- schistosomiasis (B65.–†)
- toxoplasmosis (B58.3†)

J17.8* **Pneumonia in other diseases classified elsewhere**
Pneumonia (in):
- ornithosis (A70†)
- Q fever (A78†)
- rheumatic fever (I00†)
- spirochaetal, not elsewhere classified (A69.8†)

J18   Pneumonia, organism unspecified

Excludes: abscess of lung with pneumonia (J85.1)
drug-induced interstitial lung disorders (J70.2–J70.4)
pneumonia:
- aspiration (due to):
  - NOS (J69.0)
  - anaesthesia during:
    - labour and delivery (O74.0)
    - pregnancy (O29.0)
    - puerperium (O89.0)
  - neonatal (P24.9)
  - solids and liquids (J69.–)
- congenital (P23.9)
- interstitial NOS (J84.9)
- lipid (J69.1)
pneumonitis, due to external agents (J67–J70)

J18.0   Bronchopneumonia, unspecified

Excludes: bronchiolitis (J21.–)

J18.1   Lobar pneumonia, unspecified

J18.2   Hypostatic pneumonia, unspecified

J18.8   Other pneumonia, organism unspecified

J18.9   Pneumonia, unspecified

Other acute lower respiratory infections (J20–J22)

Excludes: chronic obstructive pulmonary disease with acute:
- exacerbation NOS (J44.1)
- lower respiratory infection (J44.0)

J20 Acute bronchitis

Includes: bronchitis:
- NOS, in those under 15 years of age
- acute and subacute (with):
  - bronchospasm
  - fibrinous
  - membranous
  - purulent
  - septic
  - tracheitis
  tracheobronchitis, acute

Excludes: bronchitis:
- NOS, in those 15 years of age and above (J40)
- allergic NOS (J45.0)
- chronic:
  - NOS (J42)
  - mucopurulent (J41.1)
  - obstructive (J44.–)
  - simple (J41.0)
  tracheobronchitis:
- NOS (J40)
- chronic (J42)
  - obstructive (J44.–)

J20.0	**Acute bronchitis due to *Mycoplasma pneumoniae***
J20.1	**Acute bronchitis due to *Haemophilus influenzae***
J20.2	**Acute bronchitis due to streptococcus**
J20.3	**Acute bronchitis due to coxsackievirus**
J20.4	**Acute bronchitis due to parainfluenza virus**
J20.5	**Acute bronchitis due to respiratory syncytial virus**
J20.6	**Acute bronchitis due to rhinovirus**
J20.7	**Acute bronchitis due to echovirus**
J20.8	**Acute bronchitis due to other specified organisms**
J20.9	**Acute bronchitis, unspecified**

J21 Acute bronchiolitis
Includes: with bronchospasm

J21.0 **Acute bronchiolitis due to respiratory syncytial virus**

J21.8 **Acute bronchiolitis due to other specified organisms**

J21.9 **Acute bronchiolitis, unspecified**
Bronchiolitis (acute)

J22 Unspecified acute lower respiratory infection
Acute (lower) respiratory (tract) infection NOS
Excludes: upper respiratory infection (acute) (J06.9)

Other diseases of upper respiratory tract (J30–J39)

J30 Vasomotor and allergic rhinitis
Includes: spasmodic rhinorrhoea
Excludes: allergic rhinitis with asthma (J45.0)
rhinitis NOS (J31.0)

J30.0 **Vasomotor rhinitis**

J30.1 **Allergic rhinitis due to pollen**
Allergy NOS due to pollen
Hay fever
Pollinosis

J30.2 **Other seasonal allergic rhinitis**

J30.3 **Other allergic rhinitis**
Perennial allergic rhinitis

J30.4 **Allergic rhinitis, unspecified**

J31   Chronic rhinitis, nasopharyngitis and pharyngitis

J31.0   Chronic rhinitis
Ozena
Rhinitis (chronic):
• NOS
• atrophic
• granulomatous
• hypertrophic
• obstructive
• purulent
• ulcerative
Excludes: rhinitis:
• allergic (J30.1–J30.4)
• vasomotor (J30.0)

J31.1   Chronic nasopharyngitis
Excludes: nasopharyngitis, acute or NOS (J00)

J31.2   Chronic pharyngitis
Chronic sore throat
Pharyngitis (chronic):
• atrophic
• granular
• hypertrophic
Excludes: pharyngitis, acute or NOS (J02.9)

J32   Chronic sinusitis

Includes: abscess
empyema
infection
suppuration
} (chronic) of sinus (accessory)(nasal)

Use additional code (B95–B97), if desired, to identify infectious agent.
Excludes: acute sinusitis (J01.–)

J32.0   Chronic maxillary sinusitis
Antritis (chronic)
Maxillary sinusitis NOS

J32.1   Chronic frontal sinusitis
Frontal sinusitis NOS

J32.2 **Chronic ethmoidal sinusitis**
Ethmoidal sinusitis NOS

J32.3 **Chronic sphenoidal sinusitis**
Sphenoidal sinusitis NOS

J32.4 **Chronic pansinusitis**
Pansinusitis NOS

J32.8 **Other chronic sinusitis**
Sinusitis (chronic) involving more than one sinus but not pansinusitis

J32.9 **Chronic sinusitis, unspecified**
Sinusitis (chronic) NOS

33 ▊ Nasal polyp

Excludes: adenomatous polyps (D14.0)

J33.0 **Polyp of nasal cavity**
Polyp:
• choanal
• nasopharyngeal

J33.1 **Polypoid sinus degeneration**
Woakes' syndrome or ethmoiditis

J33.8 **Other polyp of sinus**
Polyp of sinus:
• accessory
• ethmoidal
• maxillary
• sphenoidal

J33.9 **Nasal polyp, unspecified**

34 ▊ Other disorders of nose and nasal sinuses

Excludes: varicose ulcer of nasal septum (I86.8)

J34.0 **Abscess, furuncle and carbuncle of nose**
Cellulitis ⎫
Necrosis ⎬ of nose (septum)
Ulceration ⎭

J34.1 **Cyst and mucocele of nasal sinus**

J34.2 **Deviated nasal septum**
Deflection or deviation of septum (nasal)(acquired)

J34.3 **Hypertrophy of nasal turbinates**

J34.8 **Other specified disorders of nose and nasal sinuses**
Perforation of nasal septum NOS
Rhinolith

J35 Chronic diseases of tonsils and adenoids

J35.0 **Chronic tonsillitis**
Excludes: tonsillitis:
- NOS (J03.9)
- acute (J03.–)

J35.1 **Hypertrophy of tonsils**
Enlargement of tonsils

J35.2 **Hypertrophy of adenoids**
Enlargement of adenoids

J35.3 **Hypertrophy of tonsils with hypertrophy of adenoids**

J35.8 **Other chronic diseases of tonsils and adenoids**
Adenoid vegetations
Amygdalolith
Cicatrix of tonsil (and adenoid)
Tonsillar tag
Ulcer of tonsil

J35.9 **Chronic disease of tonsils and adenoids, unspecified**
Disease (chronic) of tonsils and adenoids NOS

J36 Peritonsillar abscess

Abscess of tonsil
Peritonsillar cellulitis
Quinsy

Use additional code (B95–B97), if desired, to identify infectious agent.

Excludes: retropharyngeal abscess (J39.0)
tonsillitis:
- NOS (J03.9)
- acute (J03.–)
- chronic (J35.0)

J37 Chronic laryngitis and laryngotracheitis

Use additional code (B95–B97), if desired, to identify infectious agent.

J37.0 Chronic laryngitis

Laryngitis:
- catarrhal
- hypertrophic
- sicca

Excludes: laryngitis:
- NOS (J04.0)
- acute (J04.0)
- obstructive (acute) (J05.0)

J37.1 Chronic laryngotracheitis

Laryngitis, chronic, with tracheitis (chronic)
Tracheitis, chronic, with laryngitis

Excludes: laryngotracheitis:
- NOS (J04.2)
- acute (J04.2)
tracheitis:
- NOS (J04.1)
- acute (J04.1)
- chronic (J42)

J38 Diseases of vocal cords and larynx, not elsewhere classified

Excludes: congenital laryngeal stridor (Q31.4)
laryngitis:
- obstructive (acute) (J05.0)
- ulcerative (J04.0)
postprocedural subglottic stenosis (J95.5)
stridor (R06.1)

J38.0 Paralysis of vocal cords and larynx

Laryngoplegia
Paralysis of glottis

J38.1 Polyp of vocal cord and larynx

Excludes: adenomatous polyps (D14.1)

J38.2 Nodules of vocal cords
Chorditis (fibrinous)(nodosa)(tuberosa)
Singer's nodes
Teacher's nodes

J38.3 Other diseases of vocal cords
Abscess
Cellulitis
Granuloma   } of vocal cord(s)
Leukokeratosis
Leukoplakia

J38.4 Oedema of larynx
Oedema (of):
• glottis
• subglottic
• supraglottic
Excludes: laryngitis:
             • acute obstructive [croup] (J05.0)
             • oedematous (J04.0)

J38.5 Laryngeal spasm
Laryngismus (stridulus)

J38.6 Stenosis of larynx

J38.7 Other diseases of larynx
Abscess
Cellulitis
Disease NOS
Necrosis   } of larynx
Pachyderma
Perichondritis
Ulcer

J39 Other diseases of upper respiratory tract
Excludes: acute respiratory infection NOS (J22)
             • upper (J06.9)
             upper respiratory inflammation due to chemicals,
               gases, fumes or vapours (J68.2)

J39.0 Retropharyngeal and parapharyngeal abscess
Peripharyngeal abscess
Excludes: peritonsillar abscess (J36)

J39.1   Other abscess of pharynx
Cellulitis of pharynx
Nasopharyngeal abscess

J39.2   Other diseases of pharynx
Cyst ⎫
Oedema ⎬ of pharynx or nasopharynx
       ⎭
Excludes: pharyngitis:
 • chronic (J31.2)
 • ulcerative (J02.9)

J39.3   Upper respiratory tract hypersensitivity reaction, site unspecified

J39.8   Other specified diseases of upper respiratory tract

J39.9   Disease of upper respiratory tract, unspecified

Chronic lower respiratory diseases (J40–J47)

Excludes: cystic fibrosis (E84.–)

J40   Bronchitis, not specified as acute or chronic

Note: Bronchitis not specified as acute or chronic in those
under 15 years of age can be assumed to be of acute
nature and should be classified to J20.–.

Bronchitis:
 • NOS
 • catarrhal
 • with tracheitis NOS
Tracheobronchitis NOS

Excludes: bronchitis:
 • allergic NOS (J45.0)
 • asthmatic NOS (J45.9)
 • chemical (acute) (J68.0)

533

J41 Simple and mucopurulent chronic bronchitis

Excludes: chronic bronchitis:
- NOS (J42)
- obstructive (J44.–)

J41.0 **Simple chronic bronchitis**

J41.1 **Mucopurulent chronic bronchitis**

J41.8 **Mixed simple and mucopurulent chronic bronchitis**

J42 Unspecified chronic bronchitis

Chronic:
- bronchitis NOS
- tracheitis
- tracheobronchitis

Excludes: chronic:
- asthmatic bronchitis (J44.–)
- bronchitis:
  - simple and mucopurulent (J41.–)
  - with airways obstruction (J44.–)
- emphysematous bronchitis (J44.–)
- obstructive pulmonary disease NOS (J44.9)

J43 Emphysema

Excludes: emphysema:
- compensatory (J98.3)
- due to inhalation of chemicals, gases, fumes or vapours (J68.4)
- interstitial (J98.2)
  - neonatal (P25.0)
- mediastinal (J98.2)
- surgical (subcutaneous) (T81.8)
- traumatic subcutaneous (T79.7)
- with chronic (obstructive) bronchitis (J44.–)
emphysematous (obstructive) bronchitis (J44.–)

J43.0 **MacLeod's syndrome**
Unilateral:
- emphysema
- transparency of lung

J43.1   **Panlobular emphysema**
Panacinar emphysema

J43.2   **Centrilobular emphysema**

J43.8   **Other emphysema**

J43.9   **Emphysema, unspecified**
Emphysema (lung)(pulmonary):
- NOS
- bullous
- vesicular

Emphysematous bleb

J44   Other chronic obstructive pulmonary disease

Includes: chronic:
- bronchitis:
  - asthmatic (obstructive)
  - emphysematous
  - with:
    - airways obstruction
    - emphysema
  - obstructive:
    - asthma
    - bronchitis
    - tracheobronchitis

Excludes: asthma (J45.–)
asthmatic bronchitis NOS (J45.9)
bronchiectasis (J47)
chronic:
- bronchitis:
  - NOS (J42)
  - simple and mucopurulent (J41.–)
- tracheitis (J42)
- tracheobronchitis (J42)

emphysema (J43.–)
lung diseases due to external agents (J60–J70)

J44.0   **Chronic obstructive pulmonary disease with acute lower respiratory infection**
Excludes: with influenza (J10–J11)

J44.1   **Chronic obstructive pulmonary disease with acute exacerbation, unspecified**

J44.8 **Other specified chronic obstructive pulmonary disease**
Chronic bronchitis:
- asthmatic (obstructive) NOS
- emphysematous NOS
- obstructive NOS

J44.9 **Chronic obstructive pulmonary disease, unspecified**
Chronic obstructive:
- airway disease NOS
- lung disease NOS

J45 Asthma

Excludes: acute severe asthma (J46)
chronic asthmatic (obstructive) bronchitis (J44.–)
chronic obstructive asthma (J44.–)
eosinophilic asthma (J82)
lung diseases due to external agents (J60–J70)
status asthmaticus (J46)

J45.0 **Predominantly allergic asthma**
Allergic:
- bronchitis NOS
- rhinitis with asthma
Atopic asthma
Extrinsic allergic asthma
Hay fever with asthma

J45.1 **Nonallergic asthma**
Idiosyncratic asthma
Intrinsic nonallergic asthma

J45.8 **Mixed asthma**
Combination of conditions listed in J45.0 and J45.1

J45.9 **Asthma, unspecified**
Asthmatic bronchitis NOS
Late-onset asthma

J46 Status asthmaticus

Acute severe asthma

J47 Bronchiectasis

Bronchiolectasis

Excludes: congenital bronchiectasis (Q33.4)

tuberculous bronchiectasis (current disease) (A15–A16)

Lung diseases due to external agents (J60–J70)

Excludes: asthma classified to J45.–

J60 Coalworker's pneumoconiosis

Anthracosilicosis

Anthracosis

Coalworker's lung

Excludes: with tuberculosis (J65)

61 Pneumoconiosis due to asbestos and other mineral fibres

Asbestosis

Excludes: pleural plaque with asbestosis (J92.0)

with tuberculosis (J65)

J62 Pneumoconiosis due to dust containing silica

Includes: silicotic fibrosis (massive) of lung

Excludes: pneumoconiosis with tuberculosis (J65)

J62.0   Pneumoconiosis due to talc dust

J62.8   Pneumoconiosis due to other dust containing silica

Silicosis NOS

63 Pneumoconiosis due to other inorganic dusts

Excludes: with tuberculosis (J65)

J63.0   Aluminosis (of lung)

J63.1   Bauxite fibrosis (of lung)

J63.2   Berylliosis

J63.3   Graphite fibrosis (of lung)

J63.4   Siderosis

J63.5   Stannosis

J63.8   Pneumoconiosis due to other specified inorganic dusts

J64   Unspecified pneumoconiosis
Excludes: with tuberculosis (J65)

65   Pneumoconiosis associated with tuberculosis
Any condition in J60–J64 with tuberculosis, any type in A15–A16

J66   Airway disease due to specific organic dust
Excludes: bagassosis (J67.1)
farmer's lung (J67.0)
hypersensitivity pneumonitis due to organic dust (J67.–)
reactive airways dysfunction syndrome (J68.3)

J66.0   Byssinosis
Airway disease due to cotton dust

J66.1   Flax-dresser's disease

J66.2   Cannabinosis

J66.8   Airway disease due to other specific organic dusts

67   Hypersensitivity pneumonitis due to organic dust
Includes: allergic alveolitis and pneumonitis due to inhaled organic dust and particles of fungal, actinomycetic or other origin
Excludes: pneumonitis due to inhalation of chemicals, gases, fumes or vapours (J68.0)

J67.0 Farmer's lung
Harvester's lung
Haymaker's lung
Mouldy hay disease

J67.1 Bagassosis
Bagasse:
• disease
• pneumonitis

J67.2 Bird fancier's lung
Budgerigar fancier's disease or lung
Pigeon fancier's disease or lung

J67.3 Suberosis
Corkhandler's disease or lung
Corkworker's disease or lung

J67.4 Maltworker's lung
Alveolitis due to *Aspergillus clavatus*

J67.5 Mushroom-worker's lung

J67.6 Maple-bark-stripper's lung
Alveolitis due to *Cryptostroma corticale*
Cryptostromosis

J67.7 Air-conditioner and humidifier lung
Allergic alveolitis due to fungi, thermophilic actinomycetes and
other organisms growing in ventilation [air-conditioning]
systems

J67.8 Hypersensitivity pneumonitis due to other organic dusts
Cheese-washer's lung
Coffee-worker's lung
Fishmeal-worker's lung
Furrier's lung
Sequoiosis

**J67.9 Hypersensitivity pneumonitis due to unspecified organic
dust**
Allergic alveolitis (extrinsic) NOS
Hypersensitivity pneumonitis NOS

**J68   Respiratory conditions due to inhalation of
chemicals, gases, fumes and vapours**
Use additional external cause code (Chapter XX), if desired, to
identify cause.

J68.0   **Bronchitis and pneumonitis due to chemicals, gases, fumes and vapours**
Chemical bronchitis (acute)

J68.1   **Acute pulmonary oedema due to chemicals, gases, fumes and vapours**
Chemical pulmonary oedema (acute)

J68.2   **Upper respiratory inflammation due to chemicals, gases, fumes and vapours, not elsewhere classified**

J68.3   **Other acute and subacute respiratory conditions due to chemicals, gases, fumes and vapours**
Reactive airways dysfunction syndrome

J68.4   **Chronic respiratory conditions due to chemicals, gases, fumes and vapours**
Emphysema (diffuse)(chronic)
Obliterative bronchiolitis (chronic) (subacute)
Pulmonary fibrosis (chronic)
} due to inhalation of chemicals, gases, fumes and vapours

J68.8   **Other respiratory conditions due to chemicals, fumes and vapours**

J68.9   **Unspecified respiratory condition due to chemicals, gases, fumes and vapours**

J69   Pneumonitis due to solids and liquids

Use additional external cause code (Chapter XX), if desired, to identify cause.

Excludes: neonatal aspiration syndromes (P24.–)

J69.0   **Pneumonitis due to food and vomit**
Aspiration pneumonia (due to):
- NOS
- food (regurgitated)
- gastric secretions
- milk
- vomit

Excludes: Mendelson's syndrome (J95.4)

J69.1   **Pneumonitis due to oils and essences**
Lipid pneumonia

J69.8   **Pneumonitis due to other solids and liquids**
Pneumonitis due to aspiration of blood

J70 Respiratory conditions due to other external agents
Use additional external cause code (Chapter XX), if desired, to identify cause.

J70.0 Acute pulmonary manifestations due to radiation
Radiation pneumonitis

J70.1 Chronic and other pulmonary manifestations due to radiation
Fibrosis of lung following radiation

J70.2 Acute drug-induced interstitial lung disorders

J70.3 Chronic drug-induced interstitial lung disorders

J70.4 Drug-induced interstitial lung disorder, unspecified

J70.8 Respiratory conditions due to other specified external agents

J70.9 Respiratory conditions due to unspecified external agent

Other respiratory diseases principally affecting the interstitium
(J80–J84)

J80 Adult respiratory distress syndrome
Adult hyaline membrane disease

J81 Pulmonary oedema
Acute oedema of lung
Pulmonary congestion (passive)

Excludes: hypostatic pneumonia (J18.2)
pulmonary oedema:
- chemical (acute) (J68.1)
- due to external agents (J60–J70)
- with mention of heart disease NOS or heart failure (I50.1)

J82 Pulmonary eosinophilia, not elsewhere classified

Eosinophilic asthma
Löffler's pneumonia
Tropical (pulmonary) eosinophilia NOS
Excludes: due to:
- aspergillosis (B44.–)
- drugs (J70.2–J70.4)
- specified parasitic infection (B50–B83)
- systemic connective tissue disorders (M30–M36)

J84 Other interstitial pulmonary diseases

Excludes: drug-induced interstitial lung disorders (J70.2–J70.4)
interstitial emphysema (J98.2)
lung diseases due to external agents (J60–J70)
lymphoid interstitial pneumonitis resulting from
human immunodeficiency virus [HIV] disease
(B22.1)

J84.0 Alveolar and parietoalveolar conditions

Alveolar proteinosis
Pulmonary alveolar microlithiasis

J84.1 Other interstitial pulmonary diseases with fibrosis

Diffuse pulmonary fibrosis
Fibrosing alveolitis (cryptogenic)
Hamman–Rich syndrome
Idiopathic pulmonary fibrosis
Excludes: pulmonary fibrosis (chronic):
- due to inhalation of chemicals, gases, fumes or
vapours (J68.4)
- following radiation (J70.1)

J84.8 Other specified interstitial pulmonary diseases

J84.9 Interstitial pulmonary disease, unspecified

Interstitial pneumonia NOS

Suppurative and necrotic conditions of lower respiratory tract
(J85–J86)

J85 Abscess of lung and mediastinum

J85.0 **Gangrene and necrosis of lung**

J85.1 **Abscess of lung with pneumonia**
Excludes: with pneumonia due to specified organism (J10–J16)

J85.2 **Abscess of lung without pneumonia**
Abscess of lung NOS

J85.3 **Abscess of mediastinum**

J86 Pyothorax
Includes: abscess of:
- pleura
- thorax
empyema
pyopneumothorax

Use additional code (B95–B97), if desired, to identify infectious agent.
Excludes: due to tuberculosis (A15–A16)

J86.0 **Pyothorax with fistula**

J86.9 **Pyothorax without fistula**

Other diseases of pleura
(J90–J94)

J90 Pleural effusion, not elsewhere classified
Pleurisy with effusion
Excludes: chylous (pleural) effusion (J94.0)
pleurisy NOS (R09.1)
tuberculous (A15–A16)

J91* Pleural effusion in conditions classified elsewhere

J92 Pleural plaque

Includes: pleural thickening

J92.0 Pleural plaque with presence of asbestos

J92.9 Pleural plaque without asbestos
Pleural plaque NOS

J93 Pneumothorax

Excludes: pneumothorax:
- congenital or perinatal (P25.1)
- traumatic (S27.0)
- tuberculous (current disease) (A15–A16)
pyopneumothorax (J86.–)

J93.0 Spontaneous tension pneumothorax

J93.1 Other spontaneous pneumothorax

J93.8 Other pneumothorax

J93.9 Pneumothorax, unspecified

J94 Other pleural conditions

Excludes: pleurisy NOS (R09.1)
traumatic:
- haemopneumothorax (S27.2)
- haemothorax (S27.1)
tuberculous pleural conditions (current disease)
(A15–A16)

J94.0 Chylous effusion
Chyliform effusion

J94.1 Fibrothorax

J94.2 Haemothorax
Haemopneumothorax

J94.8 Other specified pleural conditions
Hydrothorax

J94.9 Pleural condition, unspecified

Other diseases of the respiratory system (J95–J99)

J95 Postprocedural respiratory disorders, not elsewhere classified

Excludes: emphysema (subcutaneous) resulting from a procedure (T81.8)
pulmonary manifestations due to radiation (J70.0–J70.1)

J95.0 **Tracheostomy malfunction**
Haemorrhage from tracheostomy stoma
Obstruction of tracheostomy airway
Sepsis of tracheostomy stoma
Tracheo-oesophageal fistula following tracheostomy

J95.1 **Acute pulmonary insufficiency following thoracic surgery**

J95.2 **Acute pulmonary insufficiency following nonthoracic surgery**

J95.3 **Chronic pulmonary insufficiency following surgery**

J95.4 **Mendelson's syndrome**

Excludes: complicating:
- labour and delivery (O74.0)
- pregnancy (O29.0)
- puerperium (O89.0)

J95.5 **Postprocedural subglottic stenosis**

J95.8 **Other postprocedural respiratory disorders**

J95.9 **Postprocedural respiratory disorder, unspecified**

J96 Respiratory failure, not elsewhere classified

Excludes: cardiorespiratory failure (R09.2)
postprocedural respiratory failure (J95.–)
respiratory:
- arrest (R09.2)
- distress syndrome:
  - adult (J80)
  - newborn (P22.0)

J96.0 **Acute respiratory failure**

J96.1   **Chronic respiratory failure**

J96.9   **Respiratory failure, unspecified**

J98   Other respiratory disorders

Excludes: apnoea:
- NOS (R06.8)
- newborn (P28.4)
- sleep (G47.3)
  - newborn (P28.3)

J98.0   **Diseases of bronchus, not elsewhere classified**
Broncholithiasis
Calcification ⎫
Stenosis   ⎬ of bronchus
Ulcer   ⎭
Tracheobronchial:
- collapse
- dyskinesia

J98.1   **Pulmonary collapse**
Atelectasis
Collapse of lung
Excludes: atelectasis (of):
- newborn (P28.0–P28.1)
- tuberculous (current disease) (A15–A16)

J98.2   **Interstitial emphysema**
Mediastinal emphysema
Excludes: emphysema:
- NOS (J43.9)
- in fetus and newborn (P25.0)
- surgical (subcutaneous) (T81.8)
- traumatic subcutaneous (T79.7)

J98.3   **Compensatory emphysema**

J98.4   **Other disorders of lung**
Calcification of lung
Cystic lung disease (acquired)
Lung disease NOS
Pulmolithiasis

J98.5 **Diseases of mediastinum, not elsewhere classified**
Fibrosis ⎫
Hernia ⎬ of mediastinum
Retraction ⎭
Mediastinitis

Excludes: abscess of mediastinum (J85.3)

J98.6 **Disorders of diaphragm**
Diaphragmatitis
Paralysis of diaphragm
Relaxation of diaphragm

Excludes: congenital malformation of diaphragm NEC (Q79.1)
diaphragmatic hernia (K44.–)
• congenital (Q79.0)

J98.8 **Other specified respiratory disorders**

J98.9 **Respiratory disorder, unspecified**
Respiratory disease (chronic) NOS

J99* Respiratory disorders in diseases classified elsewhere

J99.0* **Rheumatoid lung disease (M05.1†)**

J99.1* **Respiratory disorders in other diffuse connective tissue disorders**
Respiratory disorders in:
• dermatomyositis (M33.0–M33.1†)
• polymyositis (M33.2†)
• sicca syndrome [Sjögren] (M35.0†)
• systemic:
  • lupus erythematosus (M32.1†)
  • sclerosis (M34.8†)
• Wegener's granulomatosis (M31.3†)

J99.8* **Respiratory disorders in other diseases classified elsewhere**
Respiratory disorders in:
• amoebiasis (A06.5†)
• ankylosing spondylitis (M45†)
• cryoglobulinaemia (D89.1†)
• sporotrichosis (B42.0†)
• syphilis (A52.7†)

CHAPTER XI

Diseases of the digestive system (K00–K93)

Excludes: certain conditions originating in the perinatal period (P00–P96)
certain infectious and parasitic diseases (A00–B99)
complications of pregnancy, childbirth and the puerperium (O00–O99)
congenital malformations, deformations and chromosomal abnormalities (Q00–Q99)
endocrine, nutritional and metabolic diseases (E00–E90)
injury, poisoning and certain other consequences of external causes (S00–T98)
neoplasms (C00–D48)
symptoms, signs and abnormal clinical and laboratory findings, not elsewhere classified (R00–R99)

This chapter contains the following blocks:

K00–K14 Diseases of oral cavity, salivary glands and jaws
K20–K31 Diseases of oesophagus, stomach and duodenum
K35–K38 Diseases of appendix
K40–K46 Hernia
K50–K52 Noninfective enteritis and colitis
K55–K63 Other diseases of intestines
K65–K67 Diseases of peritoneum
K70–K77 Diseases of liver
K80–K87 Disorders of gallbladder, biliary tract and pancreas
K90–K93 Other diseases of the digestive system

Asterisk categories for this chapter are provided as follows:

K23* Disorders of oesophagus in diseases classified elsewhere
K67* Disorders of peritoneum in infectious diseases classified elsewhere
K77* Liver disorders in diseases classified elsewhere
K87* Disorders of gallbladder, biliary tract and pancreas in diseases classified elsewhere
K93* Disorders of other digestive organs in diseases classified elsewhere

Diseases of oral cavity, salivary glands and jaws (K00–K14)

K00 Disorders of tooth development and eruption
Excludes: embedded and impacted teeth (K01.–)

K00.0 **Anodontia**
Hypodontia
Oligodontia

K00.1 **Supernumerary teeth**
Distomolar
Fourth molar
Mesiodens
Paramolar
Supplementary teeth

K00.2 **Abnormalities of size and form of teeth**
Concrescence ⎫
Fusion ⎬ of teeth
Gemination ⎭
Dens:
• evaginatus
• in dente
• invaginatus
Enamel pearls
Macrodontia
Microdontia
Peg-shaped [conical] teeth
Taurodontism
Tuberculum paramolare
Excludes: tuberculum Carabelli, which is regarded as a normal variation and should not be coded

K00.3 **Mottled teeth**
Dental fluorosis
Mottling of enamel
Nonfluoride enamel opacities
Excludes: deposits [accretions] on teeth (K03.6)

K00.4 **Disturbances in tooth formation**
Aplasia and hypoplasia of cementum
Dilaceration of tooth
Enamel hypoplasia (neonatal)(postnatal)(prenatal)
Regional odontodysplasia
Turner's tooth

Excludes: Hutchinson's teeth and mulberry molars in congenital
syphilis (A50.5)
mottled teeth (K00.3)

K00.5 **Hereditary disturbances in tooth structure, not elsewhere classified**
Amelogenesis ⎤
Dentinogenesis ⎬ imperfecta
Odontogenesis ⎦
Dentinal dysplasia
Shell teeth

K00.6 **Disturbances in tooth eruption**
Dentia praecox
Natal ⎤
Neonatal ⎦ tooth
Premature:
• eruption of tooth
• shedding of primary [deciduous] tooth
Retained [persistent] primary tooth

K00.7 **Teething syndrome**

K00.8 **Other disorders of tooth development**
Colour changes during tooth formation
Intrinsic staining of teeth NOS

K00.9 **Disorder of tooth development, unspecified**
Disorder of odontogenesis NOS

K01 **Embedded and impacted teeth**
Excludes: embedded and impacted teeth with abnormal position
of such teeth or adjacent teeth (K07.3)

K01.0 **Embedded teeth**
An embedded tooth is a tooth that has failed to erupt without
obstruction by another tooth.

K01.1   **Impacted teeth**
An impacted tooth is a tooth that has failed to erupt because of obstruction by another tooth.

K02   Dental caries

K02.0   **Caries limited to enamel**
White spot lesions [initial caries]

K02.1   **Caries of dentine**

K02.2   **Caries of cementum**

K02.3   **Arrested dental caries**

K02.4   **Odontoclasia**
Infantile melanodontia
Melanodontoclasia

K02.8   **Other dental caries**

K02.9   **Dental caries, unspecified**

K03   Other diseases of hard tissues of teeth
Excludes: bruxism (F45.8)
dental caries (K02.–)
teeth-grinding NOS (F45.8)

K03.0   **Excessive attrition of teeth**
Wear:
• approximal ⎫
                    ⎬ of teeth
• occlusal   ⎭

K03.1   **Abrasion of teeth**
Abrasion:
• dentifrice ⎫
• habitual   ⎪
• occupational ⎬ of teeth
• ritual   ⎪
• traditional ⎪
Wedge defect NOS ⎭

K03.2   **Erosion of teeth**

Erosion of teeth:
- NOS
- due to:
  - diet
  - drugs and medicaments
  - persistent vomiting
- idiopathic
- occupational

K03.3   **Pathological resorption of teeth**

Internal granuloma of pulp
Resorption of teeth (external)

K03.4   **Hypercementosis**

Cementation hyperplasia

K03.5   **Ankylosis of teeth**

K03.6   **Deposits [accretions] on teeth**

Dental calculus:
- subgingival
- supragingival

Deposits [accretions] on teeth:
- betel
- black
- green
- materia alba
- orange
- tobacco

Staining of teeth:
- NOS
- extrinsic NOS

K03.7   **Posteruptive colour changes of dental hard tissues**

Excludes: deposits [accretions] on teeth (K03.6)

K03.8   **Other specified diseases of hard tissues of teeth**

Irradiated enamel
Sensitive dentine

Use additional external cause code (Chapter XX), if desired, to identify radiation, if radiation-induced.

K03.9   **Disease of hard tissues of teeth, unspecified**

K04 Diseases of pulp and periapical tissues

K04.0 Pulpitis
Pulpal:
- abscess
- polyp

Pulpitis:
- acute
- chronic (hyperplastic)(ulcerative)
- suppurative

K04.1 Necrosis of pulp
Pulpal gangrene

K04.2 Pulp degeneration
Denticles
Pulpal:
- calcifications
- stones

K04.3 Abnormal hard tissue formation in pulp
Secondary or irregular dentine

K04.4 Acute apical periodontitis of pulpal origin
Acute apical periodontitis NOS

K04.5 Chronic apical periodontitis
Apical or periapical granuloma
Apical periodontitis NOS

K04.6 Periapical abscess with sinus
Dental ⎫
Dentoalveolar ⎬ abscess with sinus

K04.7 Periapical abscess without sinus
Dental ⎫
Dentoalveolar ⎬ abscess NOS
Periapical ⎭

K04.8 Radicular cyst
Cyst:
- apical (periodontal)
- periapical
- residual radicular

Excludes: lateral periodontal cyst (K09.0)

K04.9 Other and unspecified diseases of pulp and periapical tissues

K05   Gingivitis and periodontal diseases

K05.0   **Acute gingivitis**
Excludes: acute necrotizing ulcerative gingivitis (A69.1)
herpesviral [herpes simplex] gingivostomatitis (B00.2)

K05.1   **Chronic gingivitis**
Gingivitis (chronic):
• NOS
• desquamative
• hyperplastic
• simple marginal
• ulcerative

K05.2   **Acute periodontitis**
Acute pericoronitis
Parodontal abscess
Periodontal abscess
Excludes: acute apical periodontitis (K04.4)
periapical abscess (K04.7)
• with sinus (K04.6)

K05.3   **Chronic periodontitis**
Chronic pericoronitis
Periodontitis:
• NOS
• complex
• simplex

K05.4   **Periodontosis**
Juvenile periodontosis

K05.5   **Other periodontal diseases**

K05.6   **Periodontal disease, unspecified**

K06   Other disorders of gingiva and edentulous alveolar ridge
Excludes: atrophy of edentulous alveolar ridge (K08.2)
gingivitis:
• NOS (K05.1)
• acute (K05.0)
• chronic (K05.1)

K06.0   Gingival recession
Gingival recession (generalized)(localized)(postinfective)(post-operative)

K06.1   Gingival enlargement
Gingival fibromatosis

K06.2   Gingival and edentulous alveolar ridge lesions associated with trauma
Irritative hyperplasia of edentulous ridge [denture hyperplasia]

Use additional external cause code (Chapter XX), if desired, to identify cause.

K06.8   Other specified disorders of gingiva and edentulous alveolar ridge
Fibrous epulis
Flabby ridge
Giant cell epulis
Peripheral giant cell granuloma
Pyogenic granuloma of gingiva

K06.9   Disorder of gingiva and edentulous alveolar ridge, unspecified

K07   Dentofacial anomalies [including malocclusion]

Excludes: hemifacial atrophy or hypertrophy (Q67.4)
            unilateral condylar hyperplasia or hypoplasia (K10.8)

K07.0   Major anomalies of jaw size
Hyperplasia, hypoplasia:
• mandibular
• maxillary
Macrognathism (mandibular)(maxillary)
Micrognathism (mandibular)(maxillary)

Excludes: acromegaly (E22.0)
            Robin's syndrome (Q87.0)

K07.1   Anomalies of jaw–cranial base relationship
Asymmetry of jaw
Prognathism (mandibular)(maxillary)
Retrognathism (mandibular)(maxillary)

K07.2 **Anomalies of dental arch relationship**

Crossbite (anterior)(posterior)

Disto-occlusion

Mesio-occlusion

Midline deviation of dental arch

Openbite (anterior)(posterior)

Overbite (excessive):

- deep
- horizontal
- vertical

Overjet

Posterior lingual occlusion of mandibular teeth

K07.3 **Anomalies of tooth position**

Crowding ⎫

Diastema ⎪

Displacement ⎬ of tooth or teeth

Rotation ⎪

Spacing, abnormal ⎪

Transposition ⎭

Impacted or embedded teeth with abnormal position of such
teeth or adjacent teeth

Excludes: embedded and impacted teeth without abnormal
position (K01.–)

K07.4 **Malocclusion, unspecified**

K07.5 **Dentofacial functional abnormalities**

Abnormal jaw closure

Malocclusion due to:

- abnormal swallowing
- mouth breathing
- tongue, lip or finger habits

Excludes: bruxism (F45.8)

teeth-grinding NOS (F45.8)

K07.6 **Temporomandibular joint disorders**

Costen's complex or syndrome

Derangement of temporomandibular joint

Snapping jaw

Temporomandibular joint-pain-dysfunction syndrome

Excludes: current temporomandibular joint:

- dislocation (S03.0)
- strain (S03.4)

K07.8   Other dentofacial anomalies

K07.9   Dentofacial anomaly, unspecified

K08   Other disorders of teeth and supporting structures

K08.0   Exfoliation of teeth due to systemic causes

K08.1   Loss of teeth due to accident, extraction or local periodontal disease

K08.2   Atrophy of edentulous alveolar ridge

K08.3   Retained dental root

K08.8   Other specified disorders of teeth and supporting structures
Enlargement of alveolar ridge NOS
Irregular alveolar process
Toothache NOS

K08.9   Disorder of teeth and supporting structures, unspecified

K09   Cysts of oral region, not elsewhere classified

Includes: lesions showing histological features both of aneurysmal cyst and of another fibro-osseous lesion

Excludes: radicular cyst (K04.8)

K09.0   Developmental odontogenic cysts
Cyst:
- dentigerous
- eruption
- follicular
- gingival
- lateral periodontal
- primordial

Keratocyst

K09.1   Developmental (nonodontogenic) cysts of oral region
Cyst (of):
- globulomaxillary
- incisive canal
- median palatal
- nasopalatine
- palatine papilla

K09.2   **Other cysts of jaw**
Cyst of jaw:
- NOS
- aneurysmal
- haemorrhagic
- traumatic

Excludes: latent bone cyst of jaw (K10.0)
Stafne's cyst (K10.0)

K09.8   **Other cysts of oral region, not elsewhere classified**
Dermoid cyst ⎫
Epidermoid cyst ⎬ of mouth
Lymphoepithelial cyst ⎭
Epstein's pearl
Nasoalveolar cyst
Nasolabial cyst

K09.9   **Cyst of oral region, unspecified**

K10   Other diseases of jaws

K10.0   **Developmental disorders of jaws**
Latent bone cyst of jaw
Stafne's cyst
Torus:
- mandibularis
- palatinus

K10.1   **Giant cell granuloma, central**
Giant cell granuloma NOS

Excludes: peripheral giant cell granuloma (K06.8)

K10.2   **Inflammatory conditions of jaws**
Osteitis ⎫
Osteomyelitis (neonatal) ⎪ of jaw (acute)(chronic)
Osteoradionecrosis ⎬ (suppurative)
Periostitis ⎭
Sequestrum of jaw bone

Use additional external cause code (Chapter XX), if desired, to identify radiation, if radiation-induced.

K10.3   **Alveolitis of jaws**
Alveolar osteitis
Dry socket

K10.8   **Other specified diseases of jaws**
Cherubism
Exostosis ⎫
Fibrous dysplasia ⎬ of jaw
Unilateral condylar: ⎭
• hyperplasia
• hypoplasia

K10.9   **Disease of jaws, unspecified**

K11   Diseases of salivary glands

K11.0   **Atrophy of salivary gland**

K11.1   **Hypertrophy of salivary gland**

K11.2   **Sialoadenitis**
Excludes: epidemic parotitis (B26.–)
uveoparotid fever [Heerfordt] (D86.8)

K11.3   **Abscess of salivary gland**

K11.4   **Fistula of salivary gland**
Excludes: congenital fistula of salivary gland (Q38.4)

K11.5   **Sialolithiasis**
Calculus ⎫
Stone ⎬ of salivary gland or duct

K11.6   **Mucocele of salivary gland**
Mucous:
• extravasation cyst ⎫
• retention cyst ⎬ of salivary gland
Ranula ⎭

K11.7   **Disturbances of salivary secretion**
Hypoptyalism
Ptyalism
Xerostomia
Excludes: dry mouth NOS (R68.2)

K11.8 **Other diseases of salivary glands**
Benign lymphoepithelial lesion of salivary gland
Mikulicz' disease
Necrotizing sialometaplasia
Sialectasia
Stenosis ⎫
Stricture ⎬ of salivary duct

Excludes: sicca syndrome [Sjögren] (M35.0)

K11.9 **Disease of salivary gland, unspecified**
Sialoadenopathy NOS

K12 Stomatitis and related lesions

Excludes: cancrum oris (A69.0)
cheilitis (K13.0)
gangrenous stomatitis (A69.0)
herpesviral [herpes simplex] gingivostomatitis (B00.2)
noma (A69.0)

K12.0 **Recurrent oral aphthae**
Aphthous stomatitis (major)(minor)
Bednar's aphthae
Periadenitis mucosa necrotica recurrens
Recurrent aphthous ulcer
Stomatitis herpetiformis

K12.1 **Other forms of stomatitis**
Stomatitis:
• NOS
• denture
• ulcerative
• vesicular

K12.2 **Cellulitis and abscess of mouth**
Cellulitis of mouth (floor)
Submandibular abscess

Excludes: abscess (of):
• periapical (K04.6–K04.7)
• periodontal (K05.2)
• peritonsillar (J36)
• salivary gland (K11.3)
• tongue (K14.0)

K13   Other diseases of lip and oral mucosa

Includes: epithelial disturbances of tongue

Excludes: certain disorders of gingiva and edentulous alveolar
ridge (K05–K06)
cysts of oral region (K09.–)
diseases of tongue (K14.–)
stomatitis and related lesions (K12.–)

K13.0   Diseases of lips
Cheilitis:
• NOS
• angular
• exfoliative
• glandular
Cheilodynia
Cheilosis
Perlèche NEC

Excludes: ariboflavinosis (E53.0)
cheilitis due to radiation-related disorders (L55–L59)
perlèche due to:
• candidiasis (B37.8)
• riboflavin deficiency (E53.0)

K13.1   Cheek and lip biting

K13.2   Leukoplakia and other disturbances of oral epithelium, including tongue
Erythroplakia ⎫
Leukoedema ⎬ of oral epithelium, including tongue
Leukokeratosis nicotina palati ⎭
Smoker's palate

Excludes: hairy leukoplakia (K13.3)

K13.3   Hairy leukoplakia

K13.4   Granuloma and granuloma-like lesions of oral mucosa
Eosinophilic granuloma ⎫
Granuloma pyogenicum ⎬ of oral mucosa
Verrucous xanthoma ⎭

K13.5   Oral submucous fibrosis
Submucous fibrosis of tongue

K13.6   Irritative hyperplasia of oral mucosa
Excludes: irritative hyperplasia of edentulous ridge [denture hyperplasia] (K06.2)

K13.7   Other and unspecified lesions of oral mucosa
Focal oral mucinosis

K14   Diseases of tongue

Excludes: erythroplakia
focal epithelial hyperplasia
leukoedema } of tongue (K13.2)
leukoplakia
hairy leukoplakia (K13.3)
macroglossia (congenital) (Q38.2)
submucous fibrosis of tongue (K13.5)

K14.0   Glossitis
Abscess
Ulceration (traumatic) } of tongue
Excludes: atrophic glossitis (K14.4)

K14.1   Geographic tongue
Benign migratory glossitis
Glossitis areata exfoliativa

K14.2   Median rhomboid glossitis

K14.3   Hypertrophy of tongue papillae
Black hairy tongue
Coated tongue
Hypertrophy of foliate papillae
Lingua villosa nigra

K14.4   Atrophy of tongue papillae
Atrophic glossitis

K14.5   Plicated tongue
Fissured
Furrowed } tongue
Scrotal
Excludes: fissured tongue, congenital (Q38.3)

K14.6   Glossodynia
Glossopyrosis
Painful tongue

K14.8   Other diseases of tongue
Atrophy
Crenated } (of) tongue
Enlargement
Hypertrophy

K14.9   Disease of tongue, unspecified
Glossopathy NOS

Diseases of oesophagus, stomach and duodenum (K20–K31)

Excludes: hiatus hernia (K44.–)

K20   Oesophagitis
Abscess of oesophagus
Oesophagitis:
- NOS
- chemical
- peptic

Use additional external cause code (Chapter XX), if desired, to identify cause.
Excludes: erosion of oesophagus (K22.1)
  reflux oesophagitis (K21.0)
  with gastro-oesophageal reflux disease (K21.0)

K21   Gastro-oesophageal reflux disease

K21.0   Gastro-oesophageal reflux disease with oesophagitis
Reflux oesophagitis

K21.9   Gastro-oesophageal reflux disease without oesophagitis
Oesophageal reflux NOS

K22   Other diseases of oesophagus
Excludes: oesophageal varices (I85.–)

K22.0   Achalasia of cardia
Achalasia NOS
Cardiospasm
Excludes: congenital cardiospasm (Q40.2)

K22.1   **Ulcer of oesophagus**
Erosion of oesophagus
Ulcer of oesophagus:
- NOS
- due to ingestion of:
  - chemicals
  - drugs and medicaments
- fungal
- peptic

Use additional external cause code (Chapter XX), if desired, to identify cause.

K22.2   **Oesophageal obstruction**
Compression ⎤
Constriction ⎢ of oesophagus
Stenosis ⎟
Stricture ⎦
Excludes: congenital stenosis or stricture of oesophagus (Q39.3)

K22.3   **Perforation of oesophagus**
Rupture of oesophagus
Excludes: traumatic perforation of (thoracic) oesophagus (S27.8)

K22.4   **Dyskinesia of oesophagus**
Corkscrew oesophagus
Diffuse oesophageal spasm
Spasm of oesophagus
Excludes: cardiospasm (K22.0)

K22.5   **Diverticulum of oesophagus, acquired**
Oesophageal pouch, acquired
Excludes: diverticulum of oesophagus (congenital) (Q39.6)

K22.6   **Gastro-oesophageal laceration-haemorrhage syndrome**
Mallory–Weiss syndrome

K22.8   **Other specified diseases of oesophagus**
Haemorrhage of oesophagus NOS

K22.9   **Disease of oesophagus, unspecified**

K23*   **Disorders of oesophagus in diseases classified elsewhere**

K23.0*   **Tuberculous oesophagitis (A18.8†)**

565

K23.1*   Megaoesophagus in Chagas' disease (B57.3†)

K23.8*   Disorders of oesophagus in other diseases classified elsewhere

The following fourth-character subdivisions are for use with categories K25–K28:

.0 Acute with haemorrhage
.1 Acute with perforation
.2 Acute with both haemorrhage and perforation
.3 Acute without haemorrhage or perforation
.4 Chronic or unspecified with haemorrhage
.5 Chronic or unspecified with perforation
.6 Chronic or unspecified with both haemorrhage and perforation
.7 Chronic without haemorrhage or perforation
.9 Unspecified as acute or chronic, without haemorrhage or perforation

K25   Gastric ulcer

[See above for subdivisions]

Includes: erosion (acute) of stomach
ulcer (peptic):
- pylorus
- stomach

Use additional external cause code (Chapter XX), if desired, to identify drug, if drug-induced.

Excludes: acute haemorrhagic erosive gastritis (K29.0)
peptic ulcer NOS (K27.–)

K26   Duodenal ulcer

[See above for subdivisions]

Includes: erosion (acute) of duodenum
ulcer (peptic):
- duodenal
- postpyloric

Use additional external cause code (Chapter XX), if desired, to identify drug, if drug-induced.

Excludes: peptic ulcer NOS (K27.–)

K27 Peptic ulcer, site unspecified

[See page 566 for subdivisions]

Includes: gastroduodenal ulcer NOS
peptic ulcer NOS

Excludes: peptic ulcer of newborn (P78.8)

K28 Gastrojejunal ulcer

[See page 566 for subdivisions]

Includes: ulcer (peptic) or erosion:
• anastomotic
• gastrocolic
• gastrointestinal
• gastrojejunal
• jejunal
• marginal
• stomal

Excludes: primary ulcer of small intestine (K63.3)

K29 Gastritis and duodenitis

Excludes: eosinophilic gastritis or gastroenteritis (K52.8)
Zollinger–Ellison syndrome (E16.8)

K29.0 Acute haemorrhagic gastritis

Acute (erosive) gastritis with haemorrhage

Excludes: erosion (acute) of stomach (K25.–)

K29.1 Other acute gastritis

K29.2 Alcoholic gastritis

K29.3 Chronic superficial gastritis

K29.4 Chronic atrophic gastritis

Gastric atrophy

K29.5 Chronic gastritis, unspecified

Chronic gastritis:
• antral
• fundal

K29.6 Other gastritis

Giant hypertrophic gastritis
Granulomatous gastritis
Ménétrier's disease

K29.7 Gastritis, unspecified

K29.8 Duodenitis

K29.9 Gastroduodenitis, unspecified

K30 Dyspepsia
Indigestion

Excludes: dyspepsia:
- nervous (F45.3)
- neurotic (F45.3)
- psychogenic (F45.3)

heartburn (R12)

K31 Other diseases of stomach and duodenum
Includes: functional disorders of stomach

Excludes: diverticulum of duodenum (K57.0–K57.1)
gastrointestinal haemorrhage (K92.0–K92.2)

K31.0 Acute dilatation of stomach
Acute distension of stomach

K31.1 Adult hypertrophic pyloric stenosis
Pyloric stenosis NOS

Excludes: congenital or infantile pyloric stenosis (Q40.0)

K31.2 Hourglass stricture and stenosis of stomach

Excludes: congenital hourglass stomach (Q40.2)
hourglass contraction of stomach (K31.8)

K31.3 Pylorospasm, not elsewhere classified

Excludes: pylorospasm:
- congenital or infantile (Q40.0)
- neurotic (F45.3)
- psychogenic (F45.3)

K31.4 Gastric diverticulum

Excludes: congenital diverticulum of stomach (Q40.2)

K31.5 Obstruction of duodenum
Constriction ⎱
Stenosis ⎰ of duodenum
Stricture ⎰
Duodenal ileus (chronic)

Excludes: congenital stenosis of duodenum (Q41.0)

K31.6   **Fistula of stomach and duodenum**
Gastrocolic fistula
Gastrojejunocolic fistula

K31.8   **Other specified diseases of stomach and duodenum**
Achlorhydria
Gastroptosis
Hourglass contraction of stomach

K31.9   **Disease of stomach and duodenum, unspecified**

Diseases of appendix
(K35–K38)

K35   Acute appendicitis

K35.0   **Acute appendicitis with generalized peritonitis**
Appendicitis (acute) with:
- perforation
- peritonitis (generalized)
- rupture

K35.1   **Acute appendicitis with peritoneal abscess**
Abscess of appendix

K35.9   **Acute appendicitis, unspecified**
Acute appendicitis without:
- perforation
- peritoneal abscess
- peritonitis
- rupture

K36   Other appendicitis
Appendicitis:
- chronic
- recurrent

K37   Unspecified appendicitis

K38 Other diseases of appendix

K38.0 **Hyperplasia of appendix**

K38.1 **Appendicular concretions**
Faecalith ⎫
Stercolith ⎭ of appendix

K38.2 **Diverticulum of appendix**

K38.3 **Fistula of appendix**

K38.8 **Other specified diseases of appendix**
Intussusception of appendix

K38.9 **Disease of appendix, unspecified**

Hernia
(K40–K46)

Note: Hernia with both gangrene and obstruction is classified to hernia
with gangrene.

Includes: hernia:
• acquired
• congenital [except diaphragmatic or hiatus]
• recurrent

K40 Inguinal hernia

Includes: bubonocele
inguinal hernia:
• NOS
• direct
• double
• indirect
• oblique
scrotal hernia

K40.0 **Bilateral inguinal hernia, with obstruction, without gangrene**

K40.1 **Bilateral inguinal hernia, with gangrene**

K40.2 **Bilateral inguinal hernia, without obstruction or gangrene**
Bilateral inguinal hernia NOS

K40.3 **Unilateral or unspecified inguinal hernia, with obstruction, without gangrene**
Inguinal hernia (unilateral):
- causing obstruction
- incarcerated
- irreducible
- strangulated

} without gangrene

K40.4 **Unilateral or unspecified inguinal hernia, with gangrene**
Inguinal hernia NOS with gangrene

K40.9 **Unilateral or unspecified inguinal hernia, without obstruction or gangrene**
Inguinal hernia (unilateral) NOS

K41 Femoral hernia

K41.0 **Bilateral femoral hernia, with obstruction, without gangrene**

K41.1 **Bilateral femoral hernia, with gangrene**

K41.2 **Bilateral femoral hernia, without obstruction or gangrene**
Bilateral femoral hernia NOS

K41.3 **Unilateral or unspecified femoral hernia, with obstruction, without gangrene**
Femoral hernia (unilateral):
- causing obstruction
- incarcerated
- irreducible
- strangulated

} without gangrene

K41.4 **Unilateral or unspecified femoral hernia, with gangrene**

K41.9 **Unilateral or unspecified femoral hernia, without obstruction or gangrene**
Femoral hernia (unilateral) NOS

K42 Umbilical hernia
Includes: paraumbilical hernia
Excludes: omphalocele (Q79.2)

K42.0 **Umbilical hernia with obstruction, without gangrene**
Umbilical hernia:
- causing obstruction ⎫
- incarcerated   ⎬ without gangrene
- irreducible   ⎪
- strangulated   ⎭

K42.1 **Umbilical hernia with gangrene**
Gangrenous umbilical hernia

K42.9 **Umbilical hernia without obstruction or gangrene**
Umbilical hernia NOS

K43 Ventral hernia

Includes: hernia:
- epigastric
- incisional

K43.0 **Ventral hernia with obstruction, without gangrene**
Ventral hernia:
- causing obstruction ⎫
- incarcerated   ⎬ without gangrene
- irreducible   ⎪
- strangulated   ⎭

K43.1 **Ventral hernia with gangrene**
Gangrenous ventral hernia

K43.9 **Ventral hernia without obstruction or gangrene**
Ventral hernia NOS

K44 Diaphragmatic hernia

Includes: hiatus hernia (oesophageal)(sliding)
paraoesophageal hernia
Excludes: congenital hernia:
- diaphragmatic (Q79.0)
- hiatus (Q40.1)

K44.0 **Diaphragmatic hernia with obstruction, without gangrene**
Diaphragmatic hernia:
- causing obstruction ⎫
- incarcerated   ⎬ without gangrene
- irreducible   ⎪
- strangulated   ⎭

K44.1 **Diaphragmatic hernia with gangrene**
Gangrenous diaphragmatic hernia

K44.9 **Diaphragmatic hernia without obstruction or gangrene**
Diaphragmatic hernia NOS

K45 Other abdominal hernia

Includes: hernia:
- abdominal, specified site NEC
- lumbar
- obturator
- pudendal
- retroperitoneal
- sciatic

K45.0 **Other specified abdominal hernia with obstruction, without gangrene**
Any condition listed under K45:
- causing obstruction ⎫
- incarcerated ⎪
- irreducible ⎬ without gangrene
- strangulated ⎭

K45.1 **Other specified abdominal hernia with gangrene**
Any condition listed under K45 specified as gangrenous

K45.8 **Other specified abdominal hernia without obstruction or gangrene**

K46 Unspecified abdominal hernia

Includes: enterocele
epiplocele
hernia:
- NOS
- interstitial
- intestinal
- intra-abdominal

Excludes: vaginal enterocele (N81.5)

K46.0   **Unspecified abdominal hernia with obstruction, without gangrene**
Any condition listed under K46:
- causing obstruction ⎫
- incarcerated   ⎪
- irreducible   ⎬ without gangrene
- strangulated   ⎭

K46.1   **Unspecified abdominal hernia with gangrene**
Any condition listed under K46 specified as gangrenous

K46.9   **Unspecified abdominal hernia without obstruction or gangrene**
Abdominal hernia NOS

Noninfective enteritis and colitis (K50–K52)

Includes: noninfective inflammatory bowel disease
Excludes: irritable bowel syndrome (K58.–)
            megacolon (K59.3)

K50   **Crohn's disease [regional enteritis]**
Includes: granulomatous enteritis
Excludes: ulcerative colitis (K51.–)

K50.0   **Crohn's disease of small intestine**
Crohn's disease [regional enteritis] of:
- duodenum
- ileum
- jejunum
Ileitis:
- regional
- terminal
Excludes: with Crohn's disease of large intestine (K50.8)

574

K50.1 **Crohn's disease of large intestine**
Colitis:
- granulomatous
- regional

Crohn's disease [regional enteritis] of:
- colon
- large bowel
- rectum

Excludes: with Crohn's disease of small intestine (K50.8)

K50.8 **Other Crohn's disease**
Crohn's disease of both small and large intestine

K50.9 **Crohn's disease, unspecified**
Crohn's disease NOS
Regional enteritis NOS

K51 Ulcerative colitis

K51.0 **Ulcerative (chronic) enterocolitis**

K51.1 **Ulcerative (chronic) ileocolitis**

K51.2 **Ulcerative (chronic) proctitis**

K51.3 **Ulcerative (chronic) rectosigmoiditis**

K51.4 **Pseudopolyposis of colon**

K51.5 **Mucosal proctocolitis**

K51.8 **Other ulcerative colitis**

K51.9 **Ulcerative colitis, unspecified**
Ulcerative enteritis NOS

K52 Other noninfective gastroenteritis and colitis

K52.0 **Gastroenteritis and colitis due to radiation**

K52.1 **Toxic gastroenteritis and colitis**
Use additional external cause code (Chapter XX), if desired, to identify toxic agent.

K52.2 **Allergic and dietetic gastroenteritis and colitis**
Food hypersensitivity gastroenteritis or colitis

K52.8 **Other specified noninfective gastroenteritis and colitis**
Eosinophilic gastritis or gastroenteritis

K52.9 **Noninfective gastroenteritis and colitis, unspecified**

Diarrhoea ⎫
Enteritis ⎪ specified as noninfective, or NOS in countries
Ileitis ⎬ where the conditions can be presumed to be
Jejunitis ⎪ of noninfectious origin
Sigmoiditis ⎭

Excludes: colitis, diarrhoea, enteritis, gastroenteritis:
- infectious (A09)
- unspecified, in countries where the condition can
be presumed to be of infectious origin (A09)
functional diarrhoea (K59.1)
neonatal diarrhoea (noninfective) (P78.3)
psychogenic diarrhoea (F45.3)

Other diseases of intestines
(K55–K63)

K55 Vascular disorders of intestine

Excludes: necrotizing enterocolitis of fetus or newborn (P77)

K55.0 **Acute vascular disorders of intestine**
Acute:
- fulminant ischaemic colitis
- intestinal infarction
- small intestine ischaemia
Mesenteric (artery)(vein):
- embolism
- infarction
- thrombosis
Subacute ischaemic colitis

K55.1 **Chronic vascular disorders of intestine**
Chronic ischaemic:
- colitis
- enteritis
- enterocolitis
Ischaemic stricture of intestine
Mesenteric:
- atherosclerosis
- vascular insufficiency

K55.2 **Angiodysplasia of colon**

K55.8 **Other vascular disorders of intestine**

K55.9 **Vascular disorder of intestine, unspecified**
Ischaemic:
- colitis
- enteritis $\Big\}$ NOS
- enterocolitis

K56 Paralytic ileus and intestinal obstruction without hernia

Excludes: congenital stricture or stenosis of intestine
(Q41–Q42)
ischaemic stricture of intestine (K55.1)
meconium ileus (E84.1)
neonatal intestinal obstructions classifiable to P76.–
obstruction of duodenum (K31.5)
postoperative intestinal obstruction (K91.3)
stenosis of anus or rectum (K62.4)
with hernia (K40–K46)

K56.0 **Paralytic ileus**
Paralysis of:
- bowel
- colon
- intestine

Excludes: gallstone ileus (K56.3)
ileus NOS (K56.7)
obstructive ileus NOS (K56.6)

K56.1 **Intussusception**
Intussusception or invagination of:
- bowel
- colon
- intestine
- rectum

Excludes: intussusception of appendix (K38.8)

K56.2 **Volvulus**
Strangulation
Torsion $\Big\}$ of colon or intestine
Twist

K56.3   **Gallstone ileus**
Obstruction of intestine by gallstone

K56.4   **Other impaction of intestine**
Enterolith
Impaction (of):
• colon
• faecal

K56.5   **Intestinal adhesions [bands] with obstruction**
Peritoneal adhesions [bands] with intestinal obstruction

K56.6   **Other and unspecified intestinal obstruction**
Enterostenosis
Obstructive ileus NOS
Occlusion ⎤
Stenosis ⎬ of colon or intestine
Stricture ⎦

K56.7   **Ileus, unspecified**

K57   Diverticular disease of intestine

Includes: diverticulitis ⎤
diverticulosis ⎬ of (small)(large) intestine
diverticulum ⎦
Excludes: congenital diverticulum of intestine (Q43.8)
diverticulum of appendix (K38.2)
Meckel's diverticulum (Q43.0)

K57.0   **Diverticular disease of small intestine with perforation and abscess**
Diverticular disease of small intestine with peritonitis
Excludes: diverticular disease of both small and large intestine
with perforation and abscess (K57.4)

K57.1   **Diverticular disease of small intestine without perforation or abscess**
Diverticular disease of small intestine NOS
Excludes: diverticular disease of both small and large intestine
without perforation or abscess (K57.5)

K57.2   **Diverticular disease of large intestine with perforation and abscess**
Diverticular disease of colon with peritonitis
Excludes: diverticular disease of both small and large intestine
with perforation and abscess (K57.4)

K57.3 **Diverticular disease of large intestine without perforation or abscess**
Diverticular disease of colon NOS
Excludes: diverticular disease of both small and large intestine
without perforation or abscess (K57.5)

K57.4 **Diverticular disease of both small and large intestine with perforation and abscess**
Diverticular disease of both small and large intestine with
peritonitis

K57.5 **Diverticular disease of both small and large intestine without perforation or abscess**
Diverticular disease of both small and large intestine NOS

K57.8 **Diverticular disease of intestine, part unspecified, with perforation and abscess**
Diverticular disease of intestine NOS with peritonitis

K57.9 **Diverticular disease of intestine, part unspecified, without perforation or abscess**
Diverticular disease of intestine NOS

K58   Irritable bowel syndrome
Includes: irritable colon

K58.0 **Irritable bowel syndrome with diarrhoea**

K58.9 **Irritable bowel syndrome without diarrhoea**
Irritable bowel syndrome NOS

K59   Other functional intestinal disorders
Excludes: change in bowel habit NOS (R19.4)
functional disorders of stomach (K31.–)
intestinal malabsorption (K90.–)
psychogenic intestinal disorders (F45.3)

K59.0 **Constipation**

K59.1 **Functional diarrhoea**

K59.2 **Neurogenic bowel, not elsewhere classified**

K59.3 **Megacolon, not elsewhere classified**
Dilatation of colon
Toxic megacolon
Use additional external cause code (Chapter XX), if desired, to
identify toxic agent.
Excludes: megacolon (in):
- Chagas' disease (B57.3)
- congenital (aganglionic) (Q43.1)
- Hirschsprung's disease (Q43.1)

K59.4 **Anal spasm**
Proctalgia fugax

K59.8 **Other specified functional intestinal disorders**
Atony of colon

K59.9 **Functional intestinal disorder, unspecified**

K60 Fissure and fistula of anal and rectal regions
Excludes: with abscess or cellulitis (K61.–)

K60.0 **Acute anal fissure**

K60.1 **Chronic anal fissure**

K60.2 **Anal fissure, unspecified**

K60.3 **Anal fistula**

K60.4 **Rectal fistula**
Fistula of rectum to skin
Excludes: fistula:
- rectovaginal (N82.3)
- vesicorectal (N32.1)

K60.5 **Anorectal fistula**

K61 Abscess of anal and rectal regions
Includes: abscess ⎫ of anal and rectal regions with or
cellulitis ⎭ without fistula

K61.0 **Anal abscess**
Perianal abscess
Excludes: intrasphincteric abscess (K61.4)

K61.1   **Rectal abscess**
Perirectal abscess
Excludes: ischiorectal abscess (K61.3)

K61.2   **Anorectal abscess**

K61.3   **Ischiorectal abscess**
Abscess of ischiorectal fossa

K61.4   **Intrasphincteric abscess**

K62   Other diseases of anus and rectum
Includes: anal canal
Excludes: colostomy and enterostomy malfunction (K91.4)
faecal incontinence (R15)
haemorrhoids (I84.–)
ulcerative proctitis (K51.2)

K62.0   **Anal polyp**

K62.1   **Rectal polyp**
Excludes: adenomatous polyp (D12.8)

K62.2   **Anal prolapse**
Prolapse of anal canal

K62.3   **Rectal prolapse**
Prolapse of rectal mucosa

K62.4   **Stenosis of anus and rectum**
Stricture of anus (sphincter)

K62.5   **Haemorrhage of anus and rectum**
Excludes: neonatal rectal haemorrhage (P54.2)

K62.6   **Ulcer of anus and rectum**
Ulcer:
• solitary
• stercoral
Excludes: fissure and fistula of anus and rectum (K60.–)
in ulcerative colitis (K51.–)

K62.7   **Radiation proctitis**

K62.8   **Other specified diseases of anus and rectum**
Perforation (nontraumatic) of rectum
Proctitis NOS

K62.9   **Disease of anus and rectum, unspecified**

K63 Other diseases of intestine

K63.0 Abscess of intestine
Excludes: abscess of:
- anal and rectal regions (K61.–)
- appendix (K35.1)

with diverticular disease (K57.–)

K63.1 Perforation of intestine (nontraumatic)
Excludes: perforation (nontraumatic) of:
- appendix (K35.0)
- duodenum (K26.–)

with diverticular disease (K57.–)

K63.2 Fistula of intestine
Excludes: fistula (of):
- anal and rectal regions (K60.–)
- appendix (K38.3)
- duodenum (K31.6)
- intestinal-genital, female (N82.2–N82.4)
- vesicointestinal (N32.1)

K63.3 Ulcer of intestine
Primary ulcer of small intestine
Excludes: ulcer (of):
- anus or rectum (K62.6)
- duodenal (K26.–)
- gastrointestinal (K28.–)
- gastrojejunal (K28.–)
- jejunal (K28.–)
- peptic, site unspecified (K27.–)

ulcerative colitis (K51.–)

K63.4 Enteroptosis

K63.8 Other specified diseases of intestine

K63.9 Disease of intestine, unspecified

Diseases of peritoneum
(K65–K67)

K65 Peritonitis

Excludes: peritonitis:
- aseptic (T81.6)
- benign paroxysmal (E85.0)
- chemical (T81.6)
- due to talc or other foreign substance (T81.6)
- neonatal (P78.0–P78.1)
- pelvic, female (N73.3–N73.5)
- periodic familial (E85.0)
- puerperal (O85)
- with or following:
  - abortion or ectopic or molar pregnancy (O00–O07, O08.0)
  - appendicitis (K35.–)
  - diverticular disease of intestine (K57.–)

K65.0 Acute peritonitis
Abscess (of):
- abdominopelvic
- mesenteric
- omentum
- peritoneum
- retrocaecal
- retroperitoneal
- subdiaphragmatic
- subhepatic
- subphrenic

Peritonitis (acute):
- generalized
- pelvic, male
- subphrenic
- suppurative

Use additional code (B95–B97), if desired, to identify infectious agent.

K65.8   Other peritonitis
Chronic proliferative peritonitis
Mesenteric:
- fat necrosis
- saponification
Peritonitis due to:
- bile
- urine

K65.9   Peritonitis, unspecified

K66   Other disorders of peritoneum
Excludes: ascites (R18)

K66.0   Peritoneal adhesions
Adhesions (of):
- abdominal (wall)
- diaphragm
- intestine
- male pelvis
- mesenteric
- omentum
- stomach
Adhesive bands
Excludes: adhesions [bands] (of):
- female pelvis (N73.6)
- with intestinal obstruction (K56.5)

K66.1   Haemoperitoneum
Excludes: traumatic haemoperitoneum (S36.8)

K66.8   Other specified disorders of peritoneum

K66.9   Disorder of peritoneum, unspecified

K67*   Disorders of peritoneum in infectious diseases classified elsewhere

K67.0*   Chlamydial peritonitis (A74.8†)

K67.1*   Gonococcal peritonitis (A54.8†)

K67.2*   Syphilitic peritonitis (A52.7†)

K67.3*   Tuberculous peritonitis (A18.3†)

K67.8* **Other disorders of peritoneum in infectious diseases classified elsewhere**

Diseases of liver (K70–K77)

Excludes: haemochromatosis (E83.1)
jaundice NOS (R17)
Reye's syndrome (G93.7)
viral hepatitis (B15–B19)
Wilson's disease (E83.0)

K70 Alcoholic liver disease

K70.0 **Alcoholic fatty liver**

K70.1 **Alcoholic hepatitis**

K70.2 **Alcoholic fibrosis and sclerosis of liver**

K70.3 **Alcoholic cirrhosis of liver**
Alcoholic cirrhosis NOS

K70.4 **Alcoholic hepatic failure**
Alcoholic hepatic failure:
• NOS
• acute
• chronic
• subacute
• with or without hepatic coma

K70.9 **Alcoholic liver disease, unspecified**

K71 Toxic liver disease

Includes: drug-induced:
• idiosyncratic (unpredictable) liver disease
• toxic (predictable) liver disease

Use additional external cause code (Chapter XX), if desired, to identify toxic agent.

Excludes: alcoholic liver disease (K70.–)
Budd–Chiari syndrome (I82.0)

K71.0 **Toxic liver disease with cholestasis**
Cholestasis with hepatocyte injury
"Pure" cholestasis

K71.1 **Toxic liver disease with hepatic necrosis**
Hepatic failure (acute)(chronic) due to drugs

K71.2 **Toxic liver disease with acute hepatitis**

K71.3 **Toxic liver disease with chronic persistent hepatitis**

K71.4 **Toxic liver disease with chronic lobular hepatitis**

K71.5 **Toxic liver disease with chronic active hepatitis**
Toxic liver disease with lupoid hepatitis

K71.6 **Toxic liver disease with hepatitis, not elsewhere classified**

K71.7 **Toxic liver disease with fibrosis and cirrhosis of liver**

K71.8 **Toxic liver disease with other disorders of liver**
Toxic liver disease with:
- focal nodular hyperplasia
- hepatic granulomas
- peliosis hepatis
- veno-occlusive disease of liver

K71.9 **Toxic liver disease, unspecified**

K72 Hepatic failure, not elsewhere classified

Includes: hepatic:
- coma NOS
- encephalopathy NOS

hepatitis:
- acute
- fulminant } NEC, with hepatic failure
- malignant

liver (cell) necrosis with hepatic failure
yellow liver atrophy or dystrophy

Excludes: alcoholic hepatic failure (K70.4)
hepatic failure complicating:
- abortion or ectopic or molar pregnancy (O00–O07, O08.8)
- pregnancy, childbirth and the puerperium (O26.6)

icterus of fetus and newborn (P55–P59)
viral hepatitis (B15–B19)
with toxic liver disease (K71.1)

K72.0	**Acute and subacute hepatic failure**
K72.1	**Chronic hepatic failure**
K72.9	**Hepatic failure, unspecified**

K73 Chronic hepatitis, not elsewhere classified

Excludes: hepatitis (chronic):
- alcoholic (K70.1)
- drug-induced (K71.–)
- granulomatous NEC (K75.3)
- reactive, nonspecific (K75.2)
- viral (B15–B19)

K73.0 Chronic persistent hepatitis, not elsewhere classified

K73.1 Chronic lobular hepatitis, not elsewhere classified

K73.2 Chronic active hepatitis, not elsewhere classified
Lupoid hepatitis NEC

K73.8 Other chronic hepatitis, not elsewhere classified

K73.9 Chronic hepatitis, unspecified

K74 Fibrosis and cirrhosis of liver

Excludes: alcoholic fibrosis of liver (K70.2)
cardiac sclerosis of liver (K76.1)
cirrhosis (of liver):
- alcoholic (K70.3)
- congenital (P78.8)
with toxic liver disease (K71.7)

K74.0 Hepatic fibrosis

K74.1 Hepatic sclerosis

K74.2 Hepatic fibrosis with hepatic sclerosis

K74.3 Primary biliary cirrhosis
Chronic nonsuppurative destructive cholangitis

K74.4 Secondary biliary cirrhosis

K74.5 Biliary cirrhosis, unspecified

K74.6   Other and unspecified cirrhosis of liver
Cirrhosis (of liver):
- NOS
- cryptogenic
- macronodular
- micronodular
- mixed type
- portal
- postnecrotic

K75   **Other inflammatory liver diseases**
Excludes: chronic hepatitis NEC (K73.–)
             hepatitis:
             - acute or subacute (K72.0)
             - viral (B15–B19)
             toxic liver disease (K71.–)

K75.0   Abscess of liver
Hepatic abscess:
- NOS
- cholangitic
- haematogenic
- lymphogenic
- pylephlebitic

Excludes: amoebic liver abscess (A06.4)
             cholangitis without liver abscess (K83.0)
             pylephlebitis without liver abscess (K75.1)

K75.1   Phlebitis of portal vein
Pylephlebitis
Excludes: pylephlebitic liver abscess (K75.0)

K75.2   Nonspecific reactive hepatitis

K75.3   Granulomatous hepatitis, not elsewhere classified

K75.8   Other specified inflammatory liver diseases

K75.9   Inflammatory liver disease, unspecified
Hepatitis NOS

K76 Other diseases of liver

Excludes: alcoholic liver disease (K70.–)
amyloid degeneration of liver (E85.–)
cystic disease of liver (congenital) (Q44.6)
hepatic vein thrombosis (I82.0)
hepatomegaly NOS (R16.0)
portal vein thrombosis (I81)
toxic liver disease (K71.–)

K76.0 **Fatty (change of) liver, not elsewhere classified**

K76.1 **Chronic passive congestion of liver**
Cardiac:
- cirrhosis (so-called) ⎫
- sclerosis ⎬ of liver
               ⎭

K76.2 **Central haemorrhagic necrosis of liver**
Excludes: liver necrosis with hepatic failure (K72.–)

K76.3 **Infarction of liver**

K76.4 **Peliosis hepatis**
Hepatic angiomatosis

K76.5 **Hepatic veno-occlusive disease**
Excludes: Budd–Chiari syndrome (I82.0)

K76.6 **Portal hypertension**

K76.7 **Hepatorenal syndrome**
Excludes: following labour and delivery (O90.4)

K76.8 **Other specified diseases of liver**
Focal nodular hyperplasia of liver
Hepatoptosis

K76.9 **Liver disease, unspecified**

K77* Liver disorders in diseases classified elsewhere

K77.0* **Liver disorders in infectious and parasitic diseases classified elsewhere**
Hepatitis:
- cytomegaloviral (B25.1†)
- herpesviral [herpes simplex] (B00.8†)
- toxoplasma (B58.1†)
Hepatosplenic schistosomiasis (B65.–†)
Portal hypertension in schistosomiasis (B65.–†)
Syphilitic liver disease (A52.7†)

K77.8* **Liver disorders in other diseases classified elsewhere**
Hepatic granulomas in:
- berylliosis (J63.2†)
- sarcoidosis (D86.8†)

Disorders of gallbladder, biliary tract and pancreas (K80–K87)

K80 Cholelithiasis

K80.0 **Calculus of gallbladder with acute cholecystitis**
Any condition listed in K80.2 with acute cholecystitis

K80.1 **Calculus of gallbladder with other cholecystitis**
Any condition listed in K80.2 with cholecystitis (chronic)
Cholecystitis with cholelithiasis NOS

K80.2 **Calculus of gallbladder without cholecystitis**
Cholecystolithiasis ⎫
Cholelithiasis ⎪
Colic (recurrent) of gallbladder ⎬ unspecified or without
Gallstone (impacted) of: ⎪ cholecystitis
- cystic duct ⎪
- gallbladder ⎭

K80.3 **Calculus of bile duct with cholangitis**
Any condition listed in K80.5 with cholangitis

K80.4 **Calculus of bile duct with cholecystitis**
Any condition listed in K80.5 with cholecystitis (with cholangitis)

K80.5   Calculus of bile duct without cholangitis or cholecystitis

Choledocholithiasis
Gallstone (impacted) of:
• bile duct NOS
• common duct   unspecified or without cholangitis
• hepatic duct   or cholecystitis
Hepatic:
• cholelithiasis
• colic (recurrent)

K80.8   Other cholelithiasis

K81   Cholecystitis

Excludes: with cholelithiasis (K80.–)

K81.0   Acute cholecystitis

Abscess of gallbladder
Angiocholecystitis
Cholecystitis:
• emphysematous (acute)
• gangrenous   without calculus
• suppurative
Empyema of gallbladder
Gangrene of gallbladder

K81.1   Chronic cholecystitis

K81.8   Other cholecystitis

K81.9   Cholecystitis, unspecified

K82   Other diseases of gallbladder

Excludes: nonvisualization of gallbladder (R93.2)
          postcholecystectomy syndrome (K91.5)

K82.0   Obstruction of gallbladder

Occlusion
Stenosis   of cystic duct or gallbladder without calculus
Stricture

Excludes: with cholelithiasis (K80.–)

K82.1   Hydrops of gallbladder

Mucocele of gallbladder

K82.2   Perforation of gallbladder
Rupture of cystic duct or gallbladder

K82.3   Fistula of gallbladder
Cholecystocolic ⎫
Cholecystoduodenal ⎬ fistula

K82.4   Cholesterolosis of gallbladder
Strawberry gallbladder

K82.8   Other specified diseases of gallbladder
Adhesions ⎫
Atrophy
Cyst
Dyskinesia   ⎬ of cystic duct or gallbladder
Hypertrophy
Nonfunctioning
Ulcer ⎭

K82.9   Disease of gallbladder, unspecified

K83   Other diseases of biliary tract

Excludes: the listed conditions involving the:
- gallbladder (K81–K82)
- cystic duct (K81–K82)
postcholecystectomy syndrome (K91.5)

K83.0   Cholangitis
Cholangitis:
- NOS
- ascending
- primary
- recurrent
- sclerosing
- secondary
- stenosing
- suppurative

Excludes: cholangitic liver abscess (K75.0)
cholangitis with choledocholithiasis (K80.3–K80.4)
chronic nonsuppurative destructive cholangitis
(K74.3)

K83.1 **Obstruction of bile duct**
Occlusion ⎫
Stenosis ⎬ of bile duct without calculus
Stricture ⎭
Excludes: with cholelithiasis (K80.–)

K83.2 **Perforation of bile duct**
Rupture of bile duct

K83.3 **Fistula of bile duct**
Choledochoduodenal fistula

K83.4 **Spasm of sphincter of Oddi**

K83.5 **Biliary cyst**

K83.8 **Other specified diseases of biliary tract**
Adhesions ⎫
Atrophy ⎬
Hypertrophy ⎬ of bile duct
Ulcer ⎭

K83.9 **Disease of biliary tract, unspecified**

K85 **Acute pancreatitis**
Abscess of pancreas
Necrosis of pancreas:
• acute
• infective
Pancreatitis:
• NOS
• acute (recurrent)
• haemorrhagic
• subacute
• suppurative

K86 **Other diseases of pancreas**
Excludes: fibrocystic disease of pancreas (E84.–)
islet cell tumour (of pancreas) (D13.7)
pancreatic steatorrhoea (K90.3)

K86.0 **Alcohol-induced chronic pancreatitis**

K86.1 **Other chronic pancreatitis**
Chronic pancreatitis:
- NOS
- infectious
- recurrent
- relapsing

K86.2 **Cyst of pancreas**

K86.3 **Pseudocyst of pancreas**

K86.8 **Other specified diseases of pancreas**
Atrophy ⎫
Calculus ⎪
Cirrhosis ⎬ of pancreas
Fibrosis ⎭
Pancreatic:
- infantilism
- necrosis:
  - NOS
  - aseptic
  - fat

K86.9 **Disease of pancreas, unspecified**

K87* **Disorders of gallbladder, biliary tract and pancreas in diseases classified elsewhere**

K87.0* **Disorders of gallbladder and biliary tract in diseases classified elsewhere**

K87.1* **Disorders of pancreas in diseases classified elsewhere**
Cytomegaloviral pancreatitis (B25.2†)
Mumps pancreatitis (B26.3†)

Other diseases of the digestive system (K90–K93)

K90 **Intestinal malabsorption**
Excludes: following gastrointestinal surgery (K91.2)

K90.0   **Coeliac disease**
Gluten-sensitive enteropathy
Idiopathic steatorrhoea
Nontropical sprue

K90.1   **Tropical sprue**
Sprue NOS
Tropical steatorrhoea

K90.2   **Blind loop syndrome, not elsewhere classified**
Blind loop syndrome NOS
Excludes: blind loop syndrome:
  • congenital (Q43.8)
  • postsurgical (K91.2)

K90.3   **Pancreatic steatorrhoea**

K90.4   **Malabsorption due to intolerance, not elsewhere classified**
Malabsorption due to intolerance to:
  • carbohydrate
  • fat
  • protein
  • starch
Excludes: gluten-sensitive enteropathy (K90.0)
            lactose intolerance (E73.–)

K90.8   **Other intestinal malabsorption**
Whipple's disease† (M14.8*)

K90.9   **Intestinal malabsorption, unspecified**

K91   Postprocedural disorders of digestive system, not elsewhere classified

Excludes: gastrojejunal ulcer (K28.–)
            radiation:
              • colitis (K52.0)
              • gastroenteritis (K52.0)
              • proctitis (K62.7)

K91.0   **Vomiting following gastrointestinal surgery**

K91.1   **Postgastric surgery syndromes**
Syndrome:
  • dumping
  • postgastrectomy
  • postvagotomy

K91.2 Postsurgical malabsorption, not elsewhere classified
Postsurgical blind loop syndrome
Excludes: malabsorption:
- osteomalacia in adults (M83.2)
- osteoporosis, postsurgical (M81.3)

K91.3 Postoperative intestinal obstruction

K91.4 Colostomy and enterostomy malfunction

K91.5 Postcholecystectomy syndrome

K91.8 Other postprocedural disorders of digestive system, not elsewhere classified

K91.9 Postprocedural disorder of digestive system, unspecified

K92 Other diseases of digestive system
Excludes: neonatal gastrointestinal haemorrhage (P54.0–P54.3)

K92.0 Haematemesis

K92.1 Melaena

K92.2 Gastrointestinal haemorrhage, unspecified
Haemorrhage:
- gastric NOS
- intestinal NOS

Excludes: acute haemorrhagic gastritis (K29.0)
haemorrhage of anus and rectum (K62.5)
with peptic ulcer (K25–K28)

K92.8 Other specified diseases of digestive system

K92.9 Disease of digestive system, unspecified

K93* Disorders of other digestive organs in diseases classified elsewhere

K93.0* Tuberculous disorders of intestines, peritoneum and mesenteric glands (A18.3†)
Excludes: tuberculous peritonitis (K67.3*)

K93.1* Megacolon in Chagas' disease (B57.3†)

K93.8* Disorders of other specified digestive organs in diseases classified elsewhere

CHAPTER XII

Diseases of the skin and subcutaneous tissue (L00–L99)

Excludes: certain conditions originating in the perinatal period (P00–P96)
certain infectious and parasitic diseases (A00–B99)
complications of pregnancy, childbirth and the puerperium (O00–O99)
congenital malformations, deformations and chromosomal abnormalities (Q00–Q99)
endocrine, nutritional and metabolic diseases (E00–E90)
injury, poisoning and certain other consequences of external causes (S00–T98)
lipomelanotic reticulosis (I89.8)
neoplasms (C00–D48)
symptoms, signs and abnormal clinical and laboratory findings, not elsewhere classified (R00–R99)
systemic connective tissue disorders (M30–M36)

This chapter contains the following blocks:

L00–L08 Infections of the skin and subcutaneous tissue
L10–L14 Bullous disorders
L20–L30 Dermatitis and eczema
L40–L45 Papulosquamous disorders
L50–L54 Urticaria and erythema
L55–L59 Radiation-related disorders of the skin and subcutaneous tissue
L60–L75 Disorders of skin appendages
L80–L99 Other disorders of the skin and subcutaneous tissue

Asterisk categories for this chapter are provided as follows:

L14* Bullous disorders in diseases classified elsewhere
L45* Papulosquamous disorders in diseases classified elsewhere
L54* Erythema in diseases classified elsewhere
L62* Nail disorders in diseases classified elsewhere
L86* Keratoderma in diseases classified elsewhere
L99* Other disorders of the skin and subcutaneous tissue in diseases classified elsewhere

Infections of the skin and subcutaneous tissue (L00–L08)

Use additional code (B95–B97), if desired, to identify infectious agent.

Excludes: hordeolum (H00.0)
infective dermatitis (L30.3)
local infections of skin classified in Chapter I, such as:
- erysipelas (A46)
- erysipeloid (A26.–)
- herpesviral [herpes simplex] infection (B00.–)
  - anogenital (A60.–)
- molluscum contagiosum (B08.1)
- mycoses (B35–B49)
- pediculosis, acariasis and other infestations (B85–B89)
- viral warts (B07)
panniculitis (of):
- NOS (M79.3)
- lupus (L93.2)
- neck and back (M54.0)
- relapsing [Weber–Christian] (M35.6)
perlèche (due to):
- NOS (K13.0)
- candidiasis (B37.–)
- riboflavin deficiency (E53.0)
pyogenic granuloma (L98.0)
zoster (B02.–)

L00   Staphylococcal scalded skin syndrome
Pemphigus neonatorum
Ritter's disease
Excludes: toxic epidermal necrolysis [Lyell] (L51.2)

L01   Impetigo
Excludes: impetigo herpetiformis (L40.1)
pemphigus neonatorum (L00)

L01.0   Impetigo [any organism] [any site]
Bockhart's impetigo

L01.1   Impetiginization of other dermatoses

L02   Cutaneous abscess, furuncle and carbuncle

Includes: boil
            furunculosis

Excludes: anal and rectal regions (K61.–)
            genital organs (external):
- female (N76.4)
- male (N48.2, N49.–)

L02.0   **Cutaneous abscess, furuncle and carbuncle of face**

Excludes: ear, external (H60.0)
            eyelid (H00.0)
            head [any part, except face] (L02.8)
            lacrimal:
- gland (H04.0)
- passages (H04.3)

            mouth (K12.2)
            nose (J34.0)
            orbit (H05.0)
            submandibular (K12.2)

L02.1   **Cutaneous abscess, furuncle and carbuncle of neck**

L02.2   **Cutaneous abscess, furuncle and carbuncle of trunk**

Abdominal wall
Back [any part, except buttock]
Chest wall
Groin
Perineum
Umbilicus

Excludes: breast (N61)
            hip (L02.4)
            omphalitis of newborn (P38)

L02.3   **Cutaneous abscess, furuncle and carbuncle of buttock**

Gluteal region

Excludes: pilonidal cyst with abscess (L05.0)

L02.4   **Cutaneous abscess, furuncle and carbuncle of limb**

Axilla
Hip
Shoulder

L02.8   **Cutaneous abscess, furuncle and carbuncle of other sites**

Head [any part, except face]
Scalp

L02.9   Cutaneous abscess, furuncle and carbuncle, unspecified
Furunculosis NOS

L03   Cellulitis

Includes: acute lymphangitis
Excludes: cellulitis of:
- anal and rectal regions (K61.–)
- external auditory canal (H60.1)
- external genital organs:
  - female (N76.4)
  - male (N48.2, N49.–)
- eyelid (H00.0)
- lacrimal apparatus (H04.3)
- mouth (K12.2)
- nose (J34.0)

eosinophilic cellulitis [Wells] (L98.3)
febrile neutrophilic dermatosis [Sweet] (L98.2)
lymphangitis (chronic)(subacute) (I89.1)

L03.0   Cellulitis of finger and toe
Infection of nail
Onychia
Paronychia
Perionychia

L03.1   Cellulitis of other parts of limb
Axilla
Hip
Shoulder

L03.2   Cellulitis of face

L03.3   Cellulitis of trunk
Abdominal wall
Back [any part]
Chest wall
Groin
Perineum
Umbilicus
Excludes: omphalitis of newborn (P38)

L03.8   Cellulitis of other sites
Head [any part, except face]
Scalp

L03.9   **Cellulitis, unspecified**

L04   Acute lymphadenitis

Includes: abscess (acute)   } any lymph node, except
lymphadenitis, acute   } mesenteric

Excludes: enlarged lymph nodes (R59.–)
human immunodeficiency virus [HIV] disease
resulting in generalized lymphadenopathy (B23.1)
lymphadenitis:
- NOS (I88.9)
- chronic or subacute, except mesenteric (I88.1)
- mesenteric, nonspecific (I88.0)

L04.0   **Acute lymphadenitis of face, head and neck**

L04.1   **Acute lymphadenitis of trunk**

L04.2   **Acute lymphadenitis of upper limb**
Axilla
Shoulder

L04.3   **Acute lymphadenitis of lower limb**
Hip

L04.8   **Acute lymphadenitis of other sites**

L04.9   **Acute lymphadenitis, unspecified**

L05   Pilonidal cyst

Includes: fistula   } coccygeal or pilonidal
sinus   }

L05.0   **Pilonidal cyst with abscess**

L05.9   **Pilonidal cyst without abscess**
Pilonidal cyst NOS

L08 **Other local infections of skin and subcutaneous tissue**

L08.0 **Pyoderma**
Dermatitis:
- purulent
- septic
- suppurative

Excludes: pyoderma gangrenosum (L88)

L08.1 **Erythrasma**

L08.8 **Other specified local infections of skin and subcutaneous tissue**

L08.9 **Local infection of skin and subcutaneous tissue, unspecified**

Bullous disorders (L10–L14)

Excludes: benign familial pemphigus [Hailey–Hailey] (Q82.8)
staphylococcal scalded skin syndrome (L00)
toxic epidermal necrolysis [Lyell] (L51.2)

L10 **Pemphigus**
Excludes: pemphigus neonatorum (L00)

L10.0 **Pemphigus vulgaris**

L10.1 **Pemphigus vegetans**

L10.2 **Pemphigus foliaceus**

L10.3 **Brazilian pemphigus [fogo selvagem]**

L10.4 **Pemphigus erythematosus**
Senear–Usher syndrome

L10.5 **Drug-induced pemphigus**
Use additional external cause code (Chapter XX), if desired, to identify drug.

L10.8 **Other pemphigus**

L10.9 **Pemphigus, unspecified**

L11 Other acantholytic disorders

L11.0 **Acquired keratosis follicularis**
Excludes: keratosis follicularis (congenital) [Darier–White]
(Q82.8)

L11.1 **Transient acantholytic dermatosis [Grover]**

L11.8 **Other specified acantholytic disorders**

L11.9 **Acantholytic disorder, unspecified**

L12 Pemphigoid
Excludes: herpes gestationis (O26.4)
impetigo herpetiformis (L40.1)

L12.0 **Bullous pemphigoid**

L12.1 **Cicatricial pemphigoid**
Benign mucous membrane pemphigoid

L12.2 **Chronic bullous disease of childhood**
Juvenile dermatitis herpetiformis

L12.3 **Acquired epidermolysis bullosa**
Excludes: epidermolysis bullosa (congenital) (Q81.–)

L12.8 **Other pemphigoid**

L12.9 **Pemphigoid, unspecified**

L13 Other bullous disorders

L13.0 **Dermatitis herpetiformis**
Duhring's disease

L13.1 **Subcorneal pustular dermatitis**
Sneddon–Wilkinson disease

L13.8 **Other specified bullous disorders**

L13.9 **Bullous disorder, unspecified**

L14* Bullous disorders in diseases classified elsewhere

Dermatitis and eczema
(L20–L30)

Note: In this block the terms dermatitis and eczema are used synonymously and interchangeably.

Excludes: chronic (childhood) granulomatous disease (D71)
dermatitis:
- dry skin (L85.3)
- factitial (L98.1)
- gangrenosa (L88)
- herpetiformis (L13.0)
- perioral (L71.0)
- stasis (I83.1–I83.2)
radiation-related disorders of the skin and subcutaneous tissue (L55–L59)

L20 Atopic dermatitis
Excludes: circumscribed neurodermatitis (L28.0)

L20.0   **Besnier's prurigo**

L20.8   **Other atopic dermatitis**
Eczema:
- flexural NEC
- infantile (acute)(chronic)
- intrinsic (allergic)
Neurodermatitis:
- atopic
- diffuse

L20.9   **Atopic dermatitis, unspecified**

L21 Seborrhoeic dermatitis
Excludes: infective dermatitis (L30.3)

L21.0   **Seborrhoea capitis**
Cradle cap

L21.1   **Seborrhoeic infantile dermatitis**

L21.8   **Other seborrhoeic dermatitis**

L21.9   **Seborrhoeic dermatitis, unspecified**

L22   Diaper [napkin] dermatitis

Diaper or napkin:
- erythema
- rash

Psoriasiform napkin rash

L23   Allergic contact dermatitis

Includes: allergic contact eczema

Excludes: allergy NOS (T78.4)
dermatitis (of):
- NOS (L30.9)
- contact NOS (L25.9)
- diaper [napkin] (L22)
- due to substances taken internally (L27.–)
- eyelid (H01.1)
- irritant contact (L24.–)
- perioral (L71.0)

eczema of external ear (H60.5)
radiation-related disorders of the skin and
subcutaneous tissue (L55–L59)

L23.0   **Allergic contact dermatitis due to metals**

Chromium
Nickel

L23.1   **Allergic contact dermatitis due to adhesives**

L23.2   **Allergic contact dermatitis due to cosmetics**

L23.3   **Allergic contact dermatitis due to drugs in contact with skin**

Use additional external cause code (Chapter XX), if desired, to
identify drug.

Excludes: allergic reaction NOS due to drugs (T88.7)
dermatitis due to ingested drugs and medicaments
(L27.0–L27.1)

L23.4   **Allergic contact dermatitis due to dyes**

L23.5   **Allergic contact dermatitis due to other chemical products**

Cement
Insecticide
Plastic
Rubber

L23.6 **Allergic contact dermatitis due to food in contact with skin**
Excludes: dermatitis due to ingested food (L27.2)

L23.7 **Allergic contact dermatitis due to plants, except food**

L23.8 **Allergic contact dermatitis due to other agents**

L23.9 **Allergic contact dermatitis, unspecified cause**
Allergic contact eczema NOS

L24 Irritant contact dermatitis

Includes: irritant contact eczema
Excludes: allergy NOS (T78.4)
dermatitis (of):
- NOS (L30.9)
- allergic contact (L23.–)
- contact NOS (L25.9)
- diaper [napkin] (L22)
- due to substances taken internally (L27.–)
- eyelid (H01.1)
- perioral (L71.0)
eczema of external ear (H60.5)
radiation-related disorders of the skin and
subcutaneous tissue (L55–L59)

L24.0 **Irritant contact dermatitis due to detergents**

L24.1 **Irritant contact dermatitis due to oils and greases**

L24.2 **Irritant contact dermatitis due to solvents**
Solvents:
- chlorocompound
- cyclohexane
- ester
- glycol
- hydrocarbon
- ketone

L24.3 **Irritant contact dermatitis due to cosmetics**

L24.4 **Irritant contact dermatitis due to drugs in contact with skin**
Use additional external cause code (Chapter XX), if desired, to
identify drug.
Excludes: allergic reaction NOS due to drugs (T88.7)
dermatitis due to ingested drugs and medicaments
(L27.0–L27.1)

L24.5   Irritant contact dermatitis due to other chemical products
Cement
Insecticide

L24.6   Irritant contact dermatitis due to food in contact with skin
Excludes: dermatitis due to ingested food (L27.2)

L24.7   Irritant contact dermatitis due to plants, except food

L24.8   Irritant contact dermatitis due to other agents
Dyes

L24.9   Irritant contact dermatitis, unspecified cause
Irritant contact eczema NOS

L25   Unspecified contact dermatitis

Includes: unspecified contact eczema
Excludes: allergy NOS (T78.4)
　　　　　dermatitis (of):
　　　　　• NOS (L30.9)
　　　　　• allergic contact (L23.–)
　　　　　• due to substances taken internally (L27.–)
　　　　　• eyelid (H01.1)
　　　　　• irritant contact (L24.–)
　　　　　• perioral (L71.0)
　　　　　eczema of external ear (H60.5)
　　　　　radiation-related disorders of the skin and
　　　　　　　subcutaneous tissue (L55–L59)

L25.0   Unspecified contact dermatitis due to cosmetics

L25.1   Unspecified contact dermatitis due to drugs in contact with skin
Use additional external cause code (Chapter XX), if desired, to identify drug.
Excludes: allergic reaction NOS due to drugs (T88.7)
　　　　　dermatitis due to ingested drugs and medicaments
　　　　　　　(L27.0–L27.1)

L25.2   Unspecified contact dermatitis due to dyes

L25.3   Unspecified contact dermatitis due to other chemical products
Cement
Insecticide

L25.4 **Unspecified contact dermatitis due to food in contact with skin**
Excludes: dermatitis due to ingested food (L27.2)

L25.5 **Unspecified contact dermatitis due to plants, except food**

L25.8 **Unspecified contact dermatitis due to other agents**

L25.9 **Unspecified contact dermatitis, unspecified cause**
Contact:
• dermatitis (occupational) NOS
• eczema (occupational) NOS

L26 Exfoliative dermatitis
Hebra's pityriasis
Excludes: Ritter's disease (L00)

L27 Dermatitis due to substances taken internally
Excludes: adverse:
• effect NOS of drugs (T88.7)
• food reaction, except dermatitis (T78.0–T78.1)
allergy NOS (T78.4)
contact dermatitis (L23–L25)
drug:
• photoallergic response (L56.1)
• phototoxic response (L56.0)
urticaria (L50.–)

L27.0 **Generalized skin eruption due to drugs and medicaments**
Use additional external cause code (Chapter XX), if desired, to identify drug.

L27.1 **Localized skin eruption due to drugs and medicaments**
Use additional external cause code (Chapter XX), if desired, to identify drug.

L27.2 **Dermatitis due to ingested food**
Excludes: dermatitis due to food in contact with skin (L23.6, L24.6, L25.4)

L27.8 **Dermatitis due to other substances taken internally**

L27.9 **Dermatitis due to unspecified substance taken internally**

L28   Lichen simplex chronicus and prurigo

L28.0   Lichen simplex chronicus
Circumscribed neurodermatitis
Lichen NOS

L28.1   Prurigo nodularis

L28.2   Other prurigo
Prurigo:
• NOS
• Hebra
• mitis
Urticaria papulosa

L29   Pruritus

Excludes: neurotic excoriation (L98.1)
        psychogenic pruritus (F45.8)

L29.0   Pruritus ani

L29.1   Pruritus scroti

L29.2   Pruritus vulvae

L29.3   Anogenital pruritus, unspecified

L29.8   Other pruritus

L29.9   Pruritus, unspecified
Itch NOS

L30   Other dermatitis

Excludes: dermatitis:
        • contact (L23–L25)
        • dry skin (L85.3)
        small plaque parapsoriasis (L41.3)
        stasis dermatitis (I83.1–I83.2)

L30.0   Nummular dermatitis

L30.1   Dyshidrosis [pompholyx]

L30.2   Cutaneous autosensitization
Candidid [levurid]
Dermatophytid
Eczematid

L30.3	**Infective dermatitis** Infectious eczematoid dermatitis
L30.4	**Erythema intertrigo**
L30.5	**Pityriasis alba**
L30.8	**Other specified dermatitis**
L30.9	**Dermatitis, unspecified** Eczema NOS

Papulosquamous disorders (L40–L45)

▉40▉ Psoriasis

L40.0	**Psoriasis vulgaris** Nummular psoriasis Plaque psoriasis
L40.1	**Generalized pustular psoriasis** Impetigo herpetiformis Von Zumbusch's disease
L40.2	**Acrodermatitis continua**
L40.3	**Pustulosis palmaris et plantaris**
L40.4	**Guttate psoriasis**
L40.5†	**Arthropathic psoriasis (M07.0–M07.3*, M09.0*)**
L40.8	**Other psoriasis** Flexural psoriasis
L40.9	**Psoriasis, unspecified**

▉41▉ Parapsoriasis
Excludes: poikiloderma vasculare atrophicans (L94.5)

L41.0	**Pityriasis lichenoides et varioliformis acuta** Mucha–Habermann disease
L41.1	**Pityriasis lichenoides chronica**
L41.2	**Lymphomatoid papulosis**

L41.3	Small plaque parapsoriasis
L41.4	Large plaque parapsoriasis
L41.5	Retiform parapsoriasis
L41.8	Other parapsoriasis
L41.9	Parapsoriasis, unspecified

L42 Pityriasis rosea

L43 Lichen planus

Excludes: lichen planopilaris (L66.1)

L43.0	Hypertrophic lichen planus
L43.1	Bullous lichen planus
L43.2	Lichenoid drug reaction

Use additional external cause code (Chapter XX), if desired, to identify drug.

| L43.3 | Subacute (active) lichen planus |

Lichen planus tropicus

| L43.8 | Other lichen planus |
| L43.9 | Lichen planus, unspecified |

L44 Other papulosquamous disorders

L44.0	Pityriasis rubra pilaris
L44.1	Lichen nitidus
L44.2	Lichen striatus
L44.3	Lichen ruber moniliformis
L44.4	Infantile papular acrodermatitis [Giannotti-Crosti]
L44.8	Other specified papulosquamous disorders
L44.9	Papulosquamous disorder, unspecified

L45* Papulosquamous disorders in diseases classified elsewhere

Urticaria and erythema (L50–L54)

Excludes: Lyme disease (A69.2)
rosacea (L71.–)

L50 Urticaria

Excludes: allergic contact dermatitis (L23.–)
angioneurotic oedema (T78.3)
hereditary angio-oedema (E88.0)
Quincke's oedema (T78.3)
urticaria:
• giant (T78.3)
• neonatorum (P83.8)
• papulosa (L28.2)
• pigmentosa (Q82.2)
• serum (T80.6)
• solar (L56.3)

L50.0 Allergic urticaria

L50.1 Idiopathic urticaria

L50.2 Urticaria due to cold and heat

L50.3 Dermatographic urticaria

L50.4 Vibratory urticaria

L50.5 Cholinergic urticaria

L50.6 Contact urticaria

L50.8 Other urticaria
Urticaria:
• chronic
• recurrent periodic

L50.9 Urticaria, unspecified

L51 Erythema multiforme

L51.0 Nonbullous erythema multiforme

L51.1 Bullous erythema multiforme
Stevens–Johnson syndrome

L51.2	**Toxic epidermal necrolysis [Lyell]**
L51.8	**Other erythema multiforme**
L51.9	**Erythema multiforme, unspecified**

L52 Erythema nodosum

L53 Other erythematous conditions

Excludes: erythema:
- ab igne (L59.0)
- due to external agents in contact with skin (L23–L25)
- intertrigo (L30.4)

L53.0 Toxic erythema
Use additional external cause code (Chapter XX), if desired, to identify external agent.
Excludes: neonatal erythema toxicum (P83.1)

L53.1 Erythema annulare centrifugum

L53.2 Erythema marginatum

L53.3 Other chronic figurate erythema

L53.8 Other specified erythematous conditions

L53.9 Erythematous condition, unspecified
Erythema NOS
Erythroderma NOS

L54* Erythema in diseases classified elsewhere

L54.0* Erythema marginatum in acute rheumatic fever (I00†)

L54.8* Erythema in other diseases classified elsewhere

Radiation-related disorders of the skin and subcutaneous tissue (L55–L59)

L55 Sunburn

L55.0 Sunburn of first degree

L55.1 Sunburn of second degree

L55.2 Sunburn of third degree

L55.8 Other sunburn

L55.9 Sunburn, unspecified

L56 Other acute skin changes due to ultraviolet radiation

L56.0 Drug phototoxic response
Use additional external cause code (Chapter XX), if desired, to identify drug.

L56.1 Drug photoallergic response
Use additional external cause code (Chapter XX), if desired, to identify drug.

L56.2 Photocontact dermatitis [berloque dermatitis]

L56.3 Solar urticaria

L56.4 Polymorphous light eruption

L56.8 Other specified acute skin changes due to ultraviolet radiation

L56.9 Acute skin change due to ultraviolet radiation, unspecified

L57 Skin changes due to chronic exposure to nonionizing radiation

L57.0 **Actinic keratosis**
Keratosis:
- NOS
- senile
- solar

L57.1 **Actinic reticuloid**

L57.2 **Cutis rhomboidalis nuchae**

L57.3 **Poikiloderma of Civatte**

L57.4 **Cutis laxa senilis**
Elastosis senilis

L57.5 **Actinic granuloma**

L57.8 **Other skin changes due to chronic exposure to nonionizing radiation**
Farmer's skin
Sailor's skin
Solar dermatitis

L57.9 **Skin changes due to chronic exposure to nonionizing radiation, unspecified**

L58 Radiodermatitis

L58.0 **Acute radiodermatitis**

L58.1 **Chronic radiodermatitis**

L58.9 **Radiodermatitis, unspecified**

L59 Other disorders of skin and subcutaneous tissue related to radiation

L59.0 **Erythema ab igne [dermatitis ab igne]**

L59.8 **Other specified disorders of skin and subcutaneous tissue related to radiation**

L59.9 **Disorder of skin and subcutaneous tissue related to radiation, unspecified**

Disorders of skin appendages (L60–L75)

Excludes: congenital malformations of integument (Q84.–)

L60 Nail disorders
Excludes: clubbing of nails (R68.3)
onychia and paronychia (L03.0)

L60.0 **Ingrowing nail**

L60.1 **Onycholysis**

L60.2 **Onychogryphosis**

L60.3 **Nail dystrophy**

L60.4 **Beau's lines**

L60.5 **Yellow nail syndrome**

L60.8 **Other nail disorders**

L60.9 **Nail disorder, unspecified**

L62* Nail disorders in diseases classified elsewhere

L62.0* **Clubbed nail pachydermoperiostosis (M89.4†)**

L62.8* **Nail disorders in other diseases classified elsewhere**

L63 Alopecia areata

L63.0 **Alopecia (capitis) totalis**

L63.1 **Alopecia universalis**

L63.2 **Ophiasis**

L63.8 **Other alopecia areata**

L63.9 **Alopecia areata, unspecified**

L64 Androgenic alopecia
Includes: male-pattern baldness

L64.0 **Drug-induced androgenic alopecia**
Use additional external cause code (Chapter XX), if desired, to identify drug.

L64.8 **Other androgenic alopecia**

L64.9 **Androgenic alopecia, unspecified**

L65 Other nonscarring hair loss
Use additional external cause code (Chapter XX), if desired, to identify drug, if drug-induced.
Excludes: trichotillomania (F63.3)

L65.0 **Telogen effluvium**

L65.1 **Anagen effluvium**

L65.2 **Alopecia mucinosa**

L65.8 **Other specified nonscarring hair loss**

L65.9 **Nonscarring hair loss, unspecified**
Alopecia NOS

L66 Cicatricial alopecia [scarring hair loss]

L66.0 **Pseudopelade**

L66.1 **Lichen planopilaris**
Follicular lichen planus

L66.2 **Folliculitis decalvans**

L66.3 **Perifolliculitis capitis abscedens**

L66.4 **Folliculitis ulerythematosa reticulata**

L66.8 **Other cicatricial alopecia**

L66.9 **Cicatricial alopecia, unspecified**

L67 Hair colour and hair shaft abnormalities
Excludes: monilethrix (Q84.1)
         pili annulati (Q84.1)
         telogen effluvium (L65.0)

L67.0 **Trichorrhexis nodosa**

L67.1 **Variations in hair colour**
Canities
Greyness, hair (premature)
Heterochromia of hair
Poliosis:
- NOS
- circumscripta, acquired

L67.8 **Other hair colour and hair shaft abnormalities**
Fragilitas crinium

L67.9 **Hair colour and hair shaft abnormality, unspecified**

L68 Hypertrichosis

Includes: excess hair
Excludes: congenital hypertrichosis (Q84.2)
persistent lanugo (Q84.2)

L68.0 **Hirsutism**
Use additional external cause code (Chapter XX), if desired, to identify drug, if drug-induced.

L68.1 **Acquired hypertrichosis lanuginosa**
Use additional external cause code (Chapter XX), if desired, to identify drug, if drug-induced.

L68.2 **Localized hypertrichosis**

L68.3 **Polytrichia**

L68.8 **Other hypertrichosis**

L68.9 **Hypertrichosis, unspecified**

L70 Acne

Excludes: acne keloid (L73.0)

L70.0 **Acne vulgaris**

L70.1 **Acne conglobata**

L70.2 **Acne varioliformis**
Acne necrotica miliaris

L70.3 **Acne tropica**

L70.4 **Infantile acne**

L70.5 **Acné excoriée des jeunes filles**

L70.8   **Other acne**

L70.9   **Acne, unspecified**

L71   Rosacea

L71.0   **Perioral dermatitis**
Use additional external cause code (Chapter XX), if desired, to identify drug, if drug-induced.

L71.1   **Rhinophyma**

L71.8   **Other rosacea**

L71.9   **Rosacea, unspecified**

L72   Follicular cysts of skin and subcutaneous tissue

L72.0   **Epidermal cyst**

L72.1   **Trichilemmal cyst**
Pilar cyst
Sebaceous cyst

L72.2   **Steatocystoma multiplex**

L72.8   **Other follicular cysts of skin and subcutaneous tissue**

L72.9   **Follicular cyst of skin and subcutaneous tissue, unspecified**

L73   Other follicular disorders

L73.0   **Acne keloid**

L73.1   **Pseudofolliculitis barbae**

L73.2   **Hidradenitis suppurativa**

L73.8   **Other specified follicular disorders**
Sycosis barbae

L73.9   **Follicular disorder, unspecified**

L74   Eccrine sweat disorders
Excludes: hyperhidrosis (R61.–)

L74.0   **Miliaria rubra**

L74.1   **Miliaria crystallina**

L74.2   **Miliaria profunda**
Miliaria tropicalis

L74.3   **Miliaria, unspecified**

L74.4   **Anhidrosis**
Hypohidrosis

L74.8   **Other eccrine sweat disorders**

L74.9   **Eccrine sweat disorder, unspecified**
Sweat gland disorder NOS

L75   Apocrine sweat disorders
Excludes: dyshidrosis [pompholyx] (L30.1)
hidradenitis suppurativa (L73.2)

L75.0   **Bromhidrosis**

L75.1   **Chromhidrosis**

L75.2   **Apocrine miliaria**
Fox–Fordyce disease

L75.8   **Other apocrine sweat disorders**

L75.9   **Apocrine sweat disorder, unspecified**

Other disorders of the skin and subcutaneous tissue (L80–L99)

L80   Vitiligo

L81   Other disorders of pigmentation
Excludes: birthmark NOS (Q82.5)
naevus—see Alphabetical Index
Peutz–Jeghers syndrome (Q85.8)

L81.0   **Postinflammatory hyperpigmentation**

L81.1   **Chloasma**

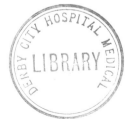

L81.2 **Freckles**

L81.3 **Café au lait spots**

L81.4 **Other melanin hyperpigmentation**
Lentigo

L81.5 **Leukoderma, not elsewhere classified**

L81.6 **Other disorders of diminished melanin formation**

L81.7 **Pigmented purpuric dermatosis**
Angioma serpiginosum

L81.8 **Other specified disorders of pigmentation**
Iron pigmentation
Tattoo pigmentation

L81.9 **Disorder of pigmentation, unspecified**

L82 Seborrhoeic keratosis
Dermatosis papulosa nigra
Leser–Trélat disease

L83 Acanthosis nigricans
Confluent and reticulated papillomatosis

L84 Corns and callosities
Callus
Clavus

L85 Other epidermal thickening
Excludes: hypertrophic disorders of skin (L91.–)

L85.0 **Acquired ichthyosis**
Excludes: congenital ichthyosis (Q80.–)

L85.1 **Acquired keratosis [keratoderma] palmaris et plantaris**
Excludes: inherited keratosis palmaris et plantaris (Q82.8)

L85.2 **Keratosis punctata (palmaris et plantaris)**

L85.3 **Xerosis cutis**
Dry skin dermatitis

L85.8   **Other specified epidermal thickening**
Cutaneous horn

L85.9   **Epidermal thickening, unspecified**

L86*   Keratoderma in diseases classified elsewhere

Follicular keratosis ⎱
Xeroderma ⎰ due to vitamin A deficiency (E50.8†)

L87   Transepidermal elimination disorders

Excludes: granuloma annulare (perforating) (L92.0)

L87.0   **Keratosis follicularis et parafollicularis in cutem penetrans [Kyrle]**
Hyperkeratosis follicularis penetrans

L87.1   **Reactive perforating collagenosis**

L87.2   **Elastosis perforans serpiginosa**

L87.8   **Other transepidermal elimination disorders**

L87.9   **Transepidermal elimination disorder, unspecified**

L88   Pyoderma gangrenosum

Dermatitis gangrenosa
Phagedenic pyoderma

L89   Decubitus ulcer

Bedsore
Plaster ulcer
Pressure ulcer
Excludes: decubitus (trophic) ulcer of cervix (uteri) (N86)

L90   Atrophic disorders of skin

L90.0   **Lichen sclerosus et atrophicus**

L90.1   **Anetoderma of Schweninger–Buzzi**

L90.2   **Anetoderma of Jadassohn–Pellizzari**

L90.3   **Atrophoderma of Pasini and Pierini**

L90.4   **Acrodermatitis chronica atrophicans**

L90.5   **Scar conditions and fibrosis of skin**
Adherent scar (skin)
Cicatrix
Disfigurement due to scar
Scar NOS
Excludes: hypertrophic scar (L91.0)
           keloid scar (L91.0)

L90.6   **Striae atrophicae**

L90.8   **Other atrophic disorders of skin**

L90.9   **Atrophic disorder of skin, unspecified**

L91   Hypertrophic disorders of skin

L91.0   **Keloid scar**
Hypertrophic scar
Keloid
Excludes: acne keloid (L73.0)
           scar NOS (L90.5)

L91.8   **Other hypertrophic disorders of skin**

L91.9   **Hypertrophic disorder of skin, unspecified**

L92   Granulomatous disorders of skin and subcutaneous tissue
Excludes: actinic granuloma (L57.5)

L92.0   **Granuloma annulare**
Perforating granuloma annulare

L92.1   **Necrobiosis lipoidica, not elsewhere classified**
Excludes: that associated with diabetes mellitus (E10–E14)

L92.2   **Granuloma faciale [eosinophilic granuloma of skin]**

L92.3   **Foreign body granuloma of skin and subcutaneous tissue**

L92.8   **Other granulomatous disorders of skin and subcutaneous tissue**

L92.9   **Granulomatous disorder of skin and subcutaneous tissue, unspecified**

L93   Lupus erythematosus

Excludes: lupus:
- exedens (A18.4)
- vulgaris (A18.4)

scleroderma (M34.–)

systemic lupus erythematosus (M32.–)

Use additional external cause code (Chapter XX), if desired, to identify drug, if drug-induced.

L93.0   **Discoid lupus erythematosus**
Lupus erythematosus NOS

L93.1   **Subacute cutaneous lupus erythematosus**

L93.2   **Other local lupus erythematosus**
Lupus:
- erythematosus profundus
- panniculitis

L94   Other localized connective tissue disorders

Excludes: systemic connective tissue disorders (M30–M36)

L94.0   **Localized scleroderma [morphea]**
Circumscribed scleroderma

L94.1   **Linear scleroderma**
En coup de sabre lesion

L94.2   **Calcinosis cutis**

L94.3   **Sclerodactyly**

L94.4   **Gottron's papules**

L94.5   **Poikiloderma vasculare atrophicans**

L94.6   **Ainhum**

L94.8   **Other specified localized connective tissue disorders**

L94.9   **Localized connective tissue disorder, unspecified**

L95 Vasculitis limited to skin, not elsewhere classified

Excludes: angioma serpiginosum (L81.7)
Henoch(–Schönlein) purpura (D69.0)
hypersensitivity angiitis (M31.0)
panniculitis (of):
- NOS (M79.3)
- lupus (L93.2)
- neck and back (M54.0)
- relapsing [Weber–Christian] (M35.6)
polyarteritis nodosa (M30.0)
rheumatoid vasculitis (M05.2)
serum sickness (T80.6)
urticaria (L50.–)
Wegener's granulomatosis (M31.3)

L95.0 Livedoid vasculitis
Atrophie blanche (en plaque)

L95.1 Erythema elevatum diutinum

L95.8 Other vasculitis limited to skin

L95.9 Vasculitis limited to skin, unspecified

L97 Ulcer of lower limb, not elsewhere classified

Excludes: decubitus ulcer (L89)
gangrene (R02)
skin infections (L00–L08)
specific infections classified to A00–B99
varicose ulcer (I83.0, I83.2)

L98 Other disorders of skin and subcutaneous tissue, not elsewhere classified

L98.0 Pyogenic granuloma

L98.1 Factitial dermatitis
Neurotic excoriation

L98.2 Febrile neutrophilic dermatosis [Sweet]

L98.3 Eosinophilic cellulitis [Wells]

L98.4 **Chronic ulcer of skin, not elsewhere classified**
Chronic ulcer of skin NOS
Tropical ulcer NOS
Ulcer of skin NOS
Excludes: decubitus ulcer (L89)
gangrene (R02)
skin infections (L00–L08)
specific infections classified to A00–B99
ulcer of lower limb NEC (L97)
varicose ulcer (I83.0, I83.2)

L98.5 **Mucinosis of skin**
Focal mucinosis
Lichen myxoedematosus
Excludes: focal oral mucinosis (K13.7)
myxoedema (E03.9)

L98.6 **Other infiltrative disorders of skin and subcutaneous tissue**
Excludes: hyalinosis cutis et mucosae (E78.8)

L98.8 **Other specified disorders of skin and subcutaneous tissue**

L98.9 **Disorder of skin and subcutaneous tissue, unspecified**

L99* **Other disorders of skin and subcutaneous tissue in diseases classified elsewhere**

L99.0* **Amyloidosis of skin (E85.–†)**
Lichen amyloidosis
Macular amyloid

L99.8* **Other specified disorders of skin and subcutaneous tissue in diseases classified elsewhere**
Syphilitic:
• alopecia (A51.3†)
• leukoderma (A51.3†, A52.7†)

CHAPTER XIII

Diseases of the musculoskeletal system and connective tissue (M00–M99)

Excludes: certain conditions originating in the perinatal period (P00–P96)
certain infectious and parasitic diseases (A00–B99)
compartment syndrome (T79.6)
complications of pregnancy, childbirth and the puerperium (O00–O99)
congenital malformations, deformations and chromosomal abnormalities (Q00–Q99)
endocrine, nutritional and metabolic diseases (E00–E90)
injury, poisoning and certain other consequences of external causes (S00–T98)
neoplasms (C00–D48)
symptoms, signs and abnormal clinical and laboratory findings, not elsewhere classified (R00–R99)

This chapter contains the following blocks:

M00–M25 Arthropathies
    M00–M03 Infectious arthropathies
    M05–M14 Inflammatory polyarthropathies
    M15–M19 Arthrosis
    M20–M25 Other joint disorders
M30–M36 Systemic connective tissue disorders
M40–M54 Dorsopathies
    M40–M43 Deforming dorsopathies
    M45–M49 Spondylopathies
    M50–M54 Other dorsopathies
M60–M79 Soft tissue disorders
    M60–M63 Disorders of muscles
    M65–M68 Disorders of synovium and tendon
    M70–M79 Other soft tissue disorders
M80–M94 Osteopathies and chondropathies
    M80–M85 Disorders of bone density and structure
    M86–M90 Other osteopathies
    M91–M94 Chondropathies
M95–M99 Other disorders of the musculoskeletal system and connective tissue

Asterisk categories for this chapter are provided as follows:

M01*   Direct infections of joint in infectious and parasitic diseases classified elsewhere

M03*   Postinfective and reactive arthropathies in diseases classified elsewhere

M07*   Psoriatic and enteropathic arthropathies

M09*   Juvenile arthritis in diseases classified elsewhere

M14*   Arthropathies in other diseases classified elsewhere

M36*   Systemic disorders of connective tissue in diseases classified elsewhere

M49*   Spondylopathies in diseases classified elsewhere

M63*   Disorders of muscle in diseases classified elsewhere

M68*   Disorders of synovium and tendon in diseases classified elsewhere

M73*   Soft tissue disorders in diseases classified elsewhere

M82*   Osteoporosis in diseases classified elsewhere

M90*   Osteopathies in diseases classified elsewhere

Site of musculoskeletal involvement

The following subclassification to indicate the site of involvement is provided for optional use with appropriate categories in Chapter XIII. As local extensions or specialty adaptations may vary in the number of characters used, it is suggested that the supplementary site subclassification be placed in an identifiably separate position (e.g. in an additional box). Different subclassifications for use with derangement of knee, dorsopathies, and biomechanical lesions not elsewhere classified are given on pages 642, 649 and 677 respectively.

0 Multiple sites

1 Shoulder region	clavicle scapula	acromioclavicular glenohumeral ⎫ joints sternoclavicular ⎭
2 Upper arm	humerus	elbow joint
3 Forearm	radius ulna	wrist joint
4 Hand	carpus fingers metacarpus	joints between these bones

5 Pelvic region and thigh	buttock femur pelvis	hip (joint) sacroiliac joint
6 Lower leg	fibula tibia	knee joint
7 Ankle and foot	metatarsus tarsus toes	ankle joint other joints in foot
8 Other	head neck ribs skull trunk vertebral column	

9 Site unspecified

Arthropathies
(M00–M25)

Disorders affecting predominantly peripheral (limb) joints

Infectious arthropathies
(M00–M03)

Note: This block comprises arthropathies due to microbiological agents. Distinction is made between the following types of etiological relationship:
(a) direct infection of joint, where organisms invade synovial tissue and microbial antigen is present in the joint;
(b) indirect infection, which may be of two types: a *reactive arthropathy*, where microbial infection of the body is established but neither organisms nor antigens can be identified in the joint, and a *postinfective arthropathy*, where microbial antigen is present but recovery of an organism is inconstant and evidence of local multiplication is lacking.

M00 Pyogenic arthritis
[See site code pages 628–629]

M00.0 **Staphylococcal arthritis and polyarthritis**

M00.1 **Pneumococcal arthritis and polyarthritis**

M00.2 **Other streptococcal arthritis and polyarthritis**

M00.8 **Arthritis and polyarthritis due to other specified bacterial agents**
Use additional code (B95–B96), if desired, to identify bacterial agent.

M00.9 **Pyogenic arthritis, unspecified**
Infective arthritis NOS

M01* Direct infections of joint in infectious and parasitic diseases classified elsewhere
[See site code pages 628–629]
Excludes: arthropathy in sarcoidosis (M14.8*)
postinfective and reactive arthropathy (M03.–*)

M01.0* **Meningococcal arthritis (A39.8†)**
Excludes: postmeningococcal arthritis (M03.0*)

M01.1* **Tuberculous arthritis (A18.0†)**
Excludes: of spine (M49.0*)

M01.2* **Arthritis in Lyme disease (A69.2†)**

M01.3* **Arthritis in other bacterial diseases classified elsewhere**
Arthritis in:
• leprosy [Hansen's disease] (A30.–†)
• localized salmonella infection (A02.2†)
• typhoid or paratyphoid fever (A01.–†)
Gonococcal arthritis (A54.4†)

M01.4* **Rubella arthritis (B06.8†)**

M01.5* **Arthritis in other viral diseases classified elsewhere**
Arthritis in:
• mumps (B26.8†)
• O'nyong-nyong fever (A92.1†)

M01.6* **Arthritis in mycoses (B35–B49†)**

M01.8* **Arthritis in other infectious and parasitic diseases classified elsewhere**

M02 Reactive arthropathies

[See site code pages 628–629]

Excludes: Behçet's disease (M35.2)
rheumatic fever (I00)

M02.0 **Arthropathy following intestinal bypass**

M02.1 **Postdysenteric arthropathy**

M02.2 **Postimmunization arthropathy**

M02.3 **Reiter's disease**

M02.8 **Other reactive arthropathies**

M02.9 **Reactive arthopathy, unspecified**

M03* Postinfective and reactive arthropathies in diseases classified elsewhere

[See site code pages 628–629]

Excludes: direct infections of joint in infectious and parasitic
diseases classified elsewhere (M01.–*)

M03.0* **Postmeningococcal arthritis (A39.8†)**

Excludes: meningococcal arthritis (M01.0*)

M03.1* **Postinfective arthropathy in syphilis**
Clutton's joints (A50.5†)

Excludes: Charcot's or tabetic arthropathy (M14.6*)

M03.2* **Other postinfectious arthropathies in diseases classified elsewhere**
Postinfectious arthropathy in:
• enteritis due to *Yersinia enterocolitica* (A04.6†)
• viral hepatitis (B15–B19†)

Excludes: viral arthropathies (M01.4–M01.5*)

M03.6* **Reactive arthropathy in other diseases classified elsewhere**
Arthropathy in infective endocarditis (I33.0†)

Inflammatory polyarthropathies (M05–M14)

M05 Seropositive rheumatoid arthritis

[See site code pages 628–629]

Excludes: rheumatic fever (I00)
rheumatoid arthritis (of):
- juvenile (M08.–)
- spine (M45)

M05.0 Felty's syndrome
Rheumatoid arthritis with splenoadenomegaly and leukopenia.

M05.1† Rheumatoid lung disease (J99.0*)

M05.2 Rheumatoid vasculitis

M05.3† Rheumatoid arthritis with involvement of other organs and systems
Rheumatoid:
- carditis (I52.8*)
- endocarditis (I39.–*)
- myocarditis (I41.8*)
- myopathy (G73.7*)
- pericarditis (I32.8*)
- polyneuropathy (G63.6*)

M05.8 Other seropositive rheumatoid arthritis

M05.9 Seropositive rheumatoid arthritis, unspecified

M06 Other rheumatoid arthritis

[See site code pages 628–629]

M06.0 Seronegative rheumatoid arthritis

M06.1 Adult-onset Still's disease
Excludes: Still's disease NOS (M08.2)

M06.2 Rheumatoid bursitis

M06.3 Rheumatoid nodule

M06.4   **Inflammatory polyarthropathy**
Excludes: polyarthritis NOS (M13.0)

M06.8   **Other specified rheumatoid arthritis**

M06.9   **Rheumatoid arthritis, unspecified**

M07*   Psoriatic and enteropathic arthropathies
[See site code pages 628–629]

Excludes: juvenile psoriatic and enteropathic arthropathies
(M09.–*)

M07.0*   **Distal interphalangeal psoriatic arthropathy (L40.5†)**

M07.1*   **Arthritis mutilans (L40.5†)**

M07.2*   **Psoriatic spondylitis (L40.5†)**

M07.3*   **Other psoriatic arthropathies (L40.5†)**

M07.4*   **Arthropathy in Crohn's disease [regional enteritis] (K50.–†)**

M07.5*   **Arthropathy in ulcerative colitis (K51.–†)**

M07.6*   **Other enteropathic arthropathies**

M08   Juvenile arthritis
[See site code pages 628–629]

Includes: arthritis in children, with onset before 16th birthday
and lasting longer than 3 months

Excludes: Felty's syndrome (M05.0)
juvenile dermatomyositis (M33.0)

M08.0   **Juvenile rheumatoid arthritis**
Juvenile rheumatoid arthritis with or without rheumatoid factor

M08.1   **Juvenile ankylosing spondylitis**
Excludes: ankylosing spondylitis in adults (M45)

M08.2   **Juvenile arthritis with systemic onset**
Still's disease NOS
Excludes: adult-onset Still's disease (M06.1)

M08.3   **Juvenile polyarthritis (seronegative)**
Chronic juvenile polyarthritis

M08.4   **Pauciarticular juvenile arthritis**

M08.8 Other juvenile arthritis

M08.9 Juvenile arthritis, unspecified

M09* Juvenile arthritis in diseases classified elsewhere
[See site code pages 628–629]

Excludes: arthropathy in Whipple's disease (M14.8*)

M09.0* Juvenile arthritis in psoriasis (L40.5†)

M09.1* Juvenile arthritis in Crohn's disease [regional enteritis] (K50.–†)

M09.2* Juvenile arthritis in ulcerative colitis (K51.–†)

M09.8* Juvenile arthritis in other diseases classified elsewhere

M10 Gout
[See site code pages 628–629]

M10.0 Idiopathic gout
Gouty bursitis
Primary gout
Urate tophus of heart† (I43.8*)

M10.1 Lead-induced gout

M10.2 Drug-induced gout
Use additional external cause code (Chapter XX), if desired, to identify drug.

M10.3 Gout due to impairment of renal function

M10.4 Other secondary gout

M10.9 Gout, unspecified

M11 Other crystal arthropathies
[See site code pages 628–629]

M11.0 Hydroxyapatite deposition disease

M11.1 Familial chondrocalcinosis

M11.2 Other chondrocalcinosis
Chondrocalcinosis NOS

M11.8   **Other specified crystal arthropathies**

M11.9   **Crystal arthropathy, unspecified**

M12   Other specific arthropathies

[See site code pages 628–629]

Excludes: arthropathy NOS (M13.9)
          arthrosis (M15–M19)
          cricoarytenoid arthropathy (J38.7)

M12.0   **Chronic postrheumatic arthropathy [Jaccoud]**

M12.1   **Kaschin–Beck disease**

M12.2   **Villonodular synovitis (pigmented)**

M12.3   **Palindromic rheumatism**

M12.4   **Intermittent hydrarthrosis**

M12.5   **Traumatic arthropathy**

Excludes: post-traumatic arthrosis (of):
- NOS (M19.1)
- first carpometacarpal joint (M18.2–M18.3)
- hip (M16.4–M16.5)
- knee (M17.2–M17.3)
- other single joints (M19.1)

M12.8   **Other specific arthropathies, not elsewhere classified**
Transient arthropathy

M13   Other arthritis

[See site code pages 628–629]

Excludes: arthrosis (M15–M19)

M13.0   **Polyarthritis, unspecified**

M13.1   **Monoarthritis, not elsewhere classified**

M13.8   **Other specified arthritis**
Allergic arthritis

M13.9   **Arthritis, unspecified**
Arthropathy NOS

635

M14* Arthropathies in other diseases classified elsewhere

Excludes: arthropathy in:
- haematological disorders (M36.2–M36.3*)
- hypersensitivity reactions (M36.4*)
- neoplastic disease (M36.1*)
  neuropathic spondylopathy (M49.4*)
  psoriatic and enteropathic arthropathies (M07.–*)
- juvenile (M09.–*)

M14.0* **Gouty arthropathy due to enzyme defects and other inherited disorders**
Gouty arthropathy in:
- Lesch–Nyhan syndrome (E79.1†)
- sickle-cell disorders (D57.–†)

M14.1* **Crystal arthropathy in other metabolic disorders**
Crystal arthropathy in hyperparathyroidism (E21.–†)

M14.2* **Diabetic arthropathy (E10–E14† with common fourth character .6)**
Excludes: diabetic neuropathic arthropathy (M14.6*)

M14.3* **Lipoid dermatoarthritis (E78.8†)**

M14.4* **Arthropathy in amyloidosis (E85.–†)**

M14.5* **Arthropathies in other endocrine, nutritional and metabolic disorders**
Arthropathy in:
- acromegaly and pituitary gigantism (E22.0†)
- haemochromatosis (E83.1†)
- hypothyroidism (E00–E03†)
- thyrotoxicosis [hyperthyroidism] (E05.–†)

M14.6* **Neuropathic arthropathy**
Charcot's or tabetic arthropathy (A52.1†)
Diabetic neuropathic arthropathy (E10–E14† with common fourth character .6)

M14.8* **Arthropathies in other specified diseases classified elsewhere**
Arthropathy in:
- erythema:
  - multiforme (L51.–†)
  - nodosum (L52†)
- sarcoidosis (D86.8†)
- Whipple's disease (K90.8†)

Arthrosis
(M15–M19)

Note: In this block the term osteoarthritis is used as a synonym for arthrosis or osteoarthrosis. The term primary has been used with its customary clinical meaning of no underlying or determining condition identified.

Excludes: osteoarthritis of spine (M47.–)

M15 Polyarthrosis

Includes: arthrosis with mention of more than one site
Excludes: bilateral involvement of single joint (M16–M19)

M15.0 **Primary generalized (osteo)arthrosis**

M15.1 **Heberden's nodes (with arthropathy)**

M15.2 **Bouchard's nodes (with arthropathy)**

M15.3 **Secondary multiple arthrosis**
Post-traumatic polyarthrosis

M15.4 **Erosive (osteo)arthrosis**

M15.8 **Other polyarthrosis**

M15.9 **Polyarthrosis, unspecified**
Generalized osteoarthritis NOS

M16 Coxarthrosis [arthrosis of hip]

M16.0 **Primary coxarthrosis, bilateral**

M16.1 **Other primary coxarthrosis**
Primary coxarthrosis:
• NOS
• unilateral

M16.2 **Coxarthrosis resulting from dysplasia, bilateral**

M16.3 **Other dysplastic coxarthrosis**
Dysplastic coxarthrosis:
• NOS
• unilateral

M16.4 **Post-traumatic coxarthrosis, bilateral**

M16.5   **Other post-traumatic coxarthrosis**
Post-traumatic coxarthrosis:
- NOS
- unilateral

M16.6   **Other secondary coxarthrosis, bilateral**

MI6.7   **Other secondary coxarthrosis**
Secondary coxarthrosis:
- NOS
- unilateral

M16.9   **Coxarthrosis, unspecified**

M17   Gonarthrosis [arthrosis of knee]

M17.0   **Primary gonarthrosis, bilateral**

M17.1   **Other primary gonarthrosis**
Primary gonarthrosis:
- NOS
- unilateral

M17.2   **Post-traumatic gonarthrosis, bilateral**

M17.3   **Other post-traumatic gonarthrosis**
Post-traumatic gonarthrosis:
- NOS
- unilateral

M17.4   **Other secondary gonarthrosis, bilateral**

M17.5   **Other secondary gonarthrosis**
Secondary gonarthrosis:
- NOS
- unilateral

M17.9   **Gonarthrosis, unspecified**

M18   Arthrosis of first carpometacarpal joint

M18.0   **Primary arthrosis of first carpometacarpal joints, bilateral**

M18.1   **Other primary arthrosis of first carpometacarpal joint**
Primary arthrosis of first carpometacarpal joint:
- NOS
- unilateral

M18.2   **Post-traumatic arthrosis of first carpometacarpal joints, bilateral**

M18.3   **Other post-traumatic arthrosis of first carpometacarpal joint**
Post-traumatic arthrosis of first carpometacarpal joint:
• NOS
• unilateral

M18.4   **Other secondary arthrosis of first carpometacarpal joints, bilateral**

M18.5   **Other secondary arthrosis of first carpometacarpal joint**
Secondary arthrosis of first carpometacarpal joint:
• NOS
• unilateral

M18.9   **Arthrosis of first carpometacarpal joint, unspecified**

M19   Other arthrosis
[See site code pages 628–629]
Excludes: arthrosis of spine (M47.–)
             hallux rigidus (M20.2)
             polyarthrosis (M15.–)

M19.0   **Primary arthrosis of other joints**
Primary arthrosis NOS

M19.1   **Post-traumatic arthrosis of other joints**
Post-traumatic arthrosis NOS

M19.2   **Secondary arthrosis of other joints**
Secondary arthrosis NOS

M19.8   **Other specified arthrosis**

M19.9   **Arthrosis, unspecified**

Other joint disorders
(M20–M25)

Excludes: joints of the spine (M40–M54)

M20 Acquired deformities of fingers and toes
Excludes: acquired absence of fingers and toes (Z89.–)
congenital:
- absence of fingers and toes (Q71.3, Q72.3)
- deformities and malformations of fingers and toes (Q66.–, Q68–Q70, Q74.–)

M20.0 Deformity of finger(s)
Boutonnière and swan-neck deformities
Excludes: clubbing of fingers (R68.3)
palmar fascial fibromatosis [Dupuytren] (M72.0)
trigger finger (M65.3)

M20.1 Hallux valgus (acquired)
Bunion

M20.2 Hallux rigidus

M20.3 Other deformity of hallux (acquired)
Hallux varus

M20.4 Other hammer toe(s) (acquired)

M20.5 Other deformities of toe(s) (acquired)

M20.6 Acquired deformity of toe(s), unspecified

M21 Other acquired deformities of limbs
[See site code pages 628–629]
Excludes: acquired absence of limb (Z89.–)
acquired deformities of fingers or toes (M20.–)
congenital:
- absence of limbs (Q71–Q73)
- deformities and malformations of limbs (Q65–Q66, Q68–Q74)
coxa plana (M91.2)

M21.0 **Valgus deformity, not elsewhere classified**
Excludes: metatarsus valgus (Q66.6)
talipes calcaneovalgus (Q66.4)

M21.1 **Varus deformity, not elsewhere classified**
Excludes: metatarsus varus (Q66.2)
tibia vara (M92.5)

M21.2 **Flexion deformity**

M21.3 **Wrist or foot drop (acquired)**

M21.4 **Flat foot [pes planus] (acquired)**
Excludes: congenital pes planus (Q66.5)

M21.5 **Acquired clawhand, clubhand, clawfoot and clubfoot**
Excludes: clubfoot, not specified as acquired (Q66.8)

M21.6 **Other acquired deformities of ankle and foot**
Excludes: deformities of toe (acquired) (M20.1–M20.6)

M21.7 **Unequal limb length (acquired)**

M21.8 **Other specified acquired deformities of limbs**

M21.9 **Acquired deformity of limb, unspecified**

M22 **Disorders of patella**
Excludes: dislocation of patella (S83.0)

M22.0 **Recurrent dislocation of patella**

M22.1 **Recurrent subluxation of patella**

M22.2 **Patellofemoral disorders**

M22.3 **Other derangements of patella**

M22.4 **Chondromalacia patellae**

M22.8 **Other disorders of patella**

M22.9 **Disorder of patella, unspecified**

M23 Internal derangement of knee

The following supplementary subclassification to indicate the site of involvement is provided for optional use with appropriate subcategories in M23.–; see also note on page 628.

0 Multiple sites

1 Anterior cruciate ligament or Anterior horn of medial meniscus

2 Posterior cruciate ligament or Posterior horn of medial meniscus

3 Medial collateral ligament or Other and unspecified medial meniscus

4 Lateral collateral ligament or Anterior horn of lateral meniscus

5 Posterior horn of lateral meniscus

6 Other and unspecified lateral meniscus

7 Capsular ligament

9 Unspecified ligament or Unspecified meniscus

Excludes: ankylosis (M24.6)

current injury—see injury to the knee and lower leg (S80–S89)

deformity of knee (M21.–)

disorders of patella (M22.–)

osteochondritis dissecans (M93.2)

recurrent dislocation or subluxation (M24.4)

• patella (M22.0–M22.1)

M23.0 Cystic meniscus

M23.1 Discoid meniscus (congenital)

M23.2 Derangement of meniscus due to old tear or injury
Old bucket-handle tear

M23.3 Other meniscus derangements
Degenerate ⎫
Detached ⎬ meniscus
Retained ⎭

M23.4 Loose body in knee

M23.5 Chronic instability of knee

M23.6 Other spontaneous disruption of ligament(s) of knee

M23.8   **Other internal derangements of knee**
Laxity of ligament of knee
Snapping knee

M23.9   **Internal derangement of knee, unspecified**

M24   **Other specific joint derangements**
[See site code pages 628–629]
Excludes: current injury—see injury of joint by body region
            ganglion (M67.4)
            snapping knee (M23.8)
            temporomandibular joint disorders (K07.6)

M24.0   **Loose body in joint**
Excludes: loose body in knee (M23.4)

M24.1   **Other articular cartilage disorders**
Excludes: chondrocalcinosis (M11.1–M11.2)
            internal derangement of knee (M23.–)
            metastatic calcification (E83.5)
            ochronosis (E70.2)

M24.2   **Disorder of ligament**
Instability secondary to old ligament injury
Ligamentous laxity NOS
Excludes: familial ligamentous laxity (M35.7)
            knee (M23.5–M23.8)

M24.3   **Pathological dislocation and subluxation of joint, not elsewhere classified**
Excludes: dislocation or displacement of joint:
            • congenital—see congenital malformations and
              deformations of the musculoskeletal system
              (Q65–Q79)
            • current injury—see injury of joints and ligaments
              by body region
            • recurrent (M24.4)

M24.4   **Recurrent dislocation and subluxation of joint**
Excludes: patella (M22.0–M22.1)
            vertebral subluxation (M43.3–M43.5)

M24.5   **Contracture of joint**
Excludes: acquired deformities of limbs (M20–M21)
              contracture of tendon (sheath) without contracture
                  of joint (M67.1)
              Dupuytren's contracture (M72.0)

M24.6   **Ankylosis of joint**
Excludes: spine (M43.2)
              stiffness of joint without ankylosis (M25.6)

M24.7   **Protrusio acetabuli**

M24.8   **Other specific joint derangements, not elsewhere classified**
Irritable hip

M24.9   **Joint derangement, unspecified**

M25 Other joint disorders, not elsewhere classified
[See site code pages 628–629]
Excludes: abnormality of gait and mobility (R26.–)
              calcification of:
              • bursa (M71.4)
              • shoulder (joint) (M75.3)
              • tendon (M65.2)
              deformities classified to M20–M21
              difficulty in walking (R26.2)

M25.0   **Haemarthrosis**
Excludes: current injury—see injury of joint by body region

M25.1   **Fistula of joint**

M25.2   **Flail joint**

M25.3   **Other instability of joint**
Excludes: instability of joint secondary to:
              • old ligament injury (M24.2)
              • removal of joint prosthesis (M96.8)

M25.4   **Effusion of joint**
Excludes: hydrarthrosis of yaws (A66.6)

M25.5   **Pain in joint**

M25.6   **Stiffness of joint, not elsewhere classified**

M25.7   **Osteophyte**

M25.8   **Other specified joint disorders**

M25.9   **Joint disorder, unspecified**

Systemic connective tissue disorders (M30–M36)

Includes: autoimmune disease:
- NOS
- systemic

collagen (vascular) disease:
- NOS
- systemic

Excludes: autoimmune disease, single organ or single cell-type (code to relevant condition category)

M30   Polyarteritis nodosa and related conditions

M30.0   **Polyarteritis nodosa**

M30.1   **Polyarteritis with lung involvement [Churg–Strauss]**
Allergic granulomatous angiitis

M30.2   **Juvenile polyarteritis**

M30.3   **Mucocutaneous lymph node syndrome [Kawasaki]**

M30.8   **Other conditions related to polyarteritis nodosa**
Polyangiitis overlap syndrome

M31   Other necrotizing vasculopathies

M31.0   **Hypersensitivity angiitis**
Goodpasture's syndrome

M31.1   **Thrombotic microangiopathy**
Thrombotic thrombocytopenic purpura

M31.2   **Lethal midline granuloma**

M31.3   **Wegener's granulomatosis**
Necrotizing respiratory granulomatosis

M31.4   **Aortic arch syndrome [Takayasu]**

M31.5   **Giant cell arteritis with polymyalgia rheumatica**

M31.6   **Other giant cell arteritis**

M31.8   **Other specified necrotizing vasculopathies**
Hypocomplementaemic vasculitis

M31.9   **Necrotizing vasculopathy, unspecified**

M32   Systemic lupus erythematosus
Excludes: lupus erythematosus (discoid)(NOS) (L93.0)

M32.0   **Drug-induced systemic lupus erythematosus**
Use additional external cause code (Chapter XX), if desired, to identify drug.

M32.1†   **Systemic lupus erythematosus with organ or system involvement**
Libman–Sacks disease (I39.–*)
Lupus pericarditis (I32.8*)
Systemic lupus erythematosus with:
• kidney involvement (N08.5*, N16.4*)
• lung involvement (J99.1*)

M32.8   **Other forms of systemic lupus erythematosus**

M32.9   **Systemic lupus erythematosus, unspecified**

M33   Dermatopolymyositis

M33.0   **Juvenile dermatomyositis**

M33.1   **Other dermatomyositis**

M33.2   **Polymyositis**

M33.9   **Dermatopolymyositis, unspecified**

M34   Systemic sclerosis
Includes: scleroderma
Excludes: scleroderma:
            • circumscribed (L94.0)
            • neonatal (P83.8)

M34.0   **Progressive systemic sclerosis**

M34.1 CR(E)ST syndrome
Combination of calcinosis, Raynaud's phenomenon, (o)eso-phageal dysfunction, sclerodactyly, telangiectasia.

M34.2 Systemic sclerosis induced by drugs and chemicals
Use additional external cause code (Chapter XX), if desired, to identify cause.

M34.8 Other forms of systemic sclerosis
Systemic sclerosis with:
- lung involvement† (J99.1*)
- myopathy† (G73.7*)

M34.9 Systemic sclerosis, unspecified

M35 Other systemic involvement of connective tissue
Excludes: reactive perforating collagenosis (L87.1)

M35.0 Sicca syndrome [Sjögren]
Sjögren's syndrome with:
- keratoconjunctivitis† (H19.3*)
- lung involvement† (J99.1*)
- myopathy† (G73.7*)
- renal tubulo-interstitial disorders† (N16.4*)

M35.1 Other overlap syndromes
Mixed connective tissue disease
Excludes: polyangiitis overlap syndrome (M30.8)

M35.2 Behçet's disease

M35.3 Polymyalgia rheumatica
Excludes: polymyalgia rheumatica with giant cell arteritis (M31.5)

M35.4 Diffuse (eosinophilic) fasciitis

M35.5 Multifocal fibrosclerosis

M35.6 Relapsing panniculitis [Weber–Christian]
Excludes: panniculitis:
- NOS (M79.3)
- lupus (L93.2)

M35.7 Hypermobility syndrome
Familial ligamentous laxity
Excludes: Ehlers–Danlos syndrome (Q79.6)
ligamentous laxity NOS (M24.2)

M35.8 **Other specified systemic involvement of connective tissue**

M35.9 **Systemic involvement of connective tissue, unspecified**
Autoimmune disease (systemic) NOS
Collagen (vascular) disease NOS

M36* Systemic disorders of connective tissue in diseases classified elsewhere

Excludes: arthropathies in diseases classified elsewhere (M14.–*)

M36.0* **Dermato(poly)myositis in neoplastic disease (C00–D48†)**

M36.1* **Arthropathy in neoplastic disease (C00–D48†)**
Arthropathy in:
- leukaemia (C91–C95†)
- malignant histiocytosis (C96.1†)
- multiple myeloma (C90.0†)

M36.2* **Haemophilic arthropathy (D66–D68†)**

M36.3* **Arthropathy in other blood disorders (D50–D76†)**
Excludes: arthropathy in Henoch(–Schönlein) purpura (M36.4*)

M36.4* **Arthropathy in hypersensitivity reactions classified elsewhere**
Arthropathy in Henoch(–Schönlein) purpura (D69.0†)

M36.8* **Systemic disorders of connective tissue in other diseases classified elsewhere**
Systemic disorders of connective tissue in:
- hypogammaglobulinaemia (D80.–†)
- ochronosis (E70.2†)

Dorsopathies
(M40–M54)

The following supplementary subclassification to indicate the site of involvement is provided for optional use with appropriate categories in the block on dorsopathies, except categories M50 and M51; see also note on page 628.

0 Multiple sites in spine

1 Occipito-atlanto-axial region

2 Cervical region

3 Cervicothoracic region

4 Thoracic region

5 Thoracolumbar region

6 Lumbar region

7 Lumbosacral region

8 Sacral and sacrococcygeal region

9 Site unspecified

Deforming dorsopathies
(M40–M43)

M40   Kyphosis and lordosis
[See site code above]
Excludes: kyphoscoliosis (M41.–)
kyphosis and lordosis:
• congenital (Q76.4)
• postprocedural (M96.–)

M40.0   **Postural kyphosis**
Excludes: osteochondrosis of spine (M42.–)

M40.1   **Other secondary kyphosis**

M40.2   **Other and unspecified kyphosis**

M40.3   **Flatback syndrome**

M40.4   **Other lordosis**
Lordosis:
- acquired
- postural

M40.5   **Lordosis, unspecified**

M41   Scoliosis
[See site code page 649]
Includes: kyphoscoliosis
Excludes: congenital scoliosis:
- NOS (Q67.5)
- due to bony malformation (Q76.3)
- postural (Q67.5)
kyphoscoliotic heart disease (I27.1)
postprocedural (M96.–)

M41.0   **Infantile idiopathic scoliosis**

M41.1   **Juvenile idiopathic scoliosis**
Adolescent scoliosis

M41.2   **Other idiopathic scoliosis**

M41.3   **Thoracogenic scoliosis**

M41.4   **Neuromuscular scoliosis**
Scoliosis secondary to cerebral palsy, Friedreich's ataxia, poliomyelitis, and other neuromuscular disorders.

M41.5   **Other secondary scoliosis**

M41.8   **Other forms of scoliosis**

M41.9   **Scoliosis, unspecified**

M42   Spinal osteochondrosis
[See site code page 649]

M42.0   **Juvenile osteochondrosis of spine**
Calvé's disease
Scheuermann's disease
Excludes: postural kyphosis (M40.0)

M42.1   **Adult osteochondrosis of spine**

M42.9   **Spinal osteochondrosis, unspecified**

M43 Other deforming dorsopathies

[See site code page 649]

Excludes: congenital spondylolysis and spondylolisthesis (Q76.2)
hemivertebra (Q76.3–Q76.4)
Klippel–Feil syndrome (Q76.1)
lumbarization and sacralization (Q76.4)
platyspondylisis (Q76.4)
spina bifida occulta (Q76.0)
spinal curvature in:
• osteoporosis (M80–M81)
• Paget's disease of bone [osteitis deformans] (M88.–)

M43.0 **Spondylolysis**

M43.1 **Spondylolisthesis**

M43.2 **Other fusion of spine**
Ankylosis of spinal joint

Excludes: ankylosing spondylitis (M45)
arthrodesis status (Z98.1)
pseudoarthrosis after fusion or arthrodesis (M96.0)

M43.3 **Recurrent atlantoaxial subluxation with myelopathy**

M43.4 **Other recurrent atlantoaxial subluxation**

M43.5 **Other recurrent vertebral subluxation**

Excludes: biomechanical lesions NEC (M99.–)

M43.6 **Torticollis**

Excludes: torticollis:
• congenital (sternomastoid) (Q68.0)
• current injury—see injury of spine by body region
• due to birth injury (P15.8)
• psychogenic (F45.8)
• spasmodic (G24.3)

M43.8 **Other specified deforming dorsopathies**

Excludes: kyphosis and lordosis (M40.–)
scoliosis (M41.–)

M43.9 **Deforming dorsopathy, unspecified**
Curvature of spine NOS

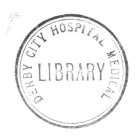

Spondylopathies
(M45–M49)

M45 Ankylosing spondylitis
[See site code page 649]
Rheumatoid arthritis of spine

Excludes: arthropathy in Reiter's disease (M02.3)
Behçet's disease (M35.2)
juvenile (ankylosing) spondylitis (M08.1)

M46 Other inflammatory spondylopathies
[See site code page 649]

M46.0 Spinal enthesopathy
Disorder of ligamentous or muscular attachments of spine

M46.1 Sacroiliitis, not elsewhere classified

M46.2 Osteomyelitis of vertebra

M46.3 Infection of intervertebral disc (pyogenic)
Use additional code (B95–B97), if desired, to identify infectious agent.

M46.4 Discitis, unspecified

M46.5 Other infective spondylopathies

M46.8 Other specified inflammatory spondylopathies

M46.9 Inflammatory spondylopathy, unspecified

M47 Spondylosis
[See site code page 649]

Includes: arthrosis or osteoarthritis of spine
degeneration of facet joints

M47.0† Anterior spinal and vertebral artery compression syndromes (G99.2*)

M47.1 Other spondylosis with myelopathy
Spondylogenic compression of spinal cord† (G99.2*)

Excludes: vertebral subluxation (M43.3–M43.5)

M47.2 **Other spondylosis with radiculopathy**

M47.8 **Other spondylosis**
Cervical spondylosis ⎫
Lumbosacral spondylosis ⎬ without myelopathy or
Thoracic spondylosis ⎭ radiculopathy

M47.9 **Spondylosis, unspecified**

M48 Other spondylopathies
[See site code page 649]

M48.0 **Spinal stenosis**
Caudal stenosis

M48.1 **Ankylosing hyperostosis [Forestier]**
Diffuse idiopathic skeletal hyperostosis [DISH]

M48.2 **Kissing spine**

M48.3 **Traumatic spondylopathy**

M48.4 **Fatigue fracture of vertebra**
Stress fracture of vertebra

M48.5 **Collapsed vertebra, not elsewhere classified**
Collapsed vertebra NOS
Wedging of vertebra NOS
Excludes: collapsed vertebra in osteoporosis (M80.–)
current injury—see injury of spine by body region

M48.8 **Other specified spondylopathies**
Ossification of posterior longitudinal ligament

M48.9 **Spondylopathy, unspecified**

M49* Spondylopathies in diseases classified elsewhere
[See site code page 649]
Excludes: psoriatic and enteropathic arthropathies (M07.–*,
M09.–*)

M49.0* **Tuberculosis of spine (A18.0†)**
Pott's curvature

M49.1* **Brucella spondylitis (A23.–†)**

M49.2* **Enterobacterial spondylitis (A01–A04†)**

M49.3* **Spondylopathy in other infectious and parasitic diseases classified elsewhere**

Excludes: neuropathic spondylopathy in tabes dorsalis (M49.4*)

M49.4* **Neuropathic spondylopathy**
Neuropathic spondylopathy in:
- syringomyelia and syringobulbia (G95.0†)
- tabes dorsalis (A52.1†)

M49.5* **Collapsed vertebra in diseases classified elsewhere**
Metastatic fracture of vertebra (C79.5†)

M49.8* **Spondylopathy in other diseases classified elsewhere**

Other dorsopathies (M50–M54)

Excludes: current injury—see injury of spine by body region
discitis NOS (M46.4)

M50 Cervical disc disorders

Includes: cervical disc disorders with cervicalgia
cervicothoracic disc disorders

M50.0† **Cervical disc disorder with myelopathy (G99.2*)**

M50.1 **Cervical disc disorder with radiculopathy**
Excludes: brachial radiculitis NOS (M54.1)

M50.2 **Other cervical disc displacement**

M50.3 **Other cervical disc degeneration**

M50.8 **Other cervical disc disorders**

M50.9 **Cervical disc disorder, unspecified**

M51 Other intervertebral disc disorders

Includes: thoracic, thoracolumbar and lumbosacral disc
disorders

M51.0† **Lumbar and other intervertebral disc disorders with myelopathy (G99.2*)**

M51.1   **Lumbar and other intervertebral disc disorders with radiculopathy**
Sciatica due to intervertebral disc disorder
Excludes: lumbar radiculitis NOS (M54.1)

M51.2   **Other specified intervertebral disc displacement**
Lumbago due to displacement of intervertebral disc

M51.3   **Other specified intervertebral disc degeneration**

M51.4   **Schmorl's nodes**

M51.8   **Other specified intervertebral disc disorders**

M51.9   **Intervertebral disc disorder, unspecified**

M53   Other dorsopathies, not elsewhere classified
[See site code page 649]

M53.0   **Cervicocranial syndrome**
Posterior cervical sympathetic syndrome

M53.1   **Cervicobrachial syndrome**
Excludes: cervical disc disorder (M50.–)
            thoracic outlet syndrome (G54.0)

M53.2   **Spinal instabilities**

M53.3   **Sacrococcygeal disorders, not elsewhere classified**
Coccygodynia

M53.8   **Other specified dorsopathies**

M53.9   **Dorsopathy, unspecified**

M54   Dorsalgia
[See site code page 649]
Excludes: psychogenic dorsalgia (F45.4)

M54.0   **Panniculitis affecting regions of neck and back**
Excludes: panniculitis:
• NOS (M79.3)
• lupus (L93.2)
• relapsing [Weber–Christian] (M35.6)

M54.1 **Radiculopathy**
Neuritis or radiculitis:
- brachial NOS
- lumbar NOS
- lumbosacral NOS
- thoracic NOS
Radiculitis NOS

Excludes: neuralgia and neuritis NOS (M79.2)
radiculopathy with:
- cervical disc disorder (M50.1)
- lumbar and other intervertebral disc disorder (M51.1)
- spondylosis (M47.2)

M54.2 **Cervicalgia**

Excludes: cervicalgia due to intervertebral cervical disc disorder (M50.–)

M54.3 **Sciatica**

Excludes: lesion of sciatic nerve (G57.0)
sciatica:
- due to intervertebral disc disorder (M51.1)
- with lumbago (M54.4)

M54.4 **Lumbago with sciatica**

Excludes: that due to intervertebral disc disorder (M51.1)

M54.5 **Low back pain**
Loin pain
Low back strain
Lumbago NOS

Excludes: lumbago:
- due to intervertebral disc displacement (M51.2)
- with sciatica (M54.4)

M54.6 **Pain in thoracic spine**

Excludes: pain due to intervertebral disc disorder (M51.–)

M54.8 **Other dorsalgia**

M54.9 **Dorsalgia, unspecified**
Backache NOS

Soft tissue disorders
(M60–M79)

Disorders of muscles
(M60–M63)

Excludes: dermatopolymyositis (M33.-)
muscular dystrophies and myopathies (G71–G72)
myopathy in:
* amyloidosis (E85.–)
* polyarteritis nodosa (M30.0)
* rheumatoid arthritis (M05.3)
* scleroderma (M34.–)
* Sjögren's syndrome (M35.0)
* systemic lupus erythematosus (M32.–)

M60 Myositis
[See site code pages 628–629]

M60.0 **Infective myositis**
Tropical pyomyositis

Use additional code (B95–B97), if desired, to identify infectious agent.

M60.1 **Interstitial myositis**

M60.2 **Foreign body granuloma of soft tissue, not elsewhere classified**

Excludes: foreign body granuloma of skin and subcutaneous tissue (L92.3)

M60.8 **Other myositis**

M60.9 **Myositis, unspecified**

M61 Calcification and ossification of muscle
[See site code pages 628–629]

M61.0 **Myositis ossificans traumatica**

M61.1 **Myositis ossificans progressiva**
Fibrodysplasia ossificans progressiva

M61.2 **Paralytic calcification and ossification of muscle**
Myositis ossificans associated with quadriplegia or paraplegia

M61.3 **Calcification and ossification of muscles associated with burns**
Myositis ossificans associated with burns

M61.4 **Other calcification of muscle**
Excludes: calcific tendinitis (M65.2)
  • of shoulder (M75.3)

M61.5 **Other ossification of muscle**

M61.9 **Calcification and ossification of muscle, unspecified**

M62 Other disorders of muscle
[See site code pages 628–629]
Excludes: cramp and spasm (R25.2)
myalgia (M79.1)
myopathy:
  • alcoholic (G72.1)
  • drug-induced (G72.0)
stiff-man syndrome (G25.8)

M62.0 **Diastasis of muscle**

M62.1 **Other rupture of muscle (nontraumatic)**
Excludes: rupture of tendon (M66.–)
traumatic rupture of muscle—see injury of muscle by body region

M62.2 **Ischaemic infarction of muscle**
Excludes: compartment syndrome (T79.6)
traumatic ischaemia of muscle (T79.6)
Volkmann's ischaemic contracture (T79.6)

M62.3 **Immobility syndrome (paraplegic)**

M62.4 **Contracture of muscle**
Excludes: contracture of joint (M24.5)

M62.5 **Muscle wasting and atrophy, not elsewhere classified**
Disuse atrophy NEC

M62.6 **Muscle strain**
Excludes: current injury—see injury of muscle by body region

M62.8 **Other specified disorders of muscle**
Muscle (sheath) hernia

M62.9   **Disorder of muscle, unspecified**

M63*   Disorders of muscle in diseases classified elsewhere
Excludes: myopathy in:
- endocrine diseases (G73.5*)
- metabolic diseases (G73.6*)

M63.0*   **Myositis in bacterial diseases classified elsewhere**
Myositis in:
- leprosy [Hansen's disease] (A30.–†)
- syphilis (A51.4†, A52.7†)

M63.1*   **Myositis in protozoal and parasitic infections classified elsewhere**
Myositis in:
- cysticercosis (B69.8†)
- schistosomiasis [bilharziasis] (B65.–†)
- toxoplasmosis (B58.8†)
- trichinellosis (B75†)

M63.2*   **Myositis in other infectious diseases classified elsewhere**
Myositis in mycosis (B35–B49†)

M63.3*   **Myositis in sarcoidosis (D86.8†)**

M63.8*   **Other disorders of muscle in diseases classified elsewhere**

Disorders of synovium and tendon (M65–M68)

M65   Synovitis and tenosynovitis
[See site code pages 628–629]
Excludes: chronic crepitant synovitis of hand and wrist (M70.0)
      current injury—see injury of ligament or tendon by body region
      soft tissue disorders related to use, overuse and pressure (M70.–)

M65.0   **Abscess of tendon sheath**
Use additional code (B95–B96), if desired, to identify bacterial agent.

M65.1   Other infective (teno)synovitis

M65.2   Calcific tendinitis
Excludes: of shoulder (M75.3)
           specified tendinitis (M75–M77)

M65.3   Trigger finger
Nodular tendinous disease

M65.4   Radial styloid tenosynovitis [de Quervain]

M65.8   Other synovitis and tenosynovitis

M65.9   Synovitis and tenosynovitis, unspecified

M66 Spontaneous rupture of synovium and tendon
[See site code pages 628–629]
Includes: rupture that occurs when a normal force is applied
           to tissues that are inferred to have less than
           normal strength
Excludes: rotator cuff syndrome (M75.1)
           rupture where an abnormal force is applied to normal
           tissue—see injury of tendon by body region

M66.0   Rupture of popliteal cyst

M66.1   Rupture of synovium
Rupture of synovial cyst
Excludes: rupture of popliteal cyst (M66.0)

M66.2   Spontaneous rupture of extensor tendons

M66.3   Spontaneous rupture of flexor tendons

M66.4   Spontaneous rupture of other tendons

M66.5   Spontaneous rupture of unspecified tendon
Rupture at musculotendinous junction, nontraumatic

M67 Other disorders of synovium and tendon

Excludes: palmar fascial fibromatosis [Dupuytren] (M72.0)
tendinitis NOS (M77.9)
xanthomatosis localized to tendons (E78.2)

M67.0 **Short Achilles tendon (acquired)**

M67.1 **Other contracture of tendon (sheath)**
Excludes: with contracture of joint (M24.5)

M67.2 **Synovial hypertrophy, not elsewhere classified**
Excludes: villonodular synovitis (pigmented) (M12.2)

M67.3 **Transient synovitis**
Toxic synovitis
Excludes: palindromic rheumatism (M12.3)

M67.4 **Ganglion**
Ganglion of joint or tendon (sheath)
Excludes: cyst of:
- bursa $\left.\right\}$ (M71.2–M71.3)
- synovium
ganglion in yaws (A66.6)

M67.8 **Other specified disorders of synovium and tendon**

M67.9 **Disorder of synovium and tendon, unspecified**

M68* Disorders of synovium and tendon in diseases classified elsewhere

M68.0* **Synovitis and tenosynovitis in bacterial diseases classified elsewhere**
Synovitis or tenosynovitis in:
- gonorrhoea (A54.4†)
- syphilis (A52.7†)
- tuberculosis (A18.0†)

M68.8* **Other disorders of synovium and tendon in diseases classified elsewhere**

Other soft tissue disorders (M70–M79)

M70 Soft tissue disorders related to use, overuse and pressure
[See site code pages 628–629]

Includes: soft tissue disorders of occupational origin

Excludes: bursitis (of):
- NOS (M71.9)
- shoulder (M75.5)

enthesopathies (M76–M77)

M70.0 Chronic crepitant synovitis of hand and wrist

M70.1 Bursitis of hand

M70.2 Olecranon bursitis

M70.3 Other bursitis of elbow

M70.4 Prepatellar bursitis

M70.5 Other bursitis of knee

M70.6 Trochanteric bursitis
Trochanteric tendinitis

M70.7 Other bursitis of hip
Ischial bursitis

M70.8 Other soft tissue disorders related to use, overuse and pressure

M70.9 Unspecified soft tissue disorder related to use, overuse and pressure

M71 Other bursopathies
[See site code pages 628–629]

Excludes: bunion (M20.1)
bursitis related to use, overuse and pressure (M70.–)
enthesopathies (M76–M77)

M71.0 Abscess of bursa

M71.1 Other infective bursitis

M71.2 Synovial cyst of popliteal space [Baker]
Excludes: with rupture (M66.0)

M71.3 **Other bursal cyst**
Synovial cyst NOS
Excludes: synovial cyst with rupture (M66.1)

M71.4 **Calcium deposit in bursa**
Excludes: of shoulder (M75.3)

M71.5 **Other bursitis, not elsewhere classified**
Excludes: bursitis (of):
- NOS (M71.9)
- shoulder (M75.5)
- tibial collateral [Pellegrini–Stieda] (M76.4)

M71.8 **Other specified bursopathies**

M71.9 **Bursopathy, unspecified**
Bursitis NOS

M72 Fibroblastic disorders
[See site code pages 628–629]
Excludes: retroperitoneal fibromatosis (D48.3)

M72.0 **Palmar fascial fibromatosis [Dupuytren]**

M72.1 **Knuckle pads**

M72.2 **Plantar fascial fibromatosis**
Plantar fasciitis

M72.3 **Nodular fasciitis**

M72.4 **Pseudosarcomatous fibromatosis**

M72.5 **Fasciitis, not elsewhere classified**
Excludes: fasciitis:
- diffuse (eosinophilic) (M35.4)
- nodular (M72.3)
- plantar (M72.2)

M72.8 **Other fibroblastic disorders**

M72.9 **Fibroblastic disorder, unspecified**

663

M73* Soft tissue disorders in diseases classified elsewhere
[See site code pages 628–629]

M73.0*   **Gonococcal bursitis (A54.4†)**

M73.1*   **Syphilitic bursitis (A52.7†)**

M73.8*   **Other soft tissue disorders in diseases classified elsewhere**

M75 Shoulder lesions
Excludes: shoulder-hand syndrome (M89.0)

M75.0   **Adhesive capsulitis of shoulder**
Frozen shoulder
Periarthritis of shoulder

M75.1   **Rotator cuff syndrome**
Rotator cuff or supraspinatus tear or rupture (complete)(incomplete), not specified as traumatic
Supraspinatus syndrome

M75.2   **Bicipital tendinitis**

M75.3   **Calcific tendinitis of shoulder**
Calcified bursa of shoulder

M75.4   **Impingement syndrome of shoulder**

M75.5   **Bursitis of shoulder**

M75.8   **Other shoulder lesions**

M75.9   **Shoulder lesion, unspecified**

M76 Enthesopathies of lower limb, excluding foot
[See site code pages 628–629]

Note: The superficially specific terms bursitis, capsulitis and tendinitis tend to be used indiscriminately for various disorders of peripheral ligamentous or muscular attachments; most of these conditions have been brought together as enthesopathies which is the generic term for lesions at these sites.

Excludes: bursitis due to use, overuse and pressure (M70.–)

M76.0   **Gluteal tendinitis**

M76.1   **Psoas tendinitis**

M76.2   **Iliac crest spur**

M76.3   **Iliotibial band syndrome**

M76.4   **Tibial collateral bursitis [Pellegrini–Stieda]**

M76.5   **Patellar tendinitis**

M76.6   **Achilles tendinitis**
Achilles bursitis

M76.7   **Peroneal tendinitis**

M76.8   **Other enthesopathies of lower limb, excluding foot**
Anterior tibial syndrome
Posterior tibial tendinitis

M76.9   **Enthesopathy of lower limb, unspecified**

M77   **Other enthesopathies**
[See site code pages 628–629]
Excludes: bursitis:
• NOS (M71.9)
• due to use, overuse and pressure (M70.–)
osteophyte (M25.7)
spinal enthesopathy (M46.0)

M77.0   **Medial epicondylitis**

M77.1   **Lateral epicondylitis**
Tennis elbow

M77.2   **Periarthritis of wrist**

M77.3   **Calcaneal spur**

M77.4   **Metatarsalgia**
Excludes: Morton's metatarsalgia (G57.6)

M77.5   **Other enthesopathy of foot**

M77.8   **Other enthesopathies, not elsewhere classified**

M77.9   **Enthesopathy, unspecified**
Bone spur NOS
Capsulitis NOS
Periarthritis NOS
Tendinitis NOS

M79 Other soft tissue disorders, not elsewhere classified
[See site code pages 628–629]

Excludes: soft tissue pain, psychogenic (F45.4)

M79.0 **Rheumatism, unspecified**
Fibromyalgia
Fibrositis
Excludes: palindromic rheumatism (M12.3)

M79.1 **Myalgia**
Excludes: myositis (M60.–)

M79.2 **Neuralgia and neuritis, unspecified**
Excludes: mononeuropathies (G56–G58)
radiculitis:
- NOS
- brachial NOS $\left.\right\}$ (M54.1)
- lumbosacral NOS
sciatica (M54.3–M54.4)

M79.3 **Panniculitis, unspecified**
Excludes: panniculitis:
- lupus (L93.2)
- neck and back (M54.0)
- relapsing [Weber–Christian] (M35.6)

M79.4 **Hypertrophy of (infrapatellar) fat pad**

M79.5 **Residual foreign body in soft tissue**
Excludes: foreign body granuloma of:
- skin and subcutaneous tissue (L92.3)
- soft tissue (M60.2)

M79.6 **Pain in limb**

M79.8 **Other specified soft tissue disorders**

M79.9 **Soft tissue disorder, unspecified**

Osteopathies and chondropathies
(M80–M94)

Disorders of bone density and structure
(M80–M85)

M80 Osteoporosis with pathological fracture
[See site code pages 628–629]

Includes: osteoporotic vertebral collapse and wedging

Excludes: collapsed vertebra NOS (M48.5)
pathological fracture NOS (M84.4)
wedging of vertebra NOS (M48.5)

M80.0 Postmenopausal osteoporosis with pathological fracture

M80.1 Postoophorectomy osteoporosis with pathological fracture

M80.2 Osteoporosis of disuse with pathological fracture

M80.3 Postsurgical malabsorption osteoporosis with pathological fracture

M80.4 Drug-induced osteoporosis with pathological fracture
Use additional external cause code (Chapter XX), if desired, to identify drug.

M80.5 Idiopathic osteoporosis with pathological fracture

M80.8 Other osteoporosis with pathological fracture

M80.9 Unspecified osteoporosis with pathological fracture

M81 Osteoporosis without pathological fracture
[See site code pages 628–629]

Excludes: osteoporosis with pathological fracture (M80.–)

M81.0 Postmenopausal osteoporosis

M81.1 Postoophorectomy osteoporosis

M81.2 Osteoporosis of disuse
Excludes: Sudeck's atrophy (M89.0)

M81.3 Postsurgical malabsorption osteoporosis

M81.4 **Drug-induced osteoporosis**
Use additional external cause code (Chapter XX), if desired, to identify drug.

M81.5 **Idiopathic osteoporosis**

M81.6 **Localized osteoporosis [Lequesne]**
Excludes: Sudeck's atrophy (M89.0)

M81.8 **Other osteoporosis**
Senile osteoporosis

M81.9 **Osteoporosis, unspecified**

M82* **Osteoporosis in diseases classified elsewhere**
[See site code pages 628–629]

M82.0* **Osteoporosis in multiple myelomatosis (C90.0†)**

M82.1* **Osteoporosis in endocrine disorders (E00–E34†)**

M82.8* **Osteoporosis in other diseases classified elsewhere**

M83 **Adult osteomalacia**
[See site code pages 628–629]
Excludes: osteomalacia:
- infantile and juvenile (E55.0)
- vitamin-D-resistant (E83.3)
renal osteodystrophy (N25.0)
rickets (active) (E55.0)
- sequelae (E64.3)
- vitamin-D-resistant (E83.3)

M83.0 **Puerperal osteomalacia**

M83.1 **Senile osteomalacia**

M83.2 **Adult osteomalacia due to malabsorption**
Postsurgical malabsorption osteomalacia in adults

M83.3 **Adult osteomalacia due to malnutrition**

M83.4 **Aluminium bone disease**

M83.5 **Other drug-induced osteomalacia in adults**
Use additional external cause code (Chapter XX), if desired, to identify drug.

M83.8   **Other adult osteomalacia**

M83.9   **Adult osteomalacia, unspecified**

M84   Disorders of continuity of bone
[See site code pages 628–629]

M84.0   **Malunion of fracture**

M84.1   **Nonunion of fracture [pseudarthrosis]**
Excludes: pseudarthrosis after fusion or arthrodesis (M96.0)

M84.2   **Delayed union of fracture**

M84.3   **Stress fracture, not elsewhere classified**
Stress fracture NOS
Excludes: stress fracture of vertebra (M48.4)

M84.4   **Pathological fracture, not elsewhere classified**
Pathological fracture NOS
Excludes: collapsed vertebra NEC (M48.5)
          pathological fracture in osteoporosis (M80.–)

M84.8   **Other disorders of continuity of bone**

M84.9   **Disorder of continuity of bone, unspecified**

M85   Other disorders of bone density and structure
[See site code pages 628–629]
Excludes: osteogenesis imperfecta (Q78.0)
          osteopetrosis (Q78.2)
          osteopoikilosis (Q78.8)
          polyostotic fibrous dysplasia (Q78.1)

M85.0   **Fibrous dysplasia (monostotic)**
Excludes: fibrous dysplasia of jaw (K10.8)

M85.1   **Skeletal fluorosis**

M85.2   **Hyperostosis of skull**

M85.3   **Osteitis condensans**

M85.4   **Solitary bone cyst**
Excludes: solitary cyst of jaw (K09.1–K09.2)

M85.5   **Aneurysmal bone cyst**
Excludes: aneurysmal cyst of jaw (K09.2)

M85.6   **Other cyst of bone**
Excludes: cyst of jaw NEC (K09.1–K09.2)
                   osteitis fibrosa cystica generalisata [von
                       Recklinghausen's disease of bone] (E21.0)

M85.8   **Other specified disorders of bone density and structure**
Hyperostosis of bones, except skull
Excludes: diffuse idiopathic skeletal hyperostosis [DISH]
                 (M48.1)

M85.9   **Disorder of bone density and structure, unspecified**

Other osteopathies
(M86–M90)

Excludes: postprocedural osteopathies (M96.–)

M86   Osteomyelitis
[See site code pages 628–629]

Use additional code (B95–B97), if desired, to identify infectious
agent.
Excludes: ostemyelitis (of):
                 • due to salmonella (A01–A02)
                 • jaw (K10.2)
                 • vertebra (M46.2)

M86.0   **Acute haematogenous osteomyelitis**

M86.1   **Other acute osteomyelitis**

M86.2   **Subacute osteomyelitis**

M86.3   **Chronic multifocal osteomyelitis**

M86.4   **Chronic osteomyelitis with draining sinus**

M86.5   **Other chronic haematogenous osteomyelitis**

M86.6   **Other chronic osteomyelitis**

M86.8   **Other osteomyelitis**
Brodie's abscess

M86.9   **Osteomyelitis, unspecified**
Infection of bone NOS
Periostitis without mention of osteomyelitis

M87   Osteonecrosis
[See site code pages 628–629]

Includes: avascular necrosis of bone
Excludes: osteochondropathies (M91–M93)

M87.0   **Idiopathic aseptic necrosis of bone**

M87.1   **Osteonecrosis due to drugs**
Use additional external cause code (Chapter XX), if desired, to identify drug.

M87.2   **Osteonecrosis due to previous trauma**

M87.3   **Other secondary osteonecrosis**

M87.8   **Other osteonecrosis**

M87.9   **Osteonecrosis, unspecified**

M88   Paget's disease of bone [osteitis deformans]
[See site code pages 628–629]

M88.0   **Paget's disease of skull**

M88.8   **Paget's disease of other bones**

M88.9   **Paget's disease of bone, unspecified**

M89   Other disorders of bone
[See site code pages 628–629]

M89.0   **Algoneurodystrophy**
Shoulder–hand syndrome
Sudeck's atrophy
Sympathetic reflex dystrophy

M89.1   **Epiphyseal arrest**

M89.2   **Other disorders of bone development and growth**

M89.3   **Hypertrophy of bone**

M89.4   **Other hypertrophic osteoarthropathy**
Marie–Bamberger disease
Pachydermoperiostosis

M89.5   **Osteolysis**

M89.6   **Osteopathy after poliomyelitis**
Use additional code (B91), if desired, to identify previous poliomyelitis.

M89.8   **Other specified disorders of bone**
Infantile cortical hyperostoses
Post-traumatic subperiosteal ossification

M89.9   **Disorder of bone, unspecified**

M90*   Osteopathies in diseases classified elsewhere
[See site code pages 628–629]

M90.0*   **Tuberculosis of bone (A18.0†)**
Excludes: tuberculosis of spine (M49.0*)

M90.1*   **Periostitis in other infectious diseases classified elsewhere**
Secondary syphilitic periostitis (A51.4†)

M90.2*   **Osteopathy in other infectious diseases classified elsewhere**
Osteomyelitis:
- echinococcal (B67.2†)
- gonococcal (A54.4†)
- salmonella (A02.2†)

Syphilitic osteopathy or osteochondropathy (A50.5†, A52.7†)

M90.3*   **Osteonecrosis in caisson disease (T70.3†)**

M90.4*   **Osteonecrosis due to haemoglobinopathy (D50–D64†)**

M90.5*   **Osteonecrosis in other diseases classified elsewhere**

M90.6*   **Osteitis deformans in neoplastic disease (C00–D48†)**
Osteitis deformans in malignant neoplasm of bone (C40–C41†)

M90.7*   **Fracture of bone in neoplastic disease (C00–D48†)**
Excludes: collapse of vertebra in neoplastic disease (M49.5*)

M90.8*   **Osteopathy in other diseases classified elsewhere**
Osteopathy in renal osteodystrophy (N25.0†)

Chondropathies
(M91–M94)

Excludes: postprocedural chondropathies (M96.–)

M91 Juvenile osteochondrosis of hip and pelvis
[See site code pages 628–629]

Excludes: slipped upper femoral epiphysis (nontraumatic) (M93.0)

M91.0 Juvenile osteochondrosis of pelvis
Osteochondrosis (juvenile) of:
- acetabulum
- iliac crest [Buchanan]
- ischiopubic synchondrosis [van Neck]
- symphisis pubis [Pierson]

M91.1 Juvenile osteochondrosis of head of femur [Legg–Calvé–Perthes]

M91.2 Coxa plana
Hip deformity due to previous juvenile osteochondrosis

M91.3 Pseudocoxalgia

M91.8 Other juvenile osteochondrosis of hip and pelvis
Juvenile osteochondrosis after reduction of congenital dislocation of hip

M91.9 Juvenile osteochondrosis of hip and pelvis, unspecified

M92 Other juvenile osteochondrosis

M92.0 Juvenile osteochondrosis of humerus
Osteochondrosis (juvenile) of:
- capitulum of humerus [Panner]
- head of humerus [Haas]

M92.1 Juvenile osteochondrosis of radius and ulna
Osteochondrosis (juvenile) of:
- lower ulna [Burns]
- radial head [Brailsford]

M92.2   Juvenile osteochondrosis of hand
Osteochondrosis (juvenile) of:
- carpal lunate [Kienböck]
- metacarpal heads [Mauclaire]

M92.3   Other juvenile osteochondrosis of upper limb

M92.4   Juvenile osteochondrosis of patella
Osteochondrosis (juvenile) of:
- primary patellar centre [Köhler]
- secondary patellar centre [Sinding Larsen]

M92.5   Juvenile osteochondrosis of tibia and fibula
Osteochondrosis (juvenile) of:
- proximal tibia [Blount]
- tibial tubercle [Osgood–Schlatter]
Tibia vara

M92.6   Juvenile osteochondrosis of tarsus
Osteochondrosis (juvenile) of:
- calcaneum [Sever]
- os tibiale externum [Haglund]
- talus [Diaz]
- tarsal navicular [Köhler]

M92.7   Juvenile osteochondrosis of metatarsus
Osteochondrosis (juvenile) of:
- fifth metatarsus [Iselin]
- second metatarsus [Freiberg]

M92.8   Other specified juvenile osteochondrosis
Calcaneal apophysitis

M92.9   Juvenile osteochondrosis, unspecified

Apophysitis
Epiphysitis   } specified as juvenile, of unspecified site
Osteochondritis
Osteochondrosis

M93   Other osteochondropathies
Excludes: osteochondrosis of spine (M42.–)

M93.0   Slipped upper femoral epiphysis (nontraumatic)

M93.1   Kienböck's disease of adults
Adult osteochondrosis of carpal lunate

M93.2   **Osteochondritis dissecans**

M93.8   **Other specified osteochondropathies**

M93.9   **Osteochondropathy, unspecified**
Apophysitis ⎫
Epiphysitis ⎪ not specified as adult or juvenile, of
Osteochondritis ⎬ unspecified site
Osteochondrosis ⎭

M94   Other disorders of cartilage
[See site code pages 628–629]

M94.0   **Chondrocostal junction syndrome [Tietze]**

M94.1   **Relapsing polychondritis**

M94.2   **Chondromalacia**
Excludes: chondromalacia patellae (M22.4)

M94.3   **Chondrolysis**

M94.8   **Other specified disorders of cartilage**

M94.9   **Disorder of cartilage, unspecified**

Other disorders of the musculoskeletal system and connective tissue
(M95–M99)

M95   Other acquired deformities of musculoskeletal system and connective tissue
Excludes: acquired:
• absence of limbs and organs (Z89–Z90)
• deformities of limbs (M20–M21)
congenital malformations and deformations of the
    musculoskeletal system (Q65–Q79)
deforming dorsopathies (M40–M43)
dentofacial anomalies [including malocclusion]
    (K07.–)
postprocedural musculoskeletal disorders (M96.–)

M95.0 **Acquired deformity of nose**
Excludes: deviated nasal septum (J34.2)

M95.1 **Cauliflower ear**
Excludes: other acquired deformities of ear (H61.1)

M95.2 **Other acquired deformity of head**

M95.3 **Acquired deformity of neck**

M95.4 **Acquired deformity of chest and rib**

M95.5 **Acquired deformity of pelvis**
Excludes: maternal care for known or suspected disproportion (O33.–)

M95.8 **Other specified acquired deformities of musculoskeletal system**

M95.9 **Acquired deformity of musculoskeletal system, unspecified**

M96 Postprocedural musculoskeletal disorders, not elsewhere classified
Excludes: arthropathy following intestinal bypass (M02.0)
disorders associated with osteoporosis (M80–M81)
presence of functional implants and other devices (Z95–Z97)

M96.0 **Pseudarthrosis after fusion or arthrodesis**

M96.1 **Postlaminectomy syndrome, not elsewhere classified**

M96.2 **Postradiation kyphosis**

M96.3 **Postlaminectomy kyphosis**

M96.4 **Postsurgical lordosis**

M96.5 **Postradiation scoliosis**

M96.6 **Fracture of bone following insertion of orthopaedic implant, joint prosthesis, or bone plate**
Excludes: complication of internal orthopaedic devices, implants or grafts (T84.–)

M96.8 **Other postprocedural musculoskeletal disorders**
Instability of joint secondary to removal of joint prosthesis

M96.9 **Postprocedural musculoskeletal disorder, unspecified**

M99 Biomechanical lesions, not elsewhere classified

Note: This category should not be used if the condition can be classified elsewhere.

The following supplementary subclassification to indicate the site of lesions is provided for optional use with appropriate subcategories in M99.–; see also note on page 628.

0	Head region	occipitocervical
1	Cervical region	cervicothoracic
2	Thoracic region	thoracolumbar
3	Lumbar region	lumbosacral
4	Sacral region	sacrococcygeal, sacroiliac
5	Pelvic region	hip, pubic
6	Lower extremity	
7	Upper extremity	acromioclavicular, sternoclavicular
8	Rib cage	costochondral, costovertebral, sternochondral
9	Abdomen and other	

M99.0	Segmental and somatic dysfunction
M99.1	Subluxation complex (vertebral)
M99.2	Subluxation stenosis of neural canal
M99.3	Osseous stenosis of neural canal
M99.4	Connective tissue stenosis of neural canal
M99.5	Intervertebral disc stenosis of neural canal
M99.6	Osseous and subluxation stenosis of intervertebral foramina
M99.7	Connective tissue and disc stenosis of intervertebral foramina
M99.8	Other biomechanical lesions
M99.9	Biomechanical lesion, unspecified

CHAPTER XIV

Diseases of the genitourinary system (N00–N99)

Excludes: certain conditions originating in the perinatal period (P00–P96)
certain infectious and parasitic diseases (A00–B99)
complications of pregnancy, childbirth and the puerperium (O00–O99)
congenital malformations, deformations and chromosomal abnormalities (Q00–Q99)
endocrine, nutritional and metabolic diseases (E00–E90)
injury, poisoning and certain other consequences of external causes (S00–T98)
neoplasms (C00–D48)
symptoms, signs and abnormal clinical and laboratory findings, not elsewhere classified (R00–R99)

This chapter contains the following blocks:

N00–N08 Glomerular diseases
N10–N16 Renal tubulo-interstitial diseases
N17–N19 Renal failure
N20–N23 Urolithiasis
N25–N29 Other disorders of kidney and ureter
N30–N39 Other diseases of the urinary system
N40–N51 Diseases of male genital organs
N60–N64 Disorders of breast
N70–N77 Inflammatory diseases of female pelvic organs
N80–N98 Noninflammatory disorders of female genital tract
N99   Other disorders of the genitourinary system

Asterisk categories for this chapter are provided as follows:

N08*   Glomerular disorders in diseases classified elsewhere
N16*   Renal tubulo-interstitial disorders in diseases classified elsewhere
N22*   Calculus of urinary tract in diseases classified elsewhere
N29*   Other disorders of kidney and ureter in diseases classified elsewhere
N33*   Bladder disorders in diseases classified elsewhere
N37*   Urethral disorders in diseases classified elsewhere
N51*   Disorders of male genital organs in diseases classified elsewhere

N74*   Female pelvic inflammatory disorders in diseases classified elsewhere

N77*   Vulvovaginal ulceration and inflammation in diseases classified elsewhere

Glomerular diseases
(N00–N08)

Use additional code, if desired, to identify external cause (Chapter XX) or presence of renal failure (N17–N19).

Excludes: hypertensive renal disease (I12.–)

The following fourth-character subdivisions classify morphological changes and are for use with categories N00–N07. Subdivisions .0–.8 should not normally be used unless these have been specifically identified (e.g. by renal biopsy or autopsy). The three-character categories relate to clinical syndromes.

.0 Minor glomerular abnormality
Minimal change lesion

.1 Focal and segmental glomerular lesions
Focal and segmental:
• hyalinosis
• sclerosis
Focal glomerulonephritis

.2 Diffuse membranous glomerulonephritis

.3 Diffuse mesangial proliferative glomerulonephritis

.4 Diffuse endocapillary proliferative glomerulonephritis

.5 Diffuse mesangiocapillary glomerulonephritis
Membranoproliferative glomerulonephritis, types 1 and 3, or NOS

.6 Dense deposit disease
Membranoproliferative glomerulonephritis, type 2

.7 Diffuse crescentic glomerulonephritis
Extracapillary glomerulonephritis

.8 Other
Proliferative glomerulonephritis NOS

.9 Unspecified

N00 Acute nephritic syndrome
[See page 680 for subdivisions]

Includes: acute:
- glomerular disease
- glomerulonephritis
- nephritis
- renal disease NOS

Excludes: acute tubulo-interstitial nephritis (N10)
nephritic syndrome NOS (N05.–)

N01 Rapidly progressive nephritic syndrome
[See page 680 for subdivisions]

Includes: rapidly progressive:
- glomerular disease
- glomerulonephritis
- nephritis

Excludes: nephritic syndrome NOS (N05.–)

N02 Recurrent and persistent haematuria
[See page 680 for subdivisions]

Includes: haematuria:
- benign (familial)(of childhood)
- with morphological lesion specified in .0–.8 on page 680

Excludes: haematuria NOS (R31)

N03 Chronic nephritic syndrome
[See page 680 for subdivisions]

Includes: chronic:
- glomerular disease
- glomerulonephritis
- nephritis
- renal disease NOS

Excludes: chronic tubulo-interstitial nephritis (N11.–)
diffuse sclerosing glomerulonephritis (N18.–)
nephritic syndrome NOS (N05.–)

N04 Nephrotic syndrome
[See page 680 for subdivisions]

Includes: congenital nephrotic syndrome
lipoid nephrosis

N05 Unspecified nephritic syndrome
[See page 680 for subdivisions]

Includes: glomerular disease
glomerulonephritis } NOS
nephritis
nephropathy NOS and renal disease NOS with
morphological lesion specified in .0–.8 on page 680

Excludes: nephropathy NOS with no stated cause (N28.9)
renal disease NOS with no stated cause (N28.9)
tubulo-interstitial nephritis NOS (N12)

N06 Isolated proteinuria with specified morphological lesion
[See page 680 for subdivisions]

Includes: proteinuria (isolated)(orthostatic)(persistent) with
morphological lesion specified in .0–.8 on page
680

Excludes: proteinuria:
• NOS (R80)
• Bence Jones (R80)
• gestational (O12.1)
• isolated NOS (R80)
• orthostatic NOS (N39.2)
• persistent NOS (N39.1)

N07 Hereditary nephropathy, not elsewhere classified
[See page 680 for subdivisions]

Excludes: Alport's syndrome (Q87.8)
hereditary amyloid nephropathy (E85.0)
nail patella syndrome (Q87.2)
non-neuropathic heredofamilial amyloidosis (E85.0)

N08* Glomerular disorders in diseases classified elsewhere

Includes: nephropathy in diseases classified elsewhere
Excludes: renal tubulo-interstitial disorders in diseases classified
elsewhere (N16.–*)

N08.0* **Glomerular disorders in infectious and parasitic diseases classified elsewhere**
Glomerular disorders in:
- *Plasmodium malariae* malaria (B52.0†)
- mumps (B26.8†)
- schistosomiasis [bilharziasis] (B65.–†)
- septicaemia (A40–A41†)
- strongyloidiasis (B78.–†)
- syphilis (A52.7†)

N08.1* **Glomerular disorders in neoplastic diseases**
Glomerular disorders in:
- multiple myeloma (C90.0†)
- Waldenström's macroglobulinaemia (C88.0†)

N08.2* **Glomerular disorders in blood diseases and disorders involving the immune mechanism**
Glomerular disorders in:
- cryoglobulinaemia (D89.1†)
- disseminated intravascular coagulation [defibrination syndrome] (D65†)
- haemolytic-uraemic syndrome (D59.3†)
- Henoch(-Schönlein) purpura (D69.0†)
- sickle-cell disorders (D57.–†)

N08.3* **Glomerular disorders in diabetes mellitus (E10–E14† with common fourth character .2)**

N08.4* **Glomerular disorders in other endocrine, nutritional and metabolic diseases**
Glomerular disorders in:
- amyloidosis (E85.–†)
- Fabry(–Anderson) disease (E75.2†)
- lecithin cholesterol acyltransferase deficiency (E78.6†)

N08.5*   **Glomerular disorders in systemic connective tissue disorders**

Glomerular disorders in:
- Goodpasture's syndrome (M31.0†)
- polyarteritis nodosa (M30.0†)
- systemic lupus erythematosus (M32.1†)
- thrombotic thrombocytopenic purpura (M31.1†)
- Wegener's granulomatosis (M31.3†)

N08.8*   **Glomerular disorders in other diseases classified elsewhere**

Glomerular disorders in subacute bacterial endocarditis (I33.0†)

Renal tubulo-interstitial diseases (N10–N16)

Includes: pyelonephritis
Excludes: pyeloureteritis cystica (N28.8)

N10   Acute tubulo-interstitial nephritis

Acute:
- infectious interstitial nephritis
- pyelitis
- pyelonephritis

Use additional code (B95–B97), if desired, to identify infectious agent.

N11   Chronic tubulo-interstitial nephritis

Includes: chronic:
- infectious interstitial nephritis
- pyelitis
- pyelonephritis

Use additional code (B95–B97), if desired, to identify infectious agent.

N11.0   **Nonobstructive reflux-associated chronic pyelonephritis**

Pyelonephritis (chronic) associated with (vesicoureteral) reflux

Excludes: vesicoureteral reflux NOS (N13.7)

N11.1 **Chronic obstructive pyelonephritis**
Pyelonephritis (chronic) associated with:
- anomaly
- kinking
- obstruction
- stricture

} of {
pelviureteric junction
pyeloureteric junction
ureter

Excludes: calculous pyelonephritis (N20.9)
obstructive uropathy (N13.–)

N11.8 **Other chronic tubulo-interstitial nephritis**
Nonobstructive chronic pyelonephritis NOS

N11.9 **Chronic tubulo-interstitial nephritis, unspecified**
Chronic:
- interstitial nephritis NOS
- pyelitis NOS
- pyelonephritis NOS

N12 Tubulo-interstitial nephritis, not specified as acute or chronic
Interstitial nephritis NOS
Pyelitis NOS
Pyelonephritis NOS
Excludes: calculous pyelonephritis (N20.9)

N13 Obstructive and reflux uropathy
Excludes: calculus of kidney and ureter without hydronephrosis
(N20.–)
congenital obstructive defects of renal pelvis and
ureter (Q62.0–Q62.3)
obstructive pyelonephritis (N11.1)

N13.0 **Hydronephrosis with ureteropelvic junction obstruction**
Excludes: with infection (N13.6)

N13.1 **Hydronephrosis with ureteral stricture, not elsewhere classified**
Excludes: with infection (N13.6)

N13.2 **Hydronephrosis with renal and ureteral calculous obstruction**
Excludes: with infection (N13.6)

N13.3 **Other and unspecified hydronephrosis**
Excludes: with infection (N13.6)

N13.4 **Hydroureter**
Excludes: with infection (N13.6)

N13.5 **Kinking and stricture of ureter without hydronephrosis**
Excludes: with infection (N13.6)

N13.6 **Pyonephrosis**
Conditions in N13.0–N13.5 with infection
Obstructive uropathy with infection

Use additional code (B95–B97), if desired, to identify infectious agent.

N13.7 **Vesicoureteral-reflux-associated uropathy**
Vesicoureteral reflux:
• NOS
• with scarring
Excludes: reflux-associated pyelonephritis (N11.0)

N13.8 **Other obstructive and reflux uropathy**

N13.9 **Obstructive and reflux uropathy, unspecified**
Urinary tract obstruction NOS

N14 Drug- and heavy-metal-induced tubulo-interstitial and tubular conditions
Use additional external cause code (Chapter XX), if desired, to identify toxic agent.

N14.0 **Analgesic nephropathy**

N14.1 **Nephropathy induced by other drugs, medicaments and biological substances**

N14.2 **Nephropathy induced by unspecified drug, medicament or biological substance**

N14.3 **Nephropathy induced by heavy metals**

N14.4 **Toxic nephropathy, not elsewhere classified**

N15 Other renal tubulo-interstitial diseases

N15.0 **Balkan nephropathy**
Balkan endemic nephropathy

N15.1   **Renal and perinephric abscess**

N15.8   **Other specified renal tubulo-interstitial diseases**

N15.9   **Renal tubulo-interstitial disease, unspecified**
Infection of kidney NOS
Excludes: urinary tract infection NOS (N39.0)

N16* Renal tubulo-interstitial disorders in diseases classified elsewhere

N16.0*   **Renal tubulo-interstitial disorders in infectious and parasitic diseases classified elsewhere**
Renal tubulo-interstitial disorders (due to)(in):
- brucellosis (A23.–†)
- diphtheria (A36.8†)
- salmonella infection (A02.2†)
- septicaemia (A40–A41†)
- toxoplasmosis (B58.8†)

N16.1*   **Renal tubulo-interstitial disorders in neoplastic diseases**
Renal tubulo-interstitial disorders in:
- leukaemia (C91–C95†)
- lymphoma (C81–C85†, C96.–†)
- multiple myeloma (C90.0†)

N16.2*   **Renal tubulo-interstitial disorders in blood diseases and disorders involving the immune mechanism**
Renal tubulo-interstitial disorders in:
- mixed cryoglobulinaemia (D89.1†)
- sarcoidosis (D86.–†)

N16.3*   **Renal tubulo-interstitial disorders in metabolic diseases**
Renal tubulo-interstitial disorders in:
- cystinosis (E72.0†)
- glycogen storage disease (E74.0†)
- Wilson's disease (E83.0†)

N16.4*   **Renal tubulo-interstitial disorders in systemic connective tissue disorders**
Renal tubulo-interstitial disorders in:
- sicca syndrome [Sjögren] (M35.0†)
- systemic lupus erythematosus (M32.1†)

N16.5*   **Renal tubulo-interstitial disorders in transplant rejection (T86.–†)**

N16.8* **Renal tubulo-interstitial disorders in other diseases classified elsewhere**

Renal failure
(N17–N19)

Use additional external cause code (Chapter XX), if desired, to identify external agent.

Excludes: congenital renal failure (P96.0)
   drug- and heavy-metal-induced tubulo-interstitial and tubular conditions (N14.–)
   extrarenal uraemia (R39.2)
   haemolytic-uraemic syndrome (D59.3)
   hepatorenal syndrome (K76.7)
   • postpartum (O90.4)
   prerenal uraemia (R39.2)
   renal failure:
   • complicating abortion or ectopic or molar pregnancy (O00–O07, O08.4)
   • following labour and delivery (O90.4)
   • postprocedural (N99.0)

N17   Acute renal failure

N17.0   **Acute renal failure with tubular necrosis**
Tubular necrosis:
• NOS
• acute
• renal

N17.1   **Acute renal failure with acute cortical necrosis**
Cortical necrosis:
• NOS
• acute
• renal

N17.2   **Acute renal failure with medullary necrosis**
Medullary [papillary] necrosis:
• NOS
• acute
• renal

N17.8   **Other acute renal failure**

N17.9   **Acute renal failure, unspecified**

N18   Chronic renal failure

Includes: chronic uraemia
diffuse sclerosing glomerulonephritis
Excludes: chronic renal failure with hypertension (I12.0)

N18.0   **End-stage renal disease**

N18.8   **Other chronic renal failure**
Uraemic:
- neuropathy† (G63.8*)
- pericarditis† (I32.8*)

N18.9   **Chronic renal failure, unspecified**

N19   Unspecified renal failure

Uraemia NOS
Excludes: renal failure with hypertension (I12.0)
uraemia of newborn (P96.0)

Urolithiasis
(N20–N23)

N20   Calculus of kidney and ureter

Excludes: with hydronephrosis (N13.2)

N20.0   **Calculus of kidney**
Nephrolithiasis NOS
Renal calculus or stone
Staghorn calculus
Stone in kidney

N20.1   **Calculus of ureter**
Ureteric stone

N20.2   **Calculus of kidney with calculus of ureter**

N20.9   **Urinary calculus, unspecified**
Calculous pyelonephritis

N21 Calculus of lower urinary tract
Includes: with cystitis and urethritis

N21.0 Calculus in bladder
Calculus in diverticulum of bladder
Urinary bladder stone
Excludes: staghorn calculus (N20.0)

N21.1 Calculus in urethra

N21.8 Other lower urinary tract calculus

N21.9 Calculus of lower urinary tract, unspecified

N22* Calculus of urinary tract in diseases classified elsewhere

N22.0* Urinary calculus in schistosomiasis [bilharziasis] (B65.–†)

N22.8* Calculus of urinary tract in other diseases classified elsewhere

N23 Unspecified renal colic

Other disorders of kidney and ureter (N25–N29)

Excludes: with urolithiasis (N20–N23)

N25 Disorders resulting from impaired renal tubular function
Excludes: metabolic disorders classifiable to E70–E90

N25.0 Renal osteodystrophy
Azotaemic osteodystrophy
Phosphate-losing tubular disorders
Renal:
• rickets
• short stature

N25.1   **Nephrogenic diabetes insipidus**

N25.8   **Other disorders resulting from impaired renal tubular function**
Lightwood–Albright syndrome
Renal tubular acidosis NOS
Secondary hyperparathyroidism of renal origin

N25.9   **Disorder resulting from impaired renal tubular function, unspecified**

N26   Unspecified contracted kidney
Atrophy of kidney (terminal)
Renal sclerosis NOS

Excludes: contracted kidney with hypertension (I12.–)
diffuse sclerosing glomerulonephritis (N18.–)
hypertensive nephrosclerosis (arteriolar)(arteriosclerotic) (I12.–)
small kidney of unknown cause (N27.–)

N27   Small kidney of unknown cause

N27.0   **Small kidney, unilateral**

N27.1   **Small kidney, bilateral**

N27.9   **Small kidney, unspecified**

N28   Other disorders of kidney and ureter, not elsewhere classified
Excludes: hydroureter (N13.4)
renal disease:
• acute NOS (N00.9)
• chronic NOS (N03.9)
ureteric kinking and stricture:
• with hydronephrosis (N13.1)
• without hydronephrosis (N13.5)

N28.0 **Ischaemia and infarction of kidney**
Renal artery:
- embolism
- obstruction
- occlusion
- thrombosis
Renal infarct
Excludes: Goldblatt's kidney (I70.1)
renal artery (extrarenal part):
- atherosclerosis (I70.1)
- congenital stenosis (Q27.1)

N28.1 **Cyst of kidney, acquired**
Cyst (multiple)(solitary) of kidney, acquired
Excludes: cystic kidney disease (congenital) (Q61.–)

N28.8 **Other specified disorders of kidney and ureter**
Hypertrophy of kidney
Megaloureter
Nephroptosis
Pyelitis
Pyeloureteritis ⎫
Ureteritis ⎬ cystica
Ureterocele ⎭

N28.9 **Disorder of kidney and ureter, unspecified**
Nephropathy NOS
Renal disease NOS
Excludes: nephropathy NOS and renal disease NOS with
morphological lesion specified in .0–.8 on
page 680 (N05.–)

N29* Other disorders of kidney and ureter in diseases classified elsewhere

N29.0* **Late syphilis of kidney (A52.7†)**

N29.1* **Other disorders of kidney and ureter in infectious and parasitic diseases classified elsewhere**
Disorders of kidney and ureter in:
- schistosomiasis [bilharziasis] (B65.–†)
- tuberculosis (A18.1†)

N29.8* **Other disorders of kidney and ureter in other diseases classified elsewhere**

Other diseases of the urinary system (N30–N39)

Excludes: urinary infection (complicating):
- abortion or ectopic or molar pregnancy (O00–O07, O08.8)
- pregnancy, childbirth and the puerperium (O23.–, O75.3, O86.2)
- with urolithiasis (N20–N23)

N30 Cystitis

Use additional code, if desired, to identify infectious agent (B95–B97) or responsible external agent (Chapter XX).

Excludes: prostatocystitis (N41.3)

N30.0 Acute cystitis

Excludes: irradiation cystitis (N30.4)
trigonitis (N30.3)

N30.1 Interstitial cystitis (chronic)

N30.2 Other chronic cystitis

N30.3 Trigonitis

Urethrotrigonitis

N30.4 Irradiation cystitis

N30.8 Other cystitis

Abscess of bladder

N30.9 Cystitis, unspecified

N31 Neuromuscular dysfunction of bladder, not elsewhere classified

Excludes: cord bladder NOS (G95.8)
due to spinal cord lesion (G95.8)
neurogenic bladder due to cauda equina syndrome (G83.4)
urinary incontinence:
- NOS (R32)
- specified (N39.3–N39.4)

N31.0 Uninhibited neuropathic bladder, not elsewhere classified

N31.1 **Reflex neuropathic bladder, not elsewhere classified**

N31.2 **Flaccid neuropathic bladder, not elsewhere classified**
Neuropathic bladder:
- atonic (motor)(sensory)
- autonomous
- nonreflex

N31.8 **Other neuromuscular dysfunction of bladder**

N31.9 **Neuromuscular dysfunction of bladder, unspecified**
Neurogenic bladder dysfunction NOS

N32 Other disorders of bladder

Excludes: calculus in bladder (N21.0)
cystocele (N81.1)
hernia or prolapse of bladder, female (N81.1)

N32.0 **Bladder-neck obstruction**
Bladder-neck stenosis (acquired)

N32.1 **Vesicointestinal fistula**
Vesicorectal fistula

N32.2 **Vesical fistula, not elsewhere classified**
Excludes: fistula between bladder and female genital tract
(N82.0–N82.1)

N32.3 **Diverticulum of bladder**
Diverticulitis of bladder
Excludes: calculus in diverticulum of bladder (N21.0)

N32.4 **Rupture of bladder, nontraumatic**

N32.8 **Other specified disorders of bladder**
Bladder:
- calcified
- contracted

N32.9 **Bladder disorder, unspecified**

N33* Bladder disorders in diseases classified elsewhere

N33.0* **Tuberculous cystitis (A18.1†)**

N33.8* **Bladder disorders in other diseases classified elsewhere**
Bladder disorder in schistosomiasis [bilharziasis] (B65.–†)

N34   Urethritis and urethral syndrome

Use additional code (B95–B97), if desired, to identify infectious agent.

Excludes: Reiter's disease (M02.3)
          urethritis in diseases with a predominantly sexual
            mode of transmission (A50–A64)
          urethrotrigonitis (N30.3)

N34.0   **Urethral abscess**

Abscess (of):
- Cowper's gland
- Littré's gland
- periurethral
- urethral (gland)

Excludes: urethral caruncle (N36.2)

N34.1   **Nonspecific urethritis**

Urethritis:
- nongonococcal
- nonvenereal

N34.2   **Other urethritis**

Meatitis, urethral
Ulcer of urethra (meatus)
Urethritis:
- NOS
- postmenopausal

N34.3   **Urethral syndrome, unspecified**

N35   Urethral stricture

Excludes: postprocedural urethral stricture (N99.1)

N35.0   **Post-traumatic urethral stricture**

Stricture of urethra as a sequela of:
- childbirth
- injury

N35.1   **Postinfective urethral stricture, not elsewhere classified**

N35.8   **Other urethral stricture**

N35.9   **Urethral stricture, unspecified**

Pinhole meatus NOS

N36   Other disorders of urethra

N36.0   **Urethral fistula**
False urethral passage
Fistula:
- urethroperineal
- urethrorectal
- urinary NOS

Excludes: fistula:
- urethroscrotal (N50.8)
- urethrovaginal (N82.1)

N36.1   **Urethral diverticulum**

N36.2   **Urethral caruncle**

N36.3   **Prolapsed urethral mucosa**
Prolapse of urethra
Urethrocele, male

Excludes: urethrocele, female (N81.0)

N36.8   **Other specified disorders of urethra**

N36.9   **Urethral disorder, unspecified**

N37*   Urethral disorders in diseases classified elsewhere

N37.0*   **Urethritis in diseases classified elsewhere**
Candidal urethritis (B37.4†)

N37.8*   **Other urethral disorders in diseases classified elsewhere**

N39   Other disorders of urinary system

Excludes: haematuria:
- NOS (R31)
- recurrent and persistent (N02.–)
- with specified morphological lesion (N02.–)

proteinuria NOS (R80)

N39.0   **Urinary tract infection, site not specified**
Use additional code (B95–B97), if desired, to identify infectious agent.

N39.1   **Persistent proteinuria, unspecified**

Excludes: complicating pregnancy, childbirth and the
puerperium (O11–O15)
with specified morphological lesion (N06.–)

N39.2   **Orthostatic proteinuria, unspecified**

Excludes: with specified morphological lesion (N06.–)

N39.3   **Stress incontinence**

N39.4   **Other specified urinary incontinence**

Overflow ⎫
Reflex   ⎬ incontinence
Urge   ⎭

Excludes: enuresis NOS (R32)
urinary incontinence (of):
• NOS (R32)
• nonorganic origin (F98.0)

N39.8   **Other specified disorders of urinary system**

N39.9   **Disorder of urinary system, unspecified**

Diseases of male genital organs (N40–N51)

N40   **Hyperplasia of prostate**

Adenofibromatous hypertrophy ⎫
Adenoma (benign)   ⎪
Enlargement (benign)   ⎪
Fibroadenoma   ⎬ of prostate
Fibroma   ⎪
Hypertrophy (benign)   ⎪
Myoma   ⎭
Median bar (prostate)
Prostatic obstruction NOS

Excludes: benign neoplasms, except adenoma, fibroma and
myoma of prostate (D29.1)

697

N41   Inflammatory diseases of prostate

Use additional code (B95–B97), if desired, to identify infectious agent.

N41.0	**Acute prostatitis**
N41.1	**Chronic prostatitis**
N41.2	**Abscess of prostate**
N41.3	**Prostatocystitis**
N41.8	**Other inflammatory diseases of prostate**
N41.9	**Inflammatory disease of prostate, unspecified**

Prostatitis NOS

N42   Other disorders of prostate

N42.0	**Calculus of prostate**

Prostatic stone

N42.1	**Congestion and haemorrhage of prostate**
N42.2	**Atrophy of prostate**
N42.8	**Other specified disorders of prostate**
N42.9	**Disorder of prostate, unspecified**

N43   Hydrocele and spermatocele

Includes: hydrocele of spermatic cord, testis or tunica vaginalis
Excludes: congenital hydrocele (P83.5)

N43.0	**Encysted hydrocele**
N43.1	**Infected hydrocele**

Use additional code (B95–B97), if desired, to identify infectious agent.

N43.2	**Other hydrocele**
N43.3	**Hydrocele, unspecified**
N43.4	**Spermatocele**

N44 Torsion of testis

Torsion of:
- epididymis
- spermatic cord
- testicle

N45 Orchitis and epididymitis

Use additional code (B95–B97), if desired, to identify infectious agent.

N45.0 Orchitis, epididymitis and epididymo-orchitis with abscess
Abscess of epididymis or testis

N45.9 Orchitis, epididymitis and epididymo-orchitis without abscess
Epididymitis NOS
Orchitis NOS

N46 Male infertility

Azoospermia NOS
Oligospermia NOS

N47 Redundant prepuce, phimosis and paraphimosis

Adherent prepuce
Tight foreskin

N48 Other disorders of penis

N48.0 Leukoplakia of penis
Kraurosis of penis

Excludes: carcinoma in situ of penis (D07.4)

N48.1 Balanoposthitis
Balanitis

Use additional code (B95–B97), if desired, to identify infectious agent.

N48.2 **Other inflammatory disorders of penis**

Abscess ⎫
Boil ⎪
Carbuncle ⎬ of corpus cavernosum and penis
Cellulitis ⎭
Cavernitis (penis)

Use additional code (B95–B97), if desired, to identify infectious agent.

N48.3 **Priapism**
Painful erection

N48.4 **Impotence of organic origin**
Use additional code, if desired, to identify cause.
Excludes: psychogenic impotence (F52.2)

N48.5 **Ulcer of penis**

N48.6 **Balanitis xerotica obliterans**
Plastic induration of penis

N48.8 **Other specified disorders of penis**
Atrophy ⎫
Hypertrophy ⎬ of corpus cavernosum and penis
Thrombosis ⎭

N48.9 **Disorder of penis, unspecified**

N49 **Inflammatory disorders of male genital organs, not elsewhere classified**
Use additional code (B95–B97), if desired, to identify infectious agent.
Excludes: inflammation of penis (N48.1–N48.2)
orchitis and epididymitis (N45.–)

N49.0 **Inflammatory disorders of seminal vesicle**
Vesiculitis NOS

N49.1 **Inflammatory disorders of spermatic cord, tunica vaginalis and vas deferens**
Vasitis

N49.2 **Inflammatory disorders of scrotum**

N49.8 **Inflammatory disorders of other specified male genital organs**
Inflammation of multiple sites in male genital organs

N49.9   **Inflammatory disorder of unspecified male genital organ**

Abscess   ⎤
Boil   ⎬ of unspecified male genital organ
Carbuncle   ⎪
Cellulitis   ⎦

N50   Other disorders of male genital organs

Excludes: torsion of testis (N44)

N50.0   **Atrophy of testis**

N50.1   **Vascular disorders of male genital organs**

Haematocele NOS   ⎤
Haemorrhage   ⎬ of male genital organs
Thrombosis   ⎦

N50.8   **Other specified disorders of male genital organs**

Atrophy   ⎤
Hypertrophy   ⎬ of scrotum, seminal vesicle, spermatic cord,
Oedema   ⎪   testis [except atrophy], tunica vaginalis and
Ulcer   ⎦   vas deferens
Chylocele, tunica vaginalis (nonfilarial) NOS
Fistula, urethroscrotal
Stricture of:
• spermatic cord
• tunica vaginalis
• vas deferens

N50.9   **Disorder of male genital organs, unspecified**

N51*   Disorders of male genital organs in diseases classified elsewhere

N51.0*   **Disorders of prostate in diseases classified elsewhere**
Prostatitis:
• gonococcal (A54.2†)
• trichomonal (A59.0†)
• tuberculous (A18.1†)

N51.1* **Disorders of testis and epididymis in diseases classified elsewhere**
Chlamydial:
- epididymitis (A56.1†)
- orchitis (A56.1†)
Gonococcal:
- epididymitis (A54.2†)
- orchitis (A54.2†)
Mumps orchitis (B26.0†)
Tuberculosis of:
- epididymis (A18.1†)
- testis (A18.1†)

N51.2* **Balanitis in diseases classified elsewhere**
Balanitis:
- amoebic (A06.8†)
- candidal (B37.4†)

N51.8* **Other disorders of male genital organs in diseases classified elsewhere**
Filarial chylocele, tunica vaginalis (B74.–†)
Herpesviral [herpes simplex] infection of male genital tract (A60.0†)
Tuberculosis of seminal vesicle (A18.1†)

Disorders of breast
(N60–N64)

Excludes: disorders of breast associated with childbirth (O91–O92)

N60 Benign mammary dysplasia
Includes: fibrocystic mastopathy

N60.0 **Solitary cyst of breast**
Cyst of breast

N60.1 **Diffuse cystic mastopathy**
Cystic breast
Excludes: with epithelial proliferation (N60.3)

N60.2 **Fibroadenosis of breast**
Excludes: fibroadenoma of breast (D24)

N60.3 **Fibrosclerosis of breast**
Cystic mastopathy with epithelial proliferation

N60.4 **Mammary duct ectasia**

N60.8 **Other benign mammary dysplasias**

N60.9 **Benign mammary dysplasia, unspecified**

N61 Inflammatory disorders of breast
Abscess (acute)(chronic)(nonpuerperal) of:
- areola
- breast

Carbuncle of breast
Mastitis (acute)(subacute)(nonpuerperal):
- NOS
- infective

Excludes: neonatal infective mastitis (P39.0)

N62 Hypertrophy of breast
Gynaecomastia
Hypertrophy of breast:
- NOS
- massive pubertal

N63 Unspecified lump in breast
Nodule(s) NOS in breast

N64 Other disorders of breast

N64.0 **Fissure and fistula of nipple**

N64.1 **Fat necrosis of breast**
Fat necrosis (segmental) of breast

N64.2 **Atrophy of breast**

N64.3 **Galactorrhoea not associated with childbirth**

N64.4 **Mastodynia**

N64.5 **Other signs and symptoms in breast**
Induration of breast
Nipple discharge
Retraction of nipple

N64.8   **Other specified disorders of breast**
Galactocele
Subinvolution of breast (postlactational)

N64.9   **Disorder of breast, unspecified**

Inflammatory diseases of female pelvic organs (N70–N77)

Excludes: those complicating:
- abortion or ectopic or molar pregnancy (O00–O07, O08.0)
- pregnancy, childbirth and the puerperium (O23.–, O75.3, O85, O86.–)

N70   Salpingitis and oophoritis

Includes: abscess (of):
- fallopian tube
- ovary
- tubo-ovarian

pyosalpinx
salpingo-oophoritis
tubo-ovarian inflammatory disease

Use additional code (B95–B97), if desired, to identify infectious agent.

N70.0   **Acute salpingitis and oophoritis**

N70.1   **Chronic salpingitis and oophoritis**
Hydrosalpinx

N70.9   **Salpingitis and oophoritis, unspecified**

N71 Inflammatory disease of uterus, except cervix

Includes: endo(myo)metritis
metritis
myometritis
pyometra
uterine abscess

Use additional code (B95–B97), if desired, to identify infectious agent.

N71.0 **Acute inflammatory disease of uterus**

N71.1 **Chronic inflammatory disease of uterus**

N71.9 **Inflammatory disease of uterus, unspecified**

N72 Inflammatory disease of cervix uteri

Cervicitis ⎫
Endocervicitis ⎬ with or without erosion or ectropion
Exocervicitis ⎭

Use additional code (B95–B97), if desired, to identify infectious agent.

Excludes: erosion and ectropion of cervix without cervicitis
(N86)

N73 Other female pelvic inflammatory diseases

Use additional code (B95–B97), if desired, to identify infectious agent.

N73.0 **Acute parametritis and pelvic cellulitis**
Abscess of:
• broad ligament ⎫
• parametrium ⎬ specified as acute
Pelvic cellulitis, female ⎭

N73.1 **Chronic parametritis and pelvic cellulitis**
Any condition in N73.0 specified as chronic

N73.2 **Unspecified parametritis and pelvic cellulitis**
Any condition in N73.0 unspecified whether acute or chronic

N73.3 **Female acute pelvic peritonitis**

N73.4 **Female chronic pelvic peritonitis**

N73.5 Female pelvic peritonitis, unspecified

N73.6 Female pelvic peritoneal adhesions
Excludes: postprocedural pelvic peritoneal adhesions (N99.4)

N73.8 Other specified female pelvic inflammatory diseases

N73.9 Female pelvic inflammatory disease, unspecified
Female pelvic infection or inflammation NOS

N74* Female pelvic inflammatory disorders in diseases classified elsewhere

N74.0* Tuberculous infection of cervix uteri (A18.1†)

N74.1* Female tuberculous pelvic inflammatory disease (A18.1†)
Tuberculous endometritis

N74.2* Female syphilitic pelvic inflammatory disease (A51.4†, A52.7†)

N74.3* Female gonococcal pelvic inflammatory disease (A54.2†)

N74.4* Female chlamydial pelvic inflammatory disease (A56.1†)

N74.8* Female pelvic inflammatory disorders in other diseases classified elsewhere

N75 Diseases of Bartholin's gland

N75.0 Cyst of Bartholin's gland

N75.1 Abscess of Bartholin's gland

N75.8 Other diseases of Bartholin's gland
Bartholinitis

N75.9 Disease of Bartholin's gland, unspecified

N76 Other inflammation of vagina and vulva
Use additional code (B95–B97), if desired, to identify infectious agent.
Excludes: senile (atrophic) vaginitis (N95.2)

N76.0   **Acute vaginitis**
Vaginitis NOS
Vulvovaginitis:
- NOS
- acute

N76.1   **Subacute and chronic vaginitis**
Vulvovaginitis:
- chronic
- subacute

N76.2   **Acute vulvitis**
Vulvitis NOS

N76.3   **Subacute and chronic vulvitis**

N76.4   **Abscess of vulva**
Furuncle of vulva

N76.5   **Ulceration of vagina**

N76.6   **Ulceration of vulva**

N76.8   **Other specified inflammation of vagina and vulva**

N77*   Vulvovaginal ulceration and inflammation in diseases classified elsewhere

N77.0*   **Ulceration of vulva in infectious and parasitic diseases classified elsewhere**
Ulceration of vulva in:
- herpesviral [herpes simplex] infection (A60.0†)
- tuberculosis (A18.1†)

N77.1*   **Vaginitis, vulvitis and vulvovaginitis in infectious and parasitic diseases classified elsewhere**
Vaginitis, vulvitis and vulvovaginitis in:
- candidiasis (B37.3†)
- herpesviral [herpes simplex] infection (A60.0†)
- pinworm infection (B80†)

N77.8*   **Vulvovaginal ulceration and inflammation in other diseases classified elsewhere**
Ulceration of vulva in Behçet's disease (M35.2†)

Noninflammatory disorders of female genital tract (N80–N98)

N80 Endometriosis

N80.0 Endometriosis of uterus
Adenomyosis

N80.1 Endometriosis of ovary

N80.2 Endometriosis of fallopian tube

N80.3 Endometriosis of pelvic peritoneum

N80.4 Endometriosis of rectovaginal septum and vagina

N80.5 Endometriosis of intestine

N80.6 Endometriosis in cutaneous scar

N80.8 Other endometriosis

N80.9 Endometriosis, unspecified

N81 Female genital prolapse

Excludes: genital prolapse complicating pregnancy, labour or
delivery (O34.5)
prolapse and hernia of ovary and fallopian tube
(N83.4)
prolapse of vaginal vault after hysterectomy (N99.3)

N81.0 Female urethrocele

Excludes: urethrocele with:
• cystocele (N81.1)
• prolapse of uterus (N81.2–N81.4)

N81.1 Cystocele
Cystocele with urethrocele
Prolapse of (anterior) vaginal wall NOS
Excludes: cystocele with prolapse of uterus (N81.2–N81.4)

N81.2 Incomplete uterovaginal prolapse
Prolapse of cervix NOS
Uterine prolapse:
• first degree
• second degree

N81.3 **Complete uterovaginal prolapse**
Procidentia (uteri) NOS
Third degree uterine prolapse

N81.4 **Uterovaginal prolapse, unspecified**
Prolapse of uterus NOS

N81.5 **Vaginal enterocele**
Excludes: enterocele with prolapse of uterus (N81.2–N81.4)

N81.6 **Rectocele**
Prolapse of posterior vaginal wall
Excludes: rectal prolapse (K62.3)
rectocele with prolapse of uterus (N81.2–N81.4)

N81.8 **Other female genital prolapse**
Deficient perineum
Old laceration of muscles of pelvic floor

N81.9 **Female genital prolapse, unspecified**

N82 Fistulae involving female genital tract
Excludes: vesicointestinal fistulae (N32.1)

N82.0 **Vesicovaginal fistula**

N82.1 **Other female urinary–genital tract fistulae**
Fistula:
• cervicovesical
• ureterovaginal
• urethrovaginal
• uteroureteric
• uterovesical

N82.2 **Fistula of vagina to small intestine**

N82.3 **Fistula of vagina to large intestine**
Rectovaginal fistula

N82.4 **Other female intestinal–genital tract fistulae**
Intestinouterine fistula

N82.5 **Female genital tract–skin fistulae**
Fistula:
• uterus to abdominal wall
• vaginoperineal

N82.8 **Other female genital tract fistulae**

N82.9 **Female genital tract fistula, unspecified**

N83 Noninflammatory disorders of ovary, fallopian tube and broad ligament

Excludes: hydrosalpinx (N70.1)

N83.0 **Follicular cyst of ovary**
Cyst of graafian follicle
Haemorrhagic follicular cyst (of ovary)

N83.1 **Corpus luteum cyst**
Haemorrhagic corpus luteum cyst

N83.2 **Other and unspecified ovarian cysts**
Retention cyst ⎫
Simple cyst ⎬ of ovary
⎭

Excludes: ovarian cyst:
• developmental (Q50.1)
• neoplastic (D27)
polycystic ovarian syndrome (E28.2)

N83.3 **Acquired atrophy of ovary and fallopian tube**

N83.4 **Prolapse and hernia of ovary and fallopian tube**

N83.5 **Torsion of ovary, ovarian pedicle and fallopian tube**
Torsion:
• accessory tube
• hydatid of Morgagni

N83.6 **Haematosalpinx**
Excludes: haematosalpinx with:
• haematocolpos (N89.7)
• haematometra (N85.7)

N83.7 **Haematoma of broad ligament**

N83.8 **Other noninflammatory disorders of ovary, fallopian tube and broad ligament**
Broad ligament laceration syndrome [Allen–Masters]

N83.9 **Noninflammatory disorder of ovary, fallopian tube and broad ligament, unspecified**

N84 Polyp of female genital tract

Excludes: adenomatous polyp (D28.–)
placental polyp (O90.8)

N84.0 Polyp of corpus uteri
Polyp of:
- endometrium
- uterus NOS

Excludes: polypoid endometrial hyperplasia (N85.0)

N84.1 Polyp of cervix uteri
Mucous polyp of cervix

N84.2 Polyp of vagina

N84.3 Polyp of vulva
Polyp of labia

N84.8 Polyp of other parts of female genital tract

N84.9 Polyp of female genital tract, unspecified

N85 Other noninflammatory disorders of uterus, except cervix

Excludes: endometriosis (N80.–)
inflammatory diseases of uterus (N71.–)
noninflammatory disorders of cervix (N86–N88)
polyp of corpus uteri (N84.0)
uterine prolapse (N81.–)

N85.0 Endometrial glandular hyperplasia
Hyperplasia of endometrium:
- NOS
- cystic
- glandular–cystic
- polypoid

N85.1 Endometrial adenomatous hyperplasia
Hyperplasia of endometrium, atypical (adenomatous)

N85.2 Hypertrophy of uterus
Bulky or enlarged uterus
Excludes: puerperal hypertrophy of uterus (O90.8)

N85.3 Subinvolution of uterus
Excludes: puerperal subinvolution of uterus (O90.8)

N85.4 **Malposition of uterus**

Anteversion ⎫

Retroflexion ⎬ of uterus

Retroversion ⎭

Excludes: that complicating pregnancy, labour or delivery
(O34.5, O65.5)

N85.5 **Inversion of uterus**

Excludes: current obstetric trauma (O71.2)
postpartum inversion of uterus (O71.2)

N85.6 **Intrauterine synechiae**

N85.7 **Haematometra**

Haematosalpinx with haematometra

Excludes: haematometra with haematocolpos (N89.7)

N85.8 **Other specified noninflammatory disorders of uterus**

Atrophy of uterus, acquired

Fibrosis of uterus NOS

N85.9 **Noninflammatory disorder of uterus, unspecified**

Disorder of uterus NOS

N86 Erosion and ectropion of cervix uteri

Decubitus (trophic) ulcer ⎫

Eversion ⎬ of cervix

Excludes: with cervicitis (N72)

N87 Dysplasia of cervix uteri

Excludes: carcinoma in situ of cervix (D06.–)

N87.0 **Mild cervical dysplasia**

Cervical intraepithelial neoplasia [CIN], grade I

N87.1 **Moderate cervical dysplasia**

Cervical intraepithelial neoplasia [CIN], grade II

N87.2 **Severe cervical dysplasia, not elsewhere classified**

Severe cervical dysplasia NOS

Excludes: cervical intraepithelial neoplasia [CIN], grade III,
with or without mention of severe dysplasia
(D06.–)

N87.9   **Dysplasia of cervix uteri, unspecified**

N88   Other noninflammatory disorders of cervix uteri

Excludes: inflammatory disease of cervix (N72)
           polyp of cervix (N84.1)

N88.0   **Leukoplakia of cervix uteri**

N88.1   **Old laceration of cervix uteri**

Adhesions of cervix

Excludes: current obstetric trauma (O71.3)

N88.2   **Stricture and stenosis of cervix uteri**

Excludes: complicating labour (O65.5)

N88.3   **Incompetence of cervix uteri**

Investigation and management of (suspected) cervical in-
     competence in a nonpregnant woman

Excludes: affecting fetus or newborn (P01.0)
           complicating pregnancy (O34.3)

N88.4   **Hypertrophic elongation of cervix uteri**

N88.8   **Other specified noninflammatory disorders of cervix uteri**

Excludes: current obstetric trauma (O71.3)

N88.9   **Noninflammatory disorder of cervix uteri, unspecified**

N89   Other noninflammatory disorders of vagina

Excludes: carcinoma in situ of vagina (D07.2)
           inflammation of vagina (N76.–)
           senile (atrophic) vaginitis (N95.2)
           trichomonal leukorrhoea (A59.0)

N89.0   **Mild vaginal dysplasia**

Vaginal intraepithelial neoplasia [VAIN], grade I

N89.1   **Moderate vaginal dysplasia**

Vaginal intraepithelial neoplasia [VAIN], grade II

N89.2   **Severe vaginal dysplasia, not elsewhere classified**

Severe vaginal dysplasia NOS

Excludes: vaginal intraepithelial neoplasia [VAIN], grade III,
           with or without mention of severe dysplasia
           (D07.2)

N89.3**Dysplasia of vagina, unspecified**

N89.4**Leukoplakia of vagina**

N89.5**Stricture and atresia of vagina**
Vaginal:
- adhesions
- stenosis

Excludes: postoperative adhesions of vagina (N99.2)

N89.6**Tight hymenal ring**
Rigid hymen
Tight introitus

Excludes: imperforate hymen (Q52.3)

N89.7**Haematocolpos**
Haematocolpos with haematometra or haematosalpinx

N89.8**Other specified noninflammatory disorders of vagina**
Leukorrhoea NOS
Old vaginal laceration
Pessary ulcer of vagina

Excludes: current obstetric trauma (O70.–, O71.4, O71.7–
O71.8)
old laceration involving muscles of pelvic floor
(N81.8)

N89.9**Noninflammatory disorder of vagina, unspecified**

N90 Other noninflammatory disorders of vulva and perineum

Excludes: carcinoma in situ of vulva (D07.1)
current obstetric trauma (O70.–, O71.7–O71.8)
inflammation of vulva (N76.–)

N90.0**Mild vulvar dysplasia**
Vulvar intraepithelial neoplasia [VIN], grade I

N90.1**Moderate vulvar dysplasia**
Vulvar intraepithelial neoplasia [VIN], grade II

N90.2**Severe vulvar dysplasia, not elsewhere classified**
Severe vulvar dysplasia NOS

Excludes: vulvar intraepithelial neoplasia [VIN], grade III, with
or without mention of severe dysplasia (D07.1)

N90.3**Dysplasia of vulva, unspecified**

N90.4   **Leukoplakia of vulva**
Dystrophy ⎫
Kraurosis ⎬ of vulva

N90.5   **Atrophy of vulva**
Stenosis of vulva

N90.6   **Hypertrophy of vulva**
Hypertrophy of labia

N90.7   **Vulvar cyst**

N90.8   **Other specified noninflammatory disorders of vulva and perineum**
Adhesions of vulva
Hypertrophy of clitoris

N90.9   **Noninflammatory disorder of vulva and perineum, unspecified**

N91   Absent, scanty and rare menstruation

Excludes: ovarian dysfunction (E28.–)

N91.0   **Primary amenorrhoea**
Failure to start menstruation at puberty.

N91.1   **Secondary amenorrhoea**
Absence of menstruation in a woman who had previously menstruated.

N91.2   **Amenorrhoea, unspecified**
Absence of menstruation NOS

N91.3   **Primary oligomenorrhoea**
Menstruation which is scanty or rare from the start.

N91.4   **Secondary oligomenorrhoea**
Scanty and rare menstruation in a woman with previously normal periods.

N91.5   **Oligomenorrhoea, unspecified**
Hypomenorrhoea NOS

N92   Excessive, frequent and irregular menstruation

Excludes: postmenopausal bleeding (N95.0)

N92.0   Excessive and frequent menstruation with regular cycle
Heavy periods NOS
Menorrhagia NOS
Polymenorrhoea

N92.1   Excessive and frequent menstruation with irregular cycle
Irregular intermenstrual bleeding
Irregular, shortened intervals between menstrual bleeding
Menometrorrhagia
Metrorrhagia

N92.2   Excessive menstruation at puberty
Excessive bleeding associated with onset of menstrual periods
Pubertal menorrhagia
Puberty bleeding

N92.3   Ovulation bleeding
Regular intermenstrual bleeding

N92.4   Excessive bleeding in the premenopausal period
Menorrhagia or metrorrhagia:
• climacteric
• menopausal
• preclimacteric
• premenopausal

N92.5   Other specified irregular menstruation

N92.6   Irregular menstruation, unspecified
Irregular:
• bleeding NOS
• periods NOS

Excludes: irregular menstruation with:
            • lengthened intervals or scanty bleeding (N91.3–
              N91.5)
            • shortened intervals or excessive bleeding (N92.1)

N93   Other abnormal uterine and vaginal bleeding
Excludes: neonatal vaginal haemorrhage (P54.6)
            pseudomenses (P54.6)

N93.0   Postcoital and contact bleeding

N93.8   Other specified abnormal uterine and vaginal bleeding
Dysfunctional or functional uterine or vaginal bleeding NOS

N93.9   Abnormal uterine and vaginal bleeding, unspecified

N94 Pain and other conditions associated with female genital organs and menstrual cycle

N94.0 **Mittelschmerz**

N94.1 **Dyspareunia**
Excludes: psychogenic dyspareunia (F52.6)

N94.2 **Vaginismus**
Excludes: psychogenic vaginismus (F52.5)

N94.3 **Premenstrual tension syndrome**

N94.4 **Primary dysmenorrhoea**

N94.5 **Secondary dysmenorrhoea**

N94.6 **Dysmenorrhoea, unspecified**

N94.8 **Other specified conditions associated with female genital organs and menstrual cycle**

N94.9 **Unspecified condition associated with female genital organs and menstrual cycle**

N95 Menopausal and other perimenopausal disorders
Excludes: excessive bleeding in the premenopausal period
(N92.4)
postmenopausal:
• osteoporosis (M81.0)
• with pathological fracture (M80.0)
• urethritis (N34.2)
premature menopause NOS (E28.3)

N95.0 **Postmenopausal bleeding**
Excludes: that associated with artificial menopause (N95.3)

N95.1 **Menopausal and female climacteric states**
Symptoms such as flushing, sleeplessness, headache, lack of concentration, associated with menopause
Excludes: those associated with artificial menopause (N95.3)

N95.2 **Postmenopausal atrophic vaginitis**
Senile (atrophic) vaginitis
Excludes: that associated with artificial menopause (N95.3)

N95.3 **States associated with artificial menopause**
Post-artificial-menopause syndrome

N95.8   **Other specified menopausal and perimenopausal disorders**

N95.9   **Menopausal and perimenopausal disorder, unspecified**

N96   Habitual aborter

Investigation or care in a nonpregnant woman
Relative infertility
Excludes: currently pregnant (O26.2)
               with current abortion (O03–O06)

N97   Female infertility

Includes: inability to achieve a pregnancy
           sterility, female NOS
Excludes: relative infertility (N96)

N97.0   **Female infertility associated with anovulation**

N97.1   **Female infertility of tubal origin**
Associated with congenital anomaly of tube
Tubal:
- block
- occlusion
- stenosis

N97.2   **Female infertility of uterine origin**
Associated with congenital anomaly of uterus
Nonimplantation of ovum

N97.3   **Female infertility of cervical origin**

N97.4   **Female infertility associated with male factors**

N97.8   **Female infertility of other origin**

N97.9   **Female infertility, unspecified**

N98   Complications associated with artificial fertilization

N98.0   **Infection associated with artificial insemination**

N98.1   **Hyperstimulation of ovaries**
Hyperstimulation of ovaries:
- NOS
- associated with induced ovulation

N98.2 **Complications of attempted introduction of fertilized ovum following in vitro fertilization**

N98.3 **Complications of attempted introduction of embryo in embryo transfer**

N98.8 **Other complications associated with artificial fertilization**
Complications of artificial insemination by:
- donor
- husband

N98.9 **Complication associated with artificial fertilization, unspecified**

Other disorders of the genitourinary system (N99)

N99 **Postprocedural disorders of genitourinary system, not elsewhere classified**
Excludes: irradiation cystitis (N30.4)
postoophorectomy osteoporosis (M81.1)
- with pathological fracture (M80.1)
states associated with artificial menopause (N95.3)

N99.0 **Postprocedural renal failure**

N99.1 **Postprocedural urethral stricture**
Postcatheterization urethral stricture

N99.2 **Postoperative adhesions of vagina**

N99.3 **Prolapse of vaginal vault after hysterectomy**

N99.4 **Postprocedural pelvic peritoneal adhesions**

N99.5 **Malfunction of external stoma of urinary tract**

N99.8 **Other postprocedural disorders of genitourinary system**
Residual ovary syndrome

N99.9 **Postprocedural disorder of genitourinary system, unspecified**

CHAPTER XV

Pregnancy, childbirth and the puerperium
(O00–O99)

Excludes: human immunodeficiency virus [HIV] disease (B20–B24)
injury, poisoning and certain other consequences of external
causes (S00–T98)
mental and behavioural disorders associated with the puerperium
(F53.–)
obstetrical tetanus (A34)
postpartum necrosis of pituitary gland (E23.0)
puerperal osteomalacia (M83.0)
supervision of:
• high-risk pregnancy (Z35.–)
• normal pregnancy (Z34.–)

This chapter contains the following blocks:

O00–O08 Pregnancy with abortive outcome
O10–O16 Oedema, proteinuria and hypertensive disorders in pregnancy,
childbirth and the puerperium
O20–O29 Other maternal disorders predominantly related to pregnancy
O30–O48 Maternal care related to the fetus and amniotic cavity and
possible delivery problems
O60–O75 Complications of labour and delivery
O80–O84 Delivery
O85–O92 Complications predominantly related to the puerperium
O95–O99 Other obstetric conditions, not elsewhere classified

Pregnancy with abortive outcome (O00–O08)

Excludes: continuing pregnancy in multiple gestation after abortion of one fetus or more (O31.1)

O00 Ectopic pregnancy

Includes: ruptured ectopic pregnancy

Use additional code from category O08.–, if desired, to identify any associated complication.

O00.0 Abdominal pregnancy
Excludes: delivery of viable fetus in abdominal pregnancy (O83.3)

maternal care for viable fetus in abdominal pregnancy (O36.7)

O00.1 Tubal pregnancy
Fallopian pregnancy
Rupture of (fallopian) tube due to pregnancy
Tubal abortion

O00.2 Ovarian pregnancy

O00.8 Other ectopic pregnancy
Pregnancy:
- cervical
- cornual
- intraligamentous
- mural

O00.9 Ectopic pregnancy, unspecified

O01 Hydatidiform mole

Use additional code from category O08.-, if desired, to identify any associated complication.

Excludes: malignant hydatidiform mole (D39.2)

O01.0 Classical hydatidiform mole

Complete hydatidiform mole

O01.1 Incomplete and partial hydatidiform mole

O01.9 Hydatidiform mole, unspecified

Trophoblastic disease NOS

Vesicular mole NOS

O02 Other abnormal products of conception

Use additional code from category O08.-, if desired, to identify any associated complication.

Excludes: papyraceous fetus (O31.0)

O02.0 Blighted ovum and nonhydatidiform mole

Mole:
- carneous
- fleshy
- intrauterine NOS

Pathological ovum

O02.1 Missed abortion

Early fetal death with retention of dead fetus.

Excludes: missed abortion with:
- blighted ovum (O02.0)
- mole:
  - hydatidiform (O01.-)
  - nonhydatidiform (O02.0)

O02.8 Other specified abnormal products of conception

Excludes: those with:
- blighted ovum (O02.0)
- mole:
  - hydatidiform (O01.-)
  - nonhydatidiform (O02.0)

O02.9 Abnormal product of conception, unspecified

The following fourth-character subdivisions are for use with categories O03–O06:

Note: Incomplete abortion includes retained products of conception following abortion.

.0 Incomplete, complicated by genital tract and pelvic infection
With conditions in O08.0

.1 Incomplete, complicated by delayed or excessive haemorrhage
With conditions in O08.1

.2 Incomplete, complicated by embolism
With conditions in O08.2

.3 Incomplete, with other and unspecified complications
With conditions in O08.3–O08.9

.4 Incomplete, without complication

.5 Complete or unspecified, complicated by genital tract and pelvic infection
With conditions in O08.0

.6 Complete or unspecified, complicated by delayed or excessive haemorrhage
With conditions in O08.1

.7 Complete or unspecified, complicated by embolism
With conditions in O08.2

.8 Complete or unspecified, with other and unspecified complications
With conditions in O08.3–O08.9

.9 Complete or unspecified, without complication

O03 Spontaneous abortion
[See above for subdivisions]
Includes: miscarriage

O04 Medical abortion
[See above for subdivisions]
Includes: termination of pregnancy:
- legal
- therapeutic
therapeutic abortion

O05 Other abortion
[See above for subdivisions]

O06 Unspecified abortion
[See page 724 for subdivisions]
Includes: induced abortion NOS

O07 Failed attempted abortion
Includes: failure of attempted induction of abortion
Excludes: incomplete abortion (O03–O06)

O07.0 **Failed medical abortion, complicated by genital tract and pelvic infection**
With conditions in O08.0

O07.1 **Failed medical abortion, complicated by delayed or excessive haemorrhage**
With conditions in O08.1

O07.2 **Failed medical abortion, complicated by embolism**
With conditions in O08.2

O07.3 **Failed medical abortion, with other and unspecified complications**
With conditions in O08.3–O08.9

O07.4 **Failed medical abortion, without complication**
Failed medical abortion NOS

O07.5 **Other and unspecified failed attempted abortion, complicated by genital tract and pelvic infection**
With conditions in O08.0

O07.6 **Other and unspecified failed attempted abortion, complicated by delayed or excessive haemorrhage**
With conditions in O08.1

O07.7 **Other and unspecified failed attempted abortion, complicated by embolism**
With conditions in O08.2

O07.8 **Other and unspecified failed attempted abortion, with other and unspecified complications**
With conditions in O08.3–O08.9

O07.9 **Other and unspecified failed attempted abortion, without complication**
Failed attempted abortion NOS

O08 Complications following abortion and ectopic and molar pregnancy

Note: This code is provided primarily for morbidity coding. For use of this category reference should be made to the morbidity coding rules and guidelines in Volume 2.

O08.0 **Genital tract and pelvic infection following abortion and ectopic and molar pregnancy**

Endometritis
Oophoritis
Parametritis
Pelvic peritonitis
Salpingitis
Salpingo-oophoritis
Sepsis
Septic shock
Septicaemia

} following conditions classifiable to O00–O07

Excludes: septic or septicopyaemic embolism (O08.2)
urinary tract infection (O08.8)

O08.1 **Delayed or excessive haemorrhage following abortion and ectopic and molar pregnancy**

Afibrinogenaemia
Defibrination syndrome
Intravascular coagulation

} following conditions classifiable to O00–O07

O08.2 **Embolism following abortion and ectopic and molar pregnancy**

Embolism:
- NOS
- air
- amniotic fluid
- blood-clot
- pulmonary
- pyaemic
- septic or septicopyaemic
- soap

} following conditions classifiable to O00–O07

O08.3 **Shock following abortion and ectopic and molar pregnancy**

Circulatory collapse
Shock (postoperative)

} following conditions classifiable to O00–O07

Excludes: septic shock (O08.0)

O08.4   **Renal failure following abortion and ectopic and molar pregnancy**

Oliguria

Renal

• failure (acute)   } following conditions classifiable to

• shutdown   } O00–O07

• tubular necrosis

Uraemia

O08.5   **Metabolic disorders following abortion and ectopic and molar pregnancy**

Electrolyte imbalance following conditions classifiable to
O00–O07

O08.6   **Damage to pelvic organs and tissues following abortion and ectopic and molar pregnancy**

Laceration, perforation, tear or chemical damage of:

• bladder

• bowel

• broad ligament   } following conditions classifiable to

• cervix   } O00–O07

• periurethral tissue

• uterus

O08.7   **Other venous complications following abortion and ectopic and molar pregnancy**

O08.8   **Other complications following abortion and ectopic and molar pregnancy**

Cardiac arrest   } following conditions classifiable to

Urinary tract infection   } O00–O07

O08.9   **Complication following abortion and ectopic and molar pregnancy, unspecified**

Unspecified complication following conditions classifiable to
O00–O07

Oedema, proteinuria and hypertensive disorders in pregnancy, childbirth and the puerperium (O10–O16)

O10   Pre-existing hypertension complicating pregnancy, childbirth and the puerperium
Includes: the listed conditions with pre-existing proteinuria
Excludes: that with increased or superimposed proteinuria (O11)

O10.0   Pre-existing essential hypertension complicating pregnancy, childbirth and the puerperium
Any condition in I10 specified as a reason for obstetric care during pregnancy, childbirth or the puerperium

O10.1   Pre-existing hypertensive heart disease complicating pregnancy, childbirth and the puerperium
Any condition in I11.– specified as a reason for obstetric care during pregnancy, childbirth or the puerperium

O10.2   Pre-existing hypertensive renal disease complicating pregnancy, childbirth and the puerperium
Any condition in I12.– specified as a reason for obstetric care during pregnancy, childbirth or the puerperium

O10.3   Pre-existing hypertensive heart and renal disease complicating pregnancy, childbirth and the puerperium
Any condition in I13.– specified as a reason for obstetric care during pregnancy, childbirth or the puerperium

O10.4   Pre-existing secondary hypertension complicating pregnancy, childbirth and the puerperium
Any condition in I15.– specified as a reason for obstetric care during pregnancy, childbirth or the puerperium

O10.9   Unspecified pre-existing hypertension complicating pregnancy, childbirth and the puerperium

O11 Pre-existing hypertensive disorder with superimposed proteinuria

Conditions in O10.– complicated by increased proteinuria
Superimposed pre-eclampsia

O12 Gestational [pregnancy-induced] oedema and proteinuria without hypertension

O12.0 Gestational oedema

O12.1 Gestational proteinuria

O12.2 Gestational oedema with proteinuria

O13 Gestational [pregnancy-induced] hypertension without significant proteinuria

Gestational hypertension NOS
Mild pre-eclampsia

O14 Gestational [pregnancy-induced] hypertension with significant proteinuria

Excludes: superimposed pre-eclampsia (O11)

O14.0 Moderate pre-eclampsia

O14.1 Severe pre-eclampsia

O14.9 Pre-eclampsia, unspecified

O15 Eclampsia

Includes: convulsions following conditions in O10–O14 and O16

O15.0 Eclampsia in pregnancy

O15.1 Eclampsia in labour

O15.2 Eclampsia in the puerperium

O15.9 Eclampsia, unspecified as to time period
Eclampsia NOS

O16 Unspecified maternal hypertension
Transient hypertension of pregnancy

Other maternal disorders predominantly related to pregnancy
(O20–O29)

Note: Categories O24.– and O25 include the listed conditions even if they occur during childbirth or the puerperium.

Excludes: maternal:
- care related to the fetus and amniotic cavity and possible delivery problems (O30–O48)
- diseases classifiable elsewhere but complicating pregnancy, labour and delivery, and the puerperium (O98–O99)

O20 Haemorrhage in early pregnancy
Excludes: pregnancy with abortive outcome (O00–O08)

O20.0 **Threatened abortion**
Haemorrhage specified as due to threatened abortion

O20.8 **Other haemorrhage in early pregnancy**

O20.9 **Haemorrhage in early pregnancy, unspecified**

O21 Excessive vomiting in pregnancy

O21.0 **Mild hyperemesis gravidarum**
Hyperemesis gravidarum, mild or unspecified, starting before the end of the 22nd week of gestation

O21.1 **Hyperemesis gravidarum with metabolic disturbance**
Hyperemesis gravidarum, starting before the end of the 22nd week of gestation, with metabolic disturbance such as:
- carbohydrate depletion
- dehydration
- electrolyte imbalance

O21.2 **Late vomiting of pregnancy**
Excessive vomiting starting after 22 completed weeks of gestation

O21.8 **Other vomiting complicating pregnancy**
Vomiting due to diseases classified elsewhere, complicating pregnancy

Use additional code, if desired, to identify cause.

O21.9 **Vomiting of pregnancy, unspecified**

O22 Venous complications in pregnancy
Excludes: obstetric pulmonary embolism (O88.–)
the listed conditions as complications of:
- abortion or ectopic or molar pregnancy (O00–O07, O08.7)
- childbirth and the puerperium (O87.–)

O22.0 **Varicose veins of lower extremity in pregnancy**
Varicose veins NOS in pregnancy

O22.1 **Genital varices in pregnancy**
Perineal ⎤
Vaginal ⎬ varices in pregnancy
Vulval ⎦

O22.2 **Superficial thrombophlebitis in pregnancy**
Thrombophlebitis of legs in pregnancy

O22.3 **Deep phlebothrombosis in pregnancy**
Deep-vein thrombosis, antepartum

O22.4 **Haemorrhoids in pregnancy**

O22.5 **Cerebral venous thrombosis in pregnancy**
Cerebrovenous sinus thrombosis in pregnancy

O22.8 **Other venous complications in pregnancy**

O22.9 **Venous complication in pregnancy, unspecified**
Gestational:
- phlebitis NOS
- phlebopathy NOS
- thrombosis NOS

O23 Infections of genitourinary tract in pregnancy

O23.0 Infections of kidney in pregnancy

O23.1 Infections of bladder in pregnancy

O23.2 Infections of urethra in pregnancy

O23.3 Infections of other parts of urinary tract in pregnancy

O23.4 Unspecified infection of urinary tract in pregnancy

O23.5 Infections of the genital tract in pregnancy

O23.9 Other and unspecified genitourinary tract infection in pregnancy
Genitourinary tract infection in pregnancy NOS

O24 Diabetes mellitus in pregnancy
Includes: in childbirth and the puerperium

O24.0 Pre-existing diabetes mellitus, insulin-dependent

O24.1 Pre-existing diabetes mellitus, non-insulin-dependent

O24.2 Pre-existing malnutrition-related diabetes mellitus

O24.3 Pre-existing diabetes mellitus, unspecified

O24.4 Diabetes mellitus arising in pregnancy
Gestational diabetes mellitus NOS

O24.9 Diabetes mellitus in pregnancy, unspecified

O25 Malnutrition in pregnancy
Malnutrition in childbirth and the puerperium

O26   Maternal care for other conditions predominantly related to pregnancy

O26.0   **Excessive weight gain in pregnancy**
Excludes: gestational oedema (O12.0, O12.2)

O26.1   **Low weight gain in pregnancy**

O26.2   **Pregnancy care of habitual aborter**
Excludes: habitual aborter:
- with current abortion (O03–O06)
- without current pregnancy (N96)

O26.3   **Retained intrauterine contraceptive device in pregnancy**

O26.4   **Herpes gestationis**

O26.5   **Maternal hypotension syndrome**
Supine hypotensive syndrome

O26.6   **Liver disorders in pregnancy, childbirth and the puerperium**
Excludes: hepatorenal syndrome following labour and delivery (O90.4)

O26.7   **Subluxation of symphysis (pubis) in pregnancy, childbirth and the puerperium**
Excludes: traumatic separation of symphysis (pubis) during childbirth (O71.6)

O26.8   **Other specified pregnancy-related conditions**
Exhaustion and fatigue ⎤
Peripheral neuritis ⎬ pregnancy-related
Renal disease ⎦

O26.9   **Pregnancy-related condition, unspecified**

O28   Abnormal findings on antenatal screening of mother
Excludes: diagnostic findings classified elsewhere—see Alphabetical Index
maternal care related to the fetus and amniotic cavity and possible delivery problems (O30–O48)

O28.0   **Abnormal haematological finding on antenatal screening of mother**

O28.1   **Abnormal biochemical finding on antenatal screening of mother**

O28.2   Abnormal cytological finding on antenatal screening of mother

O28.3   Abnormal ultrasonic finding on antenatal screening of mother

O28.4   Abnormal radiological finding on antenatal screening of mother

O28.5   Abnormal chromosomal and genetic finding on antenatal screening of mother

O28.8   Other abnormal findings on antenatal screening of mother

O28.9   Abnormal finding on antenatal screening of mother, unspecified

O29   Complications of anaesthesia during pregnancy

Includes: maternal complications arising from the administration of a general or local anaesthetic, analgesic or other sedation during pregnancy

Excludes: complications of anaesthesia during:
  • abortion or ectopic or molar pregnancy (O00–O08)
  • labour and delivery (O74.–)
  • puerperium (O89.–)

O29.0   Pulmonary complications of anaesthesia during pregnancy
Aspiration pneumonitis
Inhalation of stomach contents
    or secretions NOS   } due to anaesthesia during pregnancy
Mendelson's syndrome
Pressure collapse of lung

O29.1   Cardiac complications of anaesthesia during pregnancy
Cardiac:
  • arrest
  • failure   } due to anaesthesia during pregnancy

O29.2   Central nervous system complications of anaesthesia during pregnancy
Cerebral anoxia due to anaesthesia during pregnancy

O29.3   Toxic reaction to local anaesthesia during pregnancy

O29.4   Spinal and epidural anaesthesia-induced headache during pregnancy

O29.5   Other complications of spinal and epidural anaesthesia during pregnancy

O29.6   **Failed or difficult intubation during pregnancy**

O29.8   **Other complications of anaesthesia during pregnancy**

O29.9   **Complication of anaesthesia during pregnancy, unspecified**

Maternal care related to the fetus and amniotic cavity and possible delivery problems (O30–O48)

O30   Multiple gestation
Excludes: complications specific to multiple gestation (O31.–)

O30.0   **Twin pregnancy**

O30.1   **Triplet pregnancy**

O30.2   **Quadruplet pregnancy**

O30.8   **Other multiple gestation**

O30.9   **Multiple gestation, unspecified**
Multiple pregnancy NOS

O31   Complications specific to multiple gestation
Excludes: conjoined twins causing disproportion (O33.7)
delayed delivery of second twin, triplet, etc. (O63.2)
malpresentation of one fetus or more (O32.5)
with obstructed labour (O64–O66)

O31.0   **Papyraceous fetus**
Fetus compressus

O31.1   **Continuing pregnancy after abortion of one fetus or more**

O31.2   **Continuing pregnancy after intrauterine death of one fetus or more**

O31.8   **Other complications specific to multiple gestation**

O32 Maternal care for known or suspected malpresentation of fetus

Includes: the listed conditions as a reason for observation, hospitalization or other obstetric care of the mother, or for caesarean section before onset of labour

Excludes: the listed conditions with obstructed labour (O64.–)

O32.0 Maternal care for unstable lie

O32.1 Maternal care for breech presentation

O32.2 Maternal care for transverse and oblique lie
Presentation:
• oblique
• transverse

O32.3 Maternal care for face, brow and chin presentation

O32.4 Maternal care for high head at term
Failure of head to enter pelvic brim

O32.5 Maternal care for multiple gestation with malpresentation of one fetus or more

O32.6 Maternal care for compound presentation

O32.8 Maternal care for other malpresentation of fetus

O32.9 Maternal care for malpresentation of fetus, unspecified

O33 Maternal care for known or suspected disproportion

Includes: the listed conditions as a reason for observation, hospitalization or other obstetric care of the mother, or for caesarean section before onset of labour

Excludes: the listed conditions with obstructed labour (O65–O66)

O33.0 Maternal care for disproportion due to deformity of maternal pelvic bones
Pelvic deformity causing disproportion NOS

O33.1 Maternal care for disproportion due to generally contracted pelvis
Contracted pelvis NOS causing disproportion

O33.2   **Maternal care for disproportion due to inlet contraction of pelvis**
Inlet contraction (pelvis) causing disproportion

O33.3   **Maternal care for disproportion due to outlet contraction of pelvis**
Mid-cavity contraction (pelvis) ⎫
Outlet contraction (pelvis) ⎭ causing disproportion

O33.4   **Maternal care for disproportion of mixed maternal and fetal origin**

O33.5   **Maternal care for disproportion due to unusually large fetus**
Disproportion of fetal origin with normally formed fetus
Fetal disproportion NOS

O33.6   **Maternal care for disproportion due to hydrocephalic fetus**

O33.7   **Maternal care for disproportion due to other fetal deformities**
Conjoined twins ⎫
Fetal: ⎪
• ascites ⎪
• hydrops ⎬ causing disproportion
• meningomyelocele ⎪
• sacral teratoma ⎪
• tumour ⎭

O33.8   **Maternal care for disproportion of other origin**

O33.9   **Maternal care for disproportion, unspecified**
Cephalopelvic disproportion NOS
Fetopelvic disproportion NOS

O34   Maternal care for known or suspected abnormality of pelvic organs

Includes: the listed conditions as a reason for observation, hospitalization or other obstetric care of the mother, or for caesarean section before onset of labour
Excludes: the listed conditions with obstructed labour (O65.5)

O34.0   **Maternal care for congenital malformation of uterus**
Maternal care for:
• double uterus
• uterus bicornis

O34.1 **Maternal care for tumour of corpus uteri**
Maternal care for:
- polyp of corpus uteri
- uterine fibroid

Excludes: maternal care for tumour of cervix (O34.4)

O34.2 **Maternal care due to uterine scar from previous surgery**
Maternal care for scar from previous caesarean section

Excludes: vaginal delivery following previous caesarean section
NOS (O75.7)

O34.3 **Maternal care for cervical incompetence**
Maternal care for:
- cerclage ⎫ with or without mention of cervical
- Shirodkar suture ⎬ incompetence

O34.4 **Maternal care for other abnormalities of cervix**
Maternal care for:
- polyp of cervix
- previous surgery to cervix
- stricture or stenosis of cervix
- tumour of cervix

O34.5 **Maternal care for other abnormalities of gravid uterus**
Maternal care for:
- incarceration ⎫
- prolapse ⎬ of gravid uterus
- retroversion ⎭

O34.6 **Maternal care for abnormality of vagina**
Maternal care for:
- previous surgery to vagina
- septate vagina
- stenosis of vagina (acquired)(congenital)
- stricture of vagina
- tumour of vagina

Excludes: maternal care for vaginal varices in pregnancy
(O22.1)

O34.7 **Maternal care for abnormality of vulva and perineum**
Maternal care for:
- fibrosis of perineum
- previous surgery to perineum or vulva
- rigid perineum
- tumour of vulva

Excludes: maternal care for perineal and vulval varices in
pregnancy (O22.1)

O34.8 **Maternal care for other abnormalities of pelvic organs**
Maternal care for:
- cystocele
- pelvic floor repair (previous)
- pendulous abdomen
- rectocele
- rigid pelvic floor

O34.9 **Maternal care for abnormality of pelvic organ, unspecified**

O35 Maternal care for known or suspected fetal abnormality and damage

Includes: the listed conditions in the fetus as a reason for observation, hospitalization or other obstetric care of the mother, or for termination of pregnancy

Excludes: maternal care for known or suspected disproportion (O33.–)

O35.0 **Maternal care for (suspected) central nervous system malformation in fetus**
Maternal care for (suspected) fetal:
- anencephaly
- spina bifida

Excludes: chromosomal abnormality in fetus (O35.1)

O35.1 **Maternal care for (suspected) chromosomal abnormality in fetus**

O35.2 **Maternal care for (suspected) hereditary disease in fetus**
Excludes: chromosomal abnormality in fetus (O35.1)

O35.3 **Maternal care for (suspected) damage to fetus from viral disease in mother**
Maternal care for (suspected) damage to fetus from maternal:
- cytomegalovirus infection
- rubella

O35.4 **Maternal care for (suspected) damage to fetus from alcohol**

O35.5 **Maternal care for (suspected) damage to fetus by drugs**
Maternal care for (suspected) damage to fetus from drug addiction

Excludes: fetal distress in labour and delivery due to drug administration (O68.–)

O35.6 **Maternal care for (suspected) damage to fetus by radiation**

O35.7 **Maternal care for (suspected) damage to fetus by other medical procedures**
Maternal care for (suspected) damage to fetus by:
- amniocentesis
- biopsy procedures
- haematological investigation
- intrauterine contraceptive device
- intrauterine surgery

O35.8 **Maternal care for other (suspected) fetal abnormality and damage**
Maternal care for (suspected) damage to fetus from maternal:
- listeriosis
- toxoplasmosis

O35.9 **Maternal care for (suspected) fetal abnormality and damage, unspecified**

O36 Maternal care for other known or suspected fetal problems

Includes: the listed conditions in the fetus as a reason for observation, hospitalization or other obstetric care of the mother, or for termination of pregnancy

Excludes: labour and delivery complicated by fetal stress [distress] (O68.–)
placental transfusion syndromes (O43.0)

O36.0 **Maternal care for rhesus isoimmunization**
Anti-D [Rh] antibodies
Rh incompatibility (with hydrops fetalis)

O36.1 **Maternal care for other isoimmunization**
ABO isoimmunization
Isoimmunization NOS (with hydrops fetalis)

O36.2 **Maternal care for hydrops fetalis**
Hydrops fetalis:
- NOS
- not associated with isoimmunization

O36.3 **Maternal care for signs of fetal hypoxia**

O36.4 **Maternal care for intrauterine death**
Excludes: missed abortion (O02.1)

O36.5 **Maternal care for poor fetal growth**
Maternal care for known or suspected:
- light-for-dates
- placental insufficiency
- small-for-dates

O36.6 **Maternal care for excessive fetal growth**
Maternal care for known or suspected large-for-dates

O36.7 **Maternal care for viable fetus in abdominal pregnancy**

O36.8 **Maternal care for other specified fetal problems**

O36.9 **Maternal care for fetal problem, unspecified**

O40 Polyhydramnios
Hydramnios

O41 Other disorders of amniotic fluid and membranes
Excludes: premature rupture of membranes (O42.–)

O41.0 **Oligohydramnios**
Oligohydramnios without mention of rupture of membranes

O41.1 **Infection of amniotic sac and membranes**
Amnionitis
Chorioamnionitis
Membranitis
Placentitis

O41.8 **Other specified disorders of amniotic fluid and membranes**

O41.9 **Disorder of amniotic fluid and membranes, unspecified**

O42 Premature rupture of membranes

O42.0 **Premature rupture of membranes, onset of labour within 24 hours**

O42.1 **Premature rupture of membranes, onset of labour after 24 hours**
Excludes: with labour delayed by therapy (O42.2)

O42.2 **Premature rupture of membranes, labour delayed by therapy**

O42.9 **Premature rupture of membranes, unspecified**

O43 Placental disorders

Excludes: maternal care for poor fetal growth due to placental
insufficiency (O36.5)
placenta praevia (O44.–)
premature separation of placenta [abruptio placentae]
(O45.–)

O43.0   Placental transfusion syndromes
Transfusion:
• fetomaternal
• maternofetal
• twin-to-twin

O43.1   Malformation of placenta
Abnormal placenta NOS
Circumvallate placenta

O43.8   Other placental disorders
Placental:
• dysfunction
• infarction

O43.9   Placental disorder, unspecified

O44 Placenta praevia

O44.0   Placenta praevia specified as without haemorrhage
Low implantation of placenta specified as without haemorrhage

O44.1   Placenta praevia with haemorrhage
Low implantation of placenta, NOS or with haemorrhage
Placenta praevia:
• marginal ⎫
• partial ⎬ NOS or with haemorrhage
• total ⎭

Excludes: labour and delivery complicated by haemorrhage
from vasa praevia (O69.4)

O45 Premature separation of placenta [abruptio placentae]

O45.0 **Premature separation of placenta with coagulation defect**
Abruptio placentae with (excessive) haemorrhage associated with:
• afibrinogenaemia
• disseminated intravascular coagulation
• hyperfibrinolysis
• hypofibrinogenaemia

O45.8 **Other premature separation of placenta**

O45.9 **Premature separation of placenta, unspecified**
Abruptio placentae NOS

O46 Antepartum haemorrhage, not elsewhere classified

Excludes: haemorrhage in early pregnancy (O20.–)
intrapartum haemorrhage NEC (O67.–)
placenta praevia (O44.–)
premature separation of placenta [abruptio placentae] (O45.–)

O46.0 **Antepartum haemorrhage with coagulation defect**
Antepartum haemorrhage (excessive) associated with:
• afibrinogenaemia
• disseminated intravascular coagulation
• hyperfibrinolysis
• hypofibrinogenaemia

O46.8 **Other antepartum haemorrhage**

O46.9 **Antepartum haemorrhage, unspecified**

O47 False labour

O47.0 **False labour before 37 completed weeks of gestation**

O47.1 **False labour at or after 37 completed weeks of gestation**

O47.9 **False labour, unspecified**

O48 Prolonged pregnancy
Post-dates
Post-term

Complications of labour and delivery (O60–O75)

O60 Preterm delivery
Onset (spontaneous) of delivery before 37 completed weeks of gestation

O61 Failed induction of labour

O61.0 Failed medical induction of labour
Failed induction (of labour) by:
- oxytocin
- prostaglandins

O61.1 Failed instrumental induction of labour
Failed induction (of labour):
- mechanical
- surgical

O61.8 Other failed induction of labour

O61.9 Failed induction of labour, unspecified

O62 Abnormalities of forces of labour

O62.0 Primary inadequate contractions
Failure of cervical dilatation
Primary hypotonic uterine dysfunction

O62.1 Secondary uterine inertia
Arrested active phase of labour
Secondary hypotonic uterine dysfunction

O62.2 **Other uterine inertia**
Atony of uterus
Desultory labour
Hypotonic uterine dysfunction NOS
Irregular labour
Poor contractions
Uterine inertia NOS

O62.3 **Precipitate labour**

O62.4 **Hypertonic, incoordinate, and prolonged uterine contractions**
Contraction ring dystocia
Dyscoordinate labour
Hour-glass contraction of uterus
Hypertonic uterine dysfunction
Incoordinate uterine action
Tetanic contractions
Uterine dystocia NOS
Excludes: dystocia (fetal)(maternal) NOS (O66.9)

O62.8 **Other abnormalities of forces of labour**

O62.9 **Abnormality of forces of labour, unspecified**

O63 Long labour

O63.0 **Prolonged first stage (of labour)**

O63.1 **Prolonged second stage (of labour)**

O63.2 **Delayed delivery of second twin, triplet, etc.**

O63.9 **Long labour, unspecified**
Prolonged labour NOS

O64 Obstructed labour due to malposition and malpresentation of fetus

O64.0 **Obstructed labour due to incomplete rotation of fetal head**
Deep transverse arrest
Obstructed labour due to persistent (position):
• occipitoiliac
• occipitoposterior
• occipitosacral
• occipitotransverse

O64.1 **Obstructed labour due to breech presentation**

O64.2 **Obstructed labour due to face presentation**
Obstructed labour due to chin presentation

O64.3 **Obstructed labour due to brow presentation**

O64.4 **Obstructed labour due to shoulder presentation**
Prolapsed arm
Excludes: impacted shoulders (O66.0)
shoulder dystocia (O66.0)

O64.5 **Obstructed labour due to compound presentation**

O64.8 **Obstructed labour due to other malposition and malpresentation**

O64.9 **Obstructed labour due to malposition and malpresentation, unspecified**

O65 **Obstructed labour due to maternal pelvic abnormality**

O65.0 **Obstructed labour due to deformed pelvis**

O65.1 **Obstructed labour due to generally contracted pelvis**

O65.2 **Obstructed labour due to pelvic inlet contraction**

O65.3 **Obstructed labour due to pelvic outlet and mid-cavity contraction**

O65.4 **Obstructed labour due to fetopelvic disproportion, unspecified**
Excludes: dystocia due to abnormality of fetus (O66.2–O66.3)

O65.5 **Obstructed labour due to abnormality of maternal pelvic organs**
Obstructed labour due to conditions listed in O34.–

O65.8 **Obstructed labour due to other maternal pelvic abnormalities**

O65.9 **Obstructed labour due to maternal pelvic abnormality, unspecified**

O66 Other obstructed labour

O66.0 Obstructed labour due to shoulder dystocia
Impacted shoulders

O66.1 Obstructed labour due to locked twins

O66.2 Obstructed labour due to unusually large fetus

O66.3 Obstructed labour due to other abnormalities of fetus
Dystocia due to:
- conjoined twins
- fetal:
  - ascites
  - hydrops
  - meningomyelocele
  - sacral teratoma
  - tumour
- hydrocephalic fetus

O66.4 Failed trial of labour, unspecified
Failed trial of labour with subsequent delivery by caesarean
section

O66.5 Failed application of vacuum extractor and forceps, unspecified
Failed application of ventouse or forceps, with subsequent
delivery by forceps or caesarean section respectively

O66.8 Other specified obstructed labour

O66.9 Obstructed labour, unspecified
Dystocia:
- NOS
- fetal NOS
- maternal NOS

O67 Labour and delivery complicated by intrapartum haemorrhage, not elsewhere classified

Excludes: antepartum haemorrhage NEC (O46.–)
placenta praevia (O44.–)
postpartum haemorrhage (O72.–)
premature separation of placenta [abruptio placentae]
(O45.–)

O67.0 **Intrapartum haemorrhage with coagulation defect**
Intrapartum haemorrhage (excessive) associated with:
- afibrinogenaemia
- disseminated intravascular coagulation
- hyperfibrinolysis
- hypofibrinogenaemia

O67.8 **Other intrapartum haemorrhage**
Excessive intrapartum haemorrhage

O67.9 **Intrapartum haemorrhage, unspecified**

O68 Labour and delivery complicated by fetal stress [distress]

Includes: fetal distress in labour or delivery due to drug administration

O68.0 **Labour and delivery complicated by fetal heart rate anomaly**
Fetal:
- bradycardia
- heart rate irregularity
- tachycardia

Excludes: with meconium in amniotic fluid (O68.2)

O68.1 **Labour and delivery complicated by meconium in amniotic fluid**

Excludes: with fetal heart rate anomaly (O68.2)

O68.2 **Labour and delivery complicated by fetal heart rate anomaly with meconium in amniotic fluid**

O68.3 **Labour and delivery complicated by biochemical evidence of fetal stress**
Abnormal fetal:
- acidaemia
- acid–base balance

O68.8 **Labour and delivery complicated by other evidence of fetal stress**
Evidence of fetal distress:
- electrocardiographic
- ultrasonic

O68.9 **Labour and delivery complicated by fetal stress, unspecified**

O69 Labour and delivery complicated by umbilical cord complications

O69.0 **Labour and delivery complicated by prolapse of cord**

O69.1 **Labour and delivery complicated by cord around neck, with compression**

O69.2 **Labour and delivery complicated by other cord entanglement**
Entanglement of cords of twins in monoamniotic sac
Knot in cord

O69.3 **Labour and delivery complicated by short cord**

O69.4 **Labour and delivery complicated by vasa praevia**
Haemorrhage from vasa praevia

O69.5 **Labour and delivery complicated by vascular lesion of cord**
Cord:
• bruising
• haematoma
Thrombosis of umbilical vessels

O69.8 **Labour and delivery complicated by other cord complications**

O69.9 **Labour and delivery complicated by cord complication, unspecified**

O70 Perineal laceration during delivery
Includes: episiotomy extended by laceration
Excludes: obstetric high vaginal laceration alone (O71.4)

O70.0 **First degree perineal laceration during delivery**
Perineal laceration, rupture or tear (involving):
• fourchette
• labia
• skin
• slight } during delivery
• vagina
• vulva

O70.1 **Second degree perineal laceration during delivery**

Perineal laceration, rupture or tear as in O70.0, also involving:
- pelvic floor ⎤
- perineal muscles ⎬ during delivery
- vaginal muscles ⎦

Excludes: that involving anal sphincter (O70.2)

O70.2 **Third degree perineal laceration during delivery**

Perineal laceration, rupture or tear as in O70.1, also involving:
- anal sphincter ⎤
- rectovaginal septum ⎬ during delivery
- sphincter NOS ⎦

Excludes: that involving anal or rectal mucosa (O70.3)

O70.3 **Fourth degree perineal laceration during delivery**

Perineal laceration, rupture or tear as in O70.2, also involving:
- anal mucosa ⎤
- rectal mucosa ⎦ during delivery

O70.9 **Perineal laceration during delivery, unspecified**

O71 **Other obstetric trauma**

Includes: damage from instruments

O71.0 **Rupture of uterus before onset of labour**

O71.1 **Rupture of uterus during labour**

Rupture of uterus not stated as occurring before onset of labour

O71.2 **Postpartum inversion of uterus**

O71.3 **Obstetric laceration of cervix**

Annular detachment of cervix

O71.4 **Obstetric high vaginal laceration alone**

Laceration of vaginal wall without mention of perineal laceration

Excludes: with perineal laceration (O70.–)

O71.5 **Other obstetric injury to pelvic organs**

Obstetric injury to:
- bladder
- urethra

O71.6 **Obstetric damage to pelvic joints and ligaments**

Avulsion of inner symphyseal cartilage ⎤
Damage to coccyx ⎬ obstetric
Traumatic separation of symphysis (pubis) ⎦

O71.7 **Obstetric haematoma of pelvis**
Obstetric haematoma of:
- perineum
- vagina
- vulva

O71.8 **Other specified obstetric trauma**

O71.9 **Obstetric trauma, unspecified**

O72 Postpartum haemorrhage

Includes: haemorrhage after delivery of fetus or infant

O72.0 **Third-stage haemorrhage**
Haemorrhage associated with retained, trapped or adherent placenta
Retained placenta NOS

O72.1 **Other immediate postpartum haemorrhage**
Haemorrhage following delivery of placenta
Postpartum haemorrhage (atonic) NOS

O72.2 **Delayed and secondary postpartum haemorrhage**
Haemorrhage associated with retained portions of placenta or membranes
Retained products of conception NOS, following delivery

O72.3 **Postpartum coagulation defects**
Postpartum:
- afibrinogenaemia
- fibrinolysis

O73 Retained placenta and membranes, without haemorrhage

O73.0 **Retained placenta without haemorrhage**
Placenta accreta without haemorrhage

O73.1 **Retained portions of placenta and membranes, without haemorrhage**
Retained products of conception following delivery, without haemorrhage

O74 Complications of anaesthesia during labour and delivery

Includes: maternal complications arising from the administration of a general or local anaesthetic, analgesic or other sedation during labour and delivery

O74.0 Aspiration pneumonitis due to anaesthesia during labour and delivery

Inhalation of stomach contents or secretions NOS
Mendelson's syndrome
} due to anaesthesia during labour and delivery

O74.1 Other pulmonary complications of anaesthesia during labour and delivery

Pressure collapse of lung due to anaesthesia during labour and delivery

O74.2 Cardiac complications of anaesthesia during labour and delivery

Cardiac:
- arrest
- failure
} due to anaesthesia during labour and delivery

O74.3 Central nervous system complications of anaesthesia during labour and delivery

Cerebral anoxia due to anaesthesia during labour and delivery

O74.4 Toxic reaction to local anaesthesia during labour and delivery

O74.5 Spinal and epidural anaesthesia-induced headache during labour and delivery

O74.6 Other complications of spinal and epidural anaesthesia during labour and delivery

O74.7 Failed or difficult intubation during labour and delivery

O74.8 Other complications of anaesthesia during labour and delivery

O74.9 Complication of anaesthesia during labour and delivery, unspecified

O75 Other complications of labour and delivery, not elsewhere classified

Excludes: puerperal:
- infection (O86.–)
- sepsis (O85)

O75.0 **Maternal distress during labour and delivery**

O75.1 **Shock during or following labour and delivery**
Obstetric shock

O75.2 **Pyrexia during labour, not elsewhere classified**

O75.3 **Other infection during labour**
Septicaemia during labour

O75.4 **Other complications of obstetric surgery and procedures**

Cardiac:
- arrest
- failure
Cerebral anoxia
} following caesarean or other obstetric surgery or procedures, including delivery NOS

Excludes: complications of anaesthesia during labour and delivery (O74.–)
obstetric (surgical) wound:
- disruption (O90.0–O90.1)
- haematoma (O90.2)
- infection (O86.0)

O75.5 **Delayed delivery after artificial rupture of membranes**

O75.6 **Delayed delivery after spontaneous or unspecified rupture of membranes**
Excludes: spontaneous premature rupture of membranes (O42.–)

O75.7 **Vaginal delivery following previous caesarean section**

O75.8 **Other specified complications of labour and delivery**

O75.9 **Complication of labour and delivery, unspecified**

Delivery
(O80–O84)

Note: Codes O80–O84 are provided for morbidity coding purposes. Codes from this block should be used for primary morbidity coding only if no other condition classifiable to Chapter XV is recorded. For use of these categories reference should be made to the morbidity coding rules and guidelines in Volume 2.

O80 Single spontaneous delivery

Includes: cases with minimal or no assistance, with or without episiotomy
delivery in a completely normal case

O80.0 Spontaneous vertex delivery

O80.1 Spontaneous breech delivery

O80.8 Other single spontaneous delivery

O80.9 Single spontaneous delivery, unspecified
Spontaneous delivery NOS

O81 Single delivery by forceps and vacuum extractor

Excludes: failed application of vacuum extractor or forceps (O66.5)

O81.0 Low forceps delivery

O81.1 Mid-cavity forceps delivery

O81.2 Mid-cavity forceps with rotation

O81.3 Other and unspecified forceps delivery

O81.4 Vacuum extractor delivery
Ventouse delivery

O81.5 Delivery by combination of forceps and vacuum extractor
Forceps and ventouse delivery

O82 Single delivery by caesarean section

O82.0 Delivery by elective caesarean section
Repeat caesarean section NOS

O82.1   Delivery by emergency caesarean section

O82.2   Delivery by caesarean hysterectomy

O82.8   Other single delivery by caesarean section

O82.9   Delivery by caesarean section, unspecified

O83   Other assisted single delivery

O83.0   Breech extraction

O83.1   Other assisted breech delivery
Breech delivery NOS

O83.2   Other manipulation-assisted delivery
Version with extraction

O83.3   Delivery of viable fetus in abdominal pregnancy

O83.4   Destructive operation for delivery
Cleidotomy ⎤
Craniotomy ⎬ to facilitate delivery
Embryotomy ⎦

O83.8   Other specified assisted single delivery

O83.9   Assisted single delivery, unspecified
Assisted delivery NOS

O84   Multiple delivery
Use additional code (O80–O83), if desired, to indicate the method of delivery of each fetus or infant.

O84.0   Multiple delivery, all spontaneous

O84.1   Multiple delivery, all by forceps and vacuum extractor

O84.2   Multiple delivery, all by caesarean section

O84.8   Other multiple delivery
Multiple delivery by combination of methods

O84.9   Multiple delivery, unspecified

Complications predominantly related to the puerperium (O85–O92)

Note: Categories O88.–, O91.– and O92.– include the listed conditions even if they occur during pregnancy and childbirth.

Excludes: mental and behavioural disorders associated with the puerperium (F53.–)
obstetrical tetanus (A34)
puerperal osteomalacia (M83.0)

O85   Puerperal sepsis
Puerperal:
- endometritis
- fever
- peritonitis
- septicaemia

Use additional code (B95–B97), if desired, to identify infectious agent.

Excludes: obstetric pyaemic and septic embolism (O88.3)
septicaemia during labour (O75.3)

O86   Other puerperal infections
Excludes: infection during labour (O75.3)

O86.0   Infection of obstetric surgical wound
Infected:
- caesarean section wound   }
- perineal repair   } following delivery

O86.1   Other infection of genital tract following delivery
Cervicitis }
Vaginitis } following delivery

O86.2   Urinary tract infection following delivery
Conditions in N10–N12, N15.–, N30.–, N34.–, N39.0 following delivery

O86.3   Other genitourinary tract infections following delivery
Puerperal genitourinary tract infection NOS

O86.4 **Pyrexia of unknown origin following delivery**
Puerperal:
- infection NOS
- pyrexia NOS

Excludes: puerperal fever (O85)
pyrexia during labour (O75.2)

O86.8 **Other specified puerperal infections**

O87 Venous complications in the puerperium

Includes: in labour, delivery and the puerperium
Excludes: obstetric embolism (O88.–)
venous complications in pregnancy (O22.–)

O87.0 **Superficial thrombophlebitis in the puerperium**

O87.1 **Deep phlebothrombosis in the puerperium**
Deep-vein thrombosis, postpartum
Pelvic thrombophlebitis, postpartum

O87.2 **Haemorrhoids in the puerperium**

O87.3 **Cerebral venous thrombosis in the puerperium**
Cerebrovenous sinus thrombosis in the puerperium

O87.8 **Other venous complications in the puerperium**
Genital varices in the puerperium

O87.9 **Venous complication in the puerperium, unspecified**
Puerperal:
- phlebitis NOS
- phlebopathy NOS
- thrombosis NOS

O88 Obstetric embolism

Includes: pulmonary emboli in pregnancy, childbirth or the
puerperium
Excludes: embolism complicating abortion or ectopic or molar
pregnancy (O00–O07, O08.2)

O88.0 **Obstetric air embolism**

O88.1 **Amniotic fluid embolism**

O88.2   **Obstetric blood-clot embolism**
Obstetric (pulmonary) embolism NOS
Puerperal (pulmonary) embolism NOS

O88.3   **Obstetric pyaemic and septic embolism**

O88.8   **Other obstetric embolism**
Obstetric fat embolism

O89   Complications of anaesthesia during the puerperium

Includes: maternal complications arising from the administration of a general or local anaesthetic, analgesic or other sedation during the puerperium

O89.0   **Pulmonary complications of anaesthesia during the puerperium**
Aspiration pneumonitis
Inhalation of stomach   } due to anaesthesia during the
   contents or secretions NOS   } puerperium
Mendelson's syndrome
Pressure collapse of lung

O89.1   **Cardiac complications of anaesthesia during the puerperium**
Cardiac:
• arrest   } due to anaesthesia during the puerperium
• failure

O89.2   **Central nervous system complications of anaesthesia during the puerperium**
Cerebral anoxia due to anaesthesia during the puerperium

O89.3   **Toxic reaction to local anaesthesia during the puerperium**

O89.4   **Spinal and epidural anaesthesia-induced headache during the puerperium**

O89.5   **Other complications of spinal and epidural anaesthesia during the puerperium**

O89.6   **Failed or difficult intubation during the puerperium**

O89.8   **Other complications of anaesthesia during the puerperium**

O89.9   **Complication of anaesthesia during the puerperium, unspecified**

O90 Complications of the puerperium, not elsewhere classified

O90.0 **Disruption of caesarean section wound**

O90.1 **Disruption of perineal obstetric wound**
Disruption of wound of:
- episiotomy
- perineal laceration
Secondary perineal tear

O90.2 **Haematoma of obstetric wound**

O90.3 **Cardiomyopathy in the puerperium**
Conditions in I42.–

O90.4 **Postpartum acute renal failure**
Hepatorenal syndrome following labour and delivery

O90.5 **Postpartum thyroiditis**

O90.8 **Other complications of the puerperium, not elsewhere classified**
Placental polyp

O90.9 **Complication of the puerperium, unspecified**

O91 Infections of breast associated with childbirth

Includes: the listed conditions during pregnancy, the puerperium or lactation

O91.0 **Infection of nipple associated with childbirth**
Abscess of nipple:
- gestational
- puerperal

O91.1 **Abscess of breast associated with childbirth**
Mammary abscess ⎫
Purulent mastitis ⎬ gestational or puerperal
Subareolar abscess ⎭

O91.2 **Nonpurulent mastitis associated with childbirth**
Lymphangitis of breast ⎫
Mastitis: ⎪
- NOS ⎬ gestational or puerperal
- interstitial ⎪
- parenchymatous ⎭

O92 Other disorders of breast and lactation associated with childbirth

Includes: the listed conditions during pregnancy, the
 puerperium or lactation

O92.0 Retracted nipple associated with childbirth

O92.1 Cracked nipple associated with childbirth
Fissure of nipple, gestational or puerperal

O92.2 Other and unspecified disorders of breast associated with childbirth

O92.3 Agalactia
Primary agalactia

O92.4 Hypogalactia

O92.5 Suppressed lactation
Agalactia:
• elective
• secondary
• therapeutic

O92.6 Galactorrhoea
Excludes: galactorrhoea not associated with childbirth (N64.3)

O92.7 Other and unspecified disorders of lactation
Puerperal galactocele

Other obstetric conditions, not elsewhere classified (O95–O99)

Note: For use of categories O95–O97 reference should be made to the
 mortality coding rules and guidelines in Volume 2.

O95 Obstetric death of unspecified cause
Maternal death from unspecified cause occurring during pregnancy,
 labour and delivery, or the puerperium

O96 **Death from any obstetric cause occurring more than 42 days but less than one year after delivery**

Use additional code, if desired, to identify obstetric cause of death.

O97 **Death from sequelae of direct obstetric causes**

Death from any direct obstetric cause occurring one year or more after delivery

O98 **Maternal infectious and parasitic diseases classifiable elsewhere but complicating pregnancy, childbirth and the puerperium**

Includes: the listed conditions when complicating the pregnant state, when aggravated by the pregnancy, or as a reason for obstetric care

Use additional code (Chapter I), if desired, to identify specific condition.

Excludes: asymptomatic human immunodeficiency virus [HIV] infection status (Z21)

human immunodeficiency virus [HIV] disease (B20–B24)

laboratory evidence of human immunodeficiency virus [HIV] (R75)

obstetrical tetanus (A34)

puerperal:

- infection (O86.–)
- sepsis (O85)

when the reason for maternal care is that the disease is known or suspected to have affected the fetus (O35–O36)

O98.0 **Tuberculosis complicating pregnancy, childbirth and the puerperium**

Conditions in A15–A19

O98.1 **Syphilis complicating pregnancy, childbirth and the puerperium**

Conditions in A50–A53

O98.2 **Gonorrhoea complicating pregnancy, childbirth and the puerperium**

Conditions in A54.–

O98.3   **Other infections with a predominantly sexual mode of transmission complicating pregnancy, childbirth and the puerperium**
Conditions in A55–A64

O98.4   **Viral hepatitis complicating pregnancy, childbirth and the puerperium**
Conditions in B15–B19

O98.5   **Other viral diseases complicating pregnancy, childbirth and the puerperium**
Conditions in A80–B09, B25–B34

O98.6   **Protozoal diseases complicating pregnancy, childbirth and the puerperium**
Conditions in B50–B64

O98.8   **Other maternal infectious and parasitic diseases complicating pregnancy, childbirth and the puerperium**

O98.9   **Unspecified maternal infectious or parasitic disease complicating pregnancy, childbirth and the puerperium**

O99   Other maternal diseases classifiable elsewhere but complicating pregnancy, childbirth and the puerperium

Note: This category includes conditions which complicate the pregnant state, are aggravated by the pregnancy or are a main reason for obstetric care and for which the Alphabetical Index does not indicate a specific rubric in Chapter XV.

Use additional code, if desired, to identify specific condition.

Excludes: infectious and parasitic diseases (O98.–)
injury, poisoning and certain other consequences of external causes (S00–T98)
when the reason for maternal care is that the condition is known or suspected to have affected the fetus (O35–O36)

O99.0   **Anaemia complicating pregnancy, childbirth and the puerperium**
Conditions in D50–D64

O99.1 **Other diseases of the blood and blood-forming organs and certain disorders involving the immune mechanism complicating pregnancy, childbirth and the puerperium**
Conditions in D65–D89

Excludes: haemorrhage with coagulation defects (O46.0, O67.0, O72.3)

O99.2 **Endocrine, nutritional and metabolic diseases complicating pregnancy, childbirth and the puerperium**
Conditions in E00–E90

Excludes: diabetes mellitus (O24.–)
malnutrition (O25)
postpartum thyroiditis (O90.5)

O99.3 **Mental disorders and diseases of the nervous system complicating pregnancy, childbirth and the puerperium**
Conditions in F00–F99 and G00–G99

Excludes: postnatal depression (F53.0)
pregnancy-related peripheral neuritis (O26.8)
puerperal psychosis (F53.1)

O99.4 **Diseases of the circulatory system complicating pregnancy, childbirth and the puerperium**
Conditions in I00–I99

Excludes: cardiomyopathy in the puerperium (O90.3)
hypertensive disorders (O10–O16)
obstetric embolism (O88.–)
venous complications and cerebrovenous sinus thrombosis in:
• labour, childbirth and the puerperium (O87.–)
• pregnancy (O22.–)

O99.5 **Diseases of the respiratory system complicating pregnancy, childbirth and the puerperium**
Conditions in J00–J99

O99.6 **Diseases of the digestive system complicating pregnancy, childbirth and the puerperium**
Conditions in K00–K93

Excludes: liver disorders in pregnancy, childbirth and the puerperium (O26.6)

O99.7 **Diseases of the skin and subcutaneous tissue complicating pregnancy, childbirth and the puerperium**
Conditions in L00–L99

Excludes: herpes gestationis (O26.4)

O99.8 **Other specified diseases and conditions complicating pregnancy, childbirth and the puerperium**
Combination of conditions classifiable to O99.0–O99.7
Conditions in C00–D48, H00–H95, M00–M99, N00–N99, and Q00–Q99

Excludes: genitourinary infections in pregnancy (O23.–)
infection of genitourinary tract following delivery (O86.0–O86.3)
maternal care for known or suspected abnormality of maternal pelvic organs (O34.–)
postpartum acute renal failure (O90.4)

Certain conditions originating in the perinatal period (P00–P96)

Includes: conditions that have their origin in the perinatal period even though death or morbidity occurs later

Excludes: congenital malformations, deformations and chromosomal abnormalities (Q00–Q99)
endocrine, nutritional and metabolic diseases (E00–E90)
injury, poisoning and certain other consequences of external causes (S00–T98)
neoplasms (C00–D48)
tetanus neonatorum (A33)

This chapter contains the following blocks:

P00–P04 Fetus and newborn affected by maternal factors and by complications of pregnancy, labour and delivery
P05–P08 Disorders related to length of gestation and fetal growth
P10–P15 Birth trauma
P20–P29 Respiratory and cardiovascular disorders specific to the perinatal period
P35–P39 Infections specific to the perinatal period
P50–P61 Haemorrhagic and haematological disorders of fetus and newborn
P70–P74 Transitory endocrine and metabolic disorders specific to fetus and newborn
P75–P78 Digestive system disorders of fetus and newborn
P80–P83 Conditions involving the integument and temperature regulation of fetus and newborn
P90–P96 Other disorders originating in the perinatal period

An asterisk category for this chapter is provided as follows:

P75* Meconium ileus

Fetus and newborn affected by maternal factors and by complications of pregnancy, labour and delivery (P00–P04)

Includes: the listed maternal conditions only when specified as a cause of mortality or morbidity in fetus or newborn

P00 Fetus and newborn affected by maternal conditions that may be unrelated to present pregnancy

Excludes: fetus and newborn affected by:
- maternal complications of pregnancy (P01.–)
- maternal endocrine and metabolic disorders (P70–P74)
- noxious influences transmitted via placenta or breast milk (P04.–)

P00.0 Fetus and newborn affected by maternal hypertensive disorders

Fetus or newborn affected by maternal conditions classifiable to O10–O11, O13–O16

P00.1 Fetus and newborn affected by maternal renal and urinary tract diseases

Fetus or newborn affected by maternal conditions classifiable to N00–N39

P00.2 Fetus and newborn affected by maternal infectious and parasitic diseases

Fetus or newborn affected by maternal infectious disease classifiable to A00–B99 and J10–J11, but not itself manifesting that disease

Excludes: infections specific to the perinatal period (P35–P39)
maternal genital tract and other localized infections (P00.8)

P00.3 Fetus and newborn affected by other maternal circulatory and respiratory diseases

Fetus or newborn affected by maternal conditions classifiable to I00–I99, J00–J99, Q20–Q34 and not included in P00.0, P00.2

P00.4   Fetus and newborn affected by maternal nutritional disorders

Fetus or newborn affected by maternal disorders classifiable to E40–E64

Maternal malnutrition NOS

P00.5   Fetus and newborn affected by maternal injury

Fetus or newborn affected by maternal conditions classifiable to S00–T79

P00.6   Fetus and newborn affected by surgical procedure on mother

Excludes: caesarean section for present delivery (P03.4)
damage to placenta from amniocentesis, caesarean section or surgical induction (P02.1)
previous surgery to uterus or pelvic organs (P03.8)
termination of pregnancy, fetus (P96.4)

P00.7   Fetus and newborn affected by other medical procedures on mother, not elsewhere classified

Fetus or newborn affected by radiology on mother

Excludes: damage to placenta from amniocentesis, caesarean section or surgical induction (P02.1)
fetus or newborn affected by other complications of labour and delivery (P03.–)

P00.8   Fetus and newborn affected by other maternal conditions

Fetus or newborn affected by:
- conditions classifiable to T80–T88
- maternal genital tract and other localized infections
- maternal systemic lupus erythematosus

Excludes: transitory neonatal endocrine and metabolic disorders (P70–P74)

P00.9   Fetus and newborn affected by unspecified maternal condition

P01   Fetus and newborn affected by maternal complications of pregnancy

P01.0   Fetus and newborn affected by incompetent cervix

P01.1   Fetus and newborn affected by premature rupture of membranes

P01.2   **Fetus and newborn affected by oligohydramnios**
Excludes: when due to premature rupture of membranes
(P01.1)

P01.3   **Fetus and newborn affected by polyhydramnios**
Hydramnios

P01.4   **Fetus and newborn affected by ectopic pregnancy**
Abdominal pregnancy

P01.5   **Fetus and newborn affected by multiple pregnancy**
Triplet (pregnancy)
Twin (pregnancy)

P01.6   **Fetus and newborn affected by maternal death**

P01.7   **Fetus and newborn affected by malpresentation before labour**
Breech presentation ⎫
External version ⎪
Face presentation ⎬ before labour
Transverse lie ⎪
Unstable lie ⎭

P01.8   **Fetus and newborn affected by other maternal complications of pregnancy**
Spontaneous abortion, fetus

P01.9   **Fetus and newborn affected by maternal complication of pregnancy, unspecified**

P02   **Fetus and newborn affected by complications of placenta, cord and membranes**

P02.0   **Fetus and newborn affected by placenta praevia**

P02.1   **Fetus and newborn affected by other forms of placental separation and haemorrhage**
Abruptio placentae
Accidental haemorrhage
Antepartum haemorrhage
Damage to placenta from amniocentesis, caesarean section or surgical induction
Maternal blood loss
Premature separation of placenta

P02.2 **Fetus and newborn affected by other and unspecified morphological and functional abnormalities of placenta**
Placental:
- dysfunction
- infarction
- insufficiency

P02.3 **Fetus and newborn affected by placental transfusion syndromes**
Placental and cord abnormalities resulting in twin-to-twin or other transplacental transfusion

Use additional code, if desired, to indicate resultant condition in the fetus or newborn.

P02.4 **Fetus and newborn affected by prolapsed cord**

P02.5 **Fetus and newborn affected by other compression of umbilical cord**
Cord (tightly) around neck
Entanglement of cord
Knot in cord

P02.6 **Fetus and newborn affected by other and unspecified conditions of umbilical cord**
Short cord
Vasa praevia
Excludes: single umbilical artery (Q27.0)

P02.7 **Fetus and newborn affected by chorioamnionitis**
Amnionitis
Membranitis
Placentitis

P02.8 **Fetus and newborn affected by other abnormalities of membranes**

P02.9 **Fetus and newborn affected by abnormality of membranes, unspecified**

P03 Fetus and newborn affected by other complications of labour and delivery

P03.0 **Fetus and newborn affected by breech delivery and extraction**

P03.1 **Fetus and newborn affected by other malpresentation, malposition and disproportion during labour and delivery**
Contracted pelvis
Fetus or newborn affected by conditions classifiable to O64–O66
Persistent occipitoposterior
Transverse lie

P03.2 **Fetus and newborn affected by forceps delivery**

P03.3 **Fetus and newborn affected by delivery by vacuum extractor [ventouse]**

P03.4 **Fetus and newborn affected by caesarean delivery**

P03.5 **Fetus and newborn affected by precipitate delivery**
Rapid second stage

P03.6 **Fetus and newborn affected by abnormal uterine contractions**
Fetus or newborn affected by conditions classifiable to O62.–, except O62.3
Hypertonic labour
Uterine inertia

P03.8 **Fetus and newborn affected by other specified complications of labour and delivery**
Abnormality of maternal soft tissues
Destructive operation to facilitate delivery
Fetus or newborn affected by conditions classifiable to O60–O75 and by procedures used in labour and delivery not included in P02.– and P03.0–P03.6
Induction of labour

P03.9 **Fetus and newborn affected by complication of labour and delivery, unspecified**

P04 Fetus and newborn affected by noxious influences transmitted via placenta or breast milk

Includes: nonteratogenic effects of substances transmitted via placenta
Excludes: congenital malformations (Q00–Q99)
neonatal jaundice from other excessive haemolysis due to drugs or toxins transmitted from mother (P58.4)

P04.0 **Fetus and newborn affected by maternal anaesthesia and analgesia in pregnancy, labour and delivery**
Reactions and intoxications from maternal opiates and tranquillizers administered during labour and delivery

P04.1 **Fetus and newborn affected by other maternal medication**
Cancer chemotherapy
Cytotoxic drugs
Excludes: dysmorphism due to warfarin (Q86.2)
fetal hydantoin syndrome (Q86.1)
maternal use of drugs of addiction (P04.4)

P04.2 **Fetus and newborn affected by maternal use of tobacco**

P04.3 **Fetus and newborn affected by maternal use of alcohol**
Excludes: fetal alcohol syndrome (Q86.0)

P04.4 **Fetus and newborn affected by maternal use of drugs of addiction**
Excludes: maternal anaesthesia and analgesia (P04.0)
withdrawal symptoms from maternal use of drugs of addiction (P96.1)

P04.5 **Fetus and newborn affected by maternal use of nutritional chemical substances**

P04.6 **Fetus and newborn affected by maternal exposure to environmental chemical substances**

P04.8 **Fetus and newborn affected by other maternal noxious influences**

P04.9 **Fetus and newborn affected by maternal noxious influence, unspecified**

Disorders related to length of gestation and fetal growth
(P05–P08)

P05 Slow fetal growth and fetal malnutrition

P05.0 **Light for gestational age**
Usually referred to as weight below but length above 10th centile for gestational age.

Light-for-dates

P05.1 **Small for gestational age**
Usually referred to as weight and length below 10th centile for gestational age.

Small-for-dates
Small-and-light-for-dates

P05.2 **Fetal malnutrition without mention of light or small for gestational age**
Infant, not light or small for gestational age, showing signs of fetal malnutrition, such as dry, peeling skin and loss of subcutaneous tissue.

Excludes: fetal malnutrition with mention of:
• light for gestational age (P05.0)
• small for gestational age (P05.1)

P05.9 **Slow fetal growth, unspecified**
Fetal growth retardation NOS

P07 Disorders related to short gestation and low birth weight, not elsewhere classified

Note: When both birth weight and gestational age are available, priority of assignment should be given to birth weight.

Includes: the listed conditions, without further specification, as the cause of mortality, morbidity or additional care, in newborn

Excludes: low birth weight due to slow fetal growth and fetal malnutrition (P05.–)

P07.0 **Extremely low birth weight**
Birth weight 999 g or less.

P07.1 **Other low birth weight**
Birth weight 1000–2499 g.

P07.2 **Extreme immaturity**
Less than 28 completed weeks (less than 196 completed days) of gestation.

P07.3 **Other preterm infants**
28 completed weeks or more but less than 37 completed weeks (196 completed days but less than 259 completed days) of gestation.

Prematurity NOS

P08 Disorders related to long gestation and high birth weight

Note: When both birth weight and gestational age are available, priority of assignment should be given to birth weight.

Includes: the listed conditions, without further specification, as causes of mortality, morbidity or additional care, in fetus or newborn

P08.0 **Exceptionally large baby**
Usually implies a birth weight of 4500 g or more.

Excludes: syndrome of:
- infant of diabetic mother (P70.1)
- infant of mother with gestational diabetes (P70.0)

P08.1 **Other heavy for gestational age infants**
Other fetus or infant heavy- or large-for-dates regardless of period of gestation.

P08.2 **Post-term infant, not heavy for gestational age**
Fetus or infant with gestation period of 42 completed weeks or more (294 days or more), not heavy- or large-for-dates.

Postmaturity NOS

Birth trauma
(P10–P15)

P10 Intracranial laceration and haemorrhage due to birth injury

Excludes: intracranial haemorrhage of fetus or newborn:
- NOS (P52.9)
- due to anoxia or hypoxia (P52.–)

P10.0 **Subdural haemorrhage due to birth injury**
Subdural haematoma (localized) due to birth injury
Excludes: subdural haemorrhage accompanying tentorial tear (P10.4)

P10.1 **Cerebral haemorrhage due to birth injury**

P10.2 **Intraventricular haemorrhage due to birth injury**

P10.3 **Subarachnoid haemorrhage due to birth injury**

P10.4 **Tentorial tear due to birth injury**

P10.8 **Other intracranial lacerations and haemorrhages due to birth injury**

P10.9 **Unspecified intracranial laceration and haemorrhage due to birth injury**

P11 Other birth injuries to central nervous system

P11.0 **Cerebral oedema due to birth injury**

P11.1 **Other specified brain damage due to birth injury**

P11.2 **Unspecified brain damage due to birth injury**

P11.3 **Birth injury to facial nerve**
Facial palsy due to birth injury

P11.4 **Birth injury to other cranial nerves**

P11.5 **Birth injury to spine and spinal cord**
Fracture of spine due to birth injury

P11.9 **Birth injury to central nervous system, unspecified**

P12 Birth injury to scalp

P12.0	**Cephalhaematoma due to birth injury**
P12.1	**Chignon due to birth injury**
P12.2	**Epicranial subaponeurotic haemorrhage due to birth injury**
P12.3	**Bruising of scalp due to birth injury**
P12.4	**Monitoring injury of scalp of newborn** Sampling incision Scalp clip (electrode) injury
P12.8	**Other birth injuries to scalp**
P12.9	**Birth injury to scalp, unspecified**

P13 Birth injury to skeleton
Excludes: birth injury to spine (P11.5)

P13.0	**Fracture of skull due to birth injury**
P13.1	**Other birth injuries to skull** *Excludes:* cephalhaematoma (P12.0)
P13.2	**Birth injury to femur**
P13.3	**Birth injury to other long bones**
P13.4	**Fracture of clavicle due to birth injury**
P13.8	**Birth injuries to other parts of skeleton**
P13.9	**Birth injury to skeleton, unspecified**

P14 Birth injury to peripheral nervous system

P14.0	**Erb's paralysis due to birth injury**
P14.1	**Klumpke's paralysis due to birth injury**
P14.2	**Phrenic nerve paralysis due to birth injury**
P14.3	**Other brachial plexus birth injuries**
P14.8	**Birth injuries to other parts of peripheral nervous system**
P14.9	**Birth injury to peripheral nervous system, unspecified**

P15 Other birth injuries

P15.0   **Birth injury to liver**
Rupture of liver due to birth injury

P15.1   **Birth injury to spleen**
Rupture of spleen due to birth injury

P15.2   **Sternomastoid injury due to birth injury**

P15.3   **Birth injury to eye**
Subconjunctival haemorrhage ⎫
Traumatic glaucoma ⎬ due to birth injury
⎭

P15.4   **Birth injury to face**
Facial congestion due to birth injury

P15.5   **Birth injury to external genitalia**

P15.6   **Subcutaneous fat necrosis due to birth injury**

P15.8   **Other specified birth injuries**

P15.9   **Birth injury, unspecified**

Respiratory and cardiovascular disorders specific to the perinatal period
(P20–P29)

P20 Intrauterine hypoxia

Includes: abnormal fetal heart rate
fetal or intrauterine:
• acidosis
• anoxia
• asphyxia
• distress
• hypoxia
meconium in liquor
passage of meconium

Excludes: intracranial haemorrhage due to anoxia or hypoxia
(P52.–)

P20.0   **Intrauterine hypoxia first noted before onset of labour**

P20.1   Intrauterine hypoxia first noted during labour and delivery

P20.9   Intrauterine hypoxia, unspecified

P21   Birth asphyxia

> *Note:*   This category is not to be used for low Apgar score without mention of asphyxia or other respiratory problems.

Excludes: intrauterine hypoxia or asphyxia (P20.–)

P21.0   Severe birth asphyxia
Pulse less than 100 per minute at birth and falling or steady, respiration absent or gasping, colour poor, tone absent.

Asphyxia with 1-minute Apgar score 0–3
White asphyxia

P21.1   Mild and moderate birth asphyxia
Normal respiration not established within one minute, but heart rate 100 or above, some muscle tone present, some response to stimulation.

Asphyxia with 1-minute Apgar score 4–7
Blue asphyxia

P21.9   Birth asphyxia, unspecified
Anoxia   ⎫
Asphyxia   ⎬ NOS
Hypoxia   ⎭

P22   Respiratory distress of newborn

Excludes: respiratory failure of newborn (P28.5)

P22.0   Respiratory distress syndrome of newborn
Hyaline membrane disease

P22.1   Transient tachypnoea of newborn

P22.8   Other respiratory distress of newborn

P22.9   Respiratory distress of newborn, unspecified

P23　Congenital pneumonia

Includes: infective pneumonia acquired in utero or during birth
Excludes: neonatal pneumonia resulting from aspiration (P24.–)

P23.0　**Congenital pneumonia due to viral agent**
Excludes: congenital rubella pneumonitis (P35.0)

P23.1　**Congenital pneumonia due to *Chlamydia***

P23.2　**Congenital pneumonia due to staphylococcus**

P23.3　**Congenital pneumonia due to streptococcus, group B**

P23.4　**Congenital pneumonia due to *Escherichia coli***

P23.5　**Congenital pneumonia due to *Pseudomonas***

P23.6　**Congenital pneumonia due to other bacterial agents**
Haemophilus influenzae
Klebsiella pneumoniae
Mycoplasma
Streptococcus, except group B

P23.8　**Congenital pneumonia due to other organisms**

P23.9　**Congenital pneumonia, unspecified**

P24　Neonatal aspiration syndromes

Includes: neonatal pneumonia resulting from aspiration

P24.0　**Neonatal aspiration of meconium**

P24.1　**Neonatal aspiration of amniotic fluid and mucus**
Aspiration of liquor (amnii)

P24.2　**Neonatal aspiration of blood**

P24.3　**Neonatal aspiration of milk and regurgitated food**

P24.8　**Other neonatal aspiration syndromes**

P24.9　**Neonatal aspiration syndrome, unspecified**
Neonatal aspiration pneumonia NOS

P25　Interstitial emphysema and related conditions originating in the perinatal period

P25.0　**Interstitial emphysema originating in the perinatal period**

P25.1   Pneumothorax originating in the perinatal period

P25.2   Pneumomediastinum originating in the perinatal period

P25.3   Pneumopericardium originating in the perinatal period

P25.8   Other conditions related to interstitial emphysema originating in the perinatal period

P26 Pulmonary haemorrhage originating in the perinatal period

P26.0   Tracheobronchial haemorrhage originating in the perinatal period

P26.1   Massive pulmonary haemorrhage originating in the perinatal period

P26.8   Other pulmonary haemorrhages originating in the perinatal period

P26.9   Unspecified pulmonary haemorrhage originating in the perinatal period

P27 Chronic respiratory disease originating in the perinatal period

P27.0   Wilson–Mikity syndrome
Pulmonary dysmaturity

P27.1   Bronchopulmonary dysplasia originating in the perinatal period

P27.8   Other chronic respiratory diseases originating in the perinatal period
Congenital pulmonary fibrosis
Ventilator lung in newborn

P27.9   Unspecified chronic respiratory disease originating in the perinatal period

P28 Other respiratory conditions originating in the perinatal period

Excludes: congenital malformations of the respiratory system
(Q30–Q34)

779

P28.0   Primary atelectasis of newborn
Primary failure to expand terminal respiratory units
Pulmonary:
- hypoplasia associated with short gestation
- immaturity NOS

P28.1   Other and unspecified atelectasis of newborn
Atelectasis:
- NOS
- partial
- secondary
Resorption atelectasis without respiratory distress syndrome

P28.2   Cyanotic attacks of newborn
Excludes: apnoea of newborn (P28.3–P28.4)

P28.3   Primary sleep apnoea of newborn
Sleep apnoea of newborn NOS

P28.4   Other apnoea of newborn

P28.5   Respiratory failure of newborn

P28.8   Other specified respiratory conditions of newborn
Snuffles in newborn
Excludes: early congenital syphilitic rhinitis (A50.0)

P28.9   Respiratory condition of newborn, unspecified

P29   Cardiovascular disorders originating in the perinatal period
Excludes: congenital malformations of the circulatory system
(Q20–Q28)

P29.0   Neonatal cardiac failure

P29.1   Neonatal cardiac dysrhythmia

P29.2   Neonatal hypertension

P29.3   Persistent fetal circulation
Delayed closure of ductus arteriosus

P29.4   Transient myocardial ischaemia of newborn

P29.8   Other cardiovascular disorders originating in the perinatal period

P29.9   Cardiovascular disorder originating in the perinatal period, unspecified

Infections specific to the perinatal period (P35–P39)

Includes: infections acquired in utero or during birth

Excludes: asymptomatic human immunodeficiency virus [HIV] infection status (Z21)

congenital:
- gonococcal infection (A54.–)
- pneumonia (P23.–)
- syphilis (A50.–)

human immunodeficiency virus [HIV] disease (B20–B24)

infectious diseases acquired after birth (A00–B99, J10–J11)

intestinal infectious diseases (A00–A09)

laboratory evidence of human immunodeficiency virus [HIV] (R75)

maternal infectious disease as a cause of mortality or morbidity in fetus or newborn not itself manifesting the disease (P00.2)

tetanus neonatorum (A33)

P35 Congenital viral diseases

P35.0 **Congenital rubella syndrome**
Congenital rubella pneumonitis

P35.1 **Congenital cytomegalovirus infection**

P35.2 **Congenital herpesviral [herpes simplex] infection**

P35.3 **Congenital viral hepatitis**

P35.8 **Other congenital viral diseases**
Congenital varicella [chickenpox]

P35.9 **Congenital viral disease, unspecified**

P36 Bacterial sepsis of newborn

Includes: congenital septicaemia

P36.0 **Sepsis of newborn due to streptococcus, group B**

P36.1 **Sepsis of newborn due to other and unspecified streptococci**

P36.2	Sepsis of newborn due to *Staphylococcus aureus*
P36.3	Sepsis of newborn due to other and unspecified staphylococci
P36.4	Sepsis of newborn due to *Escherichia coli*
P36.5	Sepsis of newborn due to anaerobes
P36.8	Other bacterial sepsis of newborn
P36.9	Bacterial sepsis of newborn, unspecified

P37 Other congenital infectious and parasitic diseases

Excludes: congenital syphilis (A50.–)
necrotizing enterocolitis of fetus or newborn (P77)
neonatal diarrhoea:
• infectious (A00–A09)
• noninfective (P78.3)
ophthalmia neonatorum due to gonococcus (A54.3)
tetanus neonatorum (A33)

P37.0	Congenital tuberculosis
P37.1	Congenital toxoplasmosis
	Hydrocephalus due to congenital toxoplasmosis
P37.2	Neonatal (disseminated) listeriosis
P37.3	Congenital falciparum malaria
P37.4	Other congenital malaria
P37.5	Neonatal candidiasis
P37.8	Other specified congenital infectious and parasitic diseases
P37.9	Congenital infectious or parasitic disease, unspecified

P38 Omphalitis of newborn with or without mild haemorrhage

P39 Other infections specific to the perinatal period

| P39.0 | Neonatal infective mastitis |

Excludes: breast engorgement of newborn (P83.4)
noninfective mastitis of newborn (P83.4)

P39.1   **Neonatal conjunctivitis and dacryocystitis**
Neonatal chlamydial conjunctivitis
Ophthalmia neonatorum NOS
Excludes: gonococcal conjunctivitis (A54.3)

P39.2   **Intra-amniotic infection of fetus, not elsewhere classified**

P39.3   **Neonatal urinary tract infection**

P39.4   **Neonatal skin infection**
Neonatal pyoderma
Excludes: pemphigus neonatorum (L00)
staphylococcal scalded skin syndrome (L00)

P39.8   **Other specified infections specific to the perinatal period**

P39.9   **Infection specific to the perinatal period, unspecified**

Haemorrhagic and haematological disorders of fetus and newborn
(P50–P61)

Excludes: congenital stenosis and stricture of bile ducts (Q44.3)
Crigler–Najjar syndrome (E80.5)
Dubin–Johnson syndrome (E80.6)
Gilbert's syndrome (E80.4)
hereditary haemolytic anaemias (D55–D58)

P50   Fetal blood loss
Excludes: congenital anaemia from fetal blood loss (P61.3)

P50.0   **Fetal blood loss from vasa praevia**

P50.1   **Fetal blood loss from ruptured cord**

P50.2   **Fetal blood loss from placenta**

P50.3   **Haemorrhage into co-twin**

P50.4   **Haemorrhage into maternal circulation**

P50.5   **Fetal blood loss from cut end of co-twin's cord**

P50.8   **Other fetal blood loss**

P50.9   **Fetal blood loss, unspecified**
Fetal haemorrhage NOS

P51 Umbilical haemorrhage of newborn

Excludes: omphalitis with mild haemorrhage (P38)

P51.0 Massive umbilical haemorrhage of newborn

P51.8 Other umbilical haemorrhages of newborn
Slipped umbilical ligature NOS

P51.9 Umbilical haemorrhage of newborn, unspecified

P52 Intracranial nontraumatic haemorrhage of fetus and newborn

Includes: intracranial haemorrhage due to anoxia or hypoxia
Excludes: intracranial haemorrhage due to injury:
- birth (P10.–)
- maternal (P00.5)
- other (S06.–)

P52.0 Intraventricular (nontraumatic) haemorrhage, grade 1, of fetus and newborn
Subependymal haemorrhage (without intraventricular extension)

P52.1 Intraventricular (nontraumatic) haemorrhage, grade 2, of fetus and newborn
Subependymal haemorrhage with intraventricular extension

P52.2 Intraventricular (nontraumatic) haemorrhage, grade 3, of fetus and newborn
Subependymal haemorrhage with both intraventricular and intra-cerebral extension

P52.3 Unspecified intraventricular (nontraumatic) haemorrhage of fetus and newborn

P52.4 Intracerebral (nontraumatic) haemorrhage of fetus and newborn

P52.5 Subarachnoid (nontraumatic) haemorrhage of fetus and newborn

P52.6 Cerebellar (nontraumatic) and posterior fossa haemorrhage of fetus and newborn

P52.8 Other intracranial (nontraumatic) haemorrhages of fetus and newborn

P52.9 Intracranial (nontraumatic) haemorrhage of fetus and newborn, unspecified

P53 Haemorrhagic disease of fetus and newborn
Vitamin K deficiency of newborn

P54 Other neonatal haemorrhages
Excludes: fetal blood loss (P50.–)
pulmonary haemorrhage originating in the perinatal
period (P26.–)

P54.0 **Neonatal haematemesis**
Excludes: that due to swallowed maternal blood (P78.2)

P54.1 **Neonatal melaena**
Excludes: that due to swallowed maternal blood (P78.2)

P54.2 **Neonatal rectal haemorrhage**

P54.3 **Other neonatal gastrointestinal haemorrhage**

P54.4 **Neonatal adrenal haemorrhage**

P54.5 **Neonatal cutaneous haemorrhage**
Bruising
Ecchymoses ⎫
Petechiae ⎬ in fetus or newborn
Superficial haematomata ⎭
Excludes: bruising of scalp due to birth injury (P12.3)
cephalhaematoma due to birth injury (P12.0)

P54.6 **Neonatal vaginal haemorrhage**
Pseudomenses

P54.8 **Other specified neonatal haemorrhages**

P54.9 **Neonatal haemorrhage, unspecified**

P55 Haemolytic disease of fetus and newborn

P55.0 **Rh isoimmunization of fetus and newborn**

P55.1 **ABO isoimmunization of fetus and newborn**

P55.8 **Other haemolytic diseases of fetus and newborn**

P55.9 **Haemolytic disease of fetus and newborn, unspecified**

P56 Hydrops fetalis due to haemolytic disease

Excludes: hydrops fetalis NOS (P83.2)
- not due to haemolytic disease (P83.2)

P56.0 Hydrops fetalis due to isoimmunization

P56.9 Hydrops fetalis due to other and unspecified haemolytic disease

P57 Kernicterus

P57.0 Kernicterus due to isoimmunization

P57.8 Other specified kernicterus

Excludes: Crigler–Najjar syndrome (E80.5)

P57.9 Kernicterus, unspecified

P58 Neonatal jaundice due to other excessive haemolysis

Excludes: jaundice due to isoimmunization (P55–P57)

P58.0 Neonatal jaundice due to bruising

P58.1 Neonatal jaundice due to bleeding

P58.2 Neonatal jaundice due to infection

P58.3 Neonatal jaundice due to polycythaemia

P58.4 Neonatal jaundice due to drugs or toxins transmitted from mother or given to newborn

Use additional external cause code (Chapter XX), if desired, to identify drug, if drug-induced.

P58.5 Neonatal jaundice due to swallowed maternal blood

P58.8 Neonatal jaundice due to other specified excessive haemolysis

P58.9 Neonatal jaundice due to excessive haemolysis, unspecified

P59 Neonatal jaundice from other and unspecified causes

Excludes: due to inborn errors of metabolism (E70–E90)
kernicterus (P57.–)

P59.0 Neonatal jaundice associated with preterm delivery
Hyperbilirubinaemia of prematurity
Jaundice due to delayed conjugation associated with preterm delivery

P59.1 Inspissated bile syndrome

P59.2 Neonatal jaundice from other and unspecified hepatocellular damage
Excludes: congenital viral hepatitis (P35.3)

P59.3 Neonatal jaundice from breast milk inhibitor

P59.8 Neonatal jaundice from other specified causes

P59.9 Neonatal jaundice, unspecified
Physiological jaundice (intense)(prolonged) NOS

P60 Disseminated intravascular coagulation of fetus and newborn

Defibrination syndrome of fetus or newborn

P61 Other perinatal haematological disorders

Excludes: transient hypogammaglobulinaemia of infancy (D80.7)

P61.0 Transient neonatal thrombocytopenia
Neonatal thrombocytopenia due to:
• exchange transfusion
• idiopathic maternal thrombocytopenia
• isoimmunization

P61.1 Polycythaemia neonatorum

P61.2 Anaemia of prematurity

P61.3 Congenital anaemia from fetal blood loss

P61.4 Other congenital anaemias, not elsewhere classified
Congenital anaemia NOS

P61.5 Transient neonatal neutropenia

P61.6   Other transient neonatal disorders of coagulation

P61.8   Other specified perinatal haematological disorders

P61.9   Perinatal haematological disorder, unspecified

Transitory endocrine and metabolic disorders specific to fetus and newborn (P70–P74)

Includes: transitory endocrine and metabolic disturbances caused by the infant's response to maternal endocrine and metabolic factors, or its adjustment to extrauterine existence

P70   Transitory disorders of carbohydrate metabolism specific to fetus and newborn

P70.0   Syndrome of infant of mother with gestational diabetes

P70.1   Syndrome of infant of a diabetic mother
Maternal diabetes mellitus (pre-existing) affecting fetus or newborn (with hypoglycaemia)

P70.2   Neonatal diabetes mellitus

P70.3   Iatrogenic neonatal hypoglycaemia

P70.4   Other neonatal hypoglycaemia
Transitory neonatal hypoglycaemia

P70.8   Other transitory disorders of carbohydrate metabolism of fetus and newborn

P70.9   Transitory disorder of carbohydrate metabolism of fetus and newborn, unspecified

P71   Transitory neonatal disorders of calcium and magnesium metabolism

P71.0   Cow's milk hypocalcaemia in newborn

P71.1   Other neonatal hypocalcaemia
Excludes: neonatal hypoparathyroidism (P71.4)

P71.2   **Neonatal hypomagnesaemia**

P71.3   **Neonatal tetany without calcium or magnesium deficiency**
Neonatal tetany NOS

P71.4   **Transitory neonatal hypoparathyroidism**

P71.8   **Other transitory neonatal disorders of calcium and magnesium metabolism**

P71.9   **Transitory neonatal disorder of calcium and magnesium metabolism, unspecified**

P72   Other transitory neonatal endocrine disorders

Excludes: congenital hypothyroidism with or without goitre
(E03.0–E03.1)
dyshormogenetic goitre (E07.1)
Pendred's syndrome (E07.1)

P72.0   **Neonatal goitre, not elsewhere classified**
Transitory congenital goitre with normal function

P72.1   **Transitory neonatal hyperthyroidism**
Neonatal thyrotoxicosis

P72.2   **Other transitory neonatal disorders of thyroid function, not elsewhere classified**
Transitory neonatal hypothyroidism

P72.8   **Other specified transitory neonatal endocrine disorders**

P72.9   **Transitory neonatal endocrine disorder, unspecified**

P74   Other transitory neonatal electrolyte and metabolic disturbances

P74.0   **Late metabolic acidosis of newborn**

P74.1   **Dehydration of newborn**

P74.2   **Disturbances of sodium balance of newborn**

P74.3   **Disturbances of potassium balance of newborn**

P74.4   **Other transitory electrolyte disturbances of newborn**

P74.5   **Transitory tyrosinaemia of newborn**

P74.8   **Other transitory metabolic disturbances of newborn**

P74.9   **Transitory metabolic disturbance of newborn, unspecified**

Digestive system disorders of fetus and newborn (P75–P78)

P75* Meconium ileus (E84.1†)

P76 Other intestinal obstruction of newborn
Excludes: intestinal obstruction classifiable to K56.–

P76.0 **Meconium plug syndrome**

P76.1 **Transitory ileus of newborn**
Excludes: Hirschsprung's disease (Q43.1)

P76.2 **Intestinal obstruction due to inspissated milk**

P76.8 **Other specified intestinal obstruction of newborn**

P76.9 **Intestinal obstruction of newborn, unspecified**

P77 Necrotizing enterocolitis of fetus and newborn

P78 Other perinatal digestive system disorders
Excludes: neonatal gastrointestinal haemorrhages (P54.0–P54.3)

P78.0 **Perinatal intestinal perforation**
Meconium peritonitis

P78.1 **Other neonatal peritonitis**
Neonatal peritonitis NOS

P78.2 **Neonatal haematemesis and melaena due to swallowed maternal blood**

P78.3 **Noninfective neonatal diarrhoea**
Neonatal diarrhoea NOS
Excludes: neonatal diarrhoea NOS in countries where the
condition can be presumed to be of infectious
origin (A09)

P78.8 **Other specified perinatal digestive system disorders**
Congenital cirrhosis (of liver)
Peptic ulcer of newborn

P78.9 **Perinatal digestive system disorder, unspecified**

Conditions involving the integument and temperature regulation of fetus and newborn (P80–P83)

P80 Hypothermia of newborn

P80.0 Cold injury syndrome
Severe and usually chronic hypothermia associated with a pink flushed appearance, oedema and neurological and biochemical abnormalities.
Excludes: mild hypothermia of newborn (P80.8)

P80.8 Other hypothermia of newborn
Mild hypothermia of newborn

P80.9 Hypothermia of newborn, unspecified

P81 Other disturbances of temperature regulation of newborn

P81.0 Environmental hyperthermia of newborn

P81.8 Other specified disturbances of temperature regulation of newborn

P81.9 Disturbance of temperature regulation of newborn, unspecified
Fever of newborn NOS

P83 Other conditions of integument specific to fetus and newborn

Excludes: congenital malformations of skin and integument
(Q80–Q84)
cradle cap (L21.0)
diaper [napkin] dermatitis (L22)
hydrops fetalis due to haemolytic disease (P56.–)
neonatal skin infection (P39.4)
staphylococcal scalded skin syndrome (L00)

P83.0 Sclerema neonatorum

P83.1 Neonatal erythema toxicum

P83.2 **Hydrops fetalis not due to haemolytic disease**
Hydrops fetalis NOS

P83.3 **Other and unspecified oedema specific to fetus and newborn**

P83.4 **Breast engorgement of newborn**
Noninfective mastitis of newborn

P83.5 **Congenital hydrocele**

P83.6 **Umbilical polyp of newborn**

P83.8 **Other specified conditions of integument specific to fetus and newborn**
Bronze baby syndrome
Neonatal scleroderma
Urticaria neonatorum

P83.9 **Condition of integument specific to fetus and newborn, unspecified**

Other disorders originating in the perinatal period (P90–P96)

P90 Convulsions of newborn
Excludes: benign neonatal convulsions (familial) (G40.3)

P91 Other disturbances of cerebral status of newborn

P91.0 **Neonatal cerebral ischaemia**

P91.1 **Acquired periventricular cysts of newborn**

P91.2 **Neonatal cerebral leukomalacia**

P91.3 **Neonatal cerebral irritability**

P91.4 **Neonatal cerebral depression**

P91.5 **Neonatal coma**

P91.8 **Other specified disturbances of cerebral status of newborn**

P91.9 **Disturbance of cerebral status of newborn, unspecified**

P92   Feeding problems of newborn

P92.0	**Vomiting in newborn**
P92.1	**Regurgitation and rumination in newborn**
P92.2	**Slow feeding of newborn**
P92.3	**Underfeeding of newborn**
P92.4	**Overfeeding of newborn**
P92.5	**Neonatal difficulty in feeding at breast**
P92.8	**Other feeding problems of newborn**
P92.9	**Feeding problem of newborn, unspecified**

P93   Reactions and intoxications due to drugs administered to fetus and newborn

Grey syndrome from chloramphenicol administration in newborn

Excludes: jaundice due to drugs or toxins transmitted from
mother (P58.4)
reactions and intoxications from maternal opiates,
tranquillizers and other medication (P04.0–P04.1,
P04.4)
withdrawal symptoms from:
• maternal use of drugs of addiction (P96.1)
• therapeutic use of drugs in newborn (P96.2)

P94   Disorders of muscle tone of newborn

P94.0   **Transient neonatal myasthenia gravis**
Excludes: myasthenia gravis (G70.0)

P94.1   **Congenital hypertonia**

P94.2   **Congenital hypotonia**
Nonspecific floppy baby syndrome

P94.8   **Other disorders of muscle tone of newborn**

P94.9   **Disorder of muscle tone of newborn, unspecified**

P95 Fetal death of unspecified cause
Deadborn fetus NOS
Stillbirth NOS

P96 Other conditions originating in the perinatal period

P96.0 Congenital renal failure
Uraemia of newborn

P96.1 Neonatal withdrawal symptoms from maternal use of drugs of addiction
Drug withdrawal syndrome in infant of dependent mother
Excludes: reactions and intoxications from maternal opiates
and tranquillizers administered during labour and
delivery (P04.0)

P96.2 Withdrawal symptoms from therapeutic use of drugs in newborn

P96.3 Wide cranial sutures of newborn
Neonatal craniotabes

P96.4 Termination of pregnancy, fetus and newborn
Excludes: termination of pregnancy (mother) (O04.–)

P96.5 Complications of intrauterine procedures, not elsewhere classified

P96.8 Other specified conditions originating in the perinatal period

P96.9 Condition originating in the perinatal period, unspecified
Congenital debility NOS

Congenital malformations, deformations and chromosomal abnormalities (Q00–Q99)

Excludes: inborn errors of metabolism (E70–E90)

This chapter contains the following blocks:

Q00–Q07 Congenital malformations of the nervous system
Q10–Q18 Congenital malformations of eye, ear, face and neck
Q20–Q28 Congenital malformations of the circulatory system
Q30–Q34 Congenital malformations of the respiratory system
Q35–Q37 Cleft lip and cleft palate
Q38–Q45 Other congenital malformations of the digestive system
Q50–Q56 Congenital malformations of genital organs
Q60–Q64 Congenital malformations of the urinary system
Q65–Q79 Congenital malformations and deformations of the
  musculoskeletal system
Q80–Q89 Other congenital malformations
Q90–Q99 Chromosomal abnormalities, not elsewhere classified

Congenital malformations of the nervous system (Q00–Q07)

Q00 Anencephaly and similar malformations

Q00.0 **Anencephaly**
  Acephaly
  Acrania
  Amyelencephaly
  Hemianencephaly
  Hemicephaly

Q00.1 **Craniorachischisis**

Q00.2 **Iniencephaly**

Q01 Encephalocele

Includes: encephalomyelocele
hydroencephalocele
hydromeningocele, cranial
meningocele, cerebral
meningoencephalocele

Excludes: Meckel–Gruber syndrome (Q61.9)

Q01.0 Frontal encephalocele

Q01.1 Nasofrontal encephalocele

Q01.2 Occipital encephalocele

Q01.8 Encephalocele of other sites

Q01.9 Encephalocele, unspecified

Q02 Microcephaly

Hydromicrocephaly
Micrencephalon

Excludes: Meckel–Gruber syndrome (Q61.9)

Q03 Congenital hydrocephalus

Includes: hydrocephalus in newborn

Excludes: Arnold–Chiari syndrome (Q07.0)
hydrocephalus:
• acquired (G91.–)
• due to congenital toxoplasmosis (P37.1)
• with spina bifida (Q05.0–Q05.4)

Q03.0 Malformations of aqueduct of Sylvius
Aqueduct of Sylvius:
• anomaly
• obstruction, congenital
• stenosis

Q03.1 Atresia of foramina of Magendie and Luschka
Dandy–Walker syndrome

Q03.8 Other congenital hydrocephalus

Q03.9 Congenital hydrocephalus, unspecified

Q04 Other congenital malformations of brain

Excludes: cyclopia (Q87.0)
macrocephaly (Q75.3)

Q04.0 **Congenital malformations of corpus callosum**
Agenesis of corpus callosum

Q04.1 **Arhinencephaly**

Q04.2 **Holoprosencephaly**

Q04.3 **Other reduction deformities of brain**
Absence ⎫
Agenesis ⎬ of part of brain
Aplasia ⎪
Hypoplasia ⎭
Agyria
Hydranencephaly
Lissencephaly
Microgyria
Pachygyria
Excludes: congenital malformations of corpus callosum (Q04.0)

Q04.4 **Septo-optic dysplasia**

Q04.5 **Megalencephaly**

Q04.6 **Congenital cerebral cysts**
Porencephaly
Schizencephaly
Excludes: acquired porencephalic cyst (G93.0)

Q04.8 **Other specified congenital malformations of brain**
Macrogyria

Q04.9 **Congenital malformation of brain, unspecified**
Congenital:
• anomaly ⎫
• deformity ⎬ NOS of brain
• disease or lesion ⎪
• multiple anomalies ⎭

Q05 Spina bifida

Includes: hydromeningocele (spinal)
meningocele (spinal)
meningomyelocele
myelocele
myelomeningocele
rachischisis
spina bifida (aperta)(cystica)
syringomyelocele

Excludes: Arnold–Chiari syndrome (Q07.0)
spina bifida occulta (Q76.0)

Q05.0   **Cervical spina bifida with hydrocephalus**

Q05.1   **Thoracic spina bifida with hydrocephalus**
Spina bifida:
• dorsal ⎫
• thoracolumbar ⎬ with hydrocephalus

Q05.2   **Lumbar spina bifida with hydrocephalus**
Lumbosacral spina bifida with hydrocephalus

Q05.3   **Sacral spina bifida with hydrocephalus**

Q05.4   **Unspecified spina bifida with hydrocephalus**

Q05.5   **Cervical spina bifida without hydrocephalus**

Q05.6   **Thoracic spina bifida without hydrocephalus**
Spina bifida:
• dorsal NOS
• thoracolumbar NOS

Q05.7   **Lumbar spina bifida without hydrocephalus**
Lumbosacral spina bifida NOS

Q05.8   **Sacral spina bifida without hydrocephalus**

Q05.9   **Spina bifida, unspecified**

Q06 Other congenital malformations of spinal cord

Q06.0   **Amyelia**

Q06.1   **Hypoplasia and dysplasia of spinal cord**
Atelomyelia
Myelatelia
Myelodysplasia of spinal cord

Q06.2 **Diastematomyelia**

Q06.3 **Other congenital cauda equina malformations**

Q06.4 **Hydromyelia**
Hydrorachis

Q06.8 **Other specified congenital malformations of spinal cord**

Q06.9 **Congenital malformation of spinal cord, unspecified**
Congenital:
- anomaly
- deformity } NOS of spinal cord or meninges
- disease or lesion

Q07 Other congenital malformations of nervous system

Excludes: familial dysautonomia [Riley–Day] (G90.1)
neurofibromatosis (nonmalignant) (Q85.0)

Q07.0 **Arnold–Chiari syndrome**

Q07.8 **Other specified congenital malformations of nervous system**
Agenesis of nerve
Displacement of brachial plexus
Jaw-winking syndrome
Marcus Gunn's syndrome

Q07.9 **Congenital malformation of nervous system, unspecified**
Congenital:
- anomaly
- deformity } NOS of nervous system
- disease or lesion

Congenital malformations of eye, ear, face and neck (Q10–Q18)

Excludes: cleft lip and cleft palate (Q35–Q37)
congenital malformation of:
- cervical spine (Q05.0, Q05.5, Q67.5, Q76.0–Q76.4)
- larynx (Q31.–)
- lip NEC (Q38.0)
- nose (Q30.–)
- parathyroid gland (Q89.2)
- thyroid gland (Q89.2)

Q10 Congenital malformations of eyelid, lacrimal apparatus and orbit

Excludes: cryptophthalmos:
- NOS (Q11.2)
- syndrome (Q87.0)

Q10.0 **Congenital ptosis**

Q10.1 **Congenital ectropion**

Q10.2 **Congenital entropion**

Q10.3 **Other congenital malformations of eyelid**
Ablepharon
Absence or agenesis of:
- cilia
- eyelid
Accessory:
- eyelid
- eye muscle
Blepharophimosis, congenital
Coloboma of eyelid
Congenital malformation of eyelid NOS

Q10.4 **Absence and agenesis of lacrimal apparatus**
Absence of punctum lacrimale

Q10.5 **Congenital stenosis and stricture of lacrimal duct**

Q10.6 **Other congenital malformations of lacrimal apparatus**
Congenital malformation of lacrimal apparatus NOS

Q10.7 **Congenital malformation of orbit**

Q11 Anophthalmos, microphthalmos and macrophthalmos

Q11.0 Cystic eyeball

Q11.1 Other anophthalmos
Agenesis ⎫
Aplasia ⎬ of eye
⎭

Q11.2 Microphthalmos
Cryptophthalmos NOS
Dysplasia of eye
Hypoplasia of eye
Rudimentary eye
Excludes: cryptophthalmos syndrome (Q87.0)

Q11.3 Macrophthalmos
Excludes: macrophthalmos in congenital glaucoma (Q15.0)

Q12 Congenital lens malformations

Q12.0 Congenital cataract

Q12.1 Congenital displaced lens

Q12.2 Coloboma of lens

Q12.3 Congenital aphakia

Q12.4 Spherophakia

Q12.8 Other congenital lens malformations

Q12.9 Congenital lens malformation, unspecified

Q13 Congenital malformations of anterior segment of eye

Q13.0 Coloboma of iris
Coloboma NOS

Q13.1 Absence of iris
Aniridia

Q13.2   **Other congenital malformations of iris**
Anisocoria, congenital
Atresia of pupil
Congenital malformation of iris NOS
Corectopia

Q13.3   **Congenital corneal opacity**

Q13.4   **Other congenital corneal malformations**
Congenital malformation of cornea NOS
Microcornea
Peter's anomaly

Q13.5   **Blue sclera**

Q13.8   **Other congenital malformations of anterior segment of eye**
Rieger's anomaly

Q13.9   **Congenital malformation of anterior segment of eye, unspecified**

Q14   Congenital malformations of posterior segment of eye

Q14.0   **Congenital malformation of vitreous humour**
Congenital vitreous opacity

Q14.1   **Congenital malformation of retina**
Congenital retinal aneurysm

Q14.2   **Congenital malformation of optic disc**
Coloboma of optic disc

Q14.3   **Congenital malformation of choroid**

Q14.8   **Other congenital malformations of posterior segment of eye**
Coloboma of fundus

Q14.9   **Congenital malformation of posterior segment of eye, unspecified**

Q15   Other congenital malformations of eye

Excludes: congenital nystagmus (H55)
ocular albinism (E70.3)
retinitis pigmentosa (H35.5)

Q15.0   **Congenital glaucoma**
Buphthalmos
Glaucoma of newborn
Hydrophthalmos
Keratoglobus, congenital
Macrophthalmos in congenital glaucoma
Megalocornea

Q15.8   **Other specified congenital malformations of eye**

Q15.9   **Congenital malformation of eye, unspecified**
Congenital:
• anomaly   } NOS of eye
• deformity ∫

Q16   Congenital malformations of ear causing impairment of hearing

Excludes: congenital deafness (H90.–)

Q16.0   **Congenital absence of (ear) auricle**

Q16.1   **Congenital absence, atresia and stricture of auditory canal (external)**
Atresia or stricture of osseous meatus

Q16.2   **Absence of eustachian tube**

Q16.3   **Congenital malformation of ear ossicles**
Fusion of ear ossicles

Q16.4   **Other congenital malformations of middle ear**
Congenital malformation of middle ear NOS

Q16.5   **Congenital malformation of inner ear**
Anomaly:
• membranous labyrinth
• organ of Corti

Q16.9   **Congenital malformation of ear causing impairment of hearing, unspecified**
Congenital absence of ear NOS

Q17   Other congenital malformations of ear

Excludes: preauricular sinus (Q18.1)

Q17.0   **Accessory auricle**
Accessory tragus
Polyotia
Preauricular appendage or tag
Supernumerary:
- ear
- lobule

Q17.1   **Macrotia**

Q17.2   **Microtia**

Q17.3   **Other misshapen ear**
Pointed ear

Q17.4   **Misplaced ear**
Low-set ears
Excludes: cervical auricle (Q18.2)

Q17.5   **Prominent ear**
Bat ear

Q17.8   **Other specified congenital malformations of ear**
Congenital absence of lobe of ear

Q17.9   **Congenital malformation of ear, unspecified**
Congenital anomaly of ear NOS

Q18   Other congenital malformations of face and neck

Excludes: cleft lip and cleft palate (Q35–Q37)
conditions classified to Q67.0–Q67.4
congenital malformations of skull and face bones
(Q75.–)
cyclopia (Q87.0)
dentofacial anomalies [including malocclusion] (K07.–)
malformation syndromes affecting facial appearance
(Q87.0)
persistent thyroglossal duct (Q89.2)

Q18.0   **Sinus, fistula and cyst of branchial cleft**
Branchial vestige

Q18.1 **Preauricular sinus and cyst**
Fistula (of):
- auricle, congenital
- cervicoaural

Q18.2 **Other branchial cleft malformations**
Branchial cleft malformation NOS
Cervical auricle
Otocephaly

Q18.3 **Webbing of neck**
Pterygium colli

Q18.4 **Macrostomia**

Q18.5 **Microstomia**

Q18.6 **Macrocheilia**
Hypertrophy of lip, congenital

Q18.7 **Microcheilia**

Q18.8 **Other specified congenital malformations of face and neck**
Medial:
- cyst ⎤
- fistula ⎬ of face and neck
- sinus ⎦

Q18.9 **Congenital malformation of face and neck, unspecified**
Congenital anomaly NOS of face and neck

Congenital malformations of the circulatory system (Q20–Q28)

Q20 **Congenital malformations of cardiac chambers and connections**
Excludes: dextrocardia with situs inversus (Q89.3)
mirror-image atrial arrangement with situs inversus (Q89.3)

Q20.0 **Common arterial trunk**
Persistent truncus arteriosus

Q20.1 **Double outlet right ventricle**
Taussig–Bing syndrome

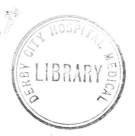

Q20.2   **Double outlet left ventricle**

Q20.3   **Discordant ventriculoarterial connection**
Dextrotransposition of aorta
Transposition of great vessels (complete)

Q20.4   **Double inlet ventricle**
Common ventricle
Cor triloculare biatriatum
Single ventricle

Q20.5   **Discordant atrioventricular connection**
Corrected transposition
Laevotransposition
Ventricular inversion

Q20.6   **Isomerism of atrial appendages**
Isomerism of atrial appendages with asplenia or polysplenia

Q20.8   **Other congenital malformations of cardiac chambers and connections**

Q20.9   **Congenital malformation of cardiac chambers and connections, unspecified**

Q21   Congenital malformations of cardiac septa
Excludes: acquired cardiac septal defect (I51.0)

Q21.0   **Ventricular septal defect**

Q21.1   **Atrial septal defect**
Coronary sinus defect
Patent or persistent:
• foramen ovale
• ostium secundum defect (type II)
Sinus venosus defect

Q21.2   **Atrioventricular septal defect**
Common atrioventricular canal
Endocardial cushion defect
Ostium primum atrial septal defect (type I)

Q21.3   **Tetralogy of Fallot**
Ventricular septal defect with pulmonary stenosis or atresia, dextroposition of aorta and hypertrophy of right ventricle.

Q21.4   **Aortopulmonary septal defect**
Aortic septal defect
Aortopulmonary window

Q21.8   Other congenital malformations of cardiac septa
Eisenmenger's syndrome
Pentalogy of Fallot

Q21.9   Congenital malformation of cardiac septum, unspecified
Septal (heart) defect NOS

Q22   Congenital malformations of pulmonary and tricuspid valves

Q22.0   Pulmonary valve atresia

Q22.1   Congenital pulmonary valve stenosis

Q22.2   Congenital pulmonary valve insufficiency
Congenital pulmonary valve regurgitation

Q22.3   Other congenital malformations of pulmonary valve
Congenital malformation of pulmonary valve NOS

Q22.4   Congenital tricuspid stenosis
Tricuspid atresia

Q22.5   Ebstein's anomaly

Q22.6   Hypoplastic right heart syndrome

Q22.8   Other congenital malformations of tricuspid valve

Q22.9   Congenital malformation of tricuspid valve, unspecified

Q23   Congenital malformations of aortic and mitral valves

Q23.0   Congenital stenosis of aortic valve
Congenital aortic:
• atresia
• stenosis
Excludes: congenital subaortic stenosis (Q24.4)
             that in hypoplastic left heart syndrome (Q23.4)

Q23.1   Congenital insufficiency of aortic valve
Bicuspid aortic valve
Congenital aortic insufficiency

Q23.2   Congenital mitral stenosis
Congenital mitral atresia

Q23.3   Congenital mitral insufficiency

Q23.4   Hypoplastic left heart syndrome
Atresia, or marked hypoplasia of aortic orifice or valve, with
hypoplasia of ascending aorta and defective development of left
ventricle (with mitral valve stenosis or atresia).

Q23.8   Other congenital malformations of aortic and mitral valves

**Q23.9   Congenital malformation of aortic and mitral valves,
unspecified**

Q24   Other congenital malformations of heart
Excludes: endocardial fibroelastosis (I42.4)

Q24.0   Dextrocardia
Excludes: dextrocardia with situs inversus (Q89.3)
isomerism of atrial appendages (with asplenia or
polysplenia) (Q20.6)
mirror-image atrial arrangement with situs inversus
(Q89.3)

Q24.1   Laevocardia

Q24.2   Cor triatriatum

Q24.3   Pulmonary infundibular stenosis

Q24.4   Congenital subaortic stenosis

Q24.5   Malformation of coronary vessels
Congenital coronary (artery) aneurysm

Q24.6   Congenital heart block

Q24.8   Other specified congenital malformations of heart
Congenital:
• diverticulum of left ventricle
• malformation of:
  • myocardium
  • pericardium
Malposition of heart
Uhl's disease

Q24.9   Congenital malformation of heart, unspecified
Congenital:
• anomaly ⎫
         ⎬ NOS of heart
• disease ⎭

Q25 Congenital malformations of great arteries

Q25.0 **Patent ductus arteriosus**
Patent ductus Botallo
Persistent ductus arteriosus

Q25.1 **Coarctation of aorta**
Coarctation of aorta (preductal)(postductal)

Q25.2 **Atresia of aorta**

Q25.3 **Stenosis of aorta**
Supravalvular aortic stenosis
Excludes: congenital aortic stenosis (Q23.0)

Q25.4 **Other congenital malformations of aorta**
Absence ⎫
Aplasia ⎪
Congenital ⎬ of aorta
• aneurysm ⎪
• dilatation ⎭
Aneurysm of sinus of Valsalva (ruptured)
Double aortic arch [vascular ring of aorta]
Hypoplasia of aorta
Persistent:
• convolutions of aortic arch
• right aortic arch
Excludes: hypoplasia of aorta in hypoplastic left heart syndrome
(Q23.4)

Q25.5 **Atresia of pulmonary artery**

Q25.6 **Stenosis of pulmonary artery**

Q25.7 **Other congenital malformations of pulmonary artery**
Aberrant pulmonary artery
Agenesis ⎫
Aneurysm ⎪
Anomaly ⎬ of pulmonary artery
Hypoplasia ⎭
Pulmonary arteriovenous aneurysm

Q25.8 **Other congenital malformations of great arteries**

Q25.9 **Congenital malformation of great arteries, unspecified**

Q26 Congenital malformations of great veins

Q26.0 **Congenital stenosis of vena cava**
Congenital stenosis of vena cava (inferior)(superior)

Q26.1 **Persistent left superior vena cava**

Q26.2 **Total anomalous pulmonary venous connection**

Q26.3 **Partial anomalous pulmonary venous connection**

Q26.4 **Anomalous pulmonary venous connection, unspecified**

Q26.5 **Anomalous portal venous connection**

Q26.6 **Portal vein–hepatic artery fistula**

Q26.8 **Other congenital malformations of great veins**
Absence of vena cava (inferior)(superior)
Azygos continuation of inferior vena cava
Persistent left posterior cardinal vein
Scimitar syndrome

Q26.9 **Congenital malformation of great vein, unspecified**
Anomaly of vena cava (inferior)(superior) NOS

Q27 Other congenital malformations of peripheral vascular system

Excludes: anomalies of:
- cerebral and precerebral vessels (Q28.0–Q28.3)
- coronary vessels (Q24.5)
- pulmonary artery (Q25.5–Q25.7)
congenital retinal aneurysm (Q14.1)
haemangioma and lymphangioma (D18.–)

Q27.0 **Congenital absence and hypoplasia of umbilical artery**
Single umbilical artery

Q27.1 **Congenital renal artery stenosis**

Q27.2 **Other congenital malformations of renal artery**
Congenital malformation of renal artery NOS
Multiple renal arteries

Q27.3 **Peripheral arteriovenous malformation**
Arteriovenous aneurysm
Excludes: acquired arteriovenous aneurysm (I77.0)

Q27.4 **Congenital phlebectasia**

Q27.8 **Other specified congenital malformations of peripheral vascular system**
Aberrant subclavian artery
Absence ⎫
Atresia ⎭ of artery or vein NEC
Congenital:
- aneurysm (peripheral)
- stricture, artery
- varix

Q27.9 **Congenital malformation of peripheral vascular system, unspecified**
Anomaly of artery or vein NOS

Q28 Other congenital malformations of circulatory system

Excludes: congenital aneurysm:
- NOS (Q27.8)
- coronary (Q24.5)
- peripheral (Q27.8)
- pulmonary (Q25.7)
- retinal (Q14.1)
ruptured:
- cerebral arteriovenous malformation (I60.8)
- malformation of precerebral vessels (I72.–)

Q28.0 **Arteriovenous malformation of precerebral vessels**
Congenital arteriovenous precerebral aneurysm (nonruptured)

Q28.1 **Other malformations of precerebral vessels**
Congenital:
- malformation of precerebral vessels NOS
- precerebral aneurysm (nonruptured)

Q28.2 **Arteriovenous malformation of cerebral vessels**
Arteriovenous malformation of brain NOS
Congenital arteriovenous cerebral aneurysm (nonruptured)

Q28.3 **Other malformations of cerebral vessels**
Congenital:
- cerebral aneurysm (nonruptured)
- malformation of cerebral vessels NOS

Q28.8   **Other specified congenital malformations of circulatory system**
Congenital aneurysm, specified site NEC

Q28.9   **Congenital malformation of circulatory system, unspecified**

Congenital malformations of the respiratory system (Q30–Q34)

Q30   Congenital malformations of nose

Excludes: congenital deviation of nasal septum (Q67.4)

Q30.0   **Choanal atresia**
Atresia
Congenital stenosis } of nares (anterior)(posterior)

Q30.1   **Agenesis and underdevelopment of nose**
Congenital absence of nose

Q30.2   **Fissured, notched and cleft nose**

Q30.3   **Congenital perforated nasal septum**

Q30.8   **Other congenital malformations of nose**
Accessory nose
Congenital anomaly of nasal sinus wall

Q30.9   **Congenital malformation of nose, unspecified**

Q31   Congenital malformations of larynx

Q31.0   **Web of larynx**
Web of larynx:
• NOS
• glottic
• subglottic

Q31.1   **Congenital subglottic stenosis**

Q31.2   **Laryngeal hypoplasia**

Q31.3   **Laryngocele**

Q31.4   **Congenital laryngeal stridor**
Congenital stridor (larynx) NOS

Q31.8 **Other congenital malformations of larynx**

Absence ⎤
Agenesis ⎬ of cricoid cartilage, epiglottis, glottis, larynx or
Atresia ⎦   thyroid cartilage
Cleft thyroid cartilage
Congenital stenosis of larynx NEC
Fissure of epiglottis
Posterior cleft of cricoid cartilage

Q31.9 **Congenital malformation of larynx, unspecified**

Q32 Congenital malformations of trachea and bronchus

Excludes: congenital bronchiectasis (Q33.4)

Q32.0 **Congenital tracheomalacia**

Q32.1 **Other congenital malformations of trachea**

Anomaly of tracheal cartilage
Atresia of trachea
Congenital:
• dilatation ⎤
• malformation ⎬ of trachea
• stenosis ⎦
• tracheocele

Q32.2 **Congenital bronchomalacia**

Q32.3 **Congenital stenosis of bronchus**

Q32.4 **Other congenital malformations of bronchus**

Absence ⎤
Agenesis ⎥
Atresia ⎬ of bronchus
Congenital malformation NOS ⎥
Diverticulum ⎦

Q33 Congenital malformations of lung

Q33.0 Congenital cystic lung
Congenital:
- honeycomb lung
- lung disease:
  - cystic
  - polycystic

Excludes: cystic lung disease, acquired or unspecified (J98.4)

Q33.1 Accessory lobe of lung

Q33.2 Sequestration of lung

Q33.3 Agenesis of lung
Absence of lung (lobe)

Q33.4 Congenital bronchiectasis

Q33.5 Ectopic tissue in lung

Q33.6 Hypoplasia and dysplasia of lung

Excludes: pulmonary hypoplasia associated with short gestation (P28.0)

Q33.8 Other congenital malformations of lung

Q33.9 Congenital malformation of lung, unspecified

Q34 Other congenital malformations of respiratory system

Q34.0 Anomaly of pleura

Q34.1 Congenital cyst of mediastinum

Q34.8 Other specified congenital malformations of respiratory system
Atresia of nasopharynx

Q34.9 Congenital malformation of respiratory system, unspecified
Congenital:
- absence
- anomaly NOS } of respiratory organ

Cleft lip and cleft palate
(Q35–Q37)

Excludes: Robin's syndrome (Q87.0)

Q35 Cleft palate
Includes: fissure of palate
palatoschisis
Excludes: cleft palate with cleft lip (Q37.–)

Q35.0 Cleft hard palate, bilateral

Q35.1 Cleft hard palate, unilateral
Cleft hard palate NOS

Q35.2 Cleft soft palate, bilateral

Q35.3 Cleft soft palate, unilateral
Cleft soft palate NOS

Q35.4 Cleft hard palate with cleft soft palate, bilateral

Q35.5 Cleft hard palate with cleft soft palate, unilateral
Cleft hard palate with cleft soft palate NOS

Q35.6 Cleft palate, medial

Q35.7 Cleft uvula

Q35.8 Cleft palate, unspecified, bilateral

Q35.9 Cleft palate, unspecified, unilateral
Cleft palate NOS

Q36 Cleft lip
Includes: cheiloschisis
congenital fissure of lip
harelip
labium leporinum
Excludes: cleft lip with cleft palate (Q37.–)

Q36.0 Cleft lip, bilateral

Q36.1 Cleft lip, medial

Q36.9 Cleft lip, unilateral
Cleft lip NOS

Q37 Cleft palate with cleft lip

Q37.0 **Cleft hard palate with cleft lip, bilateral**

Q37.1 **Cleft hard palate with cleft lip, unilateral**
Cleft hard palate with cleft lip NOS

Q37.2 **Cleft soft palate with cleft lip, bilateral**

Q37.3 **Cleft soft palate with cleft lip, unilateral**
Cleft soft palate with cleft lip NOS

Q37.4 **Cleft hard and soft palate with cleft lip, bilateral**

Q37.5 **Cleft hard and soft palate with cleft lip, unilateral**
Cleft hard and soft palate with cleft lip NOS

Q37.8 **Unspecified cleft palate with cleft lip, bilateral**

Q37.9 **Unspecified cleft palate with cleft lip, unilateral**
Cleft palate with cleft lip NOS

Other congenital malformations of the digestive system
(Q38–Q45)

Q38 Other congenital malformations of tongue, mouth and pharynx

Excludes: macrostomia (Q18.4)
microstomia (Q18.5)

Q38.0 **Congenital malformations of lips, not elsewhere classified**
Congenital:
• fistula of lip
• malformation of lip NOS
Van der Woude's syndrome

Excludes: cleft lip (Q36.–)
• with cleft palate (Q37.–)
macrocheilia (Q18.6)
microcheilia (Q18.7)

Q38.1 **Ankyloglossia**
Tongue tie

Q38.2 **Macroglossia**

Q38.3 **Other congenital malformations of tongue**
Aglossia
Bifid tongue
Congenital:
• adhesion
• fissure } of tongue
• malformation NOS
Hypoglossia
Hypoplasia of tongue
Microglossia

Q38.4 **Congenital malformations of salivary glands and ducts**
Absence
Accessory } (of) salivary gland or duct
Atresia
Congenital fistula of salivary gland

Q38.5 **Congenital malformations of palate, not elsewhere classified**
Absence of uvula
Congenital malformation of palate NOS
High arched palate
Excludes: cleft palate (Q35.–)
• with cleft lip (Q37.–)

Q38.6 **Other congenital malformations of mouth**
Congenital malformation of mouth NOS

Q38.7 **Pharyngeal pouch**
Diverticulum of pharynx
Excludes: pharyngeal pouch syndrome (D82.1)

Q38.8 **Other congenital malformations of pharynx**
Congenital malformation of pharynx NOS

Q39 **Congenital malformations of oesophagus**

Q39.0 **Atresia of oesophagus without fistula**
Atresia of oesophagus NOS

Q39.1 **Atresia of oesophagus with tracheo-oesophageal fistula**
Atresia of oesophagus with broncho-oesophageal fistula

Q39.2 **Congenital tracheo-oesophageal fistula without atresia**
Congenital tracheo-oesophageal fistula NOS

Q39.3   Congenital stenosis and stricture of oesophagus

Q39.4   Oesophageal web

Q39.5   Congenital dilatation of oesophagus

Q39.6   Diverticulum of oesophagus
Oesophageal pouch

Q39.8   Other congenital malformations of oesophagus
Absent ⎫
Congenital displacement ⎬ (of) oesophagus
Duplication ⎭

Q39.9   Congenital malformation of oesophagus, unspecified

Q40 Other congenital malformations of upper alimentary tract

Q40.0   Congenital hypertrophic pyloric stenosis
Congenital or infantile:
- constriction ⎫
- hypertrophy ⎪
- spasm ⎬ of pylorus
- stenosis ⎪
- stricture ⎭

Q40.1   Congenital hiatus hernia
Displacement of cardia through oesophageal hiatus
Excludes: congenital diaphragmatic hernia (Q79.0)

Q40.2   Other specified congenital malformations of stomach
Congenital:
- cardiospasm
- displacement of stomach
- diverticulum of stomach
- hourglass stomach
Duplication of stomach
Megalogastria
Microgastria

Q40.3   Congenital malformation of stomach, unspecified

Q40.8   Other specified congenital malformations of upper alimentary tract

Q40.9 **Congenital malformation of upper alimentary tract, unspecified**
Congenital:
- anomaly ⎫
- deformity ⎭ NOS of upper alimentary tract

Q41 Congenital absence, atresia and stenosis of small intestine

Includes: congenital obstruction, occlusion and stricture of small intestine or intestine NOS

Excludes: meconium ileus (E84.1)

Q41.0 **Congenital absence, atresia and stenosis of duodenum**

Q41.1 **Congenital absence, atresia and stenosis of jejunum**
Apple peel syndrome
Imperforate jejunum

Q41.2 **Congenital absence, atresia and stenosis of ileum**

Q41.8 **Congenital absence, atresia and stenosis of other specified parts of small intestine**

Q41.9 **Congenital absence, atresia and stenosis of small intestine, part unspecified**
Congenital absence, atresia and stenosis of intestine NOS

Q42 Congenital absence, atresia and stenosis of large intestine

Includes: congenital obstruction, occlusion and stricture of large intestine

Q42.0 **Congenital absence, atresia and stenosis of rectum with fistula**

Q42.1 **Congenital absence, atresia and stenosis of rectum without fistula**
Imperforate rectum

Q42.2 **Congenital absence, atresia and stenosis of anus with fistula**

Q42.3 **Congenital absence, atresia and stenosis of anus without fistula**
Imperforate anus

Q42.8   **Congenital absence, atresia and stenosis of other parts of large intestine**

Q42.9   **Congenital absence, atresia and stenosis of large intestine, part unspecified**

Q43   Other congenital malformations of intestine

Q43.0   **Meckel's diverticulum**
Persistent:
• omphalomesenteric duct
• vitelline duct

Q43.1   **Hirschsprung's disease**
Aganglionosis
Congenital (aganglionic) megacolon

Q43.2   **Other congenital functional disorders of colon**
Congenital dilatation of colon

Q43.3   **Congenital malformations of intestinal fixation**
Congenital adhesions [bands]:
• omental, anomalous
• peritoneal
Jackson's membrane
Malrotation of colon
Rotation:
• failure of ⎫
• incomplete ⎬ of caecum and colon
• insufficient ⎭
Universal mesentery

Q43.4   **Duplication of intestine**

Q43.5   **Ectopic anus**

Q43.6   **Congenital fistula of rectum and anus**
Excludes: congenital fistula:
        • rectovaginal (Q52.2)
        • urethrorectal (Q64.7)
        pilonidal fistula or sinus (L05.–)
        with absence, atresia and stenosis (Q42.0, Q42.2)

Q43.7   **Persistent cloaca**
Cloaca NOS

Q43.8 **Other specified congenital malformations of intestine**
Congenital:
- blind loop syndrome
- diverticulitis, colon
- diverticulum, intestine
Dolichocolon
Megaloappendix
Megaloduodenum
Microcolon
Transposition of:
- appendix
- colon
- intestine

Q43.9 **Congenital malformation of intestine, unspecified**

Q44 Congenital malformations of gallbladder, bile ducts and liver

Q44.0 **Agenesis, aplasia and hypoplasia of gallbladder**
Congenital absence of gallbladder

Q44.1 **Other congenital malformations of gallbladder**
Congenital malformation of gallbladder NOS
Intrahepatic gallbladder

Q44.2 **Atresia of bile ducts**

Q44.3 **Congenital stenosis and stricture of bile ducts**

Q44.4 **Choledochal cyst**

Q44.5 **Other congenital malformations of bile ducts**
Accessory hepatic duct
Congenital malformation of bile duct NOS
Duplication:
- biliary duct
- cystic duct

Q44.6 **Cystic disease of liver**
Fibrocystic disease of liver

821

Q44.7   **Other congenital malformations of liver**
Accessory liver
Alagille's syndrome
Congenital:
- absence of liver
- hepatomegaly
- malformation of liver NOS

Q45   **Other congenital malformations of digestive system**
Excludes: congenital:
- diaphragmatic hernia (Q79.0)
- hiatus hernia (Q40.1)

Q45.0   **Agenesis, aplasia and hypoplasia of pancreas**
Congenital absence of pancreas

Q45.1   **Annular pancreas**

Q45.2   **Congenital pancreatic cyst**

Q45.3   **Other congenital malformations of pancreas and pancreatic duct**
Accessory pancreas
Congenital malformation of pancreas or pancreatic duct NOS
Excludes: diabetes mellitus:
- congenital (E10.–)
- neonatal (P70.2)
fibrocystic disease of pancreas (E84.–)

Q45.8   **Other specified congenital malformations of digestive system**
Absence (complete)(partial) of alimentary tract NOS
Duplication
Malposition, congenital } of digestive organs NOS

Q45.9   **Congenital malformation of digestive system, unspecified**
Congenital:
- anomaly
- deformity } NOS of digestive system

Congenital malformations of genital organs (Q50–Q56)

Excludes: androgen resistance syndrome (E34.5)

syndromes associated with anomalies in the number and form of chromosomes (Q90–Q99)

testicular feminization syndrome (E34.5)

Q50 Congenital malformations of ovaries, fallopian tubes and broad ligaments

Q50.0 Congenital absence of ovary

Excludes: Turner's syndrome (Q96.–)

Q50.1 Developmental ovarian cyst

Q50.2 Congenital torsion of ovary

Q50.3 Other congenital malformations of ovary

Accessory ovary

Congenital malformation of ovary NOS

Ovarian streak

Q50.4 Embryonic cyst of fallopian tube

Fimbrial cyst

Q50.5 Embryonic cyst of broad ligament

Cyst:

• epoophoron

• Gartner's duct

• parovarian

Q50.6 Other congenital malformations of fallopian tube and broad ligament

Absence ⎫

Accessory ⎬ (of) fallopian tube or broad ligament

Atresia ⎭

Congenital malformation of fallopian tube or broad ligament NOS

Q51 Congenital malformations of uterus and cervix

Q51.0 Agenesis and aplasia of uterus

Congenital absence of uterus

Q51.1   **Doubling of uterus with doubling of cervix and vagina**

Q51.2   **Other doubling of uterus**
Doubling of uterus NOS

Q51.3   **Bicornate uterus**

Q51.4   **Unicornate uterus**

Q51.5   **Agenesis and aplasia of cervix**
Congenital absence of cervix

Q51.6   **Embryonic cyst of cervix**

Q51.7   **Congenital fistulae between uterus and digestive and urinary tracts**

Q51.8   **Other congenital malformations of uterus and cervix**
Hypoplasia of uterus and cervix

Q51.9   **Congenital malformation of uterus and cervix, unspecified**

Q52   Other congenital malformations of female genitalia

Q52.0   **Congenital absence of vagina**

Q52.1   **Doubling of vagina**
Septate vagina
Excludes: doubling of vagina with doubling of uterus and cervix (Q51.1)

Q52.2   **Congenital rectovaginal fistula**
Excludes: cloaca (Q43.7)

Q52.3   **Imperforate hymen**

Q52.4   **Other congenital malformations of vagina**
Congenital malformation of vagina NOS
Cyst:
• canal of Nuck, congenital
• embryonic vaginal

Q52.5   **Fusion of labia**

Q52.6   **Congenital malformation of clitoris**

Q52.7   **Other congenital malformations of vulva**
Congenital:
• absence ⎫
• cyst ⎬ of vulva
• malformation NOS ⎭

Q52.8   **Other specified congenital malformations of female genitalia**

Q52.9   **Congenital malformation of female genitalia, unspecified**

Q53   Undescended testicle

Q53.0   **Ectopic testis**
Unilateral or bilateral ectopic testes

Q53.1   **Undescended testicle, unilateral**

Q53.2   **Undescended testicle, bilateral**

Q53.9   **Undescended testicle, unspecified**
Cryptorchism NOS

Q54   Hypospadias
Excludes: epispadias (Q64.0)

Q54.0   **Hypospadias, balanic**
Hypospadias:
- coronal
- glandular

Q54.1   **Hypospadias, penile**

Q54.2   **Hypospadias, penoscrotal**

Q54.3   **Hypospadias, perineal**

Q54.4   **Congenital chordee**

Q54.8   **Other hypospadias**

Q54.9   **Hypospadias, unspecified**

Q55   Other congenital malformations of male genital organs
Excludes: congenital hydrocele (P83.5)
          hypospadias (Q54.–)

Q55.0   **Absence and aplasia of testis**
Monorchism

Q55.1   **Hypoplasia of testis and scrotum**
Fusion of testes

Q55.2 Other congenital malformations of testis and scrotum
Congenital malformation of testis or scrotum NOS
Polyorchism
Retractile testis
Testis migrans

Q55.3 Atresia of vas deferens

Q55.4 Other congenital malformations of vas deferens, epididymis, seminal vesicles and prostate
Absence or aplasia of:
• prostate
• spermatic cord
Congenital malformation of vas deferens, epididymis, seminal vesicles or prostate NOS

Q55.5 Congenital absence and aplasia of penis

Q55.6 Other congenital malformations of penis
Congenital malformation of penis NOS
Curvature of penis (lateral)
Hypoplasia of penis

Q55.8 Other specified congenital malformations of male genital organs

Q55.9 Congenital malformation of male genital organ, unspecified
Congenital:
• anomaly ⎫
       ⎬ NOS of male genital organ
• deformity ⎭

Q56 Indeterminate sex and pseudohermaphroditism

Excludes: pseudohermaphroditism:
        • female, with adrenocortical disorder (E25.–)
        • male, with androgen resistance (E34.5)
        • with specified chromosomal anomaly (Q96–Q99)

Q56.0 Hermaphroditism, not elsewhere classified
Ovotestis

Q56.1 Male pseudohermaphroditism, not elsewhere classified
Male pseudohermaphroditism NOS

Q56.2 Female pseudohermaphroditism, not elsewhere classified
Female pseudohermaphroditism NOS

Q56.3   **Pseudohermaphroditism, unspecified**

Q56.4   **Indeterminate sex, unspecified**
Ambiguous genitalia

Congenital malformations of the urinary system (Q60–Q64)

Q60   Renal agenesis and other reduction defects of kidney

Includes: atrophy of kidney:
- congenital
- infantile

congenital absence of kidney

Q60.0   **Renal agenesis, unilateral**

Q60.1   **Renal agenesis, bilateral**

Q60.2   **Renal agenesis, unspecified**

Q60.3   **Renal hypoplasia, unilateral**

Q60.4   **Renal hypoplasia, bilateral**

Q60.5   **Renal hypoplasia, unspecified**

Q60.6   **Potter's syndrome**

Q61   Cystic kidney disease

Excludes: acquired cyst of kidney (N28.1)
Potter's syndrome (Q60.6)

Q61.0   **Congenital single renal cyst**
Cyst of kidney (congenital)(single)

Q61.1   **Polycystic kidney, infantile type**

Q61.2   **Polycystic kidney, adult type**

Q61.3   **Polycystic kidney, unspecified**

Q61.4   **Renal dysplasia**

Q61.5   **Medullary cystic kidney**
Sponge kidney NOS

Q61.8 **Other cystic kidney diseases**
Fibrocystic:
- kidney
- renal degeneration or disease

Q61.9 **Cystic kidney disease, unspecified**
Meckel–Gruber syndrome

Q62 Congenital obstructive defects of renal pelvis and congenital malformations of ureter

Q62.0 **Congenital hydronephrosis**

Q62.1 **Atresia and stenosis of ureter**
Congenital occlusion of:
- ureter
- ureteropelvic junction
- ureterovesical orifice
Impervious ureter

Q62.2 **Congenital megaloureter**
Congenital dilatation of ureter

Q62.3 **Other obstructive defects of renal pelvis and ureter**
Congenital ureterocele

Q62.4 **Agenesis of ureter**
Absent ureter

Q62.5 **Duplication of ureter**
Accessory ⎱
Double ⎰ ureter

Q62.6 **Malposition of ureter**
Deviation ⎱
Displacement ⎮
Ectopic ⎰ (of) ureter or ureteric orifice
Implantation, anomalous ⎰

Q62.7 **Congenital vesico-uretero-renal reflux**

Q62.8 **Other congenital malformations of ureter**
Anomaly of ureter NOS

Q63   Other congenital malformations of kidney

Excludes: congenital nephrotic syndrome (N04.–)

Q63.0   Accessory kidney

Q63.1   Lobulated, fused and horseshoe kidney

Q63.2   Ectopic kidney
Congenital displaced kidney
Malrotation of kidney

Q63.3   Hyperplastic and giant kidney

Q63.8   Other specified congenital malformations of kidney
Congenital renal calculi

Q63.9   Congenital malformation of kidney, unspecified

Q64   Other congenital malformations of urinary system

Q64.0   Epispadias
Excludes: hypospadias (Q54.–)

Q64.1   Exstrophy of urinary bladder
Ectopia vesicae
Extroversion of bladder

Q64.2   Congenital posterior urethral valves

Q64.3   Other atresia and stenosis of urethra and bladder neck
Congenital:
• bladder neck obstruction
• stricture of:
  • urethra
  • urinary meatus
  • vesicourethral orifice
Impervious urethra

Q64.4   Malformation of urachus
Cyst of urachus
Patent urachus
Prolapse of urachus

Q64.5   Congenital absence of bladder and urethra

Q64.6   Congenital diverticulum of bladder

Q64.7   **Other congenital malformations of bladder and urethra**
Accessory:
• bladder
• urethra
Congenital:
• hernia of bladder
• malformation of bladder or urethra NOS
• prolapse of:
  • bladder (mucosa)
  • urethra
  • urinary meatus
• urethrorectal fistula
Double:
• urethra
• urinary meatus

Q64.8   **Other specified congenital malformations of urinary system**

Q64.9   **Congenital malformation of urinary system, unspecified**
Congenital:
• anomaly
• deformity } NOS of urinary system

Congenital malformations and deformations of the musculoskeletal system (Q65–Q79)

Q65 Congenital deformities of hip
Excludes: clicking hip (R29.4)

Q65.0   **Congenital dislocation of hip, unilateral**

Q65.1   **Congenital dislocation of hip, bilateral**

Q65.2   **Congenital dislocation of hip, unspecified**

Q65.3   **Congenital subluxation of hip, unilateral**

Q65.4   **Congenital subluxation of hip, bilateral**

Q65.5   **Congenital subluxation of hip, unspecified**

Q65.6   **Unstable hip**
Dislocatable hip
Subluxatable hip

Q65.8 **Other congenital deformities of hip**
Anteversion of femoral neck
Congenital acetabular dysplasia
Congenital coxa:
- valga
- vara

Q65.9 **Congenital deformity of hip, unspecified**

Q66 Congenital deformities of feet

Excludes: reduction defects of feet (Q72.–)
valgus deformities (acquired) (M21.0)
varus deformities (acquired) (M21.1)

Q66.0 **Talipes equinovarus**

Q66.1 **Talipes calcaneovarus**

Q66.2 **Metatarsus varus**

Q66.3 **Other congenital varus deformities of feet**
Hallux varus, congenital

Q66.4 **Talipes calcaneovalgus**

Q66.5 **Congenital pes planus**
Flat foot:
- congenital
- rigid
- spastic (everted)

Q66.6 **Other congenital valgus deformities of feet**
Metatarsus valgus

Q66.7 **Pes cavus**

Q66.8 **Other congenital deformities of feet**
Clubfoot NOS
Hammer toe, congenital
Talipes:
- NOS
- asymmetric
Tarsal coalition
Vertical talus

Q66.9 **Congenital deformity of feet, unspecified**

Q67 Congenital musculoskeletal deformities of head, face, spine and chest

Excludes: congenital malformation syndromes classified to
Q87.–
Potter's syndrome (Q60.6)

Q67.0 Facial asymmetry

Q67.1 Compression facies

Q67.2 Dolichocephaly

Q67.3 Plagiocephaly

Q67.4 Other congenital deformities of skull, face and jaw
Depressions in skull
Deviation of nasal septum, congenital
Hemifacial atrophy or hypertrophy
Squashed or bent nose, congenital

Excludes: dentofacial anomalies [including malocclusion] (K07.–)
syphilitic saddle nose (A50.5)

Q67.5 Congenital deformity of spine
Congenital scoliosis:
• NOS
• postural

Excludes: infantile idiopathic scoliosis (M41.0)
scoliosis due to congenital bony malformation (Q76.3)

Q67.6 Pectus excavatum
Congenital funnel chest

Q67.7 Pectus carinatum
Congenital pigeon chest

Q67.8 Other congenital deformities of chest
Congenital deformity of chest wall NOS

Q68 Other congenital musculoskeletal deformities

Excludes: reduction defects of limb(s) (Q71–Q73)

Q68.0 Congenital deformity of sternocleidomastoid muscle
Congenital (sternomastoid) torticollis
Contracture of sternocleidomastoid (muscle)
Sternomastoid tumour (congenital)

Q68.1 **Congenital deformity of hand**
Congenital clubfinger
Spade-like hand (congenital)

Q68.2 **Congenital deformity of knee**
Congenital:
- dislocation of knee
- genu recurvatum

Q68.3 **Congenital bowing of femur**
Excludes: anteversion of femur (neck) (Q65.8)

Q68.4 **Congenital bowing of tibia and fibula**

Q68.5 **Congenital bowing of long bones of leg, unspecified**

Q68.8 **Other specified congenital musculoskeletal deformities**
Congenital:
- deformity of:
  - clavicle
  - elbow
  - forearm
  - scapula
- dislocation of:
  - elbow
  - shoulder

Q69 Polydactyly

Q69.0 **Accessory finger(s)**

Q69.1 **Accessory thumb(s)**

Q69.2 **Accessory toe(s)**
Accessory hallux

Q69.9 **Polydactyly, unspecified**
Supernumerary digit(s) NOS

Q70 Syndactyly

Q70.0 **Fused fingers**
Complex syndactyly of fingers with synostosis

Q70.1 **Webbed fingers**
Simple syndactyly of fingers without synostosis

Q70.2 **Fused toes**
Complex syndactyly of toes with synostosis

Q70.3 **Webbed toes**
Simple syndactyly of toes without synostosis

Q70.4 **Polysyndactyly**

Q70.9 **Syndactyly, unspecified**
Symphalangy NOS

.Q71 Reduction defects of upper limb

Q71.0 **Congenital complete absence of upper limb(s)**

Q71.1 **Congenital absence of upper arm and forearm with hand present**

Q71.2 **Congenital absence of both forearm and hand**

Q71.3 **Congenital absence of hand and finger(s)**

Q71.4 **Longitudinal reduction defect of radius**
Clubhand (congenital)
Radial clubhand

Q71.5 **Longitudinal reduction defect of ulna**

Q71.6 **Lobster-claw hand**

Q71.8 **Other reduction defects of upper limb(s)**
Congenital shortening of upper limb(s)

Q71.9 **Reduction defect of upper limb, unspecified**

Q72 Reduction defects of lower limb

Q72.0 **Congenital complete absence of lower limb(s)**

Q72.1 **Congenital absence of thigh and lower leg with foot present**

Q72.2 **Congenital absence of both lower leg and foot**

Q72.3 **Congenital absence of foot and toe(s)**

Q72.4 **Longitudinal reduction defect of femur**
Proximal femoral focal deficiency

Q72.5 **Longitudinal reduction defect of tibia**

Q72.6 **Longitudinal reduction defect of fibula**

Q72.7 **Split foot**

Q72.8 **Other reduction defects of lower limb(s)**
Congenital shortening of lower limb(s)

Q72.9 **Reduction defect of lower limb, unspecified**

Q73 Reduction defects of unspecified limb

Q73.0 **Congenital absence of unspecified limb(s)**
Amelia NOS

Q73.1 **Phocomelia, unspecified limb(s)**
Phocomelia NOS

Q73.8 **Other reduction defects of unspecified limb(s)**
Longitudinal reduction deformity of unspecified limb(s)
Ectromelia NOS ⎱
Hemimelia NOS ⎰ of limb(s) NOS
Reduction defect ⎰

Q74 Other congenital malformations of limb(s)

Excludes: polydactyly (Q69.–)
reduction defect of limb (Q71–Q73)
syndactyly (Q70.–)

Q74.0 **Other congenital malformations of upper limb(s), including shoulder girdle**
Accessory carpal bones
Cleidocranial dysostosis
Congenital pseudarthrosis of clavicle
Macrodactylia (fingers)
Madelung's deformity
Radioulnar synostosis
Sprengel's deformity
Triphalangeal thumb

Q74.1   **Congenital malformation of knee**
Congenital:
- absence of patella
- dislocation of patella
- genu:
  - valgum
  - varum
Rudimentary patella

Excludes: congenital:
  - dislocation of knee (Q68.2)
  - genu recurvatum (Q68.2)
  nail patella syndrome (Q87.2)

Q74.2   **Other congenital malformations of lower limb(s), including pelvic girdle**
Congenital:
- fusion of sacroiliac joint
- malformation (of):
  - ankle (joint)
  - sacroiliac (joint)

Excludes: anteversion of femur (neck) (Q65.8)

Q74.3   **Arthrogryposis multiplex congenita**

Q74.8   **Other specified congenital malformations of limb(s)**

Q74.9   **Unspecified congenital malformation of limb(s)**
Congenital anomaly of limb(s) NOS

Q75   **Other congenital malformations of skull and face bones**

Excludes: congenital malformation of face NOS (Q18.–)
congenital malformation syndromes classified to
Q87.–
dentofacial anomalies [including malocclusion] (K07.–)
musculoskeletal deformities of head and face
(Q67.0–Q67.4)
skull defects associated with congenital anomalies of
brain such as:
  - anencephaly (Q00.0)
  - encephalocele (Q01.–)
  - hydrocephalus (Q03.–)
  - microcephaly (Q02)

Q75.0 **Craniosynostosis**
Acrocephaly
Imperfect fusion of skull
Oxycephaly
Trigonocephaly

Q75.1 **Craniofacial dysostosis**
Crouzon's disease

Q75.2 **Hypertelorism**

Q75.3 **Macrocephaly**

Q75.4 **Mandibulofacial dysostosis**

Q75.5 **Oculomandibular dysostosis**

Q75.8 **Other specified congenital malformations of skull and face bones**
Absence of skull bone, congenital
Congenital deformity of forehead
Platybasia

Q75.9 **Congenital malformation of skull and face bones, unspecified**
Congenital anomaly of:
• face bones NOS
• skull NOS

Q76 Congenital malformations of spine and bony thorax

Excludes: congenital musculoskeletal deformities of spine and chest (Q67.5–Q67.8)

Q76.0 **Spina bifida occulta**
Excludes: meningocele (spinal) (Q05.–)
spina bifida (aperta)(cystica) (Q05.–)

Q76.1 **Klippel–Feil syndrome**
Cervical fusion syndrome

Q76.2 **Congenital spondylolisthesis**
Congenital spondylolysis
Excludes: spondylolisthesis (acquired) (M43.1)
spondylolysis (acquired) (M43.0)

Q76.3 **Congenital scoliosis due to congenital bony malformation**
Hemivertebra fusion or failure of segmentation with scoliosis

Q76.4   **Other congenital malformations of spine, not associated with scoliosis**
Congenital:
- absence of vertebra
- fusion of spine
- kyphosis
- lordosis
- malformation of lumbosacral (joint) (region)
Hemivertebra
Malformation of spine
Platyspondylisis
Supernumerary vertebra

⎫ unspecified or not
⎬   associated with scoliosis
⎭

Q76.5   **Cervical rib**
Supernumerary rib in cervical region

Q76.6   **Other congenital malformations of ribs**
Accessory rib
Congenital:
- absence of rib
- fusion of ribs
- malformation of ribs NOS
Excludes: short rib syndrome (Q77.2)

Q76.7   **Congenital malformation of sternum**
Congenital absence of sternum
Sternum bifidum

Q76.8   **Other congenital malformations of bony thorax**

Q76.9   **Congenital malformation of bony thorax, unspecified**

Q77   **Osteochondrodysplasia with defects of growth of tubular bones and spine**
Excludes: mucopolysaccharidosis (E76.0–E76.3)

Q77.0   **Achondrogenesis**
Hypochondrogenesis

Q77.1   **Thanatophoric short stature**

Q77.2   **Short rib syndrome**
Asphyxiating thoracic dysplasia [Jeune]

Q77.3 **Chondrodysplasia punctata**

Q77.4 **Achondroplasia**
Hypochondroplasia

Q77.5 **Diastrophic dysplasia**

Q77.6 **Chondroectodermal dysplasia**
Ellis–van Creveld syndrome

Q77.7 **Spondyloepiphyseal dysplasia**

Q77.8 **Other osteochondrodysplasia with defects of growth of tubular bones and spine**

077.9 **Osteochondrodysplasia with defects of growth of tubular bones and spine, unspecified**

Q78 Other osteochondrodysplasias

Q78.0 **Osteogenesis imperfecta**
Fragilitas ossium
Osteopsathyrosis

Q78.1 **Polyostotic fibrous dysplasia**
Albright(–McCune)(–Sternberg) syndrome

Q78.2 **Osteopetrosis**
Albers–Schönberg syndrome

Q78.3 **Progressive diaphyseal dysplasia**
Camurati–Engelmann syndrome

Q78.4 **Enchondromatosis**
Maffucci's syndrome
Ollier's disease

Q78.5 **Metaphyseal dysplasia**
Pyle's syndrome

Q78.6 **Multiple congenital exostoses**
Diaphyseal aclasis

Q78.8 **Other specified osteochondrodysplasias**
Osteopoikilosis

Q78.9 **Osteochondrodysplasia, unspecified**
Chondrodystrophy NOS
Osteodystrophy NOS

Q79 Congenital malformations of musculoskeletal system, not elsewhere classified

Excludes: congenital (sternomastoid) torticollis (Q68.0)

Q79.0 Congenital diaphragmatic hernia

Excludes: congenital hiatus hernia (Q40.1)

Q79.1 Other congenital malformations of diaphragm
Absence of diaphragm
Congenital malformation of diaphragm NOS
Eventration of diaphragm

Q79.2 Exomphalos
Omphalocele

Excludes: umbilical hernia (K42.–)

Q79.3 Gastroschisis

Q79.4 Prune belly syndrome

Q79.5 Other congenital malformations of abdominal wall

Excludes: umbilical hernia (K42.–)

Q79.6 Ehlers–Danlos syndrome

Q79.8 Other congenital malformations of musculoskeletal system
Absence of:
• muscle
• tendon
Accessory muscle
Amyotrophia congenita
Congenital:
• constricting bands
• shortening of tendon
Poland's syndrome

Q79.9 Congenital malformation of musculoskeletal system, unspecified
Congenital:
• anomaly NOS ⎫
• deformity NOS ⎬ of musculoskeletal system NOS
⎭

Other congenital malformations (Q80–Q89)

Q80 Congenital ichthyosis

Excludes: Refsum's disease (G60.1)

Q80.0 **Ichthyosis vulgaris**

Q80.1 **X-linked ichthyosis**

Q80.2 **Lamellar ichthyosis**
Collodion baby

Q80.3 **Congenital bullous ichthyosiform erythroderma**

Q80.4 **Harlequin fetus**

Q80.8 **Other congenital ichthyosis**

Q80.9 **Congenital ichthyosis, unspecified**

Q81 Epidermolysis bullosa

Q81.0 **Epidermolysis bullosa simplex**
Excludes: Cockayne's syndrome (Q87.1)

Q81.1 **Epidermolysis bullosa letalis**
Herlitz' syndrome

Q81.2 **Epidermolysis bullosa dystrophica**

Q81.8 **Other epidermolysis bullosa**

Q81.9 **Epidermolysis bullosa, unspecified**

Q82 Other congenital malformations of skin

Excludes: acrodermatitis enteropathica (E83.2)
congenital erythropoietic porphyria (E80.0)
pilonidal cyst or sinus (L05.–)
Sturge–Weber(–Dimitri) syndrome (Q85.8)

Q82.0 **Hereditary lymphoedema**

Q82.1 **Xeroderma pigmentosum**

Q82.2 **Mastocytosis**
Urticaria pigmentosa
Excludes: malignant mastocytosis (C96.2)

Q82.3 **Incontinentia pigmenti**

Q82.4 **Ectodermal dysplasia (anhidrotic)**
Excludes: Ellis–van Creveld syndrome (Q77.6)

Q82.5 **Congenital non-neoplastic naevus**
Birthmark NOS
Naevus:
- flammeus
- portwine
- sanguineous
- strawberry
- vascular NOS
- verrucous

Excludes: café au lait spots (L81.3)
lentigo (L81.4)
naevus:
- NOS (D22.–)
- araneus (I78.1)
- melanocytic (D22.–)
- pigmented (D22.–)
- spider (I78.1)
- stellar (I78.1)

Q82.8 **Other specified congenital malformations of skin**
Abnormal palmar creases
Accessory skin tags
Benign familial pemphigus [Hailey–Hailey]
Cutis laxa (hyperelastica)
Dermatoglyphic anomalies
Inherited keratosis palmaris et plantaris
Keratosis follicularis [Darier–White]
Excludes: Ehlers–Danlos syndrome (Q79.6)

Q82.9 **Congenital malformation of skin, unspecified**

Q83 **Congenital malformations of breast**
Excludes: absence of pectoral muscle (Q79.8)

Q83.0 **Congenital absence of breast with absent nipple**

Q83.1 **Accessory breast**
Supernumerary breast

Q83.2 **Absent nipple**

Q83.3 **Accessory nipple**
Supernumerary nipple

Q83.8 **Other congenital malformations of breast**
Hypoplasia of breast

Q83.9 **Congenital malformation of breast, unspecified**

Q84 Other congenital malformations of integument

Q84.0 **Congenital alopecia**
Congenital atrichosis

Q84.1 **Congenital morphological disturbances of hair, not elsewhere classified**
Beaded hair
Monilethrix
Pili annulati
Excludes: Menkes' kinky hair syndrome (E83.0)

Q84.2 **Other congenital malformations of hair**
Congenital:
• hypertrichosis
• malformation of hair NOS
Persistent lanugo

Q84.3 **Anonychia**
Excludes: nail patella syndrome (Q87.2)

Q84.4 **Congenital leukonychia**

Q84.5 **Enlarged and hypertrophic nails**
Congenital onychauxis
Pachyonychia

Q84.6 **Other congenital malformations of nails**
Congenital:
• clubnail
• koilonychia
• malformation of nail NOS

Q84.8 **Other specified congenital malformations of integument**
Aplasia cutis congenita

Q84.9 **Congenital malformation of integument, unspecified**
Congenital:
- anomaly NOS ⎫
- deformity NOS ⎬ of integument NOS
⎭

Q85 Phakomatoses, not elsewhere classified

Excludes: ataxia telangiectasia [Louis-Bar] (G11.3)
familial dysautonomia [Riley–Day] (G90.1)

Q85.0 **Neurofibromatosis (nonmalignant)**
Von Recklinghausen's disease

Q85.1 **Tuberous sclerosis**
Bourneville's disease
Epiloia

Q85.8 **Other phakomatoses, not elsewhere classified**
Syndrome:
- Peutz–Jeghers
- Sturge–Weber(–Dimitri)
- von Hippel–Lindau
Excludes: Meckel–Gruber syndrome (Q61.9)

Q85.9 **Phakomatosis, unspecified**
Hamartosis NOS

Q86 Congenital malformation syndromes due to known exogenous causes, not elsewhere classified

Excludes: iodine-deficiency-related hypothyroidism (E00–E02)
nonteratogenic effects of substances transmitted via
placenta or breast milk (P04.–)

Q86.0 **Fetal alcohol syndrome (dysmorphic)**

Q86.1 **Fetal hydantoin syndrome**
Meadow's syndrome

Q86.2 **Dysmorphism due to warfarin**

Q86.8 **Other congenital malformation syndromes due to known exogenous causes**

Q87 Other specified congenital malformation syndromes affecting multiple systems

Q87.0 Congenital malformation syndromes predominantly affecting facial appearance
Acrocephalopolysyndactyly
Acrocephalosyndactyly [Apert]
Cryptophthalmos syndrome
Cyclopia
Syndrome:
• Goldenhar
• Moebius
• oro-facial-digital
• Robin
• Treacher Collins
Whistling face

Q87.1 Congenital malformation syndromes predominantly associated with short stature
Syndrome:
• Aarskog
• Cockayne
• De Lange
• Dubowitz
• Noonan
• Prader–Willi
• Robinow–Silverman–Smith
• Russell–Silver
• Seckel
• Smith–Lemli–Opitz
Excludes: Ellis–van Creveld syndrome (Q77.6)

Q87.2 Congenital malformation syndromes predominantly involving limbs
Syndrome:
• Holt–Oram
• Klippel–Trénaunay–Weber
• nail patella
• Rubinstein–Taybi
• sirenomelia
• thrombocytopenia with absent radius [TAR]
• VATER

Q87.3 **Congenital malformation syndromes involving early overgrowth**
Syndrome:
- Beckwith–Wiedemann
- Sotos
- Weaver

Q87.4 **Marfan's syndrome**

Q87.5 **Other congenital malformation syndromes with other skeletal changes**

Q87.8 **Other specified congenital malformation syndromes, not elsewhere classified**
Syndrome:
- Alport
- Laurence–Moon(–Bardet)–Biedl
- Zellweger

Q89 Other congenital malformations, not elsewhere classified

Q89.0 **Congenital malformations of spleen**
Asplenia (congenital)
Congenital splenomegaly
Excludes: isomerism of atrial appendages (with asplenia or polysplenia) (Q20.6)

Q89.1 **Congenital malformations of adrenal gland**
Excludes: congenital adrenal hyperplasia (E25.0)

Q89.2 **Congenital malformations of other endocrine glands**
Congenital malformation of parathyroid or thyroid gland
Persistent thyroglossal duct
Thyroglossal cyst

Q89.3 **Situs inversus**
Dextrocardia with situs inversus
Mirror-image atrial arrangement with situs inversus
Situs inversus or transversus:
- abdominalis
- thoracis
Transposition of viscera:
- abdominal
- thoracic
Excludes: dextrocardia NOS (Q24.0)

Q89.4   **Conjoined twins**
Craniopagus
Dicephaly
Double monster
Pygopagus
Thoracopagus

Q89.7   **Multiple congenital malformations, not elsewhere classified**
Monster NOS
Multiple congenital:
• anomalies NOS
• deformities NOS

Excludes: congenital malformation syndromes affecting multiple
systems (Q87.–)

Q89.8   **Other specified congenital malformations**

Q89.9   **Congenital malformation, unspecified**
Congenital:
• anomaly NOS
• deformity NOS

Chromosomal abnormalities, not elsewhere classified (Q90–Q99)

Q90   Down's syndrome

Q90.0   **Trisomy 21, meiotic nondisjunction**

Q90.1   **Trisomy 21, mosaicism (mitotic nondisjunction)**

Q90.2   **Trisomy 21, translocation**

Q90.9   **Down's syndrome, unspecified**
Trisomy 21 NOS

Q91   Edwards' syndrome and Patau's syndrome

Q91.0   **Trisomy 18, meiotic nondisjunction**

Q91.1   **Trisomy 18, mosaicism (mitotic nondisjunction)**

Q91.2   **Trisomy 18, translocation**

Q91.3 Edwards' syndrome, unspecified

Q91.4 Trisomy 13, meiotic nondisjunction

Q91.5 Trisomy 13, mosaicism (mitotic nondisjunction)

Q91.6 Trisomy 13, translocation

Q91.7 Patau's syndrome, unspecified

Q92 Other trisomies and partial trisomies of the autosomes, not elsewhere classified

Includes: unbalanced translocations and insertions
Excludes: trisomies of chromosomes 13, 18, 21 (Q90–Q91)

Q92.0 Whole chromosome trisomy, meiotic nondisjunction

Q92.1 Whole chromosome trisomy, mosaicism (mitotic nondisjunction)

Q92.2 Major partial trisomy
Whole arm or more duplicated.

Q92.3 Minor partial trisomy
Less than whole arm duplicated.

Q92.4 Duplications seen only at prometaphase

Q92.5 Duplications with other complex rearrangements

Q92.6 Extra marker chromosomes

Q92.7 Triploidy and polyploidy

Q92.8 Other specified trisomies and partial trisomies of autosomes

Q92.9 Trisomy and partial trisomy of autosomes, unspecified

Q93 Monosomies and deletions from the autosomes, not elsewhere classified

Q93.0 Whole chromosome monosomy, meiotic nondisjunction

Q93.1 Whole chromosome monosomy, mosaicism (mitotic nondisjunction)

Q93.2 Chromosome replaced with ring or dicentric

Q93.3 Deletion of short arm of chromosome 4
Wolff–Hirschorn syndrome

Q93.4   **Deletion of short arm of chromosome 5**
Cri-du-chat syndrome

Q93.5   **Other deletions of part of a chromosome**

Q93.6   **Deletions seen only at prometaphase**

Q93.7   **Deletions with other complex rearrangements**

Q93.8   **Other deletions from the autosomes**

Q93.9   **Deletion from autosomes, unspecified**

Q95   Balanced rearrangements and structural markers, not elsewhere classified

Includes: Robertsonian and balanced reciprocal translocations and insertions

Q95.0   **Balanced translocation and insertion in normal individual**

Q95.1   **Chromosome inversion in normal individual**

Q95.2   **Balanced autosomal rearrangement in abnormal individual**

Q95.3   **Balanced sex/autosomal rearrangement in abnormal individual**

Q95.4   **Individuals with marker heterochromatin**

Q95.5   **Individuals with autosomal fragile site**

Q95.8   **Other balanced rearrangements and structural markers**

Q95.9   **Balanced rearrangement and structural marker, unspecified**

Q96   Turner's syndrome

Excludes: Noonan's syndrome (Q87.1)

Q96.0   **Karyotype 45,X**

Q96.1   **Karyotype 46,X iso (Xq)**

Q96.2   **Karyotype 46,X with abnormal sex chromosome, except iso (Xq)**

Q96.3   **Mosaicism, 45,X/46,XX or XY**

Q96.4   **Mosaicism, 45,X/other cell line(s) with abnormal sex chromosome**

Q96.8   **Other variants of Turner's syndrome**

Q96.9   **Turner's syndrome, unspecified**

Q97 Other sex chromosome abnormalities, female phenotype, not elsewhere classified

Excludes: Turner's syndrome (Q96.–)

Q97.0 **Karyotype 47,XXX**

Q97.1 **Female with more than three X chromosomes**

Q97.2 **Mosaicism, lines with various numbers of X chromosomes**

Q97.3 **Female with 46,XY karyotype**

Q97.8 **Other specified sex chromosome abnormalities, female phenotype**

Q97.9 **Sex chromosome abnormality, female phenotype, unspecified**

Q98 Other sex chromosome abnormalities, male phenotype, not elsewhere classified

Q98.0 **Klinefelter's syndrome karyotype 47,XXY**

Q98.1 **Klinefelter's syndrome, male with more than two X chromosomes**

Q98.2 **Klinefelter's syndrome, male with 46,XX karyotype**

Q98.3 **Other male with 46,XX karyotype**

Q98.4 **Klinefelter's syndrome, unspecified**

Q98.5 **Karyotype 47,XYY**

Q98.6 **Male with structurally abnormal sex chromosome**

Q98.7 **Male with sex chromosome mosaicism**

Q98.8 **Other specified sex chromosome abnormalities, male phenotype**

Q98.9 **Sex chromosome abnormality, male phenotype, unspecified**

Q99 Other chromosome abnormalities, not elsewhere classified

Q99.0 **Chimera 46,XX/46,XY**
Chimera 46,XX/46,XY true hermaphrodite

Q99.1   **46,XX true hermaphrodite**
46,XX with streak gonads
46,XY with streak gonads
Pure gonadal dysgenesis

Q99.2   **Fragile X chromosome**
Fragile X syndrome

Q99.8   **Other specified chromosome abnormalities**

Q99.9   **Chromosomal abnormality, unspecified**

Symptoms, signs and abnormal clinical and laboratory findings, not elsewhere classified (R00–R99)

This chapter includes symptoms, signs, abnormal results of clinical or other investigative procedures, and ill-defined conditions regarding which no diagnosis classifiable elsewhere is recorded.

Signs and symptoms that point rather definitely to a given diagnosis have been assigned to a category in other chapters of the classification. In general, categories in this chapter include the less well-defined conditions and symptoms that, without the necessary study of the case to establish a final diagnosis, point perhaps equally to two or more diseases or to two or more systems of the body. Practically all categories in the chapter could be designated "not otherwise specified", "unknown etiology" or "transient". The Alphabetical Index should be consulted to determine which symptoms and signs are to be allocated here and which to other chapters. The residual subcategories, numbered .8, are generally provided for other relevant symptoms that cannot be allocated elsewhere in the classification.

The conditions and signs or symptoms included in categories R00–R99 consist of: (a) cases for which no more specific diagnosis can be made even after all the facts bearing on the case have been investigated; (b) signs or symptoms existing at the time of initial encounter that proved to be transient and whose causes could not be determined; (c) provisional diagnoses in a patient who failed to return for further investigation or care; (d) cases referred elsewhere for investigation or treatment before the diagnosis was made; (e) cases in which a more precise diagnosis was not available for any other reason; (f) certain symptoms, for which supplementary information is provided, that represent important problems in medical care in their own right.

Excludes: abnormal findings on antenatal screening of mother (O28.–)
certain conditions originating in the perinatal period (P00–P96)

This chapter contains the following blocks:

R00–R09 Symptoms and signs involving the circulatory and respiratory systems

Symptoms and signs involving the circulatory and respiratory systems (R00–R09)

R00   Abnormalities of heart beat

Excludes: abnormalities originating in the perinatal period
(P29.1)
specified arrhythmias (I47–I49)

R00.0   Tachycardia, unspecified
Rapid heart beat

R00.1   Bradycardia, unspecified
Slow heart beat

Use additional external cause code (Chapter XX), if desired, to identify drug, if drug-induced.

R00.2   Palpitations
Awareness of heart beat

R00.8   Other and unspecified abnormalities of heart beat

R01 Cardiac murmurs and other cardiac sounds

Excludes: those originating in the perinatal period (P29.8)

R01.0 Benign and innocent cardiac murmurs
Functional cardiac murmur

R01.1 Cardiac murmur, unspecified
Cardiac bruit NOS

R01.2 Other cardiac sounds
Cardiac dullness, increased or decreased
Precordial friction

R02 Gangrene, not elsewhere classified

Excludes: gangrene in:
- atherosclerosis (I70.2)
- diabetes mellitus (E10–E14 with common fourth character .5)
- other peripheral vascular diseases (I73.–)
gangrene of certain specified sites—see Alphabetical Index
gas gangrene (A48.0)
pyoderma gangrenosum (L88)

R03 Abnormal blood-pressure reading, without diagnosis

R03.0 Elevated blood-pressure reading, without diagnosis of hypertension

Note: This category is to be used to record an episode of elevated blood pressure in a patient in whom no formal diagnosis of hypertension has been made, or as an isolated incidental finding.

R03.1 Nonspecific low blood-pressure reading

Excludes: hypotension (I95.–)
- neurogenic orthostatic (G90.3)
maternal hypotension syndrome (O26.5)

R04   Haemorrhage from respiratory passages

R04.0   **Epistaxis**
Haemorrhage from nose
Nosebleed

R04.1   **Haemorrhage from throat**
Excludes: haemoptysis (R04.2)

R04.2   **Haemoptysis**
Blood-stained sputum
Cough with haemorrhage

R04.8   **Haemorrhage from other sites in respiratory passages**
Pulmonary haemorrhage NOS
Excludes: perinatal pulmonary haemorrhage (P26.–)

R04.9   **Haemorrhage from respiratory passages, unspecified**

R05   Cough

Excludes: cough with haemorrhage (R04.2)
psychogenic cough (F45.3)

R06   Abnormalities of breathing

Excludes: respiratory:
- arrest (R09.2)
- distress (syndrome)(of):
  - adult (J80)
  - newborn (P22.–)
- failure (J96.–)
  - of newborn (P28.5)

R06.0   **Dyspnoea**
Orthopnoea
Shortness of breath
Excludes: transient tachypnoea of newborn (P22.1)

R06.1   **Stridor**
Excludes: congenital laryngeal stridor (Q31.4)
laryngismus (stridulus) (J38.5)

R06.2   **Wheezing**

R06.3 **Periodic breathing**
Cheyne–Stokes breathing

R06.4 **Hyperventilation**
Excludes: psychogenic hyperventilation (F45.3)

R06.5 **Mouth breathing**
Snoring
Excludes: dry mouth NOS (R68.2)

R06.6 **Hiccough**
Excludes: psychogenic hiccough (F45.3)

R06.7 **Sneezing**

R06.8 **Other and unspecified abnormalities of breathing**
Apnoea NOS
Breath-holding (spells)
Choking sensation
Sighing
Excludes: apnoea (of):
  • newborn (P28.4)
  • sleep (G47.3)
    • newborn (primary) (P28.3)

R07 **Pain in throat and chest**
Excludes: dysphagia (R13)
epidemic myalgia (B33.0)
pain in:
  • breast (N64.4)
  • neck (M54.2)
sore throat (acute) NOS (J02.9)

R07.0 **Pain in throat**

R07.1 **Chest pain on breathing**
Painful respiration

R07.2 **Precordial pain**

R07.3 **Other chest pain**
Anterior chest-wall pain NOS

R07.4 **Chest pain, unspecified**

R09   Other symptoms and signs involving the circulatory and respiratory systems

Excludes: respiratory:
- distress (syndrome)(of):
  - adult (J80)
  - newborn (P22.–)
- failure (J96.–)
  - newborn (P28.5)

R09.0   **Asphyxia**

Excludes: asphyxia (due to):
- birth (P21.–)
- carbon monoxide (T58)
- foreign body in respiratory tract (T17.–)
- intrauterine (P20.–)
- traumatic (T71)

R09.1   **Pleurisy**

Excludes: pleurisy with effusion (J90)

R09.2   **Respiratory arrest**

Cardiorespiratory failure

R09.3   **Abnormal sputum**

Abnormal:
- amount
- colour   } (of) sputum
- odour

Excessive

Excludes: blood-stained sputum (R04.2)

R09.8   **Other specified symptoms and signs involving the circulatory and respiratory systems**

Bruit (arterial)

Chest:
- abnormal percussion
- friction sounds
- tympany

Rales

Weak pulse

Symptoms and signs involving the digestive system and abdomen
(R10–R19)

Excludes: gastrointestinal haemorrhage (K92.0–K92.2)
- newborn (P54.0–P54.3)

intestinal obstruction (K56.–)
- newborn (P76.–)

pylorospasm (K31.3)
- congenital or infantile (Q40.0)

symptoms and signs involving the urinary system (R30–R39)
symptoms referable to genital organs:
- female (N94.–)
- male (N48–N50)

R10   Abdominal and pelvic pain

Excludes: dorsalgia (M54.–)
flatulence and related conditions (R14)
renal colic (N23)

R10.0   **Acute abdomen**
Severe abdominal pain (generalized)(localized)(with abdominal rigidity)

R10.1   **Pain localized to upper abdomen**
Epigastric pain

R10.2   **Pelvic and perineal pain**

R10.3   **Pain localized to other parts of lower abdomen**

R10.4   **Other and unspecified abdominal pain**
Abdominal tenderness NOS
Colic:
- NOS
- infantile

R11 Nausea and vomiting

Excludes: haematemesis (K92.0)
- neonatal (P54.0)

vomiting (of):
- excessive, in pregnancy (O21.–)
- following gastrointestinal surgery (K91.0)
- newborn (P92.0)
- psychogenic (F50.5)

R12 Heartburn

Excludes: dyspepsia (K30)

R13 Dysphagia

Difficulty in swallowing

R14 Flatulence and related conditions

Abdominal distension (gaseous)
Bloating
Eructation
Gas pain
Tympanites (abdominal)(intestinal)
Excludes: psychogenic aerophagy (F45.3)

R15 Faecal incontinence

Encopresis NOS
Excludes: that of nonorganic origin (F98.1)

R16 Hepatomegaly and splenomegaly, not elsewhere classified

R16.0 Hepatomegaly, not elsewhere classified
Hepatomegaly NOS

R16.1 Splenomegaly, not elsewhere classified
Splenomegaly NOS

R16.2 Hepatomegaly with splenomegaly, not elsewhere classified
Hepatosplenomegaly NOS

R17 Unspecified jaundice

Excludes: neonatal jaundice (P55, P57–P59)

R18 Ascites

Fluid in peritoneal cavity

R19 Other symptoms and signs involving the digestive system and abdomen

Excludes: acute abdomen (R10.0)

R19.0 Intra-abdominal and pelvic swelling, mass and lump

Diffuse or generalized swelling or mass:
- intra-abdominal NOS
- pelvic NOS
- umbilical

Excludes: abdominal distension (gaseous) (R14)
ascites (R18)

R19.1 Abnormal bowel sounds

Absent bowel sounds
Hyperactive bowel sounds

R19.2 Visible peristalsis

Hyperperistalsis

R19.3 Abdominal rigidity

Excludes: that with severe abdominal pain (R10.0)

R19.4 Change in bowel habit

Excludes: constipation (K59.0)
functional diarrhoea (K59.1)

R19.5 Other faecal abnormalities

Abnormal stool colour
Bulky stools
Mucus in stools

Excludes: melaena (K92.1)
- neonatal (P54.1)

R19.6 Halitosis

R19.8 Other specified symptoms and signs involving the digestive system and abdomen

Symptoms and signs involving the skin and subcutaneous tissue (R20–R23)

R20 Disturbances of skin sensation

Excludes: dissociative anaesthesia and sensory loss (F44.6)
psychogenic disturbances (F45.8)

R20.0 Anaesthesia of skin

R20.1 Hypoaesthesia of skin

R20.2 Paraesthesia of skin
Formication
Pins and needles
Tingling skin
Excludes: acroparaesthesia (I73.8)

R20.3 Hyperaesthesia

R20.8 Other and unspecified disturbances of skin sensation

R21 Rash and other nonspecific skin eruption

R22 Localized swelling, mass and lump of skin and subcutaneous tissue

Includes: subcutaneous nodules (localized)(superficial)
Excludes: abnormal findings on diagnostic imaging (R90–R93)
enlarged lymph nodes (R59.–)
localized adiposity (E65)
mass and lump:
• breast (N63)
• intra-abdominal or pelvic (R19.0)
oedema (R60.–)
swelling (of):
• intra-abdominal or pelvic (R19.0)
• joint (M25.4)

R22.0 Localized swelling, mass and lump, head

R22.1 Localized swelling, mass and lump, neck

R22.2 Localized swelling, mass and lump, trunk

R22.3   **Localized swelling, mass and lump, upper limb**

R22.4   **Localized swelling, mass and lump, lower limb**

R22.7   **Localized swelling, mass and lump, multiple sites**

R22.9   **Localized swelling, mass and lump, unspecified**

R23   Other skin changes

R23.0   **Cyanosis**
Excludes: acrocyanosis (I73.8)
cyanotic attacks of newborn (P28.2)

R23.1   **Pallor**
Clammy skin

R23.2   **Flushing**
Excessive blushing
Excludes: menopausal and female climacteric states (N95.1)

R23.3   **Spontaneous ecchymoses**
Petechiae
Excludes: ecchymoses in fetus and newborn (P54.5)
purpura (D69.–)

R23.4   **Changes in skin texture**
Desquamation ⎱
Induration   ⎰ of skin
Scaling
Excludes: epidermal thickening NOS (L85.9)

R23.8   **Other and unspecified skin changes**

Symptoms and signs involving the nervous and musculoskeletal systems (R25–R29)

R25   Abnormal involuntary movements
Excludes: specific movement disorders (G20–G26)
stereotyped movement disorders (F98.4)
tic disorders (F95.–)

R25.0   **Abnormal head movements**

R25.1 **Tremor, unspecified**

Excludes: chorea NOS (G25.5)
 tremor:
 • essential (G25.0)
 • hysterical (F44.4)
 • intention (G25.2)

R25.2 **Cramp and spasm**

Excludes: carpopedal spasm (R29.0)
 infantile spasms (G40.4)

R25.3 **Fasciculation**
Twitching NOS

R25.8 **Other and unspecified abnormal involuntary movements**

R26 Abnormalities of gait and mobility

Excludes: ataxia:
 • NOS (R27.0)
 • hereditary (G11.–)
 • locomotor (syphilitic) (A52.1)
 immobility syndrome (paraplegic) (M62.3)

R26.0 **Ataxic gait**
Staggering gait

R26.1 **Paralytic gait**
Spastic gait

R26.2 **Difficulty in walking, not elsewhere classified**

R26.8 **Other and unspecified abnormalities of gait and mobility**
Unsteadiness on feet NOS

R27 Other lack of coordination

Excludes: ataxic gait (R26.0)
 hereditary ataxia (G11.–)
 vertigo NOS (R42)

R27.0 **Ataxia, unspecified**

R27.8 **Other and unspecified lack of coordination**

R29 Other symptoms and signs involving the nervous and musculoskeletal systems

R29.0 **Tetany**
Carpopedal spasm
Excludes: tetany:
- hysterical (F44.5)
- neonatal (P71.3)
- parathyroid (E20.9)
- post-thyroidectomy (E89.2)

R29.1 **Meningismus**

R29.2 **Abnormal reflex**
Excludes: abnormal pupillary reflex (H57.0)
hyperactive gag reflex (J39.2)
vasovagal reaction or syncope (R55)

R29.3 **Abnormal posture**

R29.4 **Clicking hip**
Excludes: congenital deformities of hip (Q65.–)

R29.8 **Other and unspecified symptoms and signs involving the nervous and musculoskeletal systems**

Symptoms and signs involving the urinary system (R30–R39)

R30 Pain associated with micturition
Excludes: psychogenic pain (F45.3)

R30.0 **Dysuria**
Strangury

R30.1 **Vesical tenesmus**

R30.9 **Painful micturition, unspecified**
Painful urination NOS

R31 Unspecified haematuria
Excludes: recurrent or persistent haematuria (N02.–)

R32 Unspecified urinary incontinence

Enuresis NOS

Excludes: nonorganic enuresis (F98.0)
   stress incontinence and other specified urinary
   incontinence (N39.3–N39.4)

R33 Retention of urine

R34 Anuria and oliguria

Excludes: that complicating:
   • abortion or ectopic or molar pregnancy (O00–O07,
     O08.4)
   • pregnancy, childbirth and the puerperium (O26.8,
     O90.4)

R35 Polyuria

Frequency of micturition
Nocturia

Excludes: psychogenic polyuria (F45.3)

R36 Urethral discharge

Penile discharge
Urethrorrhoea

R39 Other symptoms and signs involving the urinary system

R39.0 Extravasation of urine

R39.1 Other difficulties with micturition
Hesitancy of micturition
Poor urinary stream
Splitting of urinary stream

R39.2 Extrarenal uraemia
Prerenal uraemia

R39.8 Other and unspecified symptoms and signs involving the urinary system

Symptoms and signs involving cognition, perception, emotional state and behaviour (R40–R46)

Excludes: those constituting part of a pattern of mental disorder (F00–F99)

R40 Somnolence, stupor and coma

Excludes: coma:
- diabetic (E10–E14 with common fourth character .0)
- hepatic (K72.–)
- hypoglycaemic (nondiabetic) (E15)
- neonatal (P91.5)
- uraemic (N19)

R40.0 Somnolence
Drowsiness

R40.1 Stupor
Semicoma
Excludes: stupor:
- catatonic (F20.2)
- depressive (F31–F33)
- dissociative (F44.2)
- manic (F30.2)

R40.2 Coma, unspecified
Unconsciousness NOS

R41 Other symptoms and signs involving cognitive functions and awareness

Excludes: dissociative [conversion] disorders (F44.–)

R41.0 Disorientation, unspecified
Confusion NOS
Excludes: psychogenic disorientation (F44.8)

R41.1 Anterograde amnesia

R41.2 Retrograde amnesia

R41.3 **Other amnesia**
Amnesia NOS
Excludes: amnesic syndrome:
- due to psychoactive substance use (F10–F19 with common fourth character .6)
- organic (F04)
transient global amnesia (G45.4)

R41.8 **Other and unspecified symptoms and signs involving cognitive functions and awareness**

R42 Dizziness and giddiness
Light-headedness
Vertigo NOS
Excludes: vertiginous syndromes (H81.–)

R43 Disturbances of smell and taste

R43.0 **Anosmia**

R43.1 **Parosmia**

R43.2 **Parageusia**

R43.8 **Other and unspecified disturbances of smell and taste**
Mixed disturbance of smell and taste

R44 Other symptoms and signs involving general sensations and perceptions
Excludes: disturbances of skin sensation (R20.–)

R44.0 **Auditory hallucinations**

R44.1 **Visual hallucinations**

R44.2 **Other hallucinations**

R44.3 **Hallucinations, unspecified**

R44.8 **Other and unspecified symptoms and signs involving general sensations and perceptions**

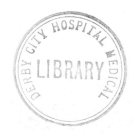

R45 Symptoms and signs involving emotional state

R45.0 **Nervousness**
Nervous tension

R45.1 **Restlessness and agitation**

R45.2 **Unhappiness**
Worries NOS

R45.3 **Demoralization and apathy**

R45.4 **Irritability and anger**

R45.5 **Hostility**

R45.6 **Physical violence**

R45.7 **State of emotional shock and stress, unspecified**

R45.8 **Other symptoms and signs involving emotional state**

R46 Symptoms and signs involving appearance and behaviour

R46.0 **Very low level of personal hygiene**

R46.1 **Bizarre personal appearance**

R46.2 **Strange and inexplicable behaviour**

R46.3 **Overactivity**

R46.4 **Slowness and poor responsiveness**
Excludes: stupor (R40.1)

R46.5 **Suspiciousness and marked evasiveness**

R46.6 **Undue concern and preoccupation with stressful events**

R46.7 **Verbosity and circumstantial detail obscuring reason for contact**

R46.8 **Other symptoms and signs involving appearance and behaviour**

Symptoms and signs involving speech and voice (R47–R49)

R47 Speech disturbances, not elsewhere classified

Excludes: autism (F84.0–F84.1)
cluttering (F98.6)
specific developmental disorders of speech and
language (F80.–)
stuttering [stammering] (F98.5)

R47.0 **Dysphasia and aphasia**

Excludes: progressive isolated aphasia (G31.0)

R47.1 **Dysarthria and anarthria**

R47.8 **Other and unspecified speech disturbances**

R48 Dyslexia and other symbolic dysfunctions, not elsewhere classified

Excludes: specific developmental disorders of scholastic skills
(F81.–)

R48.0 **Dyslexia and alexia**

R48.1 **Agnosia**

R48.2 **Apraxia**

R48.8 **Other and unspecified symbolic dysfunctions**
Acalculia
Agraphia

R49 Voice disturbances

Excludes: psychogenic voice disturbance (F44.4)

R49.0 **Dysphonia**
Hoarseness

R49.1 **Aphonia**
Loss of voice

R49.2 **Hypernasality and hyponasality**

R49.8 **Other and unspecified voice disturbances**
Change in voice NOS

General symptoms and signs (R50–R69)

R50   Fever of unknown origin

Excludes: fever of unknown origin (during)(in):
- labour (O75.2)
- newborn (P81.9)

puerperal pyrexia NOS (O86.4)

R50.0   **Fever with chills**

Fever with rigors

R50.1   **Persistent fever**

R50.9   **Fever, unspecified**

Hyperpyrexia NOS

Pyrexia NOS

Excludes: malignant hyperthermia due to anaesthesia (T88.3)

R51   Headache

Facial pain NOS

Excludes: atypical facial pain (G50.1)

migraine and other headache syndromes (G43–G44)

trigeminal neuralgia (G50.0)

R52   Pain, not elsewhere classified

Includes: pain not referable to any one organ or body region

Excludes: chronic pain personality syndrome (F62.8)

headache (R51)

pain (in):

- abdomen (R10.–)
- back (M54.9)
- breast (N64.4)
- chest (R07.1–R07.4)
- ear (H92.0)
- eye (H57.1)
- joint (M25.5)
- limb (M79.6)
- lumbar region (M54.5)
- pelvic and perineal (R10.2)
- psychogenic (F45.4)
- shoulder (M75.8)
- spine (M54.–)
- throat (R07.0)
- tongue (K14.6)
- tooth (K08.8)

renal colic (N23)

R52.0   **Acute pain**

R52.1   **Chronic intractable pain**

R52.2   **Other chronic pain**

R52.9   **Pain, unspecified**

Generalized pain NOS

R53 Malaise and fatigue

Asthenia NOS

Debility:

- NOS
- chronic
- nervous

General physical deterioration

Lethargy

Tiredness

Excludes: debility:

- congenital (P96.9)
- senile (R54)

exhaustion and fatigue (due to)(in):

- combat (F43.0)
- excessive exertion (T73.3)
- exposure (T73.2)
- heat (T67.–)
- neurasthenia (F48.0)
- pregnancy (O26.8)
- senile asthenia (R54)

fatigue syndrome (F48.0)

- postviral (G93.3)

R54 Senility

Old age
Senescence } without mention of psychosis

Senile:

- asthenia
- debility

Excludes: senile psychosis (F03)

R55 Syncope and collapse
Blackout
Fainting
Excludes: neurocirculatory asthenia (F45.3)
orthostatic hypotension (I95.1)
- neurogenic (G90.3)
shock:
- NOS (R57.9)
- cardiogenic (R57.0)
- complicating or following:
  - abortion or ectopic or molar pregnancy (O00–O07, O08.3)
  - labour and delivery (O75.1)
- postoperative (T81.1)
Stokes–Adams attack (I45.9)
syncope:
- carotid sinus (G90.0)
- heat (T67.1)
- psychogenic (F48.8)
unconsciousness NOS (R40.2)

R56 Convulsions, not elsewhere classified
Excludes: convulsions and seizures (in):
- dissociative (F44.5)
- epilepsy (G40–G41)
- newborn (P90)

R56.0 Febrile convulsions

R56.8 Other and unspecified convulsions
Fit NOS
Seizure (convulsive) NOS

R57 Shock, not elsewhere classified

Excludes: shock (due to):
- anaesthesia (T88.2)
- anaphylactic (due to):
  - NOS (T78.2)
  - adverse food reaction (T78.0)
  - serum (T80.5)
- complicating or following abortion or ectopic or molar pregnancy (O00–O07, O08.3)
- electric (T75.4)
- lightning (T75.0)
- obstetric (O75.1)
- postoperative (T81.1)
- psychic (F43.0)
- septic (A41.9)
- traumatic (T79.4)
toxic shock syndrome (A48.3)

R57.0 **Cardiogenic shock**

R57.1 **Hypovolaemic shock**

R57.8 **Other shock**
Endotoxic shock

R57.9 **Shock, unspecified**
Failure of peripheral circulation NOS

R58 Haemorrhage, not elsewhere classified
Haemorrhage NOS

R59 Enlarged lymph nodes

Includes: swollen glands
Excludes: lymphadenitis:
- NOS (I88.9)
- acute (L04.–)
- chronic (I88.1)
- mesenteric (acute)(chronic) (I88.0)

R59.0 **Localized enlarged lymph nodes**

R59.1 **Generalized enlarged lymph nodes**
Lymphadenopathy NOS
Excludes: HIV disease resulting in (persistent) generalized
lymphadenopathy (B23.1)

R59.9 **Enlarged lymph nodes, unspecified**

R60 Oedema, not elsewhere classified
Excludes: ascites (R18)
hydrops fetalis NOS (P83.2)
hydrothorax (J94.8)
oedema (of):
• angioneurotic (T78.3)
• cerebral (G93.6)
  • due to birth injury (P11.0)
• gestational (O12.0)
• hereditary (Q82.0)
• larynx (J38.4)
• malnutrition (E40–E46)
• nasopharynx (J39.2)
• newborn (P83.3)
• pharynx (J39.2)
• pulmonary (J81)

R60.0 **Localized oedema**

R60.1 **Generalized oedema**

R60.9 **Oedema, unspecified**
Fluid retention NOS

R61 Hyperhidrosis

R61.0 **Localized hyperhidrosis**

R61.1 **Generalized hyperhidrosis**

R61.9 **Hyperhidrosis, unspecified**
Excessive sweating
Night sweats

R62   Lack of expected normal physiological development

Excludes: delayed puberty (E30.0)

R62.0   **Delayed milestone**

Delayed attainment of expected physiological developmental stage

Late:
- talker
- walker

R62.8   **Other lack of expected normal physiological development**

Failure to:
- gain weight
- thrive

Infantilism NOS

Lack of growth

Physical retardation

Excludes: HIV disease resulting in failure to thrive (B22.2)
physical retardation due to malnutrition (E45)

R62.9   **Lack of expected normal physiological development, unspecified**

R63   Symptoms and signs concerning food and fluid intake

Excludes: bulimia NOS (F50.2)
eating disorders of nonorganic origin (F50.–)
malnutrition (E40–E46)

R63.0   **Anorexia**

Loss of appetite

Excludes: anorexia nervosa (F50.0)
loss of appetite of nonorganic origin (F50.8)

R63.1   **Polydipsia**

Excessive thirst

R63.2   **Polyphagia**

Excessive eating

Hyperalimentation NOS

R63.3   **Feeding difficulties and mismanagement**
Feeding problem NOS
Excludes: feeding problems of newborn (P92.–)
infant feeding disorder of nonorganic origin (F98.2)

R63.4   **Abnormal weight loss**

R63.5   **Abnormal weight gain**
Excludes: excessive weight gain in pregnancy (O26.0)
obesity (E66.–)

R63.8   **Other symptoms and signs concerning food and fluid intake**

R64   Cachexia
Excludes: HIV disease resulting in wasting syndrome (B22.2)
malignant cachexia (C80)
nutritional marasmus (E41)

R68   Other general symptoms and signs

R68.0   **Hypothermia, not associated with low environmental temperature**
Excludes: hypothermia (due to)(of):
• NOS (accidental) (T68)
• anaesthesia (T88.5)
• low environmental temperature (T68)
• newborn (P80.–)

R68.1   **Nonspecific symptoms peculiar to infancy**
Excessive crying of infant
Irritable infant
Excludes: neonatal cerebral irritability (P91.3)
teething syndrome (K00.7)

R68.2   **Dry mouth, unspecified**
Excludes: dry mouth due to:
• dehydration (E86)
• sicca syndrome [Sjögren] (M35.0)
salivary gland hyposecretion (K11.7)

R68.3   **Clubbing of fingers**
Clubbing of nails
Excludes: congenital clubfinger (Q68.1)

R68.8   Other specified general symptoms and signs

R69   Unknown and unspecified causes of morbidity
Illness NOS

Undiagnosed disease, not specified as to the site or system
involved

Abnormal findings on examination of blood, without diagnosis
(R70–R79)

Excludes: abnormalities (of)(on):
- antenatal screening of mother (O28.–)
- coagulation (D65–D68)
- lipids (E78.–)
- platelets and thrombocytes (D69.–)
- white blood cells classified elsewhere (D70–D72)

diagnostic abnormal findings classified elsewhere—see
   Alphabetical Index

haemorrhagic and haematological disorders of fetus and newborn
   (P50–P61)

R70   Elevated erythrocyte sedimentation rate and abnormality of plasma viscosity

R70.0   Elevated erythrocyte sedimentation rate

R70.1   Abnormal plasma viscosity

R71 Abnormality of red blood cells
Abnormal red-cell:
- morphology NOS
- volume NOS

Anisocytosis
Poikilocytosis

Excludes: anaemias (D50–D64)
   polycythaemia:
   - benign (familial) (D75.0)
   - neonatorum (P61.1)
   - secondary (D75.1)
   - vera (D45)

R72 Abnormality of white blood cells, not elsewhere classified
Abnormal leukocyte differential NOS

Excludes: leukocytosis (D72.8)

R73 Elevated blood glucose level
Excludes: diabetes mellitus (E10–E14)
   - in pregnancy, childbirth and the puerperium (O24.–)
   neonatal disorders (P70.0–P70.2)
   postsurgical hypoinsulinaemia (E89.1)

R73.0 Abnormal glucose tolerance test
Diabetes:
- chemical
- latent

Impaired glucose tolerance
Prediabetes

R73.9 Hyperglycaemia, unspecified

R74 Abnormal serum enzyme levels

R74.0 Elevation of levels of transaminase and lactic acid dehydrogenase [LDH]

R74.8 **Abnormal levels of other serum enzymes**
Abnormal level of:
- acid phosphatase
- alkaline phosphatase
- amylase
- lipase [triacylglycerol lipase]

R74.9 **Abnormal level of unspecified serum enzyme**

R75 Laboratory evidence of human immunodeficiency virus [HIV]
Nonconclusive HIV-test finding in infants

Excludes: asymptomatic human immunodeficiency virus [HIV] infection status (Z21)
human immunodeficiency virus [HIV] disease (B20–B24)

R76 Other abnormal immunological findings in serum

R76.0 **Raised antibody titre**
Excludes: isoimmunization, in pregnancy (O36.0–O36.1)
- affecting fetus or newborn (P55.–)

R76.1 **Abnormal reaction to tuberculin test**
Abnormal result of Mantoux test

R76.2 **False-positive serological test for syphilis**
False-positive Wassermann reaction

R76.8 **Other specified abnormal immunological findings in serum**
Raised level of immunoglobulins NOS

R76.9 **Abnormal immunological finding in serum, unspecified**

R77 Other abnormalities of plasma proteins
Excludes: disorders of plasma-protein metabolism (E88.0)

R77.0 **Abnormality of albumin**

R77.1 **Abnormality of globulin**
Hyperglobulinaemia NOS

R77.2 **Abnormality of alphafetoprotein**

R77.8 **Other specified abnormalities of plasma proteins**

R77.9   **Abnormality of plasma protein, unspecified**

R78   Findings of drugs and other substances, not normally found in blood

Excludes: mental and behavioural disorders due to psychoactive
substance use (F10–F19)

R78.0   **Finding of alcohol in blood**
Use additional external cause code (Y90.–), if desired, for detail
regarding alcohol level.

R78.1   **Finding of opiate drug in blood**

R78.2   **Finding of cocaine in blood**

R78.3   **Finding of hallucinogen in blood**

R78.4   **Finding of other drugs of addictive potential in blood**

R78.5   **Finding of psychotropic drug in blood**

R78.6   **Finding of steroid agent in blood**

R78.7   **Finding of abnormal level of heavy metals in blood**

R78.8   **Finding of other specified substances, not normally found in blood**
Finding of abnormal level of lithium in blood

R78.9   **Finding of unspecified substance, not normally found in blood**

R79   Other abnormal findings of blood chemistry

Excludes: abnormality of fluid, electrolyte or acid–base balance
(E86–E87)
asymptomatic hyperuricaemia (E79.0)
hyperglycaemia NOS (R73.9)
hypoglycaemia NOS (E16.2)
• neonatal (P70.3–P70.4)
specific findings indicating disorder of:
• amino-acid metabolism (E70–E72)
• carbohydrate metabolism (E73–E74)
• lipid metabolism (E75.–)

R79.0 **Abnormal level of blood mineral**

Abnormal blood level of:

- cobalt
- copper
- iron
- magnesium
- mineral NEC
- zinc

Excludes: abnormal level of lithium (R78.8)

disorders of mineral metabolism (E83.–)

neonatal hypomagnesaemia (P71.2)

nutritional mineral deficiency (E58–E61)

R79.8 **Other specified abnormal findings of blood chemistry**

Abnormal blood-gas level

R79.9 **Abnormal finding of blood chemistry, unspecified**

Abnormal findings on examination of urine, without diagnosis (R80–R82)

Excludes: abnormal findings on antenatal screening of mother (O28.–)

diagnostic abnormal findings classified elsewhere—see
Alphabetical Index

specific findings indicating disorder of:

- amino-acid metabolism (E70–E72)
- carbohydrate metabolism (E73–E74)

R80 **Isolated proteinuria**

Albuminuria NOS

Bence Jones proteinuria

Proteinuria NOS

Excludes: proteinuria:

- gestational (O12.1)
- isolated, with specified morphological lesion (N06.–)
- orthostatic (N39.2)
- persistent (N39.1)

R81 Glycosuria

Excludes: renal glycosuria (E74.8)

R82 Other abnormal findings in urine

Excludes: haematuria (R31)

R82.0 Chyluria

Excludes: filarial chyluria (B74.–)

R82.1 Myoglobinuria

R82.2 Biliuria

R82.3 Haemoglobinuria

Excludes: haemoglobinuria:
- due to haemolysis from external causes NEC (D59.6)
- paroxysmal nocturnal [Marchiafava–Micheli] (D59.5)

R82.4 Acetonuria

Ketonuria

R82.5 Elevated urine levels of drugs, medicaments and biological substances

Elevated urine levels of:
- catecholamines
- indoleacetic acid
- 17-ketosteroids
- steroids

R82.6 Abnormal urine levels of substances chiefly nonmedicinal as to source

Abnormal urine level of heavy metals

R82.7 Abnormal findings on microbiological examination of urine

Positive culture findings

R82.8 Abnormal findings on cytological and histological examination of urine

R82.9 Other and unspecified abnormal findings in urine

Cells and casts in urine
Crystalluria
Melanuria

Abnormal findings on examination of other body fluids, substances and tissues, without diagnosis (R83–R89)

Excludes: abnormal findings on:
- antenatal screening of mother (O28.–)
- examination of:
  - blood, without diagnosis (R70–R79)
  - urine, without diagnosis (R80–R82)

  diagnostic abnormal findings classified elsewhere—see Alphabetical Index

The following fourth-character subdivisions are for use with categories R83–R89:

.0   Abnormal level of enzymes
.1   Abnormal level of hormones
.2   Abnormal level of other drugs, medicaments and biological substances
.3   Abnormal level of substances chiefly nonmedicinal as to source
.4   Abnormal immunological findings
.5   Abnormal microbiological findings
      Positive culture findings
.6   Abnormal cytological findings
      Abnormal Papanicolaou smear
.7   Abnormal histological findings
.8   Other abnormal findings
      Abnormal chromosomal findings
.9   Unspecified abnormal finding

R83   Abnormal findings in cerebrospinal fluid

R84 Abnormal findings in specimens from respiratory organs and thorax

Abnormal findings in:
- bronchial washings
- nasal secretions
- pleural fluid
- sputum
- throat scrapings

Excludes: blood-stained sputum (R04.2)

R85 Abnormal findings in specimens from digestive organs and abdominal cavity

Abnormal findings in:
- peritoneal fluid
- saliva

Excludes: faecal abnormalities (R19.5)

R86 Abnormal findings in specimens from male genital organs

Abnormal findings in:
- prostatic secretions
- semen, seminal fluid

Abnormal spermatozoa

Excludes: azoospermia (N46)
oligospermia (N46)

R87 Abnormal findings in specimens from female genital organs

Abnormal findings in secretions and smears from:
- cervix uteri
- vagina
- vulva

Excludes: carcinoma in situ (D05–D07.3)
dysplasia of:
- cervix uteri (N87.–)
- vagina (N89.0–N89.3)
- vulva (N90.0–N90.3)

R89   Abnormal findings in specimens from other organs, systems and tissues

Abnormal findings in:
- nipple discharge
- synovial fluid
- wound secretions

Abnormal findings on diagnostic imaging and in function studies, without diagnosis (R90–R94)

Includes: nonspecific abnormal findings on diagnostic imaging by:
- computerized axial tomography [CAT scan]
- magnetic resonance imaging [MRI][NMR]
- positron emission tomography [PET scan]
- thermography
- ultrasound [echogram]
- X-ray examination

Excludes: abnormal findings on antenatal screening of mother (O28.–)
diagnostic abnormal findings classified elsewhere—see
    Alphabetical Index

R90   Abnormal findings on diagnostic imaging of central nervous system

R90.0   **Intracranial space-occupying lesion**

R90.8   **Other abnormal findings on diagnostic imaging of central nervous system**
Abnormal echoencephalogram

R91   Abnormal findings on diagnostic imaging of lung
Coin lesion NOS
Lung mass NOS

R92   Abnormal findings on diagnostic imaging of breast

R93   Abnormal findings on diagnostic imaging of other body structures

R93.0   **Abnormal findings on diagnostic imaging of skull and head, not elsewhere classified**

Excludes: intracranial space-occupying lesion (R90.0)

R93.1   **Abnormal findings on diagnostic imaging of heart and coronary circulation**

Abnormal:
- echocardiogram NOS
- heart shadow

R93.2   **Abnormal findings on diagnostic imaging of liver and biliary tract**

Nonvisualization of gallbladder

R93.3   **Abnormal findings on diagnostic imaging of other parts of digestive tract**

R93.4   **Abnormal findings on diagnostic imaging of urinary organs**

Filling defect of:
- bladder
- kidney
- ureter

Excludes: hypertrophy of kidney (N28.8)

R93.5   **Abnormal findings on diagnostic imaging of other abdominal regions, including retroperitoneum**

R93.6   **Abnormal findings on diagnostic imaging of limbs**

Excludes: abnormal finding in skin and subcutaneous tissue (R93.8)

R93.7   **Abnormal findings on diagnostic imaging of other parts of musculoskeletal system**

Excludes: abnormal findings on diagnostic imaging of skull (R93.0)

R93.8   **Abnormal findings on diagnostic imaging of other specified body structures**

Abnormal radiological finding in skin and subcutaneous tissue
Mediastinal shift

R94   Abnormal results of function studies

Includes: abnormal results of:
- radionuclide [radioisotope] uptake studies
- scintigraphy

R94.0   Abnormal results of function studies of central nervous system
Abnormal electroencephalogram [EEG]

R94.1   Abnormal results of function studies of peripheral nervous system and special senses
Abnormal:
- electromyogram [EMG]
- electro-oculogram [EOG]
- electroretinogram [ERG]
- response to nerve stimulation
- visually evoked potential [VEP]

R94.2   Abnormal results of pulmonary function studies
Reduced:
- ventilatory capacity
- vital capacity

R94.3   Abnormal results of cardiovascular function studies
Abnormal:
- electrocardiogram [ECG][EKG]
- electrophysiological intracardiac studies
- phonocardiogram
- vectorcardiogram

R94.4   Abnormal results of kidney function studies
Abnormal renal function test

R94.5   Abnormal results of liver function studies

R94.6   Abnormal results of thyroid function studies

R94.7   Abnormal results of other endocrine function studies
Excludes: abnormal glucose tolerance test (R73.0)

R94.8   Abnormal results of function studies of other organs and systems
Abnormal:
- basal metabolic rate [BMR]
- bladder function test
- splenic function test

Ill-defined and unknown causes of mortality (R95–R99)

Excludes: fetal death of unspecified cause (P95)
obstetric death NOS (O95)

R95 Sudden infant death syndrome

R96 Other sudden death, cause unknown

Excludes: sudden:
- cardiac death, so described (I46.1)
- infant death syndrome (R95)

R96.0 Instantaneous death

R96.1 Death occurring less than 24 hours from onset of symptoms, not otherwise explained
Death known not to be violent or instantaneous for which no cause can be discovered
Death without sign of disease

R98 Unattended death
Death in circumstances where the body of the deceased was found and no cause could be discovered
Found dead

R99 Other ill-defined and unspecified causes of mortality
Death NOS
Unknown cause of mortality

CHAPTER XIX

Injury, poisoning and certain other consequences of external causes (S00–T98)

Excludes: birth trauma (P10–P15)
obstetric trauma (O70–O71)

This chapter contains the following blocks:

S00–S09 Injuries to the head
S10–S19 Injuries to the neck
S20–S29 Injuries to the thorax
S30–S39 Injuries to the abdomen, lower back, lumbar spine and pelvis
S40–S49 Injuries to the shoulder and upper arm
S50–S59 Injuries to the elbow and forearm
S60–S69 Injuries to the wrist and hand
S70–S79 Injuries to the hip and thigh
S80–S89 Injuries to the knee and lower leg
S90–S99 Injuries to the ankle and foot
T00–T07 Injuries involving multiple body regions
T08–T14 Injuries to unspecified parts of trunk, limb or body region
T15–T19 Effects of foreign body entering through natural orifice
T20–T32 Burns and corrosions
T33–T35 Frostbite
T36–T50 Poisoning by drugs, medicaments and biological substances
T51–T65 Toxic effects of substances chiefly nonmedicinal as to source
T66–T78 Other and unspecified effects of external causes
T79 Certain early complications of trauma
T80–T88 Complications of surgical and medical care, not elsewhere classified
T90–T98 Sequelae of injuries, of poisoning and of other consequences of external causes

The chapter uses the S-section for coding different types of injuries related to single body regions and the T-section to cover injuries to multiple or unspecified body regions as well as poisoning and certain other consequences of external causes.

Where multiple sites of injury are specified in the titles, the word "with" indicates involvement of both sites, and the word "and" indicates involvement of either or both sites.

The principle of multiple coding of injuries should be followed wherever possible. Combination categories for multiple injuries are provided for use when there is insufficient detail as to the nature of the individual conditions, or for primary tabulation purposes when it is more convenient to record a single code; otherwise, the component injuries should be coded separately. Reference should also be made to the morbidity or mortality coding rules and guidelines in Volume 2.

The blocks of the S-section as well as T00–T14 and T90–T98 contain injuries at the three-character level classified by type as follows:

Superficial injury including:
abrasion
blister (nonthermal)
contusion, including bruise and haematoma
injury from superficial foreign body (splinter) without major open wound
insect bite (nonvenomous)

Open wound including:
animal bite
cut
laceration
puncture wound:
• NOS
• with (penetrating) foreign body

Fracture including:
Fracture:
• closed:
  • comminuted ⎤
  • depressed ⎥
  • elevated   ⎥
  • fissured   ⎥
  • greenstick ⎥
  • impacted   ⎬ with or without delayed healing
  • linear   ⎥
  • march   ⎥
  • simple   ⎥
  • slipped epiphysis ⎥
  • spiral   ⎦
• dislocated
• displaced

Fracture:
- open:
  - compound
  - infected
  - missile ⎫
  - puncture ⎬ with or without delayed healing
  - with foreign body ⎭

Excludes: fracture:
  - pathological (M84.4)
    - with osteoporosis (M80.–)
  - stress (M84.3)
  malunion of fracture (M84.0)
  nonunion of fracture [pseudoarthrosis] (M84.1)

Dislocation, sprain and strain including:
avulsion ⎫
laceration ⎪
sprain ⎪
strain ⎪
traumatic: ⎬ of ⎰ joint (capsule)
- haemarthrosis ⎪   ⎱ ligament
- rupture ⎪
- subluxation ⎪
- tear ⎭

Injury to nerves and spinal cord including:
complete or incomplete lesion of spinal cord
lesion in continuity of nerves and spinal cord
traumatic:
- division of nerve
- haematomyelia
- paralysis (transient)
- paraplegia
- quadriplegia

Injury to blood vessels including:
avulsion ⎫
cut ⎪
laceration ⎪
traumatic: ⎬ of blood vessels
- aneurysm or fistula ⎪
  (arteriovenous) ⎪
- arterial haematoma ⎪
- rupture ⎭

Injury to muscle and tendon including:

avulsion ⎫
cut ⎪
laceration ⎬ of muscle and tendon
traumatic rupture ⎭

Crushing injury

Traumatic amputation

Injury to internal organs including:

blast injuries ⎫
bruise ⎪
concussion injuries ⎪
crushing ⎪
laceration ⎪
traumatic: ⎬ of internal organs
• haematoma ⎪
• puncture ⎪
• rupture ⎪
• tear ⎭

Other and unspecified injuries

Injuries to the head
(S00–S09)

Includes: injuries of:
- ear
- eye
- face [any part]
- gum
- jaw
- mandibular joint area
- oral cavity
- palate
- periocular area
- scalp
- tongue
- tooth

Excludes: burns and corrosions (T20–T32)
         effects of foreign body:
- in:
  - ear (T16)
  - larynx (T17.3)
  - mouth (T18.0)
  - nose (T17.0–T17.1)
  - pharynx (T17.2)
- on external eye (T15.–)
frostbite (T33–T35)
insect bite or sting, venomous (T63.4)

S00   Superficial injury of head

Excludes: cerebral contusion (diffuse) (S06.2)
- focal (S06.3)
injury of eye and orbit (S05.–)

S00.0   Superficial injury of scalp

S00.1   Contusion of eyelid and periocular area
Black eye
Excludes: contusion of eyeball and orbital tissues (S05.1)

S00.2   Other superficial injuries of eyelid and periocular area
Excludes: superficial injury of conjunctiva and cornea (S05.0)

S00.3   Superficial injury of nose

S00.4   Superficial injury of ear

S00.5   Superficial injury of lip and oral cavity

S00.7   Multiple superficial injuries of head

S00.8   Superficial injury of other parts of head

S00.9   Superficial injury of head, part unspecified

S01   Open wound of head

Excludes: decapitation (S18)
injury of eye and orbit (S05.–)
traumatic amputation of part of head (S08.–)

S01.0   Open wound of scalp
Excludes: avulsion of scalp (S08.0)

S01.1	**Open wound of eyelid and periocular area**
	Open wound of eyelid and periocular area with or without involvement of lacrimal passages
S01.2	**Open wound of nose**
S01.3	**Open wound of ear**
S01.4	**Open wound of cheek and temporomandibular area**
S01.5	**Open wound of lip and oral cavity**

Excludes: tooth:
  • dislocation (S03.2)
  • fracture (S02.5)

S01.7	**Multiple open wounds of head**
S01.8	**Open wound of other parts of head**
S01.9	**Open wound of head, part unspecified**

S02 Fracture of skull and facial bones

Note: For primary coding of fracture of skull and facial bones with associated intracranial injury, reference should be made to the morbidity or mortality coding rules and guidelines in Volume 2.

The following subdivisions are provided for optional use in a supplementary character position where it is not possible or not desired to use multiple coding to identify fracture and open wound; a fracture not indicated as closed or open should be classified as closed.

0   closed
1   open

S02.0   Fracture of vault of skull
Frontal bone
Parietal bone

S02.1   **Fracture of base of skull**

Fossa:
- anterior
- middle
- posterior

Occiput

Orbital roof

Sinus:
- ethmoid
- frontal

Sphenoid

Temporal bone

Excludes: orbit NOS (S02.8)
               orbital floor (S02.3)

S02.2   **Fracture of nasal bones**

S02.3   **Fracture of orbital floor**

Excludes: orbit NOS (S02.8)
               orbital roof (S02.1)

S02.4   **Fracture of malar and maxillary bones**

Superior maxilla

Upper jaw (bone)

Zygoma

S02.5   **Fracture of tooth**

Broken tooth

S02.6   **Fracture of mandible**

Lower jaw (bone)

S02.7   **Multiple fractures involving skull and facial bones**

S02.8   **Fractures of other skull and facial bones**

Alveolus

Orbit NOS

Palate

Excludes: orbital:
            - floor (S02.3)
            - roof (S02.1)

S02.9   **Fracture of skull and facial bones, part unspecified**

S03 Dislocation, sprain and strain of joints and ligaments of head

S03.0 **Dislocation of jaw**
Jaw (cartilage)(meniscus)
Mandible
Temporomandibular (joint)

S03.1 **Dislocation of septal cartilage of nose**

S03.2 **Dislocation of tooth**

S03.3 **Dislocation of other and unspecified parts of head**

S03.4 **Sprain and strain of jaw**
Temporomandibular (joint)(ligament)

S03.5 **Sprain and strain of joints and ligaments of other and unspecified parts of head**

S04 Injury of cranial nerves

S04.0 **Injury of optic nerve and pathways**
Optic chiasm
2nd cranial nerve
Visual cortex

S04.1 **Injury of oculomotor nerve**
3rd cranial nerve

S04.2 **Injury of trochlear nerve**
4th cranial nerve

S04.3 **Injury of trigeminal nerve**
5th cranial nerve

S04.4 **Injury of abducent nerve**
6th cranial nerve

S04.5 **Injury of facial nerve**
7th cranial nerve

S04.6 **Injury of acoustic nerve**
Auditory nerve
8th cranial nerve

S04.7 **Injury of accessory nerve**
11th cranial nerve

S04.8   Injury of other cranial nerves
Glossopharyngeal [9th] nerve
Hypoglossal [12th] nerve
Olfactory [1st] nerve
Vagus [10th] nerve

S04.9   Injury of unspecified cranial nerve

S05   Injury of eye and orbit

Excludes: injury of:
- oculomotor [3rd] nerve (S04.1)
- optic [2nd] nerve (S04.0)
open wound of eyelid and periocular area (S01.1)
orbital bone fracture (S02.1, S02.3, S02.8)
superficial injury of eyelid (S00.1–S00.2)

S05.0   Injury of conjunctiva and corneal abrasion without mention of foreign body

Excludes: foreign body in:
- conjunctival sac (T15.1)
- cornea (T15.0)

S05.1   Contusion of eyeball and orbital tissues
Traumatic hyphaema

Excludes: black eye (S00.1)
contusion of eyelid and periocular area (S00.1)

S05.2   Ocular laceration and rupture with prolapse or loss of intraocular tissue

S05.3   Ocular laceration without prolapse or loss of intraocular tissue
Laceration of eye NOS

S05.4   Penetrating wound of orbit with or without foreign body

Excludes: retained (old) foreign body following penetrating wound of orbit (H05.5)

S05.5   Penetrating wound of eyeball with foreign body

Excludes: retained (old) intraocular foreign body (H44.6–H44.7)

S05.6   Penetrating wound of eyeball without foreign body
Ocular penetration NOS

S05.7   Avulsion of eye
Traumatic enucleation

S05.8   **Other injuries of eye and orbit**
Lacrimal duct injury

S05.9   **Injury of eye and orbit, part unspecified**
Injury of eye NOS

S06   Intracranial injury

Note: For primary coding of intracranial injuries with associated fractures, reference should be made to the morbidity or mortality coding rules and guidelines in Volume 2.

The following subdivisions are provided for optional use in a supplementary character position where it is not possible or not desired to use multiple coding to identify intracranial injury and open wound:

0   without open intracranial wound
1   with open intracranial wound

S06.0   **Concussion**
Commotio cerebri

S06.1   **Traumatic cerebral oedema**

S06.2   **Diffuse brain injury**
Cerebral:
• contusion NOS
• laceration NOS
Traumatic compression of brain NOS

S06.3   **Focal brain injury**
Focal:
• cerebral:
  • contusion
  • laceration
• traumatic intracerebral haemorrhage

S06.4   **Epidural haemorrhage**
Extradural haemorrhage (traumatic)

S06.5   **Traumatic subdural haemorrhage**

S06.6   **Traumatic subarachnoid haemorrhage**

S06.7   **Intracranial injury with prolonged coma**

S06.8 **Other intracranial injuries**
Traumatic haemorrhage:
- cerebellar
- intracranial NOS

S06.9 **Intracranial injury, unspecified**
Brain injury NOS
Excludes: head injury NOS (S09.9)

S07 Crushing injury of head

S07.0 **Crushing injury of face**

S07.1 **Crushing injury of skull**

S07.8 **Crushing injury of other parts of head**

S07.9 **Crushing injury of head, part unspecified**

S08 Traumatic amputation of part of head

S08.0 **Avulsion of scalp**

S08.1 **Traumatic amputation of ear**

S08.8 **Traumatic amputation of other parts of head**

S08.9 **Traumatic amputation of unspecified part of head**
Excludes: decapitation (S18)

S09 Other and unspecified injuries of head

S09.0 **Injury of blood vessels of head, not elsewhere classified**
Excludes: injury of:
- cerebral blood vessels (S06.–)
- precerebral blood vessels (S15.–)

S09.1 **Injury of muscle and tendon of head**

S09.2 **Traumatic rupture of ear drum**

S09.7 **Multiple injuries of head**
Injuries classifiable to more than one of the categories
S00–S09.2

S09.8 **Other specified injuries of head**

S09.9   **Unspecified injury of head**
Injury of:
• face NOS
• ear NOS
• nose NOS

Injuries to the neck
(S10–S19)

Includes: injuries of:
• nape
• supraclavicular region
• throat

Excludes: burns and corrosions (T20–T32)
effects of foreign body in:
• larynx (T17.3)
• oesophagus (T18.1)
• pharynx (T17.2)
• trachea (T17.4)
fracture of spine NOS (T08)
frostbite (T33–T35)
injury of:
• spinal cord NOS (T09.3)
• trunk NOS (T09.–)
insect bite or sting, venomous (T63.4)

S10   Superficial injury of neck

S10.0   **Contusion of throat**
Cervical oesophagus
Larynx
Pharynx
Trachea

S10.1   **Other and unspecified superficial injuries of throat**

S10.7   **Multiple superficial injuries of neck**

S10.8   **Superficial injury of other parts of neck**

S10.9   **Superficial injury of neck, part unspecified**

S11   Open wound of neck

Excludes: decapitation (S18)

S11.0   **Open wound involving larynx and trachea**
Trachea:
- NOS
- cervical

Excludes: thoracic trachea (S27.5)

S11.1   **Open wound involving thyroid gland**

S11.2   **Open wound involving pharynx and cervical oesophagus**

Excludes: oesophagus NOS (S27.8)

S11.7   **Multiple open wounds of neck**

S11.8   **Open wound of other parts of neck**

S11.9   **Open wound of neck, part unspecified**

S12   Fracture of neck

Includes: cervical:
- neural arch
- spine
- spinous process
- transverse process
- vertebra
- vertebral arch

The following subdivisions are provided for optional use in a supplementary character position where it is not possible or not desired to use multiple coding to identify fracture and open wound; a fracture not indicated as closed or open should be classified as closed.

0   closed
1   open

S12.0   **Fracture of first cervical vertebra**
Atlas

S12.1   **Fracture of second cervical vertebra**
Axis

S12.2   **Fracture of other specified cervical vertebra**

Excludes: multiple fractures of cervical spine (S12.7)

S12.7   **Multiple fractures of cervical spine**

S12.8   **Fracture of other parts of neck**
Hyoid bone
Larynx
Thyroid cartilage
Trachea

S12.9   **Fracture of neck, part unspecified**
Fracture of cervical:
- spine NOS
- vertebra NOS

S13   Dislocation, sprain and strain of joints and ligaments at neck level

Excludes: rupture or displacement (nontraumatic) of cervical
intervertebral disc (M50.–)

S13.0   **Traumatic rupture of cervical intervertebral disc**

S13.1   **Dislocation of cervical vertebra**
Cervical spine NOS

S13.2   **Dislocation of other and unspecified parts of neck**

S13.3   **Multiple dislocations of neck**

S13.4   **Sprain and strain of cervical spine**
Anterior longitudinal (ligament), cervical
Atlanto-axial (joints)
Atlanto-occipital (joints)
Whiplash injury

S13.5   **Sprain and strain of thyroid region**
Cricoarytenoid (joint)(ligament)
Cricothyroid (joint)(ligament)
Thyroid cartilage

S13.6   **Sprain and strain of joints and ligaments of other and unspecified parts of neck**

S14   Injury of nerves and spinal cord at neck level

S14.0   **Concussion and oedema of cervical spinal cord**

S14.1   **Other and unspecified injuries of cervical spinal cord**
Injury of cervical spinal cord NOS

S14.2   **Injury of nerve root of cervical spine**

S14.3   **Injury of brachial plexus**

S14.4   **Injury of peripheral nerves of neck**

S14.5   **Injury of cervical sympathetic nerves**

S14.6   **Injury of other and unspecified nerves of neck**

S15 Injury of blood vessels at neck level

S15.0   **Injury of carotid artery**
Carotid artery (common) (external) (internal)

S15.1   **Injury of vertebral artery**

S15.2   **Injury of external jugular vein**

S15.3   **Injury of internal jugular vein**

S15.7   **Injury of multiple blood vessels at neck level**

S15.8   **Injury of other blood vessels at neck level**

S15.9   **Injury of unspecified blood vessel at neck level**

S16 Injury of muscle and tendon at neck level

S17 Crushing injury of neck

S17.0   **Crushing injury of larynx and trachea**

S17.8   **Crushing injury of other parts of neck**

S17.9   **Crushing injury of neck, part unspecified**

S18 Traumatic amputation at neck level
Decapitation

S19   Other and unspecified injuries of neck

S19.7   **Multiple injuries of neck**
Injuries classifiable to more than one of the categories S10–S18

S19.8   **Other specified injuries of neck**

S19.9   **Unspecified injury of neck**

Injuries to the thorax
(S20–S29)

Includes: injuries of:
- breast
- chest (wall)
- interscapular area

Excludes: burns and corrosions (T20–T32)
effects of foreign body in:
- bronchus (T17.5)
- lung (T17.8)
- oesophagus (T18.1)
- trachea (T17.4)

fracture of spine NOS (T08)
frostbite (T33–T35)
injuries of:
- axilla ⎫
- clavicle ⎪
- scapular region ⎬ (S40–S49)
- shoulder ⎭
- spinal cord NOS (T09.3)
- trunk NOS (T09.–)

insect bite or sting, venomous (T63.4)

S20   Superficial injury of thorax

S20.0   **Contusion of breast**

S20.1   **Other and unspecified superficial injuries of breast**

S20.2   **Contusion of thorax**

S20.3   **Other superficial injuries of front wall of thorax**

S20.4   **Other superficial injuries of back wall of thorax**

S20.7   **Multiple superficial injuries of thorax**

S20.8   **Superficial injury of other and unspecified parts of thorax**
Thoracic wall NOS

S21   Open wound of thorax

Excludes: traumatic:
- haemopneumothorax (S27.2)
- haemothorax (S27.1)
- pneumothorax (S27.0)

S21.0   **Open wound of breast**

S21.1   **Open wound of front wall of thorax**

S21.2   **Open wound of back wall of thorax**

S21.7   **Multiple open wounds of thoracic wall**

S21.8   **Open wound of other parts of thorax**

S21.9   **Open wound of thorax, part unspecified**
Thoracic wall NOS

S22   Fracture of rib(s), sternum and thoracic spine

Includes: thoracic:
- neural arch
- spinous process
- transverse process
- vertebra
- vertebral arch

The following subdivisions are provided for optional use in a supplementary character position where it is not possible or not desired to use multiple coding to identify fracture and open wound; a fracture not indicated as closed or open should be classified as closed.

0   closed
1   open

Excludes: fracture of:
- clavicle (S42.0)
- scapula (S42.1)

S22.0   **Fracture of thoracic vertebra**
Fracture of thoracic spine NOS

S22.1   **Multiple fractures of thoracic spine**

S22.2   **Fracture of sternum**

S22.3   **Fracture of rib**

S22.4   **Multiple fractures of ribs**

S22.5   **Flail chest**

S22.8   **Fracture of other parts of bony thorax**

S22.9   **Fracture of bony thorax, part unspecified**

S23 Dislocation, sprain and strain of joints and ligaments of thorax

Excludes: dislocation, sprain and strain of sternoclavicular joint (S43.2, S43.6)
rupture or displacement (nontraumatic) of thoracic intervertebral disc (M51.–)

S23.0   **Traumatic rupture of thoracic intervertebral disc**

S23.1   **Dislocation of thoracic vertebra**
Thoracic spine NOS

S23.2   **Dislocation of other and unspecified parts of thorax**

S23.3   **Sprain and strain of thoracic spine**

S23.4   **Sprain and strain of ribs and sternum**

S23.5   **Sprain and strain of other and unspecified parts of thorax**

S24 Injury of nerves and spinal cord at thorax level

Excludes: injury of brachial plexus (S14.3)

S24.0   **Concussion and oedema of thoracic spinal cord**

S24.1   **Other and unspecified injuries of thoracic spinal cord**

S24.2   **Injury of nerve root of thoracic spine**

S24.3   **Injury of peripheral nerves of thorax**

S24.4　**Injury of thoracic sympathetic nerves**
Cardiac plexus
Oesophageal plexus
Pulmonary plexus
Stellate ganglion
Thoracic sympathetic ganglion

S24.5　**Injury of other nerves of thorax**

S24.6　**Injury of unspecified nerve of thorax**

S25　Injury of blood vessels of thorax

S25.0　**Injury of thoracic aorta**
Aorta NOS

S25.1　**Injury of innominate or subclavian artery**

S25.2　**Injury of superior vena cava**
Vena cava NOS

S25.3　**Injury of innominate or subclavian vein**

S25.4　**Injury of pulmonary blood vessels**

S25.5　**Injury of intercostal blood vessels**

S25.7　**Injury of multiple blood vessels of thorax**

S25.8　**Injury of other blood vessels of thorax**
Azygos vein
Mammary artery or vein

S25.9　**Injury of unspecified blood vessel of thorax**

S26　Injury of heart

Includes:　contusion
laceration
puncture　　} of heart
traumatic rupture

The following subdivisions are provided for optional use in a supplementary character position where it is not possible or not desired to use multiple coding:

0　without open wound into thoracic cavity
1　with open wound into thoracic cavity

S26.0　**Injury of heart with haemopericardium**

S26.8   **Other injuries of heart**

S26.9   **Injury of heart, unspecified**

S27   Injury of other and unspecified intrathoracic organs

The following subdivisions are provided for optional use in a supplementary character position where it is not possible or not desired to use multiple coding:

0   without open wound into thoracic cavity
1   with open wound into thoracic cavity

Excludes: injury of:
- cervical oesophagus (S10–S19)
- trachea (cervical) (S10–S19)

S27.0   **Traumatic pneumothorax**

S27.1   **Traumatic haemothorax**

S27.2   **Traumatic haemopneumothorax**

S27.3   **Other injuries of lung**

S27.4   **Injury of bronchus**

S27.5   **Injury of thoracic trachea**

S27.6   **Injury of pleura**

S27.7   **Multiple injuries of intrathoracic organs**

S27.8   **Injury of other specified intrathoracic organs**
Diaphragm
Lymphatic thoracic duct
Oesophagus (thoracic part)
Thymus gland

S27.9   **Injury of unspecified intrathoracic organ**

S28   Crushing injury of thorax and traumatic amputation of part of thorax

S28.0   **Crushed chest**
Excludes: flail chest (S22.5)

S28.1   **Traumatic amputation of part of thorax**
Excludes: transection of thorax (T05.8)

S29   Other and unspecified injuries of thorax

S29.0   **Injury of muscle and tendon at thorax level**

S29.7   **Multiple injuries of thorax**
Injuries classifiable to more than one of the categories
S20–S29.0

S29.8   **Other specified injuries of thorax**

S29.9   **Unspecified injury of thorax**

Injuries to the abdomen, lower back, lumbar spine and pelvis (S30–S39)

Includes: abdominal wall
anus
buttock
external genitalia
flank
groin

Excludes: burns and corrosions (T20–T32)
effects of foreign body in:
• anus and rectum (T18.5)
• genitourinary tract (T19.–)
• stomach, small intestine and colon (T18.2–T18.4)
fracture of spine NOS (T08)
frostbite (T33–T35)
injuries of:
• back NOS (T09.–)
• spinal cord NOS (T09.3)
• trunk NOS (T09.–)
insect bite or sting, venomous (T63.4)

S30   Superficial injury of abdomen, lower back and pelvis

Excludes: superficial injury of hip (S70.–)

S30.0   **Contusion of lower back and pelvis**
Buttock

S30.1 **Contusion of abdominal wall**
Flank
Groin

S30.2 **Contusion of external genital organs**
Labium (majus)(minus)
Penis
Perineum
Scrotum
Testis
Vagina
Vulva

S30.7 **Multiple superficial injuries of abdomen, lower back and pelvis**

S30.8 **Other superficial injuries of abdomen, lower back and pelvis**

S30.9 **Superficial injury of abdomen, lower back and pelvis, part unspecified**

S31 Open wound of abdomen, lower back and pelvis
Excludes: open wound of hip (S71.0)
traumatic amputation of part of abdomen, lower back and pelvis (S38.2–S38.3)

S31.0 **Open wound of lower back and pelvis**
Buttock

S31.1 **Open wound of abdominal wall**
Flank
Groin

S31.2 **Open wound of penis**

S31.3 **Open wound of scrotum and testes**

S31.4 **Open wound of vagina and vulva**

S31.5 **Open wound of other and unspecified external genital organs**
Excludes: traumatic amputation of external genital organs (S38.2)

S31.7 **Multiple open wounds of abdomen, lower back and pelvis**

S31.8 **Open wound of other and unspecified parts of abdomen**

S32 Fracture of lumbar spine and pelvis

Includes: lumbosacral:
- neural arch
- spinous process
- transverse process
- vertebra
- vertebral arch

The following subdivisions are provided for optional use in a supplementary character position where it is not possible or not desired to use multiple coding to identify fracture and open wound; a fracture not indicated as closed or open should be classified as closed.

0   closed
1   open

Excludes: fracture of hip NOS (S72.0)

S32.0   Fracture of lumbar vertebra
Fracture of lumbar spine

S32.1   Fracture of sacrum

S32.2   Fracture of coccyx

S32.3   Fracture of ilium

S32.4   Fracture of acetabulum

S32.5   Fracture of pubis

S32.7   Multiple fractures of lumbar spine and pelvis

S32.8   Fracture of other and unspecified parts of lumbar spine and pelvis
Fracture of:
- ischium
- lumbosacral spine NOS
- pelvis NOS

S33 Dislocation, sprain and strain of joints and ligaments of lumbar spine and pelvis

Excludes: dislocation, sprain and strain of joint and ligaments of hip (S73.–)
obstetric damage to pelvic joints and ligaments (O71.6)
rupture or displacement (nontraumatic) of lumbar intervertebral disc (M51.–)

S33.0 Traumatic rupture of lumbar intervertebral disc

S33.1 Dislocation of lumbar vertebra
Dislocation of lumbar spine NOS

S33.2 Dislocation of sacroiliac and sacrococcygeal joint

S33.3 Dislocation of other and unspecified parts of lumbar spine and pelvis

S33.4 Traumatic rupture of symphysis pubis

S33.5 Sprain and strain of lumbar spine

S33.6 Sprain and strain of sacroiliac joint

S33.7 Sprain and strain of other and unspecified parts of lumbar spine and pelvis

S34 Injury of nerves and lumbar spinal cord at abdomen, lower back and pelvis level

S34.0 Concussion and oedema of lumbar spinal cord

S34.1 Other injury of lumbar spinal cord

S34.2 Injury of nerve root of lumbar and sacral spine

S34.3 Injury of cauda equina

S34.4 Injury of lumbosacral plexus

S34.5 Injury of lumbar, sacral and pelvic sympathetic nerves
Coeliac ganglion or plexus
Hypogastric plexus
Mesenteric plexus (inferior)(superior)
Splanchnic nerve

S34.6 Injury of peripheral nerve(s) of abdomen, lower back and pelvis

S34.8 **Injury of other and unspecified nerves at abdomen, lower back and pelvis level**

S35 Injury of blood vessels at abdomen, lower back and pelvis level

S35.0 **Injury of abdominal aorta**
Excludes: aorta NOS (S25.0)

S35.1 **Injury of inferior vena cava**
Hepatic vein
Excludes: vena cava NOS (S25.2)

S35.2 **Injury of coeliac or mesenteric artery**
Gastric artery
Gastroduodenal artery
Hepatic artery
Mesenteric artery (inferior)(superior)
Splenic artery

S35.3 **Injury of portal or splenic vein**
Mesenteric vein (inferior)(superior)

S35.4 **Injury of renal blood vessels**
Renal artery or vein

S35.5 **Injury of iliac blood vessels**
Hypogastric artery or vein
Iliac artery or vein
Uterine artery or vein

S35.7 **Injury of multiple blood vessels at abdomen, lower back and pelvis level**

S35.8 **Injury of other blood vessels at abdomen, lower back and pelvis level**
Ovarian artery or vein

S35.9 **Injury of unspecified blood vessel at abdomen, lower back and pelvis level**

S36 Injury of intra-abdominal organs

The following subdivisions are provided for optional use in a supplementary character position where it is not possible or not desired to use multiple coding:

0   without open wound into cavity
1   with open wound into cavity

S36.0   Injury of spleen

S36.1   Injury of liver or gallbladder
Bile duct

S36.2   Injury of pancreas

S36.3   Injury of stomach

S36.4   Injury of small intestine

S36.5   Injury of colon

S36.6   Injury of rectum

S36.7   Injury of multiple intra-abdominal organs

S36.8   Injury of other intra-abdominal organs
Peritoneum
Retroperitoneum

S36.9   Injury of unspecified intra-abdominal organ

S37 Injury of pelvic organs

The following subdivisions are provided for optional use in a supplementary character position where it is not possible or not desired to use multiple coding:

0   without open wound into cavity
1   with open wound into cavity

Excludes: peritoneum and retroperitoneum (S36.8)

S37.0   Injury of kidney

S37.1   Injury of ureter

S37.2   Injury of bladder

S37.3   Injury of urethra

S37.4   Injury of ovary

S37.5   Injury of fallopian tube

S37.6   **Injury of uterus**

S37.7   **Injury of multiple pelvic organs**

S37.8   **Injury of other pelvic organs**
Adrenal gland
Prostate
Seminal vesicle
Vas deferens

S37.9   **Injury of unspecified pelvic organ**

S38   Crushing injury and traumatic amputation of part of abdomen, lower back and pelvis

S38.0   **Crushing injury of external genital organs**

S38.1   **Crushing injury of other and unspecified parts of abdomen, lower back and pelvis**

S38.2   **Traumatic amputation of external genital organs**
Labium (majus)(minus)
Penis
Scrotum
Testis
Vulva

S38.3   **Traumatic amputation of other and unspecified parts of abdomen, lower back and pelvis**
Excludes: transection of abdomen (T05.8)

S39   Other and unspecified injuries of abdomen, lower back and pelvis

S39.0   **Injury of muscle and tendon of abdomen, lower back and pelvis**

S39.6   **Injury of intra-abdominal organ(s) with pelvic organ(s)**

S39.7   **Other multiple injuries of abdomen, lower back and pelvis**
Injuries classifiable to more than one of the categories
   S30–S39.6
Excludes: injuries in S36.– with injuries in S37.– (S39.6)

S39.8   Other specified injuries of abdomen, lower back and pelvis

S39.9   Unspecified injury of abdomen, lower back and pelvis

Injuries to the shoulder and upper arm (S40–S49)

Includes: injuries of:
- axilla
- scapular region

Excludes: bilateral involvement of shoulder and upper arm (T00–T07)
burns and corrosions (T20–T32)
frostbite (T33–T35)
injuries of:
- arm, level unspecified (T10–T11)
- elbow (S50–S59)

insect bite or sting, venomous (T63.4)

S40   Superficial injury of shoulder and upper arm

S40.0   Contusion of shoulder and upper arm

S40.7   Multiple superficial injuries of shoulder and upper arm

S40.8   Other superficial injuries of shoulder and upper arm

S40.9   Superficial injury of shoulder and upper arm, unspecified

S41   Open wound of shoulder and upper arm

Excludes: traumatic amputation of shoulder and upper arm (S48.–)

S41.0   Open wound of shoulder

S41.1   Open wound of upper arm

S41.7   Multiple open wounds of shoulder and upper arm

S41.8   Open wound of other and unspecified parts of shoulder girdle

S42 Fracture of shoulder and upper arm

The following subdivisions are provided for optional use in a supplementary character position where it is not possible or not desired to use multiple coding to identify fracture and open wound; a fracture not indicated as closed or open should be classified as closed.

0   closed
1   open

S42.0   Fracture of clavicle
Clavicle:
• acromial end
• shaft
Collar bone

S42.1   Fracture of scapula
Acromial process
Acromion (process)
Scapula (body)(glenoid cavity)(neck)
Shoulder blade

S42.2   Fracture of upper end of humerus
Anatomical neck
Great tuberosity
Proximal end
Surgical neck
Upper epiphysis

S42.3   Fracture of shaft of humerus
Humerus NOS
Upper arm NOS

S42.4   Fracture of lower end of humerus
Articular process
Distal end
External condyle
Intercondylar
Internal epicondyle
Lower epiphysis
Supracondylar
Excludes: fracture of elbow NOS (S52.0)

S42.7   Multiple fractures of clavicle, scapula and humerus

S42.8   Fracture of other parts of shoulder and upper arm

S42.9   **Fracture of shoulder girdle, part unspecified**
Fracture of shoulder NOS

S43   Dislocation, sprain and strain of joints and ligaments of shoulder girdle

S43.0   **Dislocation of shoulder joint**
Glenohumeral joint

S43.1   **Dislocation of acromioclavicular joint**

S43.2   **Dislocation of sternoclavicular joint**

S43.3   **Dislocation of other and unspecified parts of shoulder girdle**
Dislocation of shoulder girdle NOS

S43.4   **Sprain and strain of shoulder joint**
Coracohumeral (ligament)
Rotator cuff (capsule)

S43.5   **Sprain and strain of acromioclavicular joint**
Acromioclavicular ligament

S43.6   **Sprain and strain of sternoclavicular joint**

S43.7   **Sprain and strain of other and unspecified parts of shoulder girdle**
Sprain and strain of shoulder girdle NOS

S44   Injury of nerves at shoulder and upper arm level

Excludes: injury of brachial plexus (S14.3)

S44.0   **Injury of ulnar nerve at upper arm level**
Excludes: ulnar nerve NOS (S54.0)

S44.1   **Injury of median nerve at upper arm level**
Excludes: median nerve NOS (S54.1)

S44.2   **Injury of radial nerve at upper arm level**
Excludes: radial nerve NOS (S54.2)

S44.3   **Injury of axillary nerve**

S44.4   **Injury of musculocutaneous nerve**

S44.5   **Injury of cutaneous sensory nerve at shoulder and upper arm level**

S44.7   Injury of multiple nerves at shoulder and upper arm level

S44.8   Injury of other nerves at shoulder and upper arm level

S44.9   Injury of unspecified nerve at shoulder and upper arm level

S45   Injury of blood vessels at shoulder and upper arm level

Excludes: injury of subclavian:
- artery (S25.1)
- vein (S25.3)

S45.0   Injury of axillary artery

S45.1   Injury of brachial artery

S45.2   Injury of axillary or brachial vein

S45.3   Injury of superficial vein at shoulder and upper arm level

S45.7   Injury of multiple blood vessels at shoulder and upper arm level

S45.8   Injury of other blood vessels at shoulder and upper arm level

S45.9   Injury of unspecified blood vessel at shoulder and upper arm level

S46   Injury of muscle and tendon at shoulder and upper arm level

Excludes: injury of muscle and tendon at or below elbow (S56.–)

S46.0   Injury of tendon of the rotator cuff of shoulder

S46.1   Injury of muscle and tendon of long head of biceps

S46.2   Injury of muscle and tendon of other parts of biceps

S46.3   Injury of muscle and tendon of triceps

S46.7   Injury of multiple muscles and tendons at shoulder and upper arm level

S46.8   Injury of other muscles and tendons at shoulder and upper arm level

S46.9   Injury of unspecified muscle and tendon at shoulder and upper arm level

S47   Crushing injury of shoulder and upper arm
Excludes: crushing injury of elbow (S57.0)

S48   Traumatic amputation of shoulder and upper arm
Excludes: traumatic amputation:
- at elbow level (S58.0)
- of arm, level unspecified (T11.6)

S48.0   Traumatic amputation at shoulder joint

S48.1   Traumatic amputation at level between shoulder and elbow

S48.9   Traumatic amputation of shoulder and upper arm, level unspecified

S49   Other and unspecified injuries of shoulder and upper arm

S49.7   Multiple injuries of shoulder and upper arm
Injuries classifiable to more than one of the categories S40–S48

S49.8   Other specified injuries of shoulder and upper arm

S49.9   Unspecified injury of shoulder and upper arm

Injuries to the elbow and forearm (S50–S59)

Excludes: bilateral involvement of elbow and forearm (T00–T07)
burns and corrosions (T20–T32)
frostbite (T33–T35)
injuries of:
- arm, level unspecified (T10–T11)
- wrist and hand (S60–S69)
insect bite or sting, venomous (T63.4)

S50   Superficial injury of forearm
Excludes: superficial injury of wrist and hand (S60.–)

S50.0   **Contusion of elbow**

S50.1   **Contusion of other and unspecified parts of forearm**

S50.7   **Multiple superficial injuries of forearm**

S50.8   **Other superficial injuries of forearm**

S50.9   **Superficial injury of forearm, unspecified**
Superficial injury of elbow NOS

S51 Open wound of forearm
Excludes: open wound of wrist and hand (S61.–)
traumatic amputation of forearm (S58.–)

S51.0   **Open wound of elbow**

S51.7   **Multiple open wounds of forearm**

S51.8   **Open wound of other parts of forearm**

S51.9   **Open wound of forearm, part unspecified**

S52 Fracture of forearm
The following subdivisions are provided for optional use in a supplementary character position where it is not possible or not desired to use multiple coding to identify fracture and open wound; a fracture not indicated as closed or open should be classified as closed.

0   closed
1   open

Excludes: fracture at wrist and hand level (S62.–)

S52.0   **Fracture of upper end of ulna**
Coronoid process
Elbow NOS
Monteggia's fracture-dislocation
Olecranon process
Proximal end

S52.1   **Fracture of upper end of radius**
Head
Neck
Proximal end

S52.2   **Fracture of shaft of ulna**

S52.3   **Fracture of shaft of radius**

S52.4   **Fracture of shafts of both ulna and radius**

S52.5   **Fracture of lower end of radius**
Colles' fracture
Smith's fracture

S52.6   **Fracture of lower end of both ulna and radius**

S52.7   **Multiple fractures of forearm**
Excludes: fractures of both ulna and radius:
- lower end (S52.6)
- shafts (S52.4)

S52.8   **Fracture of other parts of forearm**
Lower end of ulna
Head of ulna

S52.9   **Fracture of forearm, part unspecified**

S53   Dislocation, sprain and strain of joints and ligaments of elbow

S53.0   **Dislocation of radial head**
Radiohumeral joint
Excludes: Monteggia's fracture-dislocation (S52.0)

S53.1   **Dislocation of elbow, unspecified**
Ulnohumeral joint
Excludes: dislocation of radial head alone (S53.0)

S53.2   **Traumatic rupture of radial collateral ligament**

S53.3   **Traumatic rupture of ulnar collateral ligament**

S53.4   **Sprain and strain of elbow**

S54   Injury of nerves at forearm level
Excludes: injury of nerves at wrist and hand level (S64.–)

S54.0   **Injury of ulnar nerve at forearm level**
Ulnar nerve NOS

S54.1   **Injury of median nerve at forearm level**
Median nerve NOS

S54.2   **Injury of radial nerve at forearm level**
Radial nerve NOS

S54.3　Injury of cutaneous sensory nerve at forearm level

S54.7　Injury of multiple nerves at forearm level

S54.8　Injury of other nerves at forearm level

S54.9　Injury of unspecified nerve at forearm level

S55　Injury of blood vessels at forearm level

Excludes: injury of:
- blood vessels at wrist and hand level (S65.–)
- brachial vessels (S45.1–S45.2)

S55.0　Injury of ulnar artery at forearm level

S55.1　Injury of radial artery at forearm level

S55.2　Injury of vein at forearm level

S55.7　Injury of multiple blood vessels at forearm level

S55.8　Injury of other blood vessels at forearm level

S55.9　Injury of unspecified blood vessel at forearm level

S56　Injury of muscle and tendon at forearm level

Excludes: injury of muscle and tendon at or below wrist (S66.–)

S56.0　Injury of flexor muscle and tendon of thumb at forearm level

S56.1　Injury of flexor muscle and tendon of other finger(s) at forearm level

S56.2　Injury of other flexor muscle and tendon at forearm level

S56.3　Injury of extensor or abductor muscles and tendons of thumb at forearm level

S56.4　Injury of extensor muscle and tendon of other finger(s) at forearm level

S56.5　Injury of other extensor muscle and tendon at forearm level

S56.7　Injury of multiple muscles and tendons at forearm level

S56.8　Injury of other and unspecified muscles and tendons at forearm level

S57 Crushing injury of forearm

Excludes: crushing injury of wrist and hand (S67.–)

S57.0 Crushing injury of elbow

S57.8 Crushing injury of other parts of forearm

S57.9 Crushing injury of forearm, part unspecified

S58 Traumatic amputation of forearm

Excludes: traumatic amputation of wrist and hand (S68.–)

S58.0 Traumatic amputation at elbow level

S58.1 Traumatic amputation at level between elbow and wrist

S58.9 Traumatic amputation of forearm, level unspecified

S59 Other and unspecified injuries of forearm

Excludes: other and unspecified injuries of wrist and hand (S69.–)

S59.7 Multiple injuries of forearm
Injuries classifiable to more than one of the categories S50–S58

S59.8 Other specified injuries of forearm

S59.9 Unspecified injury of forearm

Injuries to the wrist and hand
(S60–S69)

Excludes: bilateral involvement of wrist and hand (T00–T07)
burns and corrosions (T20–T32)
frostbite (T33–T35)
injuries of arm, level unspecified (T10–T11)
insect bite or sting, venomous (T63.4)

S60   Superficial injury of wrist and hand

S60.0   **Contusion of finger(s) without damage to nail**
Contusion of finger(s) NOS
Excludes: contusion involving nail (matrix) (S60.1)

S60.1   **Contusion of finger(s) with damage to nail**

S60.2   **Contusion of other parts of wrist and hand**

S60.7   **Multiple superficial injuries of wrist and hand**

S60.8   **Other superficial injuries of wrist and hand**

S60.9   **Superficial injury of wrist and hand, unspecified**

S61   Open wound of wrist and hand

Excludes: traumatic amputation of wrist and hand (S68.–)

S61.0   **Open wound of finger(s) without damage to nail**
Open wound of finger(s) NOS
Excludes: open wound involving nail (matrix) (S61.1)

S61.1   **Open wound of finger(s) with damage to nail**

S61.7   **Multiple open wounds of wrist and hand**

S61.8   **Open wound of other parts of wrist and hand**

S61.9   **Open wound of wrist and hand part, part unspecified**

S62   Fracture at wrist and hand level

The following subdivisions are provided for optional use in a supplementary character position where it is not possible or not desired to use multiple coding to identify fracture and open wound; a fracture not indicated as closed or open should be classified as closed.

0   closed
1   open

Excludes: fracture of distal parts of ulna and radius (S52.–)

S62.0   **Fracture of navicular [scaphoid] bone of hand**

S62.1 **Fracture of other carpal bone(s)**
Capitate [os magnum]
Hamate [unciform]
Lunate [semilunar]
Pisiform
Trapezium [greater multangular]
Trapezoid [lesser multangular]
Triquetrum [cuneiform of carpus]

S62.2 **Fracture of first metacarpal bone**
Bennett's fracture

S62.3 **Fracture of other metacarpal bone**

S62.4 **Multiple fractures of metacarpal bones**

S62.5 **Fracture of thumb**

S62.6 **Fracture of other finger**

S62.7 **Multiple fractures of fingers**

S62.8 **Fracture of other and unspecified parts of wrist and hand**

S63 Dislocation, sprain and strain of joints and ligaments at wrist and hand level

S63.0 **Dislocation of wrist**
Carpal (bone)
Carpometacarpal (joint)
Metacarpal (bone), proximal end
Midcarpal (joint)
Radiocarpal (joint)
Radioulnar (joint), distal
Radius, distal end
Ulna, distal end

S63.1 **Dislocation of finger**
Interphalangeal (joint), hand
Metacarpal (bone), distal end
Metacarpophalangeal (joint)
Phalanx, hand
Thumb

S63.2 **Multiple dislocations of fingers**

S63.3   **Traumatic rupture of ligament of wrist and carpus**
Collateral, wrist
Radiocarpal (ligament)
Ulnocarpal (palmar)

S63.4   **Traumatic rupture of ligament of finger at metacarpophalangeal and interphalangeal joint(s)**
Collateral
Palmar
Volar plate

S63.5   **Sprain and strain of wrist**
Carpal (joint)
Radiocarpal (joint) (ligament)

S63.6   **Sprain and strain of finger(s)**
Interphalangeal (joint), hand
Metacarpophalangeal (joint)
Phalanx, hand
Thumb

S63.7   **Sprain and strain of other and unspecified parts of hand**

S64   Injury of nerves at wrist and hand level

S64.0   Injury of ulnar nerve at wrist and hand level

S64.1   Injury of median nerve at wrist and hand level

S64.2   Injury of radial nerve at wrist and hand level

S64.3   Injury of digital nerve of thumb

S64.4   Injury of digital nerve of other finger

S64.7   Injury of multiple nerves at wrist and hand level

S64.8   Injury of other nerves at wrist and hand level

S64.9   Injury of unspecified nerve at wrist and hand level

S65   Injury of blood vessels at wrist and hand level

S65.0   Injury of ulnar artery at wrist and hand level

S65.1   Injury of radial artery at wrist and hand level

S65.2   Injury of superficial palmar arch

S65.3   Injury of deep palmar arch

S65.4   Injury of blood vessel(s) of thumb

S65.5   Injury of blood vessel(s) of other finger

S65.7   Injury of multiple blood vessels at wrist and hand level

S65.8   Injury of other blood vessels at wrist and hand level

S65.9   Injury of unspecified blood vessel at wrist and hand level

S66 Injury of muscle and tendon at wrist and hand level

S66.0   Injury of long flexor muscle and tendon of thumb at wrist and hand level

S66.1   Injury of flexor muscle and tendon of other finger at wrist and hand level

S66.2   Injury of extensor muscle and tendon of thumb at wrist and hand level

S66.3   Injury of extensor muscle and tendon of other finger at wrist and hand level

S66.4   Injury of intrinsic muscle and tendon of thumb at wrist and hand level

S66.5   Injury of intrinsic muscle and tendon of other finger at wrist and hand level

S66.6   Injury of multiple flexor muscles and tendons at wrist and hand level

S66.7   Injury of multiple extensor muscles and tendons at wrist and hand level

S66.8   Injury of other muscles and tendons at wrist and hand level

S66.9   Injury of unspecified muscle and tendon at wrist and hand level

S67 Crushing injury of wrist and hand

S67.0   Crushing injury of thumb and other finger(s)

S67.8   Crushing injury of other and unspecified parts of wrist and hand

S68   Traumatic amputation of wrist and hand

S68.0   **Traumatic amputation of thumb (complete)(partial)**

S68.1   **Traumatic amputation of other single finger (complete)(partial)**

S68.2   **Traumatic amputation of two or more fingers alone (complete)(partial)**

S68.3   **Combined traumatic amputation of (part of) finger(s) with other parts of wrist and hand**

S68.4   **Traumatic amputation of hand at wrist level**

S68.8   **Traumatic amputation of other parts of wrist and hand**

S68.9   **Traumatic amputation of wrist and hand, level unspecified**

S69   Other and unspecified injuries of wrist and hand

S69.7   **Multiple injuries of wrist and hand**
Injuries classifiable to more than one of the categories S60–S68

S69.8   **Other specified injuries of wrist and hand**

S69.9   **Unspecified injury of wrist and hand**

Injuries to the hip and thigh
(S70–S79)

Excludes: bilateral involvement of hip and thigh (T00–T07)
            burns and corrosions (T20–T32)
            frostbite (T33–T35)
            injuries of leg, level unspecified (T12–T13)
            insect bite or sting, venomous (T63.4)

S70   Superficial injury of hip and thigh

S70.0   **Contusion of hip**

S70.1   **Contusion of thigh**

S70.7   **Multiple superficial injuries of hip and thigh**

S70.8   Other superficial injuries of hip and thigh

S70.9   Superficial injury of hip and thigh, unspecified

S71   Open wound of hip and thigh

Excludes: traumatic amputation of hip and thigh (S78.–)

S71.0   Open wound of hip

S71.1   Open wound of thigh

S71.7   Multiple open wounds of hip and thigh

S71.8   Open wound of other and unspecified parts of pelvic girdle

S72   Fracture of femur

The following subdivisions are provided for optional use in a supplementary character position where it is not possible or not desired to use multiple coding to identify fracture and open wound; a fracture not indicated as closed or open should be classified as closed.

0   closed
1   open

S72.0   **Fracture of neck of femur**
Fracture of hip NOS

S72.1   **Pertrochanteric fracture**
Intertrochanteric fracture
Trochanteric fracture

S72.2   Subtrochanteric fracture

S72.3   Fracture of shaft of femur

S72.4   Fracture of lower end of femur

S72.7   Multiple fractures of femur

S72.8   Fractures of other parts of femur

S72.9   Fracture of femur, part unspecified

S73 Dislocation, sprain and strain of joint and ligaments of hip

S73.0 Dislocation of hip

S73.1 Sprain and strain of hip

S74 Injury of nerves at hip and thigh level

S74.0 Injury of sciatic nerve at hip and thigh level

S74.1 Injury of femoral nerve at hip and thigh level

S74.2 Injury of cutaneous sensory nerve at hip and thigh level

S74.7 Injury of multiple nerves at hip and thigh level

S74.8 Injury of other nerves at hip and thigh level

S74.9 Injury of unspecified nerve at hip and thigh level

S75 Injury of blood vessels at hip and thigh level
Excludes: popliteal artery (S85.0)

S75.0 Injury of femoral artery

S75.1 Injury of femoral vein at hip and thigh level

S75.2 Injury of greater saphenous vein at hip and thigh level
Excludes: greater saphenous vein NOS (S85.3)

S75.7 Injury of multiple blood vessels at hip and thigh level

S75.8 Injury of other blood vessels at hip and thigh level

S75.9 Injury of unspecified blood vessel at hip and thigh level

S76 Injury of muscle and tendon at hip and thigh level

S76.0 Injury of muscle and tendon of hip

S76.1 Injury of quadriceps muscle and tendon

S76.2 Injury of adductor muscle and tendon of thigh

S76.3 Injury of muscle and tendon of the posterior muscle group at thigh level

S76.4 Injury of other and unspecified muscles and tendons at thigh level

S76.7   **Injury of multiple muscles and tendons at hip and thigh level**

S77   Crushing injury of hip and thigh

S77.0   **Crushing injury of hip**

S77.1   **Crushing injury of thigh**

S77.2   **Crushing injury of hip with thigh**

S78   Traumatic amputation of hip and thigh

Excludes: traumatic amputation of leg, level unspecified (T13.6)

S78.0   **Traumatic amputation at hip joint**

S78.1   **Traumatic amputation at level between hip and knee**

S78.9   **Traumatic amputation of hip and thigh, level unspecified**

S79   Other and unspecified injuries of hip and thigh

S79.7   **Multiple injuries of hip and thigh**
Injuries classifiable to more than one of the categories S70–S78

S79.8   **Other specified injuries of hip and thigh**

S79.9   **Unspecified injury of hip and thigh**

Injuries to the knee and lower leg (S80–S89)

Includes: fracture of ankle and malleolus

Excludes: bilateral involvement of knee and lower leg (T00–T07)
burns and corrosions (T20–T32)
frostbite (T33–T35)
injuries of:
• ankle and foot, except fracture of ankle and malleolus (S90–S99)
• leg, level unspecified (T12–T13)
insect bite or sting, venomous (T63.4)

S80 Superficial injury of lower leg

Excludes: superficial injury of ankle and foot (S90.–)

S80.0 Contusion of knee

S80.1 Contusion of other and unspecified parts of lower leg

S80.7 Multiple superficial injuries of lower leg

S80.8 Other superficial injuries of lower leg

S80.9 Superficial injury of lower leg, unspecified

S81 Open wound of lower leg

Excludes: open wound of ankle and foot (S91.–)
traumatic amputation of lower leg (S88.–)

S81.0 Open wound of knee

S81.7 Multiple open wounds of lower leg

S81.8 Open wound of other parts of lower leg

S81.9 Open wound of lower leg, part unspecified

S82 Fracture of lower leg, including ankle

Includes: malleolus

The following subdivisions are provided for optional use in a supplementary character position where it is not possible or not desired to use multiple coding to identify fracture and open wound; a fracture not indicated as closed or open should be classified as closed.

0 closed
1 open

Excludes: fracture of foot, except ankle (S92.–)

S82.0 Fracture of patella
Knee cap

S82.1   Fracture of upper end of tibia
Tibial:
- condyles
- head   ⎤ with or without mention of fracture of
- proximal end ⎬ fibula
- tuberosity   ⎦

S82.2   Fracture of shaft of tibia
With or without mention of fracture of fibula

S82.3   Fracture of lower end of tibia
With or without mention of fracture of fibula
Excludes: medial malleolus (S82.5)

S82.4   Fracture of fibula alone
Excludes: lateral malleolus (S82.6)

S82.5   Fracture of medial malleolus
Tibia involving:
- ankle
- malleolus

S82.6   Fracture of lateral malleolus
Fibula involving:
- ankle
- malleolus

S82.7   Multiple fractures of lower leg
Excludes: fractures of both tibia and fibula:
- lower end (S82.3)
- shafts (S82.2)
- upper end (S82.1)

S82.8   Fractures of other parts of lower leg
Fracture (of):
- ankle NOS
- bimalleolar
- trimalleolar

S82.9   Fracture of lower leg, part unspecified

S83 Dislocation, sprain and strain of joints and ligaments of knee

Excludes: derangement of:
- knee, internal (M23.–)
- patella (M22.0–M22.3)
  dislocation of knee:
- old (M24.3)
- pathological (M24.3)
- recurrent (M24.4)

S83.0 **Dislocation of patella**

S83.1 **Dislocation of knee**
Tibiofibular (joint)

S83.2 **Tear of meniscus, current**
Bucket-handle tear (of):
- NOS
- lateral meniscus
- medial meniscus

Excludes: old bucket-handle tear (M23.2)

S83.3 **Tear of articular cartilage of knee, current**

S83.4 **Sprain and strain involving (fibular)(tibial) collateral ligament of knee**

S83.5 **Sprain and strain involving (anterior)(posterior) cruciate ligament of knee**

S83.6 **Sprain and strain of other and unspecified parts of knee**
Patellar ligament
Tibiofibular joint and ligament, superior

S83.7 **Injury to multiple structures of knee**
Injury to (lateral)(medial) meniscus in combination with (collateral)(cruciate) ligaments

S84 Injury of nerves at lower leg level

Excludes: injury of nerves at ankle and foot level (S94.–)

S84.0 **Injury of tibial nerve at lower leg level**

S84.1 **Injury of peroneal nerve at lower leg level**

S84.2 **Injury of cutaneous sensory nerve at lower leg level**

S84.7   Injury of multiple nerves at lower leg level

S84.8   Injury of other nerves at lower leg level

S84.9   Injury of unspecified nerve at lower leg level

S85   Injury of blood vessels at lower leg level
Excludes: injury of blood vessels at ankle and foot level (S95.–)

S85.0   Injury of popliteal artery

S85.1   Injury of (anterior)(posterior) tibial artery

S85.2   Injury of peroneal artery

S85.3   Injury of greater saphenous vein at lower leg level
Greater saphenous vein NOS

S85.4   Injury of lesser saphenous vein at lower leg level

S85.5   Injury of popliteal vein

S85.7   Injury of multiple blood vessels at lower leg level

S85.8   Injury of other blood vessels at lower leg level

S85.9   Injury of unspecified blood vessel at lower leg level

S86   Injury of muscle and tendon at lower leg level
Excludes: injury of muscle and tendon at or below ankle (S96.–)

S86.0   Injury of Achilles tendon

S86.1   Injury of other muscle(s) and tendon(s) of posterior muscle group at lower leg level

S86.2   Injury of muscle(s) and tendon(s) of anterior muscle group at lower leg level

S86.3   Injury of muscle(s) and tendon(s) of peroneal muscle group at lower leg level

S86.7   Injury of multiple muscles and tendons at lower leg level

S86.8   Injury of other muscles and tendons at lower leg level

S86.9   Injury of unspecified muscle and tendon at lower leg level

S87 Crushing injury of lower leg

Excludes: crushing injury of ankle and foot (S97.–)

S87.0 **Crushing injury of knee**

S87.8 **Crushing injury of other and unspecified parts of lower leg**

S88 Traumatic amputation of lower leg

Excludes: traumatic amputation of:
- ankle and foot (S98.–)
- leg, level unspecified (T13.6)

S88.0 **Traumatic amputation at knee level**

S88.1 **Traumatic amputation at level between knee and ankle**

S88.9 **Traumatic amputation of lower leg, level unspecified**

S89 Other and unspecified injuries of lower leg

Excludes: other and unspecified injuries of ankle and foot
(S99.–)

S89.7 **Multiple injuries of lower leg**
Injuries classifiable to more than one of the categories S80–S88

S89.8 **Other specified injuries of lower leg**

S89.9 **Unspecified injury of lower leg**

Injuries to the ankle and foot
(S90–S99)

Excludes: bilateral involvement of ankle and foot (T00–T07)
burns and corrosions (T20–T32)
fracture of ankle and malleolus (S82.–)
frostbite (T33–T35)
injuries of leg, level unspecified (T12–T13)
insect bite or sting, venomous (T63.4)

S90 Superficial injury of ankle and foot

S90.0 **Contusion of ankle**

S90.1 **Contusion of toe(s) without damage to nail**
Contusion of toe(s) NOS

S90.2 **Contusion of toe(s) with damage to nail**

S90.3 **Contusion of other and unspecified parts of foot**

S90.7 **Multiple superficial injuries of ankle and foot**

S90.8 **Other superficial injuries of ankle and foot**

S90.9 **Superficial injury of ankle and foot, unspecified**

S91 Open wound of ankle and foot
Excludes: traumatic amputation of ankle and foot (S98.–)

S91.0 **Open wound of ankle**

S91.1 **Open wound of toe(s) without damage to nail**
Open wound of toe(s) NOS

S91.2 **Open wound of toe(s) with damage to nail**

S91.3 **Open wound of other parts of foot**
Open wound of foot NOS

S91.7 **Multiple open wounds of ankle and foot**

S92 Fracture of foot, except ankle
The following subdivisions are provided for optional use in a supplementary character position where it is not possible or not desired to use multiple cause coding to identify fracture and open wound; a fracture not indicated as closed or open should be classified as closed.
0   closed
1   open

Excludes: ankle (S82.–)
malleolus (S82.–)

S92.0 **Fracture of calcaneus**
Heel bone
Os calcis

S92.1 **Fracture of talus**
Astragalus

S92.2 **Fracture of other tarsal bone(s)**
Cuboid
Cuneiform, foot (intermediate)(lateral)(medial)
Navicular, foot

S92.3 **Fracture of metatarsal bone**

S92.4 **Fracture of great toe**

S92.5 **Fracture of other toe**

S92.7 **Multiple fractures of foot**

S92.9 **Fracture of foot, unspecified**

S93 Dislocation, sprain and strain of joints and ligaments at ankle and foot level

S93.0 **Dislocation of ankle joint**
Astragalus
Fibula, lower end
Talus
Tibia, lower end

S93.1 **Dislocation of toe(s)**
Interphalangeal (joint(s))
Metatarsophalangeal (joint(s))

S93.2 **Rupture of ligaments at ankle and foot level**

S93.3 **Dislocation of other and unspecified parts of foot**
Navicular, foot
Tarsal (joint(s))
Tarsometatarsal (joint(s))

S93.4 **Sprain and strain of ankle**
Calcaneofibular (ligament)
Deltoid (ligament)
Internal collateral (ligament)
Talofibular (ligament)
Tibiofibular (ligament), distal
Excludes: injury of Achilles tendon (S86.0)

S93.5 **Sprain and strain of toe(s)**
Interphalangeal (joint(s))
Metatarsophalangeal (joint(s))

S93.6   Sprain and strain of other and unspecified parts of foot
Tarsal (ligament)
Tarsometatarsal (ligament)

S94   Injury of nerves at ankle and foot level

S94.0   Injury of lateral plantar nerve

S94.1   Injury of medial plantar nerve

S94.2   Injury of deep peroneal nerve at ankle and foot level
Terminal, lateral branch of deep peroneal nerve

S94.3   Injury of cutaneous sensory nerve at ankle and foot level

S94.7   Injury of multiple nerves at ankle and foot level

S94.8   Injury of other nerves at ankle and foot level

S94.9   Injury of unspecified nerve at ankle and foot level

S95   Injury of blood vessels at ankle and foot level
Excludes: injury of posterior tibial artery and vein (S85.–)

S95.0   Injury of dorsal artery of foot

S95.1   Injury of plantar artery of foot

S95.2   Injury of dorsal vein of foot

S95.7   Injury of multiple blood vessels at ankle and foot level

S95.8   Injury of other blood vessels at ankle and foot level

S95.9   Injury of unspecified blood vessel at ankle and foot level

S96   Injury of muscle and tendon at ankle and foot level
Excludes: injury of Achilles tendon (S86.0)

S96.0   Injury of muscle and tendon of long flexor muscle of toe at ankle and foot level

S96.1   Injury of muscle and tendon of long extensor muscle of toe at ankle and foot level

S96.2   Injury of intrinsic muscle and tendon at ankle and foot level

S96.7 Injury of multiple muscles and tendons at ankle and foot level

S96.8 Injury of other muscles and tendons at ankle and foot level

S96.9 Injury of unspecified muscle and tendon at ankle and foot level

S97 Crushing injury of ankle and foot

S97.0 Crushing injury of ankle

S97.1 Crushing injury of toe(s)

S97.8 Crushing injury of other parts of ankle and foot
Crushing injury of foot NOS

S98 Traumatic amputation of ankle and foot

S98.0 Traumatic amputation of foot at ankle level

S98.1 Traumatic amputation of one toe

S98.2 Traumatic amputation of two or more toes

S98.3 Traumatic amputation of other parts of foot
Combined traumatic amputation of toe(s) and other parts of foot

S98.4 Traumatic amputation of foot, level unspecified

S99 Other and unspecified injuries of ankle and foot

S99.7 Multiple injuries of ankle and foot
Injuries classifiable to more than one of the categories S90–S98

S99.8 Other specified injuries of ankle and foot

S99.9 Unspecified injury of ankle and foot

Injuries involving multiple body regions (T00–T07)

Includes: bilateral involvement of limbs of the same body region
injuries by type involving two or more body regions classifiable
within S00–S99

Excludes: burns and corrosions (T20–T32)
frostbite (T33–T35)
insect bite or sting, venomous (T63.4)
multiple injuries involving only one body region—see S-section
sunburn (L55.–)

T00 Superficial injuries involving multiple body regions

T00.0 **Superficial injuries involving head with neck**
Superficial injuries of sites classifiable to S00.– and S10.–
Excludes: with involvement of other body region(s) (T00.8)

T00.1 **Superficial injuries involving thorax with abdomen, lower back and pelvis**
Superficial injuries of sites classifiable to S20.–, S30.– and T09.0
Excludes: with involvement of other body region(s) (T00.8)

T00.2 **Superficial injuries involving multiple regions of upper limb(s)**
Superficial injuries of sites classifiable to S40.–, S50.–, S60.– and T11.0
Excludes: with involvement of:
- lower limb(s) (T00.6)
- thorax, abdomen, lower back and pelvis (T00.8)

T00.3 **Superficial injuries involving multiple regions of lower limb(s)**
Superficial injuries of sites classifiable to S70.–, S80.–, S90.– and T13.0
Excludes: with involvement of:
- thorax, abdomen, lower back and pelvis (T00.8)
- upper limb(s) (T00.6)

T00.6 **Superficial injuries involving multiple regions of upper limb(s) with lower limb(s)**
Superficial injuries of sites classifiable to T00.2 and T00.3

Excludes: with involvement of thorax, abdomen, lower back and pelvis (T00.8)

T00.8 **Superficial injuries involving other combinations of body regions**

T00.9 **Multiple superficial injuries, unspecified**
Multiple:
- abrasions
- blisters (nonthermal)
- bruises   } NOS
- contusions
- haematomas
- insect bites (nonvenomous)

T01 Open wounds involving multiple body regions

Excludes: traumatic amputations involving multiple body regions (T05.–)

T01.0 **Open wounds involving head with neck**
Open wounds of sites classifiable to S01.– and S11.–

Excludes: with involvement of other body region(s) (T01.8)

T01.1 **Open wounds involving thorax with abdomen, lower back and pelvis**
Open wounds of sites classifiable to S21.–, S31.– and T09.1

Excludes: with involvement of other body region(s) (T01.8)

T01.2 **Open wounds involving multiple regions of upper limb(s)**
Open wounds of sites classifiable to S41.–, S51.–, S61.– and T11.1

Excludes: with involvement of:
- lower limb(s) (T01.6)
- thorax, abdomen, lower back and pelvis (T01.8)

T01.3 **Open wounds involving multiple regions of lower limb(s)**
Open wounds of sites classifiable to S71.–, S81.–, S91.– and T13.1

Excludes: with involvement of:
- thorax, abdomen, lower back and pelvis (T01.8)
- upper limb(s) (T01.6)

T01.6 **Open wounds involving multiple regions of upper limb(s) with lower limb(s)**
Open wounds of sites classifiable to T01.2 and T01.3
Excludes: with involvement of thorax, abdomen, lower back and pelvis (T01.8)

T01.8 **Open wounds involving other combinations of body regions**

T01.9 **Multiple open wounds, unspecified**
Multiple:
- animal bites
- cuts
- lacerations
- puncture wounds

} NOS

T02 Fractures involving multiple body regions
The following subdivisions are provided for optional use in a supplementary character position where it is not possible or not desired to use multiple coding to identify fracture and open wound; a fracture not indicated as closed or open should be classified as closed.

0 closed
1 open

T02.0 **Fractures involving head with neck**
Fractures of sites classifiable to S02.– and S12.–
Excludes: with involvement of other body region(s) (T02.8)

T02.1 **Fractures involving thorax with lower back and pelvis**
Fractures of sites classifiable to S22.–, S32.– and T08
Excludes: when combined with fractures of:
- limb(s) (T02.7)
- other body regions (T02.8)

T02.2 **Fractures involving multiple regions of one upper limb**
Fractures of sites classifiable to S42.–, S52.–, S62.– and T10 of one upper limb
Excludes: when combined with fractures of:
- lower limb(s) (T02.6)
- other upper limb (T02.4)
- thorax, lower back and pelvis (T02.7)

T02.3 **Fractures involving multiple regions of one lower limb**
Fractures of sites classifiable to S72.–, S82.–, S92.– and T12 of one lower limb

Excludes: when combined with fractures of:
- other lower limb (T02.5)
- thorax, lower back and pelvis (T02.7)
- upper limb(s) (T02.6)

T02.4 **Fractures involving multiple regions of both upper limbs**
Fractures of sites classifiable to S42.–, S52.–, S62.– and T10 specified as bilateral

Excludes: when combined with fractures of:
- lower limb(s) (T02.6)
- thorax, lower back and pelvis (T02.7)

T02.5 **Fractures involving multiple regions of both lower limbs**
Fractures of sites classifiable to S72.–, S82.–, S92.– and T12 specified as bilateral

Excludes: when combined with fractures of:
- thorax, lower back and pelvis (T02.7)
- upper limb(s) (T02.6)

T02.6 **Fractures involving multiple regions of upper limb(s) with lower limb(s)**

Excludes: when combined with fractures of thorax, lower back and pelvis (T02.7)

T02.7 **Fractures involving thorax with lower back and pelvis with limb(s)**

T02.8 **Fractures involving other combinations of body regions**

T02.9 **Multiple fractures, unspecified**

T03 Dislocations, sprains and strains involving multiple body regions

T03.0 **Dislocations, sprains and strains involving head with neck**
Dislocations, sprains and strains of sites classifiable to S03.– and S13.–

Excludes: when combined with dislocations, sprains and strains of other body region(s) (T03.8)

T03.1 **Dislocations, sprains and strains involving thorax with lower back and pelvis**
Dislocations, sprains and strains of sites classifiable to S23.–, S33.– and T09.2
Excludes: when combined with dislocations, sprains and strains of other body region(s) (T03.8)

T03.2 **Dislocations, sprains and strains involving multiple regions of upper limb(s)**
Dislocations, sprains and strains of sites classifiable to S43.–, S53.–, S63.– and T11.2
Excludes: when combined with dislocations, sprains and strains of:
- lower limb(s) (T03.4)
- thorax, lower back and pelvis (T03.8)

T03.3 **Dislocations, sprains and strains involving multiple regions of lower limb(s)**
Dislocations, sprains and strains of sites classifiable to S73.–, S83.–, S93.– and T13.2
Excludes: when combined with dislocations, sprains and strains of:
- thorax, lower back and pelvis (T03.8)
- upper limb(s) (T03.4)

T03.4 **Dislocations, sprains and strains involving multiple regions of upper limb(s) with lower limb(s)**
Excludes: when combined with dislocations, sprains and strains of thorax, lower back and pelvis (T03.8)

T03.8 **Dislocations, sprains and strains involving other combinations of body regions**

T03.9 **Multiple dislocations, sprains and strains, unspecified**

T04 Crushing injuries involving multiple body regions

T04.0 **Crushing injuries involving head with neck**
Crushing injuries of sites classifiable to S07.– and S17.–
Excludes: with involvement of other body region(s) (T04.8)

T04.1   **Crushing injuries involving thorax with abdomen, lower back and pelvis**
Crushing injury of:
• sites classifiable to S28.– and S38.–
• trunk NOS
Excludes: with involvement of:
  • limbs (T04.7)
  • other body regions (T04.8)

T04.2   **Crushing injuries involving multiple regions of upper limb(s)**
Crushing injury of:
• sites classifiable to S47.–, S57.– and S67.–
• upper limb NOS
Excludes: with involvement of:
  • lower limb(s) (T04.4)
  • thorax, abdomen, lower back and pelvis (T04.7)

T04.3   **Crushing injuries involving multiple regions of lower limb(s)**
Crushing injury of:
• lower limb NOS
• sites classifiable to S77.–, S87.– and S97.–
Excludes: with involvement of:
  • thorax, abdomen, lower back and pelvis (T04.7)
  • upper limb(s) (T04.4)

T04.4   **Crushing injuries involving multiple regions of upper limb(s) with lower limb(s)**
Excludes: with involvement of thorax, abdomen, lower back and pelvis (T04.7)

T04.7   **Crushing injuries of thorax with abdomen, lower back and pelvis with limb(s)**

T04.8   **Crushing injuries involving other combinations of body regions**

T04.9   **Multiple crushing injuries, unspecified**

T05   Traumatic amputations involving multiple body regions

Includes: avulsion involving multiple body regions

Excludes: decapitation (S18)

open wounds involving multiple body regions (T01.–)

traumatic amputation of:
- arm NOS (T11.6)
- leg NOS (T13.6)
- trunk NOS (T09.6)

T05.0   **Traumatic amputation of both hands**

T05.1   **Traumatic amputation of one hand and other arm [any level, except hand]**

T05.2   **Traumatic amputation of both arms [any level]**

T05.3   **Traumatic amputation of both feet**

T05.4   **Traumatic amputation of one foot and other leg [any level, except foot]**

T05.5   **Traumatic amputation of both legs [any level]**

T05.6   **Traumatic amputation of upper and lower limbs, any combination [any level]**

T05.8   **Traumatic amputations involving other combinations of body regions**

Transection of:
- abdomen
- thorax

T05.9   **Multiple traumatic amputations, unspecified**

T06   Other injuries involving multiple body regions, not elsewhere classified

T06.0   **Injuries of brain and cranial nerves with injuries of nerves and spinal cord at neck level**

Injuries classifiable to S04.– and S06.– with injuries classifiable to S14.–

T06.1   **Injuries of nerves and spinal cord involving other multiple body regions**

T06.2   **Injuries of nerves involving multiple body regions**

Multiple injuries of nerves NOS

Excludes: with spinal cord involvement (T06.0–T06.1)

T06.3   **Injuries of blood vessels involving multiple body regions**

T06.4   **Injuries of muscles and tendons involving multiple body regions**

T06.5   **Injuries of intrathoracic organs with intra-abdominal and pelvic organs**

T06.8   **Other specified injuries involving multiple body regions**

T07   Unspecified multiple injuries

Excludes: injury NOS (T14.9)

Injuries to unspecified part of trunk, limb or body region (T08–T14)

Excludes: burns and corrosions (T20–T32)
frostbite (T33–T35)
injuries involving multiple body regions (T00–T07)
insect bite or sting, venomous (T63.4)

T08   Fracture of spine, level unspecified

The following subdivisions are provided for optional use in a supplementary character position where it is not possible or not desired to use multiple coding to identify fracture and open wound; a fracture not indicated as closed or open should be classified as closed.

0   closed
1   open

Excludes: multiple fractures of spine, level unspecified (T02.1)

T09   Other injuries of spine and trunk, level unspecified

Excludes: crushing injury of trunk NOS (T04.1)
multiple injuries of trunk (T00–T06)
transection of trunk (T05.8)

T09.0   **Superficial injury of trunk, level unspecified**

T09.1   **Open wound of trunk, level unspecified**

T09.2   Dislocation, sprain and strain of unspecified joint and ligament of trunk

T09.3   Injury of spinal cord, level unspecified

T09.4   Injury of unspecified nerve, spinal nerve root and plexus of trunk

T09.5   Injury of unspecified muscle and tendon of trunk

T09.6   Traumatic amputation of trunk, level unspecified

T09.8   Other specified injuries of trunk, level unspecified

T09.9   Unspecified injury of trunk, level unspecified

T10   Fracture of upper limb, level unspecified

Broken arm NOS
Fracture of arm NOS

The following subdivisions are provided for optional use in a supplementary character position where it is not possible or not desired to use multiple coding to identify fracture and open wound; a fracture not indicated as closed or open should be classified as closed.

0   closed
1   open

Excludes: multiple fractures of arm, level unspecified (T02.–)

T11   Other injuries of upper limb, level unspecified

Excludes: crushing injury of upper limb NOS (T04.2)
           fracture of upper limb, level unspecified (T10)
           injuries involving multiple body regions (T00–T06)

T11.0   Superficial injury of upper limb, level unspecified

T11.1   Open wound of upper limb, level unspecified

T11.2   Dislocation, sprain and strain of unspecified joint and ligament of upper limb, level unspecified

T11.3   Injury of unspecified nerve of upper limb, level unspecified

T11.4   Injury of unspecified blood vessel of upper limb, level unspecified

T11.5   Injury of unspecified muscle and tendon of upper limb, level unspecified

T11.6 **Traumatic amputation of upper limb, level unspecified**
Traumatic amputation of arm NOS

T11.8 **Other specified injuries of upper limb, level unspecified**

T11.9 **Unspecified injury of upper limb, level unspecified**
Injury of arm NOS

T12 Fracture of lower limb, level unspecified
Broken leg NOS
Fracture of leg NOS

The following subdivisions are provided for optional use in a supplementary character position where it is not possible or not desired to use multiple coding to identify fracture and open wound; a fracture not indicated as closed or open should be classified as closed.

0 closed
1 open

Excludes: multiple fractures of leg, level unspecified (T02.–)

T13 Other injuries of lower limb, level unspecified
Excludes: crushing injury of lower limb NOS (T04.3)
fracture of lower limb, level unspecified (T12)
injuries involving multiple body regions (T00–T06)

T13.0 **Superficial injury of lower limb, level unspecified**

T13.1 **Open wound of lower limb, level unspecified**

T13.2 **Dislocation, sprain and strain of unspecified joint and ligament of lower limb, level unspecified**

T13.3 **Injury of unspecified nerve of lower limb, level unspecified**

T13.4 **Injury of unspecified blood vessel of lower limb, level unspecified**

T13.5 **Injury of unspecified muscle and tendon of lower limb, level unspecified**

T13.6 **Traumatic amputation of lower limb, level unspecified**
Traumatic amputation of leg NOS

T13.8 **Other specified injuries of lower limb, level unspecified**

T13.9 **Unspecified injury of lower limb, level unspecified**
Injury of leg NOS

T14 Injury of unspecified body region

Excludes: injuries involving multiple body regions (T00–T07)

T14.0   Superficial injury of unspecified body region

Abrasion
Blister (nonthermal)
Bruise
Contusion
Haematoma   } NOS
Injury from superficial foreign body
   (splinter) without major open wound
Insect bite (nonvenomous)
Superficial injury

Excludes: multiple superficial injuries NOS (T00.9)

T14.1   Open wound of unspecified body region

Animal bite
Cut
Laceration   } NOS
Open wound
Puncture wound with (penetrating) foreign body

Excludes: multiple:
- open wounds NOS (T01.9)
- traumatic amputations NOS (T05.9)

traumatic amputation NOS (T14.7)

T14.2   Fracture of unspecified body region

The following subdivisions are provided for optional use in a supplementary character position where it is not possible or not desired to use multiple coding to identify fracture and open wound; a fracture not indicated as closed or open should be classified as closed.

0   closed
1   open

Fracture:
- NOS
- closed NOS
- dislocated NOS
- displaced NOS
- open NOS

Excludes: multiple fractures NOS (T02.9)

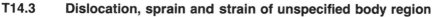

T14.3 **Dislocation, sprain and strain of unspecified body region**

Avulsion
Laceration
Sprain
Strain
Traumatic: } of { joint (capsule) } NOS
• haemarthrosis   { ligament
• rupture
• subluxation
• tear

Excludes: multiple dislocations, sprains and strains NOS (T03.9)

T14.4 **Injury of nerve(s) of unspecified body region**

Injury of nerve
Traumatic:
• division of nerve } NOS
• haematomyelia
• paralysis (transient)

Excludes: multiple injuries of nerves NOS (T06.2)

T14.5 **Injury of blood vessel(s) of unspecified body region**

Avulsion
Cut
Injury
Laceration
Traumatic: } of blood vessel(s) NOS
• aneurysm or fistula
  (arteriovenous)
• arterial haematoma
• rupture

Excludes: multiple injuries of blood vessels NOS (T06.3)

T14.6 **Injury of tendons and muscles of unspecified body region**

Avulsion
Cut
Injury } of muscle(s) NOS and tendon(s) NOS
Laceration
Traumatic rupture

Excludes: multiple injuries of muscles and tendons NOS (T06.4)

T14.7   **Crushing injury and traumatic amputation of unspecified body region**
Crushing injury NOS
Traumatic amputation NOS
Excludes: multiple:
- crushing injuries NOS (T04.9)
- traumatic amputations NOS (T05.9)

T14.8   **Other injuries of unspecified body region**

T14.9   **Injury, unspecified**
Excludes: multiple injuries NOS (T07)

Effects of foreign body entering through natural orifice
(T15–T19)

Excludes: foreign body:
- accidentally left in operation wound (T81.5)
- in puncture wound—see open wound by body region
- residual, in soft tissue (M79.5)
splinter, without major open wound—see superficial injury by body region

T15   Foreign body on external eye
Excludes: foreign body in penetrating wound of:
- orbit and eyeball (S05.4–S05.5)
  - retained (old) (H05.5, H44.6–H44.7)
retained foreign body in eyelid (H02.8)

T15.0   **Foreign body in cornea**

T15.1   **Foreign body in conjunctival sac**

T15.8   **Foreign body in other and multiple parts of external eye**
Foreign body in lacrimal punctum

T15.9   **Foreign body on external eye, part unspecified**

T16   Foreign body in ear
Auditory canal

T17 Foreign body in respiratory tract

Includes: asphyxia due to foreign body
choked on:
- food (regurgitated)
- phlegm

inhalation of liquid or vomitus NOS

T17.0 Foreign body in nasal sinus

T17.1 Foreign body in nostril
Nose NOS

T17.2 Foreign body in pharynx
Nasopharynx
Throat NOS

T17.3 Foreign body in larynx

T17.4 Foreign body in trachea

T17.5 Foreign body in bronchus

T17.8 Foreign body in other and multiple parts of respiratory tract
Bronchioles
Lung

T17.9 Foreign body in respiratory tract, part unspecified

T18 Foreign body in alimentary tract

Excludes: foreign body in pharynx (T17.2)

T18.0 Foreign body in mouth

T18.1 Foreign body in oesophagus

T18.2 Foreign body in stomach

T18.3 Foreign body in small intestine

T18.4 Foreign body in colon

T18.5 Foreign body in anus and rectum
Rectosigmoid (junction)

T18.8 Foreign body in other and multiple parts of alimentary tract

T18.9 Foreign body in alimentary tract, part unspecified
Digestive system NOS
Swallowed foreign body NOS

T19　Foreign body in genitourinary tract

Excludes: contraceptive device (intrauterine)(vaginal):
- mechanical complication of (T83.3)
- presence of (Z97.5)

T19.0　**Foreign body in urethra**

T19.1　**Foreign body in bladder**

T19.2　**Foreign body in vulva and vagina**

T19.3　**Foreign body in uterus [any part]**

T19.8　**Foreign body in other and multiple parts of genitourinary tract**

T19.9　**Foreign body in genitourinary tract, part unspecified**

Burns and corrosions
(T20–T32)

Includes: burns (thermal) from:
- electrical heating appliances
- electricity
- flame
- friction
- hot air and hot gases
- hot objects
- lightning
- radiation

chemical burns [corrosions] (external)(internal)
scalds

Excludes: erythema [dermatitis] ab igne (L59.0)
radiation-related disorders of the skin and subcutaneous tissue (L55–L59)
sunburn (L55.–)

Burns and corrosions of external body surface, specified by site (T20–T25)

Includes: burns and corrosions of:
- first degree [erythema]
- second degree [blisters] [epidermal loss]
- third degree [deep necrosis of underlying tissue] [full-thickness skin loss]

T20   Burn and corrosion of head and neck

Includes: ear [any part]
eye with other parts of face, head and neck
lip
nose (septum)
scalp [any part]
temple (region)

Excludes: burn and corrosion (of):
- confined to eye and adnexa (T26.–)
- mouth and pharynx (T28.–)

T20.0   **Burn of unspecified degree of head and neck**

T20.1   **Burn of first degree of head and neck**

T20.2   **Burn of second degree of head and neck**

T20.3   **Burn of third degree of head and neck**

T20.4   **Corrosion of unspecified degree of head and neck**

T20.5   **Corrosion of first degree of head and neck**

T20.6   **Corrosion of second degree of head and neck**

T20.7   **Corrosion of third degree of head and neck**

T21 Burn and corrosion of trunk

Includes: abdominal wall
anus
back [any part]
breast
buttock
chest wall
flank
groin
interscapular region
labium (majus)(minus)
penis
perineum
scrotum
testis
vulva

Excludes: burn and corrosion of:
- axilla (T22.–)
- scapular region (T22.–)

T21.0   **Burn of unspecified degree of trunk**

T21.1   **Burn of first degree of trunk**

T21.2   **Burn of second degree of trunk**

T21.3   **Burn of third degree of trunk**

T21.4   **Corrosion of unspecified degree of trunk**

T21.5   **Corrosion of first degree of trunk**

T21.6   **Corrosion of second degree of trunk**

T21.7   **Corrosion of third degree of trunk**

T22 Burn and corrosion of shoulder and upper limb, except wrist and hand

Includes: arm [any part, except wrist and hand alone]
axilla
scapular region

Excludes: burn and corrosion of:
- interscapular region (T21.–)
- wrist and hand alone (T23.–)

T22.0   Burn of unspecified degree of shoulder and upper limb, except wrist and hand

T22.1   Burn of first degree of shoulder and upper limb, except wrist and hand

T22.2   Burn of second degree of shoulder and upper limb, except wrist and hand

T22.3   Burn of third degree of shoulder and upper limb, except wrist and hand

T22.4   Corrosion of unspecified degree of shoulder and upper limb, except wrist and hand

T22.5   Corrosion of first degree of shoulder and upper limb, except wrist and hand

T22.6   Corrosion of second degree of shoulder and upper limb, except wrist and hand

T22.7   Corrosion of third degree of shoulder and upper limb, except wrist and hand

T23   Burn and corrosion of wrist and hand

Includes: finger (nail)
palm
thumb (nail)

T23.0   Burn of unspecified degree of wrist and hand

T23.1   Burn of first degree of wrist and hand

T23.2   Burn of second degree of wrist and hand

T23.3   Burn of third degree of wrist and hand

T23.4   Corrosion of unspecified degree of wrist and hand

T23.5   Corrosion of first degree of wrist and hand

T23.6   Corrosion of second degree of wrist and hand

T23.7   Corrosion of third degree of wrist and hand

T24   Burn and corrosion of hip and lower limb, except ankle and foot

Includes: leg [any part, except ankle and foot alone]
Excludes: burn and corrosion of ankle and foot alone (T25.–)

T24.0	Burn of unspecified degree of hip and lower limb, except ankle and foot
T24.1	Burn of first degree of hip and lower limb, except ankle and foot
T24.2	Burn of second degree of hip and lower limb, except ankle and foot
T24.3	Burn of third degree of hip and lower limb, except ankle and foot
T24.4	Corrosion of unspecified degree of hip and lower limb, except ankle and foot
T24.5	Corrosion of first degree of hip and lower limb, except ankle and foot
T24.6	Corrosion of second degree of hip and lower limb, except ankle and foot
T24.7	Corrosion of third degree of hip and lower limb, except ankle and foot

T25 Burn and corrosion of ankle and foot

Includes: toe(s)

T25.0	Burn of unspecified degree of ankle and foot
T25.1	Burn of first degree of ankle and foot
T25.2	Burn of second degree of ankle and foot
T25.3	Burn of third degree of ankle and foot
T25.4	Corrosion of unspecified degree of ankle and foot
T25.5	Corrosion of first degree of ankle and foot
T25.6	Corrosion of second degree of ankle and foot
T25.7	Corrosion of third degree of ankle and foot

Burns and corrosions confined to eye and internal organs (T26–T28)

26 Burn and corrosion confined to eye and adnexa

T26.0	Burn of eyelid and periocular area
T26.1	Burn of cornea and conjunctival sac
T26.2	Burn with resulting rupture and destruction of eyeball
T26.3	Burn of other parts of eye and adnexa
T26.4	Burn of eye and adnexa, part unspecified
T26.5	Corrosion of eyelid and periocular area
T26.6	Corrosion of cornea and conjunctival sac
T26.7	Corrosion with resulting rupture and destruction of eyeball
T26.8	Corrosion of other parts of eye and adnexa
T26.9	Corrosion of eye and adnexa, part unspecified

27 Burn and corrosion of respiratory tract

T27.0	Burn of larynx and trachea
T27.1	Burn involving larynx and trachea with lung
	Excludes: blast injury syndrome (T70.8)
T27.2	Burn of other parts of respiratory tract
	Thoracic cavity
T27.3	Burn of respiratory tract, part unspecified
T27.4	Corrosion of larynx and trachea
T27.5	Corrosion involving larynx and trachea with lung
T27.6	Corrosion of other parts of respiratory tract
T27.7	Corrosion of respiratory tract, part unspecified

28 Burn and corrosion of other internal organs

T28.0	Burn of mouth and pharynx

T28.1	Burn of oesophagus
T28.2	Burn of other parts of alimentary tract
T28.3	Burn of internal genitourinary organs
T28.4	Burn of other and unspecified internal organs
T28.5	Corrosion of mouth and pharynx
T28.6	Corrosion of oesophagus
T28.7	Corrosion of other parts of alimentary tract
T28.8	Corrosion of internal genitourinary organs
T28.9	Corrosion of other and unspecified internal organs

Burns and corrosions of multiple and unspecified body regions (T29–T32)

T29 Burns and corrosions of multiple body regions

Includes: burns and corrosions classifiable to more than one of the categories T20–T28

T29.0	Burns of multiple regions, unspecified degree
	Multiple burns NOS
T29.1	Burns of multiple regions, no more than first-degree burns mentioned
T29.2	Burns of multiple regions, no more than second-degree burns mentioned
T29.3	Burns of multiple regions, at least one burn of third degree mentioned
T29.4	Corrosions of multiple regions, unspecified degree
	Multiple corrosions NOS
T29.5	Corrosions of multiple regions, no more than first-degree corrosions mentioned
T29.6	Corrosions of multiple regions, no more than second-degree corrosions mentioned
T29.7	Corrosions of multiple regions, at least one corrosion of third degree mentioned

T30 Burn and corrosion, body region unspecified

Excludes: burn and corrosion with statement of the extent of body surface involved (T31–T32)

T30.0 **Burn of unspecified body region, unspecified degree**
Burn NOS

T30.1 **Burn of first degree, body region unspecified**
First-degree burn NOS

T30.2 **Burn of second degree, body region unspecified**
Second-degree burn NOS

T30.3 **Burn of third degree, body region unspecified**
Third-degree burn NOS

T30.4 **Corrosion of unspecified body region, unspecified degree**
Corrosion NOS

T30.5 **Corrosion of first degree, body region unspecified**
First-degree corrosion NOS

T30.6 **Corrosion of second degree, body region unspecified**
Second-degree corrosion NOS

T30.7 **Corrosion of third degree, body region unspecified**
Third-degree corrosion NOS

T31 Burns classified according to extent of body surface involved

Note: This category is to be used as the primary code only when the site of the burn is unspecified. It may be used as a supplementary code, if desired, with categories T20–T29 when the site is specified.

T31.0 **Burns involving less than 10% of body surface**

T31.1 **Burns involving 10–19% of body surface**

T31.2 **Burns involving 20–29% of body surface**

T31.3 **Burns involving 30–39% of body surface**

T31.4 **Burns involving 40–49% of body surface**

T31.5 **Burns involving 50–59% of body surface**

T31.6 **Burns involving 60–69% of body surface**

T31.7 **Burns involving 70–79% of body surface**

T31.8	Burns involving 80–89% of body surface
T31.9	Burns involving 90% or more of body surface

T32 Corrosions classified according to extent of body surface involved

Note: This category is to be used as the primary code only when the site of the corrosion is unspecified. It may be used as a supplementary code, if desired, with categories T20–T29 when the site is specified.

T32.0	Corrosions involving less than 10% of body surface
T32.1	Corrosions involving 10–19% of body surface
T32.2	Corrosions involving 20–29% of body surface
T32.3	Corrosions involving 30–39% of body surface
T32.4	Corrosions involving 40–49% of body surface
T32.5	Corrosions involving 50–59% of body surface
T32.6	Corrosions involving 60–69% of body surface
T32.7	Corrosions involving 70–79% of body surface
T32.8	Corrosions involving 80–89% of body surface
T32.9	Corrosions involving 90% or more of body surface

Frostbite
(T33–T35)

Excludes: hypothermia and other effects of reduced temperature (T68–T69)

T33 Superficial frostbite

Includes: frostbite with partial-thickness skin loss
Excludes: superficial frostbite involving multiple body regions (T35.0)

T33.0	Superficial frostbite of head
T33.1	Superficial frostbite of neck

T33.2   **Superficial frostbite of thorax**

T33.3   **Superficial frostbite of abdominal wall, lower back and pelvis**

T33.4   **Superficial frostbite of arm**

Excludes: superficial frostbite of wrist and hand alone (T33.5)

T33.5   **Superficial frostbite of wrist and hand**

T33.6   **Superficial frostbite of hip and thigh**

T33.7   **Superficial frostbite of knee and lower leg**

Excludes: superficial frostbite of ankle and foot alone (T33.8)

T33.8   **Superficial frostbite of ankle and foot**

T33.9   **Superficial frostbite of other and unspecified sites**
Superficial frostbite (of):
- NOS
- leg NOS
- trunk NOS

T34   Frostbite with tissue necrosis

Excludes: frostbite with tissue necrosis involving multiple body regions (T35.1)

T34.0   **Frostbite with tissue necrosis of head**

T34.1   **Frostbite with tissue necrosis of neck**

T34.2   **Frostbite with tissue necrosis of thorax**

T34.3   **Frostbite with tissue necrosis of abdominal wall, lower back and pelvis**

T34.4   **Frostbite with tissue necrosis of arm**

Excludes: frostbite with tissue necrosis of wrist and hand alone (T34.5)

T34.5   **Frostbite with tissue necrosis of wrist and hand**

T34.6   **Frostbite with tissue necrosis of hip and thigh**

T34.7   **Frostbite with tissue necrosis of knee and lower leg**

Excludes: frostbite with tissue necrosis of ankle and foot alone (T34.8)

T34.8   **Frostbite with tissue necrosis of ankle and foot**

T34.9 **Frostbite with tissue necrosis of other and unspecified sites**
Frostbite with tissue necrosis (of):
• NOS
• leg NOS
• trunk NOS

T35 Frostbite involving multiple body regions and unspecified frostbite

T35.0 **Superficial frostbite involving multiple body regions**
Multiple superficial frostbite NOS

T35.1 **Frostbite with tissue necrosis involving multiple body regions**
Multiple frostbite with tissue necrosis NOS

T35.2 **Unspecified frostbite of head and neck**

T35.3 **Unspecified frostbite of thorax, abdomen, lower back and pelvis**
Frostbite of trunk NOS

T35.4 **Unspecified frostbite of upper limb**

T35.5 **Unspecified frostbite of lower limb**

T35.6 **Unspecified frostbite involving multiple body regions**
Multiple frostbite NOS

T35.7 **Unspecified frostbite of unspecified site**
Frostbite NOS

Poisoning by drugs, medicaments and biological substances
(T36–T50)

Includes: overdose of these substances
wrong substance given or taken in error

Excludes: abuse of non-dependence-producing substances (F55)
adverse effects ["hypersensitivity", "reaction", etc.] of correct
substance properly administered; such cases are to be
classified according to the nature of the adverse effect, such
as:
- aspirin gastritis (K29.–)
- blood disorders (D50–D76)
- dermatitis:
  - contact (L23–L25)
  - due to substances taken internally (L27.–)
- nephropathy (N14.0–N14.2)
- unspecified adverse effect of drug (T88.7)
drug dependence and related mental and behavioural disorders
due to psychoactive substance use (F10–F19)
drug reaction and poisoning affecting the fetus and newborn
(P00–P96)
pathological drug intoxication (F10–F19)

T36   Poisoning by systemic antibiotics

Excludes: antibiotics:
- antineoplastic (T45.1)
- locally applied NEC (T49.0)
- topically used for:
  - ear, nose and throat (T49.6)
  - eye (T49.5)

T36.0   **Penicillins**

T36.1   **Cefalosporins and other β-lactam antibiotics**

T36.2   **Chloramphenicol group**

T36.3   **Macrolides**

T36.4   **Tetracyclines**

T36.5   **Aminoglycosides**
Streptomycin

T36.6   **Rifamycins**

T36.7   **Antifungal antibiotics, systemically used**

T36.8   **Other systemic antibiotics**

T36.9   **Systemic antibiotic, unspecified**

T37 Poisoning by other systemic anti-infectives and antiparasitics

Excludes: anti-infectives:
- locally applied NEC (T49.0)
- topically used for:
  - ear, nose and throat (T49.6)
  - eye (T49.5)

T37.0   **Sulfonamides**

T37.1   **Antimycobacterial drugs**

Excludes: rifamycins (T36.6)
            streptomycin (T36.5)

T37.2   **Antimalarials and drugs acting on other blood protozoa**

Excludes: hydroxyquinoline derivatives (T37.8)

T37.3   **Other antiprotozoal drugs**

T37.4   **Anthelminthics**

T37.5   **Antiviral drugs**

Excludes: amantadine (T42.8)
            cytarabine (T45.1)

T37.8   **Other specified systemic anti-infectives and antiparasitics**
Hydroxyquinoline derivatives

Excludes: antimalarial drugs (T37.2)

T37.9   **Systemic anti-infective and antiparasitic, unspecified**

T38 Poisoning by hormones and their synthetic substitutes and antagonists, not elsewhere classified

Excludes: mineralocorticoids and their antagonists (T50.0)
            oxytocic hormones (T48.0)
            parathyroid hormones and derivatives (T50.9)

T38.0 Glucocorticoids and synthetic analogues
Excludes: glucocorticoids, topically used (T49.–)

T38.1 Thyroid hormones and substitutes

T38.2 Antithyroid drugs

T38.3 Insulin and oral hypoglycaemic [antidiabetic] drugs

T38.4 Oral contraceptives
Multiple- and single-ingredient preparations

T38.5 Other estrogens and progestogens
Mixtures and substitutes

T38.6 Antigonadotrophins, antiestrogens, antiandrogens, not elsewhere classified
Tamoxifen

T38.7 Androgens and anabolic congeners

T38.8 Other and unspecified hormones and their synthetic substitutes
Anterior pituitary [adenohypophyseal] hormones

T38.9 Other and unspecified hormone antagonists

T39 Poisoning by nonopioid analgesics, antipyretics and antirheumatics

T39.0 Salicylates

T39.1 4-Aminophenol derivatives

T39.2 Pyrazolone derivatives

T39.3 Other nonsteroidal anti-inflammatory drugs [NSAID]

T39.4 Antirheumatics, not elsewhere classified
Excludes: glucocorticoids (T38.0)
salicylates (T39.0)

T39.8 Other nonopioid analgesics and antipyretics, not elsewhere classified

T39.9 Nonopioid analgesic, antipyretic and antirheumatic, unspecified

T40   Poisoning by narcotics and psychodysleptics [hallucinogens]

Excludes: drug dependence and related mental and behavioural disorders due to psychoactive substance use (F10–F19)

T40.0   **Opium**

T40.1   **Heroin**

T40.2   **Other opioids**
Codeine
Morphine

T40.3   **Methadone**

T40.4   **Other synthetic narcotics**
Pethidine

T40.5   **Cocaine**

T40.6   **Other and unspecified narcotics**

T40.7   **Cannabis (derivatives)**

T40.8   **Lysergide [LSD]**

T40.9   **Other and unspecified psychodysleptics [hallucinogens]**
Mescaline
Psilocin
Psilocybine

T41   Poisoning by anaesthetics and therapeutic gases

Excludes: benzodiazepines (T42.4)
cocaine (T40.5)
opioids (T40.0–T40.2)

T41.0   **Inhaled anaesthetics**
Excludes: oxygen (T41.5)

T41.1   **Intravenous anaesthetics**
Thiobarbiturates

T41.2   **Other and unspecified general anaesthetics**

T41.3   **Local anaesthetics**

T41.4   **Anaesthetic, unspecified**

T41.5 **Therapeutic gases**
Carbon dioxide
Oxygen

T42 Poisoning by antiepileptic, sedative–hypnotic and antiparkinsonism drugs

Excludes: drug dependence and related mental and behavioural disorders due to psychoactive substance use (F10–F19)

T42.0 **Hydantoin derivatives**

T42.1 **Iminostilbenes**
Carbamazepine

T42.2 **Succinimides and oxazolidinediones**

T42.3 **Barbiturates**
Excludes: thiobarbiturates (T41.1)

T42.4 **Benzodiazepines**

T42.5 **Mixed antiepileptics, not elsewhere classified**

T42.6 **Other antiepileptic and sedative–hypnotic drugs**
Methaqualone
Valproic acid
Excludes: carbamazepine (T42.1)

T42.7 **Antiepileptic and sedative–hypnotic drugs, unspecified**
Sleeping:
- draught
- drug   } NOS
- tablet

T42.8 **Antiparkinsonism drugs and other central muscle-tone depressants**
Amantadine

T43   Poisoning by psychotropic drugs, not elsewhere classified

Excludes: appetite depressants (T50.5)
barbiturates (T42.3)
benzodiazepines (T42.4)
drug dependence and related mental and behavioural
disorders due to psychoactive substance use
(F10–F19)
methaqualone (T42.6)
psychodysleptics [hallucinogens] (T40.7–T40.9)

T43.0   **Tricyclic and tetracyclic antidepressants**

T43.1   **Monoamine-oxidase-inhibitor antidepressants**

T43.2   **Other and unspecified antidepressants**

T43.3   **Phenothiazine antipsychotics and neuroleptics**

T43.4   **Butyrophenone and thioxanthene neuroleptics**

T43.5   **Other and unspecified antipsychotics and neuroleptics**
Excludes: rauwolfia (T46.5)

T43.6   **Psychostimulants with abuse potential**
Excludes: cocaine (T40.5)

T43.8   **Other psychotropic drugs, not elsewhere classified**

T43.9   **Psychotropic drug, unspecified**

T44   Poisoning by drugs primarily affecting the autonomic nervous system

T44.0   **Anticholinesterase agents**

T44.1   **Other parasympathomimetics [cholinergics]**

T44.2   **Ganglionic blocking drugs, not elsewhere classified**

T44.3   **Other parasympatholytics [anticholinergics and antimuscarinics] and spasmolytics, not elsewhere classified**
Papaverine

T44.4   **Predominantly α-adrenoreceptor agonists, not elsewhere classified**
Metaraminol

T44.5 **Predominantly β-adrenoreceptor agonists, not elsewhere classified**
Excludes: salbutamol (T48.6)

T44.6 **α-Adrenoreceptor antagonists, not elsewhere classified**
Excludes: ergot alkaloids (T48.0)

T44.7 **β-Adrenoreceptor antagonists, not elsewhere classified**

T44.8 **Centrally acting and adrenergic-neuron-blocking agents, not elsewhere classified**
Excludes: clonidine (T46.5)
guanethidine (T46.5)

T44.9 **Other and unspecified drugs primarily affecting the autonomic nervous system**
Drug stimulating both α- and β-adrenoreceptors

T45 Poisoning by primarily systemic and haematological agents, not elsewhere classified

T45.0 **Antiallergic and antiemetic drugs**
Excludes: phenothiazine-based neuroleptics (T43.3)

T45.1 **Antineoplastic and immunosuppressive drugs**
Antineoplastic antibiotics
Cytarabine
Excludes: tamoxifen (T38.6)

T45.2 **Vitamins, not elsewhere classified**
Excludes: nicotinic acid (derivatives) (T46.7)
vitamin K (T45.7)

T45.3 **Enzymes, not elsewhere classified**

T45.4 **Iron and its compounds**

T45.5 **Anticoagulants**

T45.6 **Fibrinolysis-affecting drugs**

T45.7 **Anticoagulant antagonists, vitamin K and other coagulants**

T45.8 **Other primarily systemic and haematological agents**
Liver preparations and other antianaemic agents
Natural blood and blood products
Plasma substitute
Excludes: immunoglobulin (T50.9)
iron (T45.4)

T45.9   Primarily systemic and haematological agent, unspecified

T46   Poisoning by agents primarily affecting the cardiovascular system
Excludes: metaraminol (T44.4)

T46.0   Cardiac-stimulant glycosides and drugs of similar action

T46.1   Calcium-channel blockers

T46.2   Other antidysrhythmic drugs, not elsewhere classified
Excludes: β-adrenoreceptor antagonists (T44.7)

T46.3   Coronary vasodilators, not elsewhere classified
Dipyridamole
Excludes: β-adrenoreceptor antagonists (T44.7)
    calcium-channel blockers (T46.1)

T46.4   Angiotensin-converting-enzyme inhibitors

T46.5   Other antihypertensive drugs, not elsewhere classified
Clonidine
Guanethidine
Rauwolfia
Excludes: β-adrenoreceptor antagonists (T44.7)
    calcium-channel blockers (T46.1)
    diuretics (T50.0–T50.2)

T46.6   Antihyperlipidaemic and antiarteriosclerotic drugs

T46.7   Peripheral vasodilators
Nicotinic acid (derivatives)
Excludes: papaverine (T44.3)

T46.8   Antivaricose drugs, including sclerosing agents

T46.9   Other and unspecified agents primarily affecting the cardiovascular system

T47   Poisoning by agents primarily affecting the gastrointestinal system

T47.0   Histamine H_2-receptor antagonists

T47.1   Other antacids and anti-gastric-secretion drugs

T47.2   Stimulant laxatives

T47.3   **Saline and osmotic laxatives**

T47.4   **Other laxatives**
Intestinal atonia drugs

T47.5   **Digestants**

T47.6   **Antidiarrhoeal drugs**
Excludes: systemic antibiotics and other anti-infectives
(T36–T37)

T47.7   **Emetics**

T47.8   **Other agents primarily affecting the gastrointestinal system**

T47.9   **Agent primarily affecting the gastrointestinal system, unspecified**

T48   Poisoning by agents primarily acting on smooth and skeletal muscles and the respiratory system

T48.0   **Oxytocic drugs**
Excludes: estrogens, progestogens and antagonists
(T38.4–T38.6)

T48.1   **Skeletal muscle relaxants [neuromuscular blocking agents]**

T48.2   **Other and unspecified agents primarily acting on muscles**

T48.3   **Antitussives**

T48.4   **Expectorants**

T48.5   **Anti-common-cold drugs**

T48.6   **Antiasthmatics, not elsewhere classified**
Salbutamol
Excludes: β-adrenoreceptor agonists (T44.5)
anterior pituitary [adenohypophyseal] hormones
(T38.8)

T48.7   **Other and unspecified agents primarily acting on the respiratory system**

T49 Poisoning by topical agents primarily affecting skin and mucous membrane and by ophthalmological, otorhinolaryngological and dental drugs

Includes: glucocorticoids, topically used

T49.0 **Local antifungal, anti-infective and anti-inflammatory drugs, not elsewhere classified**

T49.1 **Antipruritics**

T49.2 **Local astringents and local detergents**

T49.3 **Emollients, demulcents and protectants**

T49.4 **Keratolytics, keratoplastics and other hair treatment drugs and preparations**

T49.5 **Ophthalmological drugs and preparations**
Eye anti-infectives

T49.6 **Otorhinolaryngological drugs and preparations**
Ear, nose and throat anti-infectives

T49.7 **Dental drugs, topically applied**

T49.8 **Other topical agents**
Spermicides

T49.9 **Topical agent, unspecified**

T50 Poisoning by diuretics and other and unspecified drugs, medicaments and biological substances

T50.0 **Mineralocorticoids and their antagonists**

T50.1 **Loop [high-ceiling] diuretics**

T50.2 **Carbonic-anhydrase inhibitors, benzothiadiazides and other diuretics**
Acetazolamide

T50.3 **Electrolytic, caloric and water-balance agents**
Oral rehydration salts

T50.4 **Drugs affecting uric acid metabolism**

T50.5 **Appetite depressants**

T50.6 **Antidotes and chelating agents, not elsewhere classified**
Alcohol deterrents

T50.7   **Analeptics and opioid receptor antagonists**

T50.8   **Diagnostic agents**

T50.9   **Other and unspecified drugs, medicaments and biological substances**
Acidifying agents
Alkalizing agents
Immunoglobulin
Immunologicals
Lipotropic drugs
Parathyroid hormones and derivatives

Toxic effects of substances chiefly nonmedicinal as to source
(T51–T65)

Excludes: corrosions (T20–T32)
localized toxic effects classified elsewhere (A00–R99)
respiratory conditions due to external agents (J60–J70)

T51   Toxic effect of alcohol

T51.0   **Ethanol**
Ethyl alcohol
Excludes: acute alcohol intoxication or "hangover" effects (F10.0)
drunkenness (F10.0)
pathological alcohol intoxication (F10.0)

T51.1   **Methanol**
Methyl alcohol

T51.2   **2-Propanol**
Isopropyl alcohol

T51.3   **Fusel oil**
Alcohol:
• amyl
• butyl [1-butanol]
• propyl [1-propanol]

T51.8   **Other alcohols**

T51.9   **Alcohol, unspecified**

T52   Toxic effect of organic solvents
Excludes: halogen derivatives of aliphatic and aromatic
hydrocarbons (T53.–)

T52.0   **Petroleum products**
Gasoline [petrol]
Kerosine [paraffin oil]
Paraffin wax
Petroleum:
- ether
- naphtha
- spirits

T52.1   **Benzene**
Excludes: homologues of benzene (T52.2)
nitroderivatives and aminoderivatives of benzene and
its homologues (T65.3)

T52.2   **Homologues of benzene**
Toluene [methylbenzene]
Xylene [dimethylbenzene]

T52.3   **Glycols**

T52.4   **Ketones**

T52.8   **Other organic solvents**

T52.9   **Organic solvent, unspecified**

T53   Toxic effect of halogen derivatives of aliphatic and aromatic hydrocarbons

T53.0   **Carbon tetrachloride**
Tetrachloromethane

T53.1   **Chloroform**
Trichloromethane

T53.2   **Trichloroethylene**
Trichloroethene

T53.3   **Tetrachloroethylene**
Perchloroethylene
Tetrachloroethene

T53.4 **Dichloromethane**
Methylene chloride

T53.5 **Chlorofluorocarbons**

T53.6 **Other halogen derivatives of aliphatic hydrocarbons**

T53.7 **Other halogen derivatives of aromatic hydrocarbons**

T53.9 **Halogen derivative of aliphatic and aromatic hydrocarbons, unspecified**

54 Toxic effect of corrosive substances

T54.0 **Phenol and phenol homologues**

T54.1 **Other corrosive organic compounds**

T54.2 **Corrosive acids and acid-like substances**
Acid:
- hydrochloric
- sulfuric

T54.3 **Corrosive alkalis and alkali-like substances**
Potassium hydroxide
Sodium hydroxide

T54.9 **Corrosive substance, unspecified**

T55 Toxic effect of soaps and detergents

56 Toxic effect of metals

Includes: fumes and vapours of metals
metals from all sources, except medicinal substances
Excludes: arsenic and its compounds (T57.0)
manganese and its compounds (T57.2)
thallium (T60.4)

T56.0 **Lead and its compounds**

T56.1 **Mercury and its compounds**

T56.2 **Chromium and its compounds**

T56.3 **Cadmium and its compounds**

T56.4 **Copper and its compounds**

T56.5	Zinc and its compounds
T56.6	Tin and its compounds
T56.7	Beryllium and its compounds
T56.8	Other metals
T56.9	Metal, unspecified

57 Toxic effect of other inorganic substances

T57.0	Arsenic and its compounds
T57.1	Phosphorus and its compounds
	Excludes: organophosphate insecticides (T60.0)
T57.2	Manganese and its compounds
T57.3	Hydrogen cyanide
T57.8	Other specified inorganic substances
T57.9	Inorganic substance, unspecified

T58 Toxic effect of carbon monoxide
From all sources

59 Toxic effect of other gases, fumes and vapours
Includes: aerosol propellants
Excludes: chlorofluorocarbons (T53.5)

T59.0	Nitrogen oxides
T59.1	Sulfur dioxide
T59.2	Formaldehyde
T59.3	Lacrimogenic gas
	Tear gas
T59.4	Chlorine gas
T59.5	Fluorine gas and hydrogen fluoride
T59.6	Hydrogen sulfide
T59.7	Carbon dioxide
T59.8	Other specified gases, fumes and vapours

T59.9   Gases, fumes and vapours, unspecified

T60 Toxic effect of pesticides

Includes: wood preservatives

T60.0   Organophosphate and carbamate insecticides

T60.1   Halogenated insecticides

Excludes: chlorinated hydrocarbons (T53.–)

T60.2   Other insecticides

T60.3   Herbicides and fungicides

T60.4   Rodenticides

Thallium

Excludes: strychnine and its salts (T65.1)

T60.8   Other pesticides

T60.9   Pesticide, unspecified

T61 Toxic effect of noxious substances eaten as seafood

Excludes: allergic reaction to food, such as:
- anaphylactic shock due to adverse food reaction (T78.0)
- dermatitis (L23.6, L25.4, L27.2)
- gastroenteritis (noninfective) (K52.–)

bacterial foodborne intoxications (A05.–)

toxic effect of food contaminants, such as:
- aflatoxin and other mycotoxins (T64)
- cyanides (T65.0)
- hydrogen cyanide (T57.3)
- mercury (T56.1)

T61.0   Ciguatera fish poisoning

T61.1   Scombroid fish poisoning

Histamine-like syndrome

T61.2   Other fish and shellfish poisoning

T61.8   Toxic effect of other seafoods

T61.9   Toxic effect of unspecified seafood

T62   Toxic effect of other noxious substances eaten as food

Excludes: allergic reaction to food, such as:
- anaphylactic shock due to adverse food reaction (T78.0)
- dermatitis (L23.6, L25.4, L27.2)
- gastroenteritis (noninfective) (K52.–)

bacterial foodborne intoxications (A05.–)

toxic effect of food contaminants, such as:
- aflatoxin and other mycotoxins (T64)
- cyanides (T65.0)
- hydrogen cyanide (T57.3)
- mercury (T56.1)

T62.0   **Ingested mushrooms**

T62.1   **Ingested berries**

T62.2   **Other ingested (parts of) plant(s)**

T62.8   **Other specified noxious substances eaten as food**

T62.9   **Noxious substance eaten as food, unspecified**

T63   Toxic effect of contact with venomous animals

T63.0   **Snake venom**
Sea-snake venom

T63.1   **Venom of other reptiles**
Lizard venom

T63.2   **Venom of scorpion**

T63.3   **Venom of spider**

T63.4   **Venom of other arthropods**
Insect bite or sting, venomous

T63.5   **Toxic effect of contact with fish**
Excludes: poisoning by ingestion of fish (T61.0–T61.2)

T63.6   **Toxic effect of contact with other marine animals**
Jellyfish
Sea anemone
Shellfish
Starfish
Excludes: poisoning by ingestion of shellfish (T61.2)
                      sea-snake venom (T63.0)

T63.8   **Toxic effect of contact with other venomous animals**
Venom of amphibian

T63.9   **Toxic effect of contact with unspecified venomous animal**

T64   Toxic effect of aflatoxin and other mycotoxin food contaminants

T65   Toxic effect of other and unspecified substances

T65.0   **Cyanides**
Excludes: hydrogen cyanide (T57.3)

T65.1   **Strychnine and its salts**

T65.2   **Tobacco and nicotine**

T65.3   **Nitroderivatives and aminoderivatives of benzene and its homologues**
Aniline [benzenamine]
Nitrobenzene
Trinitrotoluene

T65.4   **Carbon disulfide**

T65.5   **Nitroglycerin and other nitric acids and esters**
1,2,3-Propanetriol trinitrate

T65.6   **Paints and dyes, not elsewhere classified**

T65.8   **Toxic effect of other specified substances**

T65.9   **Toxic effect of unspecified substance**
Poisoning NOS

Other and unspecified effects of external causes (T66–T78)

T66   Unspecified effects of radiation

Radiation sickness

Excludes: specified adverse effects of radiation, such as:
- burns (T20–T31)
- leukaemia (C91–C95)
- radiation:
  - gastroenteritis and colitis (K52.0)
  - pneumonitis (J70.0)
  - related disorders of the skin and subcutaneous tissue (L55–L59)
- sunburn (L55.–)

T67   Effects of heat and light

Excludes: burns (T20–T31)
erythema [dermatitis] ab igne (L59.0)
malignant hyperthermia due to anaesthesia (T88.3)
radiation-related disorders of the skin and subcutaneous tissue (L55–L59)
sunburn (L55.–)
sweat disorders due to heat (L74–L75)

T67.0   Heatstroke and sunstroke

Heat:
- apoplexy
- pyrexia

Siriasis

Thermoplegia

T67.1   Heat syncope

Heat collapse

T67.2   Heat cramp

T67.3   Heat exhaustion, anhydrotic

Heat prostration due to water depletion

Excludes: heat exhaustion due to salt depletion (T67.4)

T67.4   Heat exhaustion due to salt depletion

Heat prostration due to salt (and water) depletion

T67.5 Heat exhaustion, unspecified
Heat prostration NOS

T67.6 Heat fatigue, transient

T67.7 Heat oedema

T67.8 Other effects of heat and light

T67.9 Effect of heat and light, unspecified

T68 Hypothermia

Accidental hypothermia

Excludes: frostbite (T33–T35)
  hypothermia (of):
  • following anaesthesia (T88.5)
  • newborn (P80.–)
  • not associated with low environmental temperature
    (R68.0)

T69 Other effects of reduced temperature

Excludes: frostbite (T33–T35)

T69.0 Immersion hand and foot
Trench foot

T69.1 Chilblains

T69.8 Other specified effects of reduced temperature

T69.9 Effect of reduced temperature, unspecified

T70 Effects of air pressure and water pressure

T70.0 Otitic barotrauma
Aero-otitis media
Effects of change in ambient atmospheric pressure or water
  pressure on ears

T70.1 Sinus barotrauma
Aerosinusitis
Effects of change in ambient atmospheric pressure on sinuses

T70.2 **Other and unspecified effects of high altitude**
Alpine sickness
Anoxia due to high altitude
Barotrauma NOS
Hypobaropathy
Mountain sickness
Excludes: polycythaemia due to high altitude (D75.1)

T70.3 **Caisson disease [decompression sickness]**
Compressed-air disease
Diver's palsy or paralysis

T70.4 **Effects of high-pressure fluids**
Traumatic jet injection (industrial)

T70.8 **Other effects of air pressure and water pressure**
Blast injury syndrome

T70.9 **Effect of air pressure and water pressure, unspecified**

T71 Asphyxiation
Suffocation (by strangulation)
Systemic oxygen deficiency due to:
- low oxygen content in ambient air
- mechanical threat to breathing
Excludes: anoxia due to high altitude (T70.2)
asphyxia from:
- carbon monoxide (T58)
- inhalation of food or foreign body (T17.–)
- other gases, fumes and vapours (T59.–)
respiratory distress (syndrome) in:
- adult (J80)
- newborn (P22.–)

T73 Effects of other deprivation

T73.0 **Effects of hunger**
Deprivation of food
Starvation

T73.1 **Effects of thirst**
Deprivation of water

T73.2 **Exhaustion due to exposure**

T73.3   **Exhaustion due to excessive exertion**
Overexertion

T73.8   **Other effects of deprivation**

T73.9   **Effect of deprivation, unspecified**

T74   Maltreatment syndromes

Use additional code, if desired, to identify current injury.

T74.0   **Neglect or abandonment**

T74.1   **Physical abuse**
Battered:
- baby or child syndrome NOS
- spouse syndrome NOS

T74.2   **Sexual abuse**

T74.3   **Psychological abuse**

T74.8   **Other maltreatment syndromes**
Mixed forms

T74.9   **Maltreatment syndrome, unspecified**
Effects of:
- abuse of adult NOS
- child abuse NOS

T75   Effects of other external causes

Excludes: adverse effects NEC (T78.–)
burns (electric) (T20–T31)

T75.0   **Effects of lightning**
Shock from lightning
Struck by lightning NOS

T75.1   **Drowning and nonfatal submersion**
Immersion
Swimmer's cramp

T75.2   **Effects of vibration**
Pneumatic hammer syndrome
Traumatic vasospastic syndrome
Vertigo from infrasound

T75.3   **Motion sickness**
Airsickness
Seasickness
Travel sickness

T75.4   **Effects of electric current**
Electrocution
Shock from electric current

T75.8   **Other specified effects of external causes**
Effects of:
• abnormal gravitational [G] forces
• weightlessness

T78   Adverse effects, not elsewhere classified

Note: This category is to be used as the primary code to identify the effects, not elsewhere classifiable, of unknown, undetermined or ill-defined causes. For multiple coding purposes this category may be used as an additional code to identify the effects of conditions classified elsewhere.

Excludes: complications of surgical and medical care NEC (T80–T88)

T78.0   **Anaphylactic shock due to adverse food reaction**

T78.1   **Other adverse food reactions, not elsewhere classified**
Excludes: bacterial foodborne intoxications (A05.–)
dermatitis due to food (L27.2)
• in contact with the skin (L23.6, L24.6, L25.4)

T78.2   **Anaphylactic shock, unspecified**
Allergic shock
Anaphylactic reaction } NOS
Anaphylaxis
Excludes: anaphylactic shock due to:
• adverse effect of correct medicinal substance properly administered (T88.6)
• adverse food reaction (T78.0)
• serum (T80.5)

T78.3   **Angioneurotic oedema**
Giant urticaria
Quincke's oedema
Excludes: urticaria (L50.–)
   • serum (T80.6)

T78.4   **Allergy, unspecified**
Allergic reaction NOS
Hypersensitivity NOS
Idiosyncracy NOS
Excludes: allergic reaction NOS to correct medicinal substance
      properly administered (T88.7)
   specified types of allergic reaction such as:
   • allergic gastroenteritis and colitis (K52.2)
   • dermatitis (L23–L25, L27.–)
   • hay fever (J30.1)

T78.8   **Other adverse effects, not elsewhere classified**

T78.9   **Adverse effect, unspecified**
Excludes: adverse effect of surgical and medical care NOS
      (T88.9)

Certain early complications of trauma (T79)

T79   **Certain early complications of trauma, not elsewhere classified**
Excludes: complications of surgical and medical care NEC
      (T80–T88)
   respiratory distress syndrome of:
   • adult (J80)
   • newborn (P22.0)
   when occurring during or following medical
      procedures (T80–T88)

T79.0   **Air embolism (traumatic)**
Excludes: air embolism complicating:
   • abortion or ectopic or molar pregnancy (O00–O07,
      O08.2)
   • pregnancy, childbirth and the puerperium (O88.0)

T79.1   Fat embolism (traumatic)
Excludes: fat embolism complicating:
- abortion or ectopic or molar pregnancy (O00–O07, O08.2)
- pregnancy, childbirth and the puerperium (O88.8)

T79.2   Traumatic secondary and recurrent haemorrhage

T79.3   Post-traumatic wound infection, not elsewhere classified
Use additional code (B95–B97), if desired, to identify infectious agent.

T79.4   Traumatic shock
Shock (immediate)(delayed) following injury
Excludes: shock:
- anaesthetic (T88.2)
- anaphylactic:
  - NOS (T78.2)
  - due to:
    - adverse food reaction (T78.0)
    - correct medicinal substance properly administered (T88.6)
    - serum (T80.5)
- complicating abortion or ectopic or molar pregnancy (O00–O07, O08.3)
- electric (T75.4)
- lightning (T75.0)
- nontraumatic NEC (R57.–)
- obstetric (O75.1)
- postoperative (T81.1)

T79.5   Traumatic anuria
Crush syndrome
Renal failure following crushing

T79.6   Traumatic ischaemia of muscle
Compartment syndrome
Volkmann's ischaemic contracture
Excludes: anterior tibial syndrome (M76.8)

T79.7   Traumatic subcutaneous emphysema
Excludes: emphysema (subcutaneous) resulting from a procedure (T81.8)

T79.8   Other early complications of trauma

T79.9   Unspecified early complication of trauma

Complications of surgical and medical care, not elsewhere classified
(T80–T88)

Use additional external cause code (Chapter XX), if desired, to identify devices involved and details of circumstances.

Use additional code (B95–B97), if desired, to identify infectious agent.

Excludes: adverse effects of drugs and medicaments (A00–R99, T78.–)
any encounters with medical care for postoperative conditions
in which no complications are present, such as:
- artificial opening status (Z93.–)
- closure of external stoma (Z43.–)
- fitting and adjustment of external prosthetic device (Z44.–)
burns and corrosions from local applications and irradiation
(T20–T32)
complications of surgical procedures during pregnancy, childbirth
and the puerperium (O00–O99)
poisoning and toxic effects of drugs and chemicals (T36–T65)
specified complications classified elsewhere, such as:
- cerebrospinal fluid leak from spinal puncture (G97.0)
- colostomy malfunction (K91.4)
- disorders of fluid and electrolyte balance (E86–E87)
- functional disturbances following cardiac surgery (I97.0–I97.1)
- postgastric surgery syndromes (K91.1)
- postlaminectomy syndrome NEC (M96.1)
- postmastectomy lymphoedema syndrome (I97.2)
- postsurgical blind-loop syndrome (K91.2)

T80   Complications following infusion, transfusion and therapeutic injection
Includes: perfusion
Excludes: bone-marrow transplant rejection (T86.0)

T80.0   Air embolism following infusion, transfusion and therapeutic injection

T80.1   Vascular complications following infusion, transfusion and therapeutic injection

Phlebitis ⎱
Thromboembolism ⎰ following infusion, transfusion and
Thrombophlebitis ⎰ therapeutic injection

Excludes: the listed conditions when specified as:
- due to prosthetic devices, implants and grafts (T82.8, T83.8, T84.8, T85.8)
- postprocedural (T81.7)

T80.2   Infections following infusion, transfusion and therapeutic injection

Infection ⎱
Sepsis ⎰ following infusion, transfusion and therapeutic
Septicaemia ⎰ injection
Septic shock ⎰

Excludes: the listed conditions when specified as:
- due to prosthetic devices, implants and grafts (T82.6–T82.7, T83.5–T83.6, T84.5–T84.7, T85.7)
- postprocedural (T81.4)

T80.3   ABO incompatibility reaction

Incompatible blood transfusion
Reaction to blood-group incompatibility in infusion or transfusion

T80.4   Rh incompatibility reaction

Reaction due to Rh factor in infusion or transfusion

T80.5   Anaphylactic shock due to serum

Excludes: shock:
- allergic NOS (T78.2)
- anaphylactic:
  - NOS (T78.2)
  - due to adverse effect of correct medicinal substance properly administered (T88.6)

T80.6   Other serum reactions

Intoxication by serum
Protein sickness
Serum:
- rash
- sickness
- urticaria

Excludes: serum hepatitis (B16.–)

T80.8   Other complications following infusion, transfusion and therapeutic injection

T80.9 **Unspecified complication following infusion, transfusion and therapeutic injection**
Transfusion reaction NOS

T81 Complications of procedures, not elsewhere classified

Excludes: adverse effect of drug NOS (T88.7)
complication following:
- immunization (T88.0–T88.1)
- infusion, transfusion and therapeutic injection (T80.–)
specified complications classified elsewhere, such as:
- complications of prosthetic devices, implants and grafts (T82–T85)
- dermatitis due to drugs and medicaments (L23.3, L24.4, L25.1, L27.0–L27.1)
- poisoning and toxic effects of drugs and chemicals (T36–T65)

T81.0 **Haemorrhage and haematoma complicating a procedure, not elsewhere classified**
Haemorrhage at any site resulting from a procedure
Excludes: haematoma of obstetric wound (O90.2)
haemorrhage due to prosthetic devices, implants and grafts (T82.8, T83.8, T84.8, T85.8)

T81.1   Shock during or resulting from a procedure, not elsewhere classified

Collapse NOS
Shock (endotoxic) (hypovolaemic) (septic)   } during or following a procedure
Postoperative shock NOS

Excludes: shock:
  • anaesthetic (T88.2)
  • anaphylactic:
    • NOS (T78.2)
    • due to:
      • correct medicinal substance properly administered (T88.6)
      • serum (T80.5)
  • electric (T75.4)
  • following abortion or ectopic or molar pregnancy (O00–O07, O08.3)
  • obstetric (O75.1)
  • traumatic (T79.4)

T81.2   Accidental puncture and laceration during a procedure, not elsewhere classified

Accidental perforation of:

  • blood vessel
  • nerve   } by { catheter / endoscope / instrument / probe } during a procedure
  • organ

Excludes: damage from instruments during delivery (O70–O71)
         perforation, puncture or laceration caused by device or implant intentionally left in operation wound (T82–T85)
         specified complications classified elsewhere, such as broad ligament laceration syndrome [Allen–Masters] (N83.8)

T81.3   Disruption of operation wound, not elsewhere classified

Dehiscence
Rupture   } of operation wound

Excludes: disruption of:
  • caesarean-section wound (O90.0)
  • perineal obstetric wound (O90.1)

T81.4   **Infection following a procedure, not elsewhere classified**

Abscess:
- intra-abdominal
- stitch
- subphrenic } postprocedural
- wound

Septicaemia

Excludes: infection due to:
- infusion, transfusion and therapeutic injection (T80.2)
- prosthetic devices, implants and grafts (T82.6–T82.7, T83.5–T83.6, T84.5–T84.7, T85.7)

obstetric surgical wound infection (O86.0)

T81.5   **Foreign body accidentally left in body cavity or operation wound following a procedure**

Adhesions
Obstruction } due to foreign body accidentally left in operation wound or body cavity
Perforation

Excludes: obstruction or perforation due to prosthetic devices and implants intentionally left in body (T82.0–T82.5, T83.0–T83.4, T84.0–T84.4, T85.0–T85.6)

T81.6   **Acute reaction to foreign substance accidentally left during a procedure**

Peritonitis:
- aseptic
- chemical

T81.7   **Vascular complications following a procedure, not elsewhere classified**

Air embolism following procedure NEC

Excludes: embolism:
- complicating:
  - abortion or ectopic or molar pregnancy (O00–O07, O08.2)
  - pregnancy, childbirth and the puerperium (O88.–)
- due to prosthetic devices, implants and grafts (T82.8, T83.8, T84.8, T85.8)
- following infusion, transfusion and therapeutic injection (T80.0)
- traumatic (T79.0)

T81.8 **Other complications of procedures, not elsewhere classified**
Complication of inhalation therapy
Emphysema (subcutaneous) resulting from a procedure
Persistent postoperative fistula
Excludes: hypothermia following anaesthesia (T88.5)
malignant hyperthermia due to anaesthesia (T88.3)

T81.9 **Unspecified complication of procedure**

T82 Complications of cardiac and vascular prosthetic devices, implants and grafts

Excludes: failure and rejection of transplanted organs and tissues (T86.–)

T82.0 **Mechanical complication of heart valve prosthesis**
Breakdown (mechanical)
Displacement
Leakage
Malposition ⎫ due to heart valve prosthesis
Obstruction, mechanical
Perforation
Protrusion

T82.1 **Mechanical complication of cardiac electronic device**
Conditions listed in T82.0 due to:
• electrodes
• pulse generator (battery)

T82.2 **Mechanical complication of coronary artery bypass and valve grafts**
Conditions listed in T82.0 due to coronary artery bypass and valve grafts

T82.3 **Mechanical complication of other vascular grafts**
Conditions listed in T82.0 due to:
• aortic (bifurcation) graft (replacement)
• arterial (carotid) (femoral) graft (bypass)

T82.4 **Mechanical complication of vascular dialysis catheter**
Conditions listed in T82.0 due to vascular dialysis catheter
Excludes: mechanical complication of intraperitoneal dialysis catheter (T85.6)

T82.5 **Mechanical complication of other cardiac and vascular devices and implants**
Conditions listed in T82.0 due to:
- arteriovenous:
  - fistula ⎫
  - shunt ⎬ surgically created
- artificial heart
- balloon (counterpulsation) device
- infusion catheter
- umbrella device

Excludes: mechanical complication of epidural and subdural infusion catheter (T85.6)

T82.6 **Infection and inflammatory reaction due to cardiac valve prosthesis**

T82.7 **Infection and inflammatory reaction due to other cardiac and vascular devices, implants and grafts**

T82.8 **Other complications of cardiac and vascular prosthetic devices, implants and grafts**
Complication ⎫
Embolism ⎪
Fibrosis ⎪
Haemorrhage ⎬ due to cardiac and vascular prosthetic devices,
Pain ⎪ implants and grafts
Stenosis ⎪
Thrombosis ⎭

T82.9 **Unspecified complication of cardiac and vascular prosthetic device, implant and graft**

T83 Complications of genitourinary prosthetic devices, implants and grafts

Excludes: failure and rejection of transplanted organs and tissues (T86.–)

T83.0 **Mechanical complication of urinary (indwelling) catheter**
Conditions listed in T82.0 due to:
- catheter:
  - cystostomy
  - urethral, indwelling

T83.1   **Mechanical complication of other urinary devices and implants**
Conditions listed in T82.0 due to:
- urinary:
  - electronic stimulator device
  - sphincter implant
  - stent

T83.2   **Mechanical complication of graft of urinary organ**
Conditions listed in T82.0 due to graft of urinary organ

T83.3   **Mechanical complication of intrauterine contraceptive device**
Conditions listed in T82.0 due to intrauterine contraceptive device

T83.4   **Mechanical complication of other prosthetic devices, implants and grafts in genital tract**
Conditions listed in T82.0 due to (implanted) penile prosthesis

T83.5   **Infection and inflammatory reaction due to prosthetic device, implant and graft in urinary system**

T83.6   **Infection and inflammatory reaction due to prosthetic device, implant and graft in genital tract**

T83.8   **Other complications of genitourinary prosthetic devices, implants and grafts**
Conditions listed in T82.8 due to genitourinary prosthetic devices, implants and grafts

T83.9   **Unspecified complication of genitourinary prosthetic device, implant and graft**

T84   **Complications of internal orthopaedic prosthetic devices, implants and grafts**

Excludes: failure and rejection of transplanted organs and tissues (T86.–)
fracture of bone following insertion of orthopaedic implant, joint prosthesis or bone plate (M96.6)

T84.0   **Mechanical complication of internal joint prosthesis**
Conditions listed in T82.0 due to joint prosthesis

T84.1   **Mechanical complication of internal fixation device of bones of limb**
Conditions listed in T82.0 due to internal fixation device of bones of limb

T84.2   **Mechanical complication of internal fixation device of other bones**
Conditions listed in T82.0 due to internal fixation device of other bones

T84.3   **Mechanical complication of other bone devices, implants and grafts**
Conditions listed in T82.0 due to:
- bone graft
- electronic bone stimulator

T84.4   **Mechanical complication of other internal orthopaedic devices, implants and grafts**
Conditions listed in T82.0 due to muscle and tendon graft

T84.5   **Infection and inflammatory reaction due to internal joint prosthesis**

T84.6   **Infection and inflammatory reaction due to internal fixation device [any site]**

T84.7   **Infection and inflammatory reaction due to other internal orthopaedic prosthetic devices, implants and grafts**

T84.8   **Other complications of internal orthopaedic prosthetic devices, implants and grafts**
Conditions listed in T82.8 due to internal orthopaedic prosthetic devices, implants and grafts

T84.9   **Unspecified complication of internal orthopaedic prosthetic device, implant and graft**

T85   Complications of other internal prosthetic devices, implants and grafts

Excludes: failure and rejection of transplanted organs and tissues (T86.–)

T85.0   **Mechanical complication of ventricular intracranial (communicating) shunt**
Conditions listed in T82.0 due to ventricular intracranial (communicating) shunt

T85.1   **Mechanical complication of implanted electronic stimulator of nervous system**
Conditions listed in T82.0 due to electronic neurostimulator (electrode) of:
- brain
- peripheral nerve
- spinal cord

T85.2   **Mechanical complication of intraocular lens**
Conditions listed in T82.0 due to intraocular lens

T85.3   **Mechanical complication of other ocular prosthetic devices, implants and grafts**
Conditions listed in T82.0 due to:
- corneal graft
- prosthetic orbit of eye

T85.4   **Mechanical complication of breast prosthesis and implant**
Conditions listed in T82.0 due to breast prosthesis and implant

T85.5   **Mechanical complication of gastrointestinal prosthetic devices, implants and grafts**
Conditions listed in T82.0 due to:
- bile-duct prosthesis
- oesophageal anti-reflux device

T85.6   **Mechanical complication of other specified internal prosthetic devices, implants and grafts**
Conditions listed in T82.0 due to:
- epidural and subdural infusion catheter
- intraperitoneal dialysis catheter
- nonabsorbable surgical material NOS
- permanent sutures

Excludes: mechanical complication of permanent (wire) suture used in bone repair (T84.1–T84.2)

T85.7   **Infection and inflammatory reaction due to other internal prosthetic devices, implants and grafts**

T85.8   **Other complications of internal prosthetic devices, implants and grafts, not elsewhere classified**
Conditions listed in T82.8 due to internal prosthetic devices, implants and grafts NEC

T85.9   **Unspecified complication of internal prosthetic device, implant and graft**
Complication of internal prosthetic device, implant and graft NOS

T86 Failure and rejection of transplanted organs and tissues

T86.0 **Bone-marrow transplant rejection**
Graft-versus-host reaction or disease

T86.1 **Kidney transplant failure and rejection**

T86.2 **Heart transplant failure and rejection**
Excludes: complication of:
- artificial heart device (T82.5)
- heart–lung transplant (T86.3)

T86.3 **Heart–lung transplant failure and rejection**

T86.4 **Liver transplant failure and rejection**

T86.8 **Failure and rejection of other transplanted organs and tissues**
Transplant failure or rejection of:
- bone
- intestine
- lung
- pancreas
- skin (allograft) (autograft)

T86.9 **Failure and rejection of unspecified transplanted organ and tissue**

T87 Complications peculiar to reattachment and amputation

T87.0 **Complications of reattached (part of) upper extremity**

T87.1 **Complications of reattached (part of) lower extremity**

T87.2 **Complications of other reattached body part**

T87.3 **Neuroma of amputation stump**

T87.4 **Infection of amputation stump**

T87.5 **Necrosis of amputation stump**

T87.6 **Other and unspecified complications of amputation stump**
Amputation stump:
- contracture (flexion)(of next proximal joint)
- haematoma
- oedema

Excludes: phantom limb syndrome (G54.6–G54.7)

T88 Other complications of surgical and medical care, not elsewhere classified

Excludes: accidental puncture or laceration during a procedure
(T81.2)
complications following:
- infusion, transfusion and therapeutic injection
(T80.–)
- procedure NEC (T81.–)
specified complications classified elsewhere, such as:
- complications of:
  - anaesthesia in:
    - labour and delivery (O74.–)
    - pregnancy (O29.–)
    - puerperium (O89.–)
  - devices, implants and grafts (T82–T85)
  - obstetric surgery and procedures (O75.4)
- dermatitis due to drugs and medicaments
(L23.3, L24.4, L25.1, L27.0–L27.1)
- poisoning and toxic effects of drugs and chemicals
(T36–T65)

T88.0 **Infection following immunization**
Sepsis ⎫
Septicaemia ⎭ following immunization

T88.1 **Other complications following immunization, not elsewhere classified**
Rash following immunization

Excludes: anaphylactic shock due to serum (T80.5)
other serum reactions (T80.6)
postimmunization:
- arthropathy (M02.2)
- encephalitis (G04.0)

T88.2 **Shock due to anaesthesia**

Shock due to anaesthesia in which the correct substance was
properly administered

Excludes: complications of anaesthesia (in):
- from overdose or wrong substance given (T36–
  T50)
- labour and delivery (O74.–)
- pregnancy (O29.–)
- puerperium (O89.–)

postoperative shock NOS (T81.1)

T88.3 **Malignant hyperthermia due to anaesthesia**

T88.4 **Failed or difficult intubation**

T88.5 **Other complications of anaesthesia**

Hypothermia following anaesthesia

T88.6 **Anaphylactic shock due to adverse effect of correct drug
or medicament properly administered**

Excludes: anaphylactic shock due to serum (T80.5)

T88.7 **Unspecified adverse effect of drug or medicament**

Adverse effect of ⎤
Allergic reaction to ⎫ correct drug or medicament properly
Hypersensitivity to ⎬ administered
Idiosyncracy to ⎭

Drug:
- hypersensitivity NOS
- reaction NOS

Excludes: specified adverse effects of drugs and medicaments
(A00–R99, T80–T88.6, T88.8)

T88.8 **Other specified complications of surgical and medical care,
not elsewhere classified**

T88.9 **Complication of surgical and medical care, unspecified**

Excludes: adverse effect NOS (T78.9)

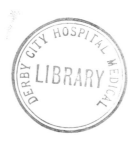

Sequelae of injuries, of poisoning and of other consequences of external causes (T90–T98)

Note: These categories are to be used to indicate conditions in S00–S99 and T00–T88 as the cause of late effects, which are themselves classified elsewhere. The "sequelae" include those specified as such, or as late effects, and those present one year or more after the acute injury.

T90 Sequelae of injuries of head

T90.0 Sequelae of superficial injury of head
Sequelae of injury classified to S00.–

T90.1 Sequelae of open wound of head
Sequelae of injury classifiable to S01.–

T90.2 Sequelae of fracture of skull and facial bones
Sequelae of injury classifiable to S02.–

T90.3 Sequelae of injury of cranial nerves
Sequelae of injury classifiable to S04.–

T90.4 Sequelae of injury of eye and orbit
Sequelae of injury classifiable to S05.–

T90.5 Sequelae of intracranial injury
Sequelae of injury classifiable to S06.–

T90.8 Sequelae of other specified injuries of head
Sequelae of injury classifiable to S03.–, S07–S08 and S09.0–S09.8

T90.9 Sequelae of unspecified injury of head
Sequelae of injury classifiable to S09.9

T91 Sequelae of injuries of neck and trunk

T91.0 Sequelae of superficial injury and open wound of neck and trunk
Sequelae of injury classifiable to S10–S11, S20–S21, S30–S31 and T09.0–T09.1

T91.1 **Sequelae of fracture of spine**
Sequelae of injury classifiable to S12.–, S22.0–S22.1, S32.0, S32.7 and T08

T91.2 **Sequelae of other fracture of thorax and pelvis**
Sequelae of injury classifiable to S22.2–S22.9, S32.1–S32.5 and S32.8

T91.3 **Sequelae of injury of spinal cord**
Sequelae of injury classifiable to S14.0–S14.1, S24.0–S24.1, S34.0– S34.1 and T09.3

T91.4 **Sequelae of injury of intrathoracic organs**
Sequelae of injury classifiable to S26–S27

T91.5 **Sequelae of injury of intra-abdominal and pelvic organs**
Sequelae of injury classifiable to S36–S37

T91.8 **Sequelae of other specified injuries of neck and trunk**
Sequelae of injury classifiable to S13.–, S14.2–S14.6, S15–S18, S19.7–S19.8, S23.–, S24.2–S24.6, S25.–, S28.–, S29.0–S29.8, S33.–, S34.2–S34.8, S35.–, S38.–, S39.0–S39.8, T09.2 and T09.4–T09.8

T91.9 **Sequelae of unspecified injury of neck and trunk**
Sequelae of injury classifiable to S19.9, S29.9, S39.9 and T09.9

T92 **Sequelae of injuries of upper limb**

T92.0 **Sequelae of open wound of upper limb**
Sequelae of injury classifiable to S41.–, S51.–, S61.– and T11.1

T92.1 **Sequelae of fracture of arm**
Sequelae of injury classifiable to S42.–, S52.– and T10

T92.2 **Sequelae of fracture at wrist and hand level**
Sequelae of injury classifiable to S62.–

T92.3 **Sequelae of dislocation, sprain and strain of upper limb**
Sequelae of injury classifiable to S43.–, S53.–, S63.– and T11.2

T92.4 **Sequelae of injury of nerve of upper limb**
Sequelae of injury classifiable to S44.–, S54.–, S64.– and T11.3

T92.5 **Sequelae of injury of muscle and tendon of upper limb**
Sequelae of injury classifiable to S46.–, S56.–, S66.– and T11.5

T92.6 **Sequelae of crushing injury and traumatic amputation of upper limb**
Sequelae of injury classifiable to S47–S48, S57–S58, S67–S68 and T11.6

T92.8 **Sequelae of other specified injuries of upper limb**
Sequelae of injury classifiable to S40.–, S45.–, S49.7–S49.8, S50.–, S55.–, S59.7–S59.8, S60.–, S65.–, S69.7–S69.8, T11.0, T11.4 and T11.8

T92.9 **Sequelae of unspecified injury of upper limb**
Sequelae of injury classifiable to S49.9, S59.9, S69.9 and T11.9

T93 Sequelae of injuries of lower limb

T93.0 **Sequelae of open wound of lower limb**
Sequelae of injury classifiable to S71.–, S81.–, S91.– and T13.1

T93.1 **Sequelae of fracture of femur**
Sequelae of injury classifiable S72.–

T93.2 **Sequelae of other fractures of lower limb**
Sequelae of injury classifiable to S82.–, S92.– and T12

T93.3 **Sequelae of dislocation, sprain and strain of lower limb**
Sequelae of injury classifiable to S73.–, S83.–, S93.– and T13.2

T93.4 **Sequelae of injury of nerve of lower limb**
Sequelae of injury classifiable to S74.–, S84.–, S94.– and T13.3

T93.5 **Sequelae of injury of muscle and tendon of lower limb**
Sequelae of injury classifiable to S76.–, S86.–, S96.– and T13.5

T93.6 **Sequelae of crushing injury and traumatic amputation of lower limb**
Sequelae of injury classifiable to S77–S78, S87–S88, S97–S98 and T13.6

T93.8 **Sequelae of other specified injuries of lower limb**
Sequelae of injury classifiable to S70.–, S75.–, S79.7–S79.8, S80.–, S85.–, S89.7–S89.8, S90.–, S95.–, S99.7–S99.8, T13.0, T13.4 and T13.8

T93.9 **Sequelae of unspecified injury of lower limb**
Sequelae of injury classifiable to S79.9, S89.9, S99.9 and T13.9

T94 Sequelae of injuries involving multiple and unspecified body regions

T94.0 **Sequelae of injuries involving multiple body regions**
Sequelae of injury classifiable to T00–T07

T94.1   **Sequelae of injuries, not specified by body region**
Sequelae of injury classifiable to T14.–

T95   Sequelae of burns, corrosions and frostbite

T95.0   **Sequelae of burn, corrosion and frostbite of head and neck**
Sequelae of injury classifiable to T20.–, T33.0–T33.1,
T34.0–T34.1 and T35.2

T95.1   **Sequelae of burn, corrosion and frostbite of trunk**
Sequelae of injury classifiable to T21.–, T33.2–T33.3,
T34.2–T34.3 and T35.3

T95.2   **Sequelae of burn, corrosion and frostbite of upper limb**
Sequelae of injury classifiable to T22–T23, T33.4–T33.5,
T34.4–T34.5 and T35.4

T95.3   **Sequelae of burn, corrosion and frostbite of lower limb**
Sequelae of injury classifiable to T24–T25, T33.6–T33.8,
T34.6–T34.8 and T35.5

T95.4   **Sequelae of burn and corrosion classifiable only according to extent of body surface involved**
Sequelae of injury classifiable to T31–T32

T95.8   **Sequelae of other specified burn, corrosion and frostbite**
Sequelae of injury classifiable T26–T29, T35.0–T35.1 and T35.6

T95.9   **Sequelae of unspecified burn, corrosion and frostbite**
Sequelae of injury classifiable to T30.–, T33.9, T34.9 and T35.7

T96   Sequelae of poisoning by drugs, medicaments and biological substances

Sequelae of poisoning classifiable to T36–T50

T97   Sequelae of toxic effects of substances chiefly nonmedicinal as to source

Sequelae of toxic effects classifiable to T51–T65

T98 Sequelae of other and unspecified effects of external causes

T98.0 **Sequelae of effects of foreign body entering through natural orifice**
Sequelae of effects classifiable to T15–T19

T98.1 **Sequelae of other and unspecified effects of external causes**
Sequelae of effects classifiable to T66–T78

T98.2 **Sequelae of certain early complications of trauma**
Sequelae of complications classifiable to T79.–

T98.3 **Sequelae of complications of surgical and medical care, not elsewhere classified**
Sequelae of complications classifiable to T80–T88

CHAPTER XX

External causes of morbidity and mortality (V01–Y98)

This chapter, which in previous revisions of ICD constituted a supplementary classification, permits the classification of environmental events and circumstances as the cause of injury, poisoning and other adverse effects. Where a code from this section is applicable, it is intended that it shall be used in addition to a code from another chapter of the Classification indicating the nature of the condition. Most often, the condition will be classifiable to Chapter XIX, Injury, poisoning and certain other consequences of external causes (S00–T98). Causes of death should preferably be tabulated according to both Chapter XIX and Chapter XX, but if only one code is tabulated then the code from Chapter XX should be used in preference. Other conditions that may be stated to be due to external causes are classified in Chapters I to XVIII. For these conditions, codes from Chapter XX should be used to provide additional information for multiple-condition analysis only.

Categories for sequelae of external causes of morbidity and mortality are included at Y85–Y89.

This chapter contains the following blocks:

V01–X59 Accidents

        V01–V99 Transport accidents

                V01–V09 Pedestrian injured in transport accident

                V10–V19 Pedal cyclist injured in transport accident

                V20–V29 Motorcycle rider injured in transport accident

                V30–V39 Occupant of three-wheeled motor vehicle injured in transport accident

                V40–V49 Car occupant injured in transport accident

                V50–V59 Occupant of pick-up truck or van injured in transport accident

                V60–V69 Occupant of heavy transport vehicle injured in transport accident

                V70–V79 Bus occupant injured in transport accident

                V80–V89 Other land transport accidents

                V90–V94 Water transport accidents

V95–V97 Air and space transport accidents
V98–V99 Other and unspecified transport accidents

W00–X59 Other external causes of accidental injury
W00–W19 Falls
W20–W49 Exposure to inanimate mechanical forces
W50–W64 Exposure to animate mechanical forces
W65–W74 Accidental drowning and submersion
W75–W84 Other accidental threats to breathing
W85–W99 Exposure to electric current, radiation and extreme ambient air temperature and pressure
X00–X09 Exposure to smoke, fire and flames
X10–X19 Contact with heat and hot substances
X20–X29 Contact with venomous animals and plants
X30–X39 Exposure to forces of nature
X40–X49 Accidental poisoning by and exposure to noxious substances
X50–X57 Overexertion, travel and privation
X58–X59 Accidental exposure to other and unspecified factors

X60–X84 Intentional self-harm

X85–Y09 Assault

Y10–Y34 Event of undetermined intent

Y35–Y36 Legal intervention and operations of war

Y40–Y84 Complications of medical and surgical care
Y40–Y59 Drugs, medicaments and biological substances causing adverse effects in therapeutic use
Y60–Y69 Misadventures to patients during surgical and medical care
Y70–Y82 Medical devices associated with adverse incidents in diagnostic and therapeutic use
Y83–Y84 Surgical and other medical procedures as the cause of abnormal reaction of the patient, or of later complication, without mention of misadventure at the time of the procedure

Y85–Y89 Sequelae of external causes of morbidity and mortality

Y90–Y98 Supplementary factors related to causes of morbidity and mortality classified elsewhere

Place of occurrence code

The following fourth-character subdivisions are for use with categories W00–Y34 except Y06.– and Y07.– to identify the place of occurrence of the external cause where relevant:

.0 Home
Apartment
Boarding-house
Caravan [trailer] park, residential
Farmhouse
Home premises
House (residential)
Noninstitutional place of residence
Private:
• driveway to home
• garage
• garden to home
• yard to home
Swimming-pool in private house or garden

Excludes: abandoned or derelict house (.8)
home under construction but not yet occupied (.6)
institutional place of residence (.1)

.1 Residential institution
Children's home
Dormitory
Home for the sick
Hospice
Military camp
Nursing home
Old people's home
Orphanage
Pensioner's home
Prison
Reform school

.2 School, other institution and public administrative area
Building (including adjacent grounds) used by the general public or by
a particular group of the public such as:
- assembly hall
- campus
- church
- cinema
- clubhouse
- college
- court-house
- dancehall
- day nursery
- gallery
- hospital
- institute for higher education
- kindergarten
- library
- movie-house
- museum
- music-hall
- opera-house
- post office
- public hall
- school (private)(public)(state)
- theatre
- university
- youth centre

Excludes: building under construction (.6)
           residential institution (.1)
           sports and athletics area (.3)

.3 Sports and athletics area
Baseball field
Basketball-court
Cricket ground
Football field
Golf-course
Gymnasium
Hockey field
Riding-school
Skating-rink
Squash-court
Stadium

Swimming-pool, public
Tennis-court

Excludes: swimming-pool or tennis-court in private home or garden
(.0)

.4 Street and highway
Freeway
Motorway
Pavement
Road
Sidewalk

.5 Trade and service area
Airport
Bank
Café
Casino
Garage (commercial)
Gas station
Hotel
Market
Office building
Petrol station
Radio or television station
Restaurant
Service station
Shop (commercial)
Shopping mall
Station (bus)(railway)
Store
Supermarket
Warehouse

Excludes: garage in private home (.0)

.6 Industrial and construction area
Building [any] under construction
Dockyard
Dry dock
Factory:
• building
• premises
Gasworks
Industrial yard
Mine
Oil rig and other offshore installations
Pit (coal)(gravel)(sand)
Power-station (coal)(nuclear)(oil)
Shipyard
Tunnel under construction
Workshop

.7 Farm
Farm:
• buildings
• land under cultivation
Ranch

Excludes: farmhouse and home premises of farm (.0)

.8 Other specified places
Beach
Campsite
Canal
Caravan site NOS
Derelict house
Desert
Dock NOS
Forest
Harbour
Hill
Lake
Marsh
Military training ground
Mountain
Park (amusement) (public)
Parking-lot and parking-place
Pond or pool
Prairie
Public place NOS

Railway line
River
Sea
Seashore
Stream
Swamp
Water reservoir
Zoo

.9 Unspecified place

Activity code

The following subclassification is provided for optional use in a supplementary character position with categories V01–Y34 to indicate the activity of the injured person at the time the event occurred. This subclassification should not be confused with, or be used instead of, the recommended fourth-character subdivisions provided to indicate the place of occurrence of events classifiable to W00–Y34.

0 While engaged in sports activity
Physical exercise with a described functional element such as:
- golf
- jogging
- riding
- school athletics
- skiing
- swimming
- trekking
- water-skiing

1 While engaged in leisure activity
Hobby activities
Leisure-time activities with an entertainment element such as going to the cinema, to a dance or to a party
Participation in sessions and activities of voluntary organizations

Excludes: sports activities (0)

2 While working for income
Paid work (manual)(professional)
Transportation (time) to and from such activities
Work for salary, bonus and other types of income

3   While engaged in other types of work
Domestic duties such as:
- caring for children and relatives
- cleaning
- cooking
- gardening
- household maintenance

Duties for which one would not normally gain an income
Learning activities, e.g. attending school session or lesson
Undergoing education

4   While resting, sleeping, eating or engaging in other vital activities
Personal hygiene

8   While engaged in other specified activities

9   During unspecified activity

Transport accidents (V01–V99)

Note: This section is structured in 12 groups. Those relating to land transport accidents (V01–V89) reflect the victim's mode of transport and are subdivided to identify the victim's "counterpart" or the type of event. The vehicle of which the injured person is an occupant is identified in the first two characters since it is seen as the most important factor to identify for prevention purposes.

Excludes: assault by crashing of motor vehicle (Y03.–)
event of undetermined intent (Y32–Y33)
intentional self-harm (X82–X83)
transport accidents due to cataclysm (X34–X38)

Definitions related to transport accidents

(a)   A *transport accident* (V01–V99) is any accident involving a device designed primarily for, or being used at the time primarily for, conveying persons or goods from one place to another.

(b)   A *public highway* [trafficway] or *street* is the entire width between property lines (or other boundary lines) of land open to the public as a matter of right or custom for purposes of moving persons or property from one place to another. A *roadway* is that part of the public highway designed, improved and customarily used for vehicular traffic.

(c) A *traffic accident* is any vehicle accident occurring on the public highway [i.e. originating on, terminating on, or involving a vehicle partially on the highway]. A vehicle accident is assumed to have occurred on the public highway unless another place is specified, except in the case of accidents involving only off-road motor vehicles, which are classified as nontraffic accidents unless the contrary is stated.

(d) A *nontraffic accident* is any vehicle accident that occurs entirely in any place other than a public highway.

(e) A *pedestrian* is any person involved in an accident who was not at the time of the accident riding in or on a motor vehicle, railway train, streetcar or animal-drawn or other vehicle, or on a pedal cycle or animal.

   Includes: person:
   - changing wheel of vehicle
   - making adjustment to motor of vehicle
   - on foot

   user of a pedestrian conveyance such as:
   - baby carriage
   - ice-skates
   - perambulator
   - push-cart
   - push-chair
   - roller-skates
   - scooter
   - skateboard
   - skis
   - sled
   - wheelchair (powered)

(f) A *driver* is an occupant of a transport vehicle who is operating or intending to operate it.

(g) A *passenger* is any occupant of a transport vehicle other than the driver.

   Excludes: person travelling on outside of vehicle—see definition (h)

1019

(h)   A *person on outside of vehicle* is any person being transported by a vehicle but not occupying the space normally reserved for the driver or passengers, or the space intended for the transport of property.

Includes: person (travelling on):
- bodywork
- bumper [fender]
- hanging on outside
- roof (rack)
- running-board
- step

(i)   A *pedal cycle* is any land transport vehicle operated solely by pedals.

Includes: bicycle
tricycle

Excludes: motorized bicycle—see definition (k)

(j)   A *pedal cyclist* is any person riding on a pedal cycle or in a sidecar or trailer attached to such a vehicle.

(k)   A *motorcycle* is a two-wheeled motor vehicle with one or two riding saddles and sometimes with a third wheel for the support of a sidecar. The sidecar is considered part of the motorcycle.

Includes: moped
motor scooter
motorcycle:
- NOS
- combination
- with sidecar
motorized bicycle
speed-limited motor-driven cycle

Excludes: motor-driven tricycle—see definition (m)

(l)   A *motorcycle rider* is any person riding on a motorcycle or in a sidecar or trailer attached to such a vehicle.

(m) A *three-wheeled motor vehicle* is a motorized tricycle designed primarily for on-road use.

Includes: motor-driven tricycle
motorized rickshaw
three-wheeled motor car

Excludes: motorcycle with sidecar—see definition (k)
special all-terrain vehicle—see definition (w)

(n) A *car* [*automobile*] is a four-wheeled motor vehicle designed primarily for carrying up to 10 persons.

Includes: minibus

(o) A *pick-up truck* or *van* is a four- or six-wheeled motor vehicle designed primarily for carrying property, weighing less than the local limit for classification as a heavy goods vehicle, and not requiring a special driver's licence.

(p) A *heavy transport vehicle* is a motor vehicle designed primarily for carrying property, meeting local criteria for classification as a heavy goods vehicle in terms of kerbside weight (usually above 3500 kg), and requiring a special driver's licence.

(q) A *bus* is a motor vehicle designed or adapted primarily for carrying more than 10 persons, and requiring a special driver's licence.

Includes: coach

(r) A *railway train* or *railway vehicle* is any device, with or without cars coupled to it, designed for traffic on a railway.

Includes: interurban:
- electric car ⎱ (operated chiefly on its own right-of-way,
- streetcar ⎰   not open to other traffic)

railway train, any power [diesel] [electric] [steam]:
- funicular
- monorail or two-rail
- subterranean or elevated

other vehicle designed to run on a railway track

Excludes: interurban electric cars [streetcars] specified to be operating on a right-of-way that forms part of the public street or highway—see definition (s)

(s) A *streetcar* is a device designed and used primarily for transporting persons within a municipality, running on rails, usually subject to normal traffic control signals, and operated principally on a right-of-way that forms part of the roadway. A trailer being towed by a streetcar is considered a part of the streetcar.

Includes: interurban electric car or streetcar, when specified to be operating on a street or public highway

tram (car)

trolley (car)

(t) A *special vehicle mainly used on industrial premises* is a motor vehicle designed primarily for use within the buildings and premises of industrial or commercial establishments.

Includes: battery-powered:
- airport passenger vehicle
- truck (baggage)(mail)

coal-car in mine
forklift (truck)
logging car
self-propelled truck, industrial
station baggage truck (powered)
tram, truck or tub (powered) in mine or quarry

(u) A *special vehicle mainly used in agriculture* is a motor vehicle designed specifically for use in farming and agriculture (horticulture), for example to work the land, tend and harvest crops and transport materials on the farm.

Includes: combine harvester
self-propelled farm machinery
tractor (and trailer)

(v) A *special construction vehicle* is a motor vehicle designed specifically for use in the construction (and demolition) of roads, buildings and other structures.

Includes: bulldozer
digger
dumper truck
earth-leveller
mechanical shovel
road-roller

(w) A *special all-terrain vehicle* is a motor vehicle of special design to enable it to negotiate rough or soft terrain or snow. Examples of special design are high construction, special wheels and tyres, tracks, and support on a cushion of air.

Includes: hovercraft on land or swamp
snowmobile

Excludes: hovercraft on open water—see definition (x)

(x) A *watercraft* is any device for transporting passengers or goods on water.

Includes: hovercraft NOS

(y) An *aircraft* is any device for transporting passengers or goods in the air.

Classification and coding instructions for transport accidents

1. If an event is unspecified as to whether it was a traffic or a nontraffic accident, it is assumed to be:

    (a) A traffic accident when the event is classifiable to categories V10–V82 and V87.

    (b) A nontraffic accident when the event is classifiable to categories V83–V86. For these categories the victim is either a pedestrian, or an occupant of a vehicle designed primarily for off-road use.

2. When accidents involving more than one kind of transport are reported, the following order of precedence should be used:

    aircraft and spacecraft (V95–V97)
    watercraft (V90–V94)
    other modes of transport (V01–V89, V98–V99)

3. Where transport accident descriptions do not specify the victim as being a vehicle occupant and the victim is described as:

crushed dragged hit injured killed knocked down run over	by any vehicle including	animal being ridden animal-drawn vehicle bicycle bulldozer bus car motorcycle motorized tricycle pick-up (truck) recreational vehicle streetcar tractor train tram truck van

classify the victim as a pedestrian (categories V01–V09).

4. Where transport accident descriptions do not indicate the victim's role, such as:

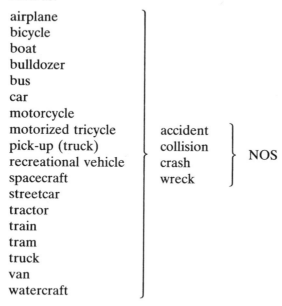

airplane
bicycle
boat
bulldozer
bus
car
motorcycle
motorized tricycle   accident
pick-up (truck)   collision
recreational vehicle   crash   NOS
spacecraft   wreck
streetcar
tractor
train
tram
truck
van
watercraft

classify the victim as an occupant or rider of the vehicle mentioned.

If more than one vehicle is mentioned, do not make any assumption as to which vehicle was occupied by the victim unless the vehicles are the same. Instead, code to the appropriate categories V87–V88, V90–V94, V95–V97, taking into account the order of precedence given in note 2 above.

5. Where a transport accident, such as:

vehicle (motor)(nonmotor):
- failing to make curve
- going out of control (due to):
  - burst tyre [blowout]
  - driver falling asleep
  - driver inattention
  - excessive speed
  - failure of mechanical part

resulted in a subsequent collision, classify the accident as a collision. If an accident other than a collision resulted, classify it as a noncollision accident according to the vehicle type involved.

6. Where a transport accident involving a vehicle in motion, such as:

accidental poisoning from exhaust gas generated by
breakage of any part of
explosion of any part of
fall, jump or being accidentally pushed from
fire starting in } vehicle in
hit by object thrown into or onto motion
injured by being thrown against some part of, or
   object in
injury from moving part of
object falling in or on

resulted in a subsequent collision, classify the accident as a collision. If
an accident other than a collision resulted, classify it as a noncollision
accident according to the vehicle type involved.

7. Land transport accidents described as:

collision (due to loss of control)(on highway) between vehicle and:

abutment (bridge)(overpass)
fallen stone
guard rail or boundary fence
inter-highway divider
landslide (not moving) } are included in V17.–,
object thrown in front of motor vehicle   V27.–, V37.–, V47.–,
safety island   V57.–, V67.– and V77.–
tree
traffic sign or marker (temporary)
utility pole
wall of cut made for road
other object, fixed, movable or moving

overturning (without collision) are included in V18.–, V28.–, V38.–,
   V48.–, V58.–, V68.–, and V78.–

collision with animal (herded)(unattended) are included in V10.–, V20.–,
   V30.–, V40.–, V50.–, V60.– and V70.–

collision with animal-drawn vehicle or animal being ridden are included
   in V16.–, V26.–, V36.–, V46.–, V56.–, V66.– and V76.–

Pedestrian injured in transport accident (V01–V09)

Excludes: collision of pedestrian (conveyance) with other pedestrian (conveyance) (W51.–)
  • with subsequent fall (W03.–)

The following fourth-character subdivisions are for use with categories V01–V06:
  .0 Nontraffic accident
  .1 Traffic accident
  .9 Unspecified whether traffic or nontraffic accident

V01 **Pedestrian injured in collision with pedal cycle**

V02 **Pedestrian injured in collision with two- or three-wheeled motor vehicle**

V03 **Pedestrian injured in collision with car, pick-up truck or van**

V04 **Pedestrian injured in collision with heavy transport vehicle or bus**

V05 **Pedestrian injured in collision with railway train or railway vehicle**

V06 **Pedestrian injured in collision with other nonmotor vehicle**

  Includes: collision with animal-drawn vehicle, animal being ridden, streetcar

V09 Pedestrian injured in other and unspecified transport accidents

Includes: pedestrian injured by special vehicle

V09.0 Pedestrian injured in nontraffic accident involving other and unspecified motor vehicles

V09.1 Pedestrian injured in unspecified nontraffic accident

V09.2 Pedestrian injured in traffic accident involving other and unspecified motor vehicles

V09.3 Pedestrian injured in unspecified traffic accident

V09.9 Pedestrian injured in unspecified transport accident

Pedal cyclist injured in transport accident (V10–V19)

The following fourth-character subdivisions are for use with categories V10–V18:

.0 Driver injured in nontraffic accident
.1 Passenger injured in nontraffic accident
.2 Unspecified pedal cyclist injured in nontraffic accident
.3 Person injured while boarding or alighting
.4 Driver injured in traffic accident
.5 Passenger injured in traffic accident
.9 Unspecified pedal cyclist injured in traffic accident

V10 Pedal cyclist injured in collision with pedestrian or animal

Excludes: collision with animal-drawn vehicle or animal being ridden (V16.–)

V11 Pedal cyclist injured in collision with other pedal cycle

V12 Pedal cyclist injured in collision with two- or three-wheeled motor vehicle

V13 Pedal cyclist injured in collision with car, pick-up truck or van

V14 Pedal cyclist injured in collision with heavy transport vehicle or bus

V15 Pedal cyclist injured in collision with railway train or railway vehicle

V16 Pedal cyclist injured in collision with other nonmotor vehicle

Includes: collision with animal-drawn vehicle, animal being ridden, streetcar

V17 Pedal cyclist injured in collision with fixed or stationary object

V18 Pedal cyclist injured in noncollision transport accident

Includes: fall or thrown from pedal cycle (without antecedent collision)
overturning:
- NOS
- without collision

V19 Pedal cyclist injured in other and unspecified transport accidents

V19.0 Driver injured in collision with other and unspecified motor vehicles in nontraffic accident

V19.1 Passenger injured in collision with other and unspecified motor vehicles in nontraffic accident

V19.2 Unspecified pedal cyclist injured in collision with other and unspecified motor vehicles in nontraffic accident
Pedal cycle collision NOS, nontraffic

V19.3 **Pedal cyclist [any] injured in unspecified nontraffic accident**
Pedal cycle accident NOS, nontraffic
Pedal cyclist injured in nontraffic accident NOS

V19.4 **Driver injured in collision with other and unspecified motor vehicles in traffic accident**

V19.5 **Passenger injured in collision with other and unspecified motor vehicles in traffic accident**

V19.6 **Unspecified pedal cyclist injured in collision with other and unspecified motor vehicles in traffic accident**
Pedal cycle collision NOS (traffic)

V19.8 **Pedal cyclist [any] injured in other specified transport accidents**
Trapped by part of pedal cycle

V19.9 **Pedal cyclist [any] injured in unspecified traffic accident**
Pedal cycle accident NOS

Motorcycle rider injured in transport accident (V20–V29)

Includes: moped
motorcycle with sidecar
motorized bicycle
motor scooter

Excludes: three-wheeled motor vehicle (V30–V39)

The following fourth-character subdivisions are for use with categories V20–V28:

.0 Driver injured in nontraffic accident
.1 Passenger injured in nontraffic accident
.2 Unspecified motorcycle rider injured in nontraffic accident
.3 Person injured while boarding or alighting
.4 Driver injured in traffic accident
.5 Passenger injured in traffic accident
.9 Unspecified motorcycle rider injured in traffic accident

V20 **Motorcycle rider injured in collision with pedestrian or animal**

Excludes: collision with animal-drawn vehicle or animal being ridden (V26.–)

V21 **Motorcycle rider injured in collision with pedal cycle**

V22 **Motorcycle rider injured in collision with two- or three-wheeled motor vehicle**

V23 **Motorcycle rider injured in collision with car, pick-up truck or van**

V24 **Motorcycle rider injured in collision with heavy transport vehicle or bus**

V25 **Motorcycle rider injured in collision with railway train or railway vehicle**

V26 **Motorcycle rider injured in collision with other nonmotor vehicle**

Includes: collision with animal-drawn vehicle, animal being ridden, streetcar

V27 **Motorcycle rider injured in collision with fixed or stationary object**

V28 **Motorcycle rider injured in noncollision transport accident**

Includes: fall or thrown from motorcycle (without antecedent collision)
overturning:
- NOS
- without collision

V29 Motorcycle rider injured in other and unspecified transport accidents

V29.0 **Driver injured in collision with other and unspecified motor vehicles in nontraffic accident**

V29.1 **Passenger injured in collision with other and unspecified motor vehicles in nontraffic accident**

V29.2 **Unspecified motorcycle rider injured in collision with other and unspecified motor vehicles in nontraffic accident**
Motorcycle collision NOS, nontraffic

V29.3 **Motorcycle rider [any] injured in unspecified nontraffic accident**
Motorcycle accident NOS, nontraffic
Motorcycle rider injured in nontraffic accident NOS

V29.4 **Driver injured in collision with other and unspecified motor vehicles in traffic accident**

V29.5 **Passenger injured in collision with other and unspecified motor vehicles in traffic accident**

V29.6 **Unspecified motorcycle rider injured in collision with other and unspecified motor vehicles in traffic accident**
Motorcycle collision NOS (traffic)

V29.8 **Motorcycle rider [any] injured in other specified transport accidents**
Trapped by part of motorcycle

V29.9 **Motorcycle rider [any] injured in unspecified traffic accident**
Motorcycle accident NOS

Occupant of three-wheeled motor vehicle injured in transport accident (V30–V39)

Includes: motorized tricycle
Excludes: motorcycle with sidecar (V20–V29)
vehicle designed primarily for off-road use (V86.–)

The following fourth-character subdivisions are for use with categories V30–V38:

.0 Driver injured in nontraffic accident
.1 Passenger injured in nontraffic accident
.2 Person on outside of vehicle injured in nontraffic accident
.3 Unspecified occupant of three-wheeled motor vehicle injured in nontraffic accident
.4 Person injured while boarding or alighting
.5 Driver injured in traffic accident
.6 Passenger injured in traffic accident
.7 Person on outside of vehicle injured in traffic accident
.9 Unspecified occupant of three-wheeled motor vehicle injured in traffic accident

V30 Occupant of three-wheeled motor vehicle injured in collision with pedestrian or animal

Excludes: collision with animal-drawn vehicle or animal being ridden (V36.–)

V31 Occupant of three-wheeled motor vehicle injured in collision with pedal cycle

V32 Occupant of three-wheeled motor vehicle injured in collision with two- or three-wheeled motor vehicle

V33 Occupant of three-wheeled motor vehicle injured in collision with car, pick-up truck or van·

V34 Occupant of three-wheeled motor vehicle injured in collision with heavy transport vehicle or bus

V35 Occupant of three-wheeled motor vehicle injured in collision with railway train or railway vehicle

V36 Occupant of three-wheeled motor vehicle injured in collision with other nonmotor vehicle

Includes: collision with animal-drawn vehicle, animal being ridden, streetcar

V37 Occupant of three-wheeled motor vehicle injured in collision with fixed or stationary object

V38 Occupant of three-wheeled motor vehicle injured in noncollision transport accident

Includes: fall or thrown from three-wheeled motor vehicle overturning:
- NOS
- without collision

V39 Occupant of three-wheeled motor vehicle injured in other and unspecified transport accidents

V39.0 Driver injured in collision with other and unspecified motor vehicles in nontraffic accident

V39.1 Passenger injured in collision with other and unspecified motor vehicles in nontraffic accident

V39.2 Unspecified occupant of three-wheeled motor vehicle injured in collision with other and unspecified motor vehicles in nontraffic accident
Collision NOS involving three-wheeled motor vehicle, nontraffic

V39.3 Occupant [any] of three-wheeled motor vehicle injured in unspecified nontraffic accident
Accident NOS involving three-wheeled motor vehicle, nontraffic
Occupant of three-wheeled motor vehicle injured in nontraffic accident NOS

V39.4 Driver injured in collision with other and unspecified motor vehicles in traffic accident

V39.5 Passenger injured in collision with other and unspecified motor vehicles in traffic accident

V39.6 **Unspecified occupant of three-wheeled motor vehicle injured in collision with other and unspecified motor vehicles in traffic accident**
Collision NOS involving three-wheeled motor vehicle (traffic)

V39.8 **Occupant [any] of three-wheeled motor vehicle injured in other specified transport accidents**
Trapped by door or other part of three-wheeled motor vehicle

V39.9 **Occupant [any] of three-wheeled motor vehicle injured in unspecified traffic accident**
Accident NOS involving three-wheeled motor vehicle

Car occupant injured in transport accident (V40–V49)

Includes: minibus

The following fourth-character subdivisions are for use with categories V40–V48:

    .0 Driver injured in nontraffic accident
    .1 Passenger injured in nontraffic accident
    .2 Person on outside of vehicle injured in nontraffic accident
    .3 Unspecified car occupant injured in nontraffic accident
    .4 Person injured while boarding or alighting
    .5 Driver injured in traffic accident
    .6 Passenger injured in traffic accident
    .7 Person on outside of vehicle injured in traffic accident
    .9 Unspecified car occupant injured in traffic accident

V40 **Car occupant injured in collision with pedestrian or animal**
Excludes: collision with animal-drawn vehicle or animal being ridden (V46.–)

V41 Car occupant injured in collision with pedal cycle

V42 Car occupant injured in collision with two- or three-wheeled motor vehicle

V43 Car occupant injured in collision with car, pick-up truck or van

V44 Car occupant injured in collision with heavy transport vehicle or bus

V45 Car occupant injured in collision with railway train or railway vehicle

V46 Car occupant injured in collision with other nonmotor vehicle

Includes: collision with animal-drawn vehicle, animal being ridden, streetcar

V47 Car occupant injured in collision with fixed or stationary object

V48 Car occupant injured in noncollision transport accident

Includes: overturning:
- NOS
- without collision

V49 Car occupant injured in other and unspecified transport accidents

V49.0 Driver injured in collision with other and unspecified motor vehicles in nontraffic accident

V49.1   **Passenger injured in collision with other and unspecified motor vehicles in nontraffic accident**

V49.2   **Unspecified car occupant injured in collision with other and unspecified motor vehicles in nontraffic accident**
Car collision NOS, nontraffic

V49.3   **Car occupant [any] injured in unspecified nontraffic accident**
Car accident NOS, nontraffic
Car occupant injured in nontraffic accident NOS

V49.4   **Driver injured in collision with other and unspecified motor vehicles in traffic accident**

V49.5   **Passenger injured in collision with other and unspecified motor vehicles in traffic accident**

V49.6   **Unspecified car occupant injured in collision with other and unspecified motor vehicles in traffic accident**
Car collision NOS (traffic)

V49.8   **Car occupant [any] injured in other specified transport accidents**
Trapped by door or other part of car

V49.9   **Car occupant [any] injured in unspecified traffic accident**
Car accident NOS

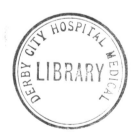

Occupant of pick-up truck or van injured in transport accident
(V50–V59)

Excludes: heavy transport vehicle (V60–V69)

The following fourth-character subdivisions are for use with categories V50–V58:

.0 Driver injured in nontraffic accident
.1 Passenger injured in nontraffic accident
.2 Person on outside of vehicle injured in nontraffic accident
.3 Unspecified occupant of pick-up truck or van injured in nontraffic accident
.4 Person injured while boarding or alighting
.5 Driver injured in traffic accident
.6 Passenger injured in traffic accident
.7 Person on outside of vehicle injured in traffic accident
.9 Unspecified occupant of pick-up truck or van injured in traffic accident

V50 Occupant of pick-up truck or van injured in collision with pedestrian or animal
Excludes: collision with animal-drawn vehicle or animal being ridden (V56.–)

V51 Occupant of pick-up truck or van injured in collision with pedal cycle

V52 Occupant of pick-up truck or van injured in collision with two- or three-wheeled motor vehicle

V53 Occupant of pick-up truck or van injured in collision with car, pick-up truck or van

V54 Occupant of pick-up truck or van injured in collision with heavy transport vehicle or bus

V55 Occupant of pick-up truck or van injured in collision with railway train or railway vehicle

V56 Occupant of pick-up truck or van injured in collision with other nonmotor vehicle

Includes: collision with animal-drawn vehicle, animal being ridden, streetcar

V57 Occupant of pick-up truck or van injured in collision with fixed or stationary object

V58 Occupant of pick-up truck or van injured in noncollision transport accident

Includes: overturning:
- NOS
- without collision

V59 Occupant of pick-up truck or van injured in other and unspecified transport accidents

V59.0 Driver injured in collision with other and unspecified motor vehicles in nontraffic accident

V59.1 Passenger injured in collision with other and unspecified motor vehicles in nontraffic accident

V59.2 Unspecified occupant of pick-up truck or van injured in collision with other and unspecified motor vehicles in nontraffic accident

Collision NOS involving pick-up truck or van, nontraffic

V59.3 Occupant [any] of pick-up truck or van injured in unspecified nontraffic accident

Accident NOS involving pick-up truck or van, nontraffic
Occupant of pick-up truck or van injured in nontraffic accident NOS

V59.4 Driver injured in collision with other and unspecified motor vehicles in traffic accident

V59.5 Passenger injured in collision with other and unspecified motor vehicles in traffic accident

V59.6   **Unspecified occupant of pick-up truck or van injured in collision with other and unspecified motor vehicles in traffic accident**
Collision NOS involving pick-up truck or van (traffic)

V59.8   **Occupant [any] of pick-up truck or van injured in other specified transport accidents**
Trapped by door or other part of pick-up truck or van

V59.9   **Occupant [any] of pick-up truck or van injured in unspecified traffic accident**
Accident NOS involving pick-up truck or van

Occupant of heavy transport vehicle injured in transport accident (V60–V69)

The following fourth-character subdivisions are for use with categories V60–V68:

.0   Driver injured in nontraffic accident
.1   Passenger injured in nontraffic accident
.2   Person on outside of vehicle injured in nontraffic accident
.3   Unspecified occupant of heavy transport vehicle injured in nontraffic accident
.4   Person injured while boarding or alighting
.5   Driver injured in traffic accident
.6   Passenger injured in traffic accident
.7   Person on outside of vehicle injured in traffic accident
.9   Unspecified occupant of heavy transport vehicle injured in traffic accident

V60   **Occupant of heavy transport vehicle injured in collision with pedestrian or animal**
Excludes: collision with animal-drawn vehicle or animal being ridden (V66.–)

V61   **Occupant of heavy transport vehicle injured in collision with pedal cycle**

V62 Occupant of heavy transport vehicle injured in collision with two- or three-wheeled motor vehicle

V63 Occupant of heavy transport vehicle injured in collision with car, pick-up truck or van

V64 Occupant of heavy transport vehicle injured in collision with heavy transport vehicle or bus

V65 Occupant of heavy transport vehicle injured in collision with railway train or railway vehicle

V66 Occupant of heavy transport vehicle injured in collision with other nonmotor vehicle

Includes: collision with animal-drawn vehicle, animal being ridden, streetcar

V67 Occupant of heavy transport vehicle injured in collision with fixed or stationary object

V68 Occupant of heavy transport vehicle injured in noncollision transport accident

Includes: overturning:
- NOS
- without collision

V69 Occupant of heavy transport vehicle injured in other and unspecified transport accidents

V69.0 Driver injured in collision with other and unspecified motor vehicles in nontraffic accident

V69.1 Passenger injured in collision with other and unspecified motor vehicles in nontraffic accident

V69.2 **Unspecified occupant of heavy transport vehicle injured in collision with other and unspecified motor vehicles in nontraffic accident**

Collision NOS involving heavy transport vehicle, nontraffic

V69.3 **Occupant [any] of heavy transport vehicle injured in unspecified nontraffic accident**

Accident NOS involving heavy transport vehicle, nontraffic

Occupant of heavy transport vehicle injured in nontraffic accident NOS

V69.4 **Driver injured in collision with other and unspecified motor vehicles in traffic accident**

V69.5 **Passenger injured in collision with other and unspecified motor vehicles in traffic accident**

V69.6 **Unspecified occupant of heavy transport vehicle injured in collision with other and unspecified motor vehicles in traffic accident**

Collision NOS involving heavy transport vehicle (traffic)

V69.8 **Occupant [any] of heavy transport vehicle injured in other specified transport accidents**

Trapped by door or other part of heavy transport vehicle

V69.9 **Occupant [any] of heavy transport vehicle injured in unspecified traffic accident**

Accident NOS involving heavy transport vehicle

Bus occupant injured in transport accident (V70–V79)

Excludes: minibus (V40–V49)

The following fourth-character subdivisions are for use with categories V70-V78:

.0 Driver injured in nontraffic accident
.1 Passenger injured in nontraffic accident
.2 Person on outside of vehicle injured in nontraffic accident
.3 Unspecified bus occupant injured in nontraffic accident
.4 Person injured while boarding or alighting
.5 Driver injured in traffic accident
.6 Passenger injured in traffic accident
.7 Person on outside of vehicle injured in traffic accident
.9 Unspecified bus occupant injured in traffic accident

V70 Bus occupant injured in collision with pedestrian or animal
Excludes: collision with animal-drawn vehicle or animal being ridden (V76.–)

V71 Bus occupant injured in collision with pedal cycle

V72 Bus occupant injured in collision with two- or three-wheeled motor vehicle

V73 Bus occupant injured in collision with car, pick-up truck or van

V74 Bus occupant injured in collision with heavy transport vehicle or bus

V75 Bus occupant injured in collision with railway train or railway vehicle

V76 Bus occupant injured in collision with other nonmotor vehicle

Includes: collision with animal-drawn vehicle, animal being ridden, streetcar

V77 Bus occupant injured in collision with fixed or stationary object

V78 Bus occupant injured in noncollision transport accident

Includes: overturning:
- NOS
- without collision

V79 Bus occupant injured in other and unspecified transport accidents

V79.0 Driver injured in collision with other and unspecified motor vehicles in nontraffic accident

V79.1 Passenger injured in collision with other and unspecified motor vehicles in nontraffic accident

V79.2 Unspecified bus occupant injured in collision with other and unspecified motor vehicles in nontraffic accident
Bus collision NOS, nontraffic

V79.3 Bus occupant [any] injured in unspecified nontraffic accident
Bus accident NOS, nontraffic
Bus occupant injured in nontraffic accident NOS

V79.4 Driver injured in collision with other and unspecified motor vehicles in traffic accident

V79.5 Passenger injured in collision with other and unspecified motor vehicles in traffic accident

V79.6 Unspecified bus occupant injured in collision with other and unspecified motor vehicles in traffic accident
Bus collision NOS (traffic)

1043

V79.8 **Bus occupant [any] injured in other specified transport accidents**
Trapped by door or other part of bus

V79.9 **Bus occupant [any] injured in unspecified traffic accident**
Bus accident NOS

Other land transport accidents (V80–V89)

V80 **Animal-rider or occupant of animal-drawn vehicle injured in transport accident**

V80.0 **Rider or occupant injured by fall from or being thrown from animal or animal-drawn vehicle in noncollision accident**
Overturning:
• NOS
• without collision

V80.1 **Rider or occupant injured in collision with pedestrian or animal**
Excludes: collision with animal-drawn vehicle or animal being ridden (V80.7)

V80.2 **Rider or occupant injured in collision with pedal cycle**

V80.3 **Rider or occupant injured in collision with two- or three-wheeled motor vehicle**

V80.4 **Rider or occupant injured in collision with car, pick-up truck, van, heavy transport vehicle or bus**

V80.5 **Rider or occupant injured in collision with other specified motor vehicle**

V80.6 **Rider or occupant injured in collision with railway train or railway vehicle**

V80.7 **Rider or occupant injured in collision with other nonmotor vehicle**
Collision with:
• animal being ridden
• animal-drawn vehicle
• streetcar

V80.8   **Rider or occupant injured in collision with fixed or stationary object**

V80.9   **Rider or occupant injured in other and unspecified transport accidents**
Animal-drawn vehicle accident NOS
Animal-rider accident NOS

V81   Occupant of railway train or railway vehicle injured in transport accident
Includes: person on outside of train

V81.0   **Occupant of railway train or railway vehicle injured in collision with motor vehicle in nontraffic accident**

V81.1   **Occupant of railway train or railway vehicle injured in collision with motor vehicle in traffic accident**

V81.2   **Occupant of railway train or railway vehicle injured in collision with or hit by rolling stock**

V81.3   **Occupant of railway train or railway vehicle injured in collision with other object**
Railway collision NOS

V81.4   **Person injured while boarding or alighting from railway train or railway vehicle**

V81.5   **Occupant of railway train or railway vehicle injured by fall in railway train or railway vehicle**
Excludes: fall:
- during derailment:
  - with antecedent collision (V81.0–V81.3)
  - without antecedent collision (V81.7)
- while boarding or alighting (V81.4)

V81.6   **Occupant of railway train or railway vehicle injured by fall from railway train or railway vehicle**
Excludes: fall:
- during derailment:
  - with antecedent collision (V81.0–V81.3)
  - without antecedent collision (V81.7)
- while boarding or alighting (V81.4)

V81.7   **Occupant of railway train or railway vehicle injured in derailment without antecedent collision**

V81.8 **Occupant of railway train or railway vehicle injured in other specified railway accidents**
Explosion or fire
Hit by falling:
- earth
- rock
- tree

Excludes: derailment:
- with antecedent collision (V81.0–V81.3)
- without antecedent collision (V81.7)

V81.9 **Occupant of railway train or railway vehicle injured in unspecified railway accident**
Railway accident NOS

V82 Occupant of streetcar injured in transport accident

Includes: person on outside of streetcar

V82.0 **Occupant of streetcar injured in collision with motor vehicle in nontraffic accident**

V82.1 **Occupant of streetcar injured in collision with motor vehicle in traffic accident**

V82.2 **Occupant of streetcar injured in collision with or hit by rolling stock**

V82.3 **Occupant of streetcar injured in collision with other object**

Excludes: collision with animal-drawn vehicle or animal being ridden (V82.8)

V82.4 **Person injured while boarding or alighting from streetcar**

V82.5 **Occupant of streetcar injured by fall in streetcar**

Excludes: fall:
- while boarding or alighting (V82.4)
- with antecedent collision (V82.0–V82.3)

V82.6 **Occupant of streetcar injured by fall from streetcar**

Excludes: fall:
- while boarding or alighting (V82.4)
- with antecedent collision (V82.0–V82.3)

V82.7 **Occupant of streetcar injured in derailment without antecedent collision**

V82.8 **Occupant of streetcar injured in other specified transport accidents**
Collision with train or other nonmotor vehicle

V82.9 **Occupant of streetcar injured in unspecified traffic accident**
Streetcar accident NOS

V83 Occupant of special vehicle mainly used on industrial premises injured in transport accident

Excludes: vehicle in stationary use or maintenance (W31.–)

V83.0 **Driver of special industrial vehicle injured in traffic accident**

V83.1 **Passenger of special industrial vehicle injured in traffic accident**

V83.2 **Person on outside of special industrial vehicle injured in traffic accident**

V83.3 **Unspecified occupant of special industrial vehicle injured in traffic accident**

V83.4 **Person injured while boarding or alighting from special industrial vehicle**

V83.5 **Driver of special industrial vehicle injured in nontraffic accident**

V83.6 **Passenger of special industrial vehicle injured in nontraffic accident**

V83.7 **Person on outside of special industrial vehicle injured in nontraffic accident**

V83.9 **Unspecified occupant of special industrial vehicle injured in nontraffic accident**
Special-industrial-vehicle accident NOS

V84 Occupant of special vehicle mainly used in agriculture injured in transport accident

Excludes: vehicle in stationary use or maintenance (W30.–)

V84.0 **Driver of special agricultural vehicle injured in traffic accident**

V84.1 **Passenger of special agricultural vehicle injured in traffic accident**

V84.2 Person on outside of special agricultural vehicle injured in traffic accident

V84.3 Unspecified occupant of special agricultural vehicle injured in traffic accident

V84.4 Person injured while boarding or alighting from special agricultural vehicle

V84.5 Driver of special agricultural vehicle injured in nontraffic accident

V84.6 Passenger of special agricultural vehicle injured in nontraffic accident

V84.7 Person on outside of special agricultural vehicle injured in nontraffic accident

V84.9 Unspecified occupant of special agricultural vehicle injured in nontraffic accident

Special-agricultural-vehicle accident NOS

V85 Occupant of special construction vehicle injured in transport accident

Excludes: vehicle in stationary use or maintenance (W31.–)

V85.0 Driver of special construction vehicle injured in traffic accident

V85.1 Passenger of special construction vehicle injured in traffic accident

V85.2 Person on outside of special construction vehicle injured in traffic accident

V85.3 Unspecified occupant of special construction vehicle injured in traffic accident

V85.4 Person injured while boarding or alighting from special construction vehicle

V85.5 Driver of special construction vehicle injured in nontraffic accident

V85.6 Passenger of special construction vehicle injured in nontraffic accident

V85.7 Person on outside of special construction vehicle injured in nontraffic accident

V85.9 **Unspecified occupant of special construction vehicle injured in nontraffic accident**
Special-construction-vehicle accident NOS

V86 **Occupant of special all-terrain or other motor vehicle designed primarily for off-road use, injured in transport accident**
Excludes: vehicle in stationary use or maintenance (W31.–)

V86.0 **Driver of all-terrain or other off-road motor vehicle injured in traffic accident**

V86.1 **Passenger of all-terrain or other off-road motor vehicle injured in traffic accident**

V86.2 **Person on outside of all-terrain or other off-road motor vehicle injured in traffic accident**

V86.3 **Unspecified occupant of all-terrain or other off-road motor vehicle injured in traffic accident**

V86.4 **Person injured while boarding or alighting from all-terrain or other off-road motor vehicle**

V86.5 **Driver of all-terrain or other off-road motor vehicle injured in nontraffic accident**

V86.6 **Passenger of all-terrain or other off-road motor vehicle injured in nontraffic accident**

V86.7 **Person on outside of all-terrain or other off-road motor vehicle injured in nontraffic accident**

V86.9 **Unspecified occupant of all-terrain or other off-road motor vehicle injured in nontraffic accident**
All-terrain motor-vehicle accident NOS
Off-road motor-vehicle accident NOS

V87 **Traffic accident of specified type but victim's mode of transport unknown**
Excludes: collision involving:
- pedal cyclist (V10–V19)
- pedestrian (V01–V09)

V87.0 **Person injured in collision between car and two- or three-wheeled motor vehicle (traffic)**

V87.1 Person injured in collision between other motor vehicle and two- or three-wheeled motor vehicle (traffic)

V87.2 Person injured in collision between car and pick-up truck or van (traffic)

V87.3 Person injured in collision between car and bus (traffic)

V87.4 Person injured in collision between car and heavy transport vehicle (traffic)

V87.5 Person injured in collision between heavy transport vehicle and bus (traffic)

V87.6 Person injured in collision between railway train or railway vehicle and car (traffic)

V87.7 Person injured in collision between other specified motor vehicles (traffic)

V87.8 Person injured in other specified noncollision transport accidents involving motor vehicle (traffic)

V87.9 Person injured in other specified (collision)(noncollision) transport accidents involving nonmotor vehicle (traffic)

V88 Nontraffic accident of specified type but victim's mode of transport unknown

Excludes: collision involving:
- pedal cyclist (V10–V19)
- pedestrian (V01–V09)

V88.0 Person injured in collision between car and two- or three-wheeled motor vehicle, nontraffic

V88.1 Person injured in collision between other motor vehicle and two- or three-wheeled motor vehicle, nontraffic

V88.2 Person injured in collision between car and pick-up truck or van, nontraffic

V88.3 Person injured in collision between car and bus, nontraffic

V88.4 Person injured in collision between car and heavy transport vehicle, nontraffic

V88.5 Person injured in collision between heavy transport vehicle and bus, nontraffic

V88.6 Person injured in collision between railway train or railway vehicle and car, nontraffic

V88.7 **Person injured in collision between other specified motor vehicles, nontraffic**

V88.8 **Person injured in other specified noncollision transport accidents involving motor vehicle, nontraffic**

V88.9 **Person injured in other specified (collision)(noncollision) transport accidents involving nonmotor vehicle, nontraffic**

V89 Motor- or nonmotor-vehicle accident, type of vehicle unspecified

V89.0 **Person injured in unspecified motor-vehicle accident, nontraffic**
Motor-vehicle accident NOS, nontraffic

V89.1 **Person injured in unspecified nonmotor-vehicle accident, nontraffic**
Nonmotor-vehicle accident NOS (nontraffic)

V89.2 **Person injured in unspecified motor-vehicle accident, traffic**
Motor-vehicle accident [MVA] NOS
Road (traffic) accident [RTA] NOS

V89.3 **Person injured in unspecified nonmotor-vehicle accident, traffic**
Nonmotor-vehicle traffic accident NOS

V89.9 **Person injured in unspecified vehicle accident**
Collision NOS

Water transport accidents (V90–V94)

Includes: watercraft accidents in the course of recreational activities

The following fourth-character subdivisions are for use with categories V90–V94:

.0 **Merchant ship**
.1 **Passenger ship**
Ferry-boat
Liner
.2 **Fishing boat**
.3 **Other powered watercraft**
Hovercraft (on open water)
Jet skis
.4 **Sailboat**
Yacht
.5 **Canoe or kayak**
.6 **Inflatable craft (nonpowered)**
.7 **Water-skis**
.8 **Other unpowered watercraft**
Surf-board
Windsurfer
.9 **Unspecified watercraft**
Boat NOS
Ship NOS
Watercraft NOS

V90 Accident to watercraft causing drowning and submersion

Includes: drowning and submersion due to:
- boat:
  - overturning
  - sinking
- falling or jumping from:
  - burning ship
  - crushed watercraft
- other accident to watercraft

Excludes: water-transport-related drowning or submersion without accident to watercraft (V92.–)

V91   Accident to watercraft causing other injury

Includes: any injury except drowning and submersion as a
result of an accident to watercraft
burned while ship on fire
crushed between colliding ships
crushed by lifeboat after abandoning ship
fall due to collision or other accident to watercraft
hit by falling object as a result of accident to
watercraft
injured in watercraft accident involving collision of
watercraft
struck by boat or part thereof after falling or jumping
from damaged boat

Excludes: burns from localized fire or explosion on board ship
(V93.–)

V92   Water-transport-related drowning and submersion without accident to watercraft

Includes: drowning and submersion as a result of an accident,
such as:
- fall:
  - from gangplank
  - from ship
  - overboard
- thrown overboard by motion of ship
- washed overboard

Excludes: drowning or submersion of swimmer or diver who
voluntarily jumps from boat not involved in an
accident (W69.–, W73.–)

V93 **Accident on board watercraft without accident to watercraft, not causing drowning and submersion**

Includes: accidental poisoning by gases or fumes on ship
atomic reactor malfunction in watercraft
crushed by falling object on ship
excessive heat in:
- boiler room
- engine room
- evaporator room
- fire room

explosion of boiler on steamship
fall from one level to another in watercraft
fall on stairs or ladders in watercraft
injuries in watercraft caused by:
- deck
- engine room
- galley } machinery
- laundry
- loading

localized fire on ship
machinery accident in watercraft

V94 **Other and unspecified water transport accidents**

Includes: accident to nonoccupant of watercraft
hit by boat while water-skiing

Air and space transport accidents (V95–V97)

V95 Accident to powered aircraft causing injury to occupant

Includes: collision with any object,
    fixed, movable or
      moving
    crash
    explosion
    fire
    forced landing
        } of or on (powered) aircraft

V95.0 Helicopter accident injuring occupant

V95.1 Ultralight, microlight or powered-glider accident injuring occupant

V95.2 Accident to other private fixed-wing aircraft, injuring occupant

V95.3 Accident to commercial fixed-wing aircraft, injuring occupant

V95.4 Spacecraft accident injuring occupant

V95.8 Other aircraft accidents injuring occupant

V95.9 Unspecified aircraft accident injuring occupant
Aircraft accident NOS
Air transport accident NOS

V96 Accident to nonpowered aircraft causing injury to occupant

Includes: collision with any object,
    fixed, movable or
      moving
    crash
    explosion
    fire
    forced landing
        } of or on nonpowered aircraft

V96.0 Balloon accident injuring occupant

V96.1 **Hang-glider accident injuring occupant**

V96.2 **Glider (nonpowered) accident injuring occupant**

V96.8 **Other nonpowered-aircraft accidents injuring occupant**
Kite carrying a person

V96.9 **Unspecified nonpowered-aircraft accident injuring occupant**
Nonpowered-aircraft accident NOS

V97 Other specified air transport accidents

Includes: accidents to nonoccupants of aircraft

V97.0 **Occupant of aircraft injured in other specified air transport accidents**
Fall in, on or from aircraft in air transport accident
Excludes: accident while boarding or alighting (V97.1)

V97.1 **Person injured while boarding or alighting from aircraft**

V97.2 **Parachutist injured in air transport accident**
Excludes: person making descent after accident to aircraft
(V95–V96)

V97.3 **Person on ground injured in air transport accident**
Hit by object falling from aircraft
Injured by rotating propeller
Sucked into jet

V97.8 **Other air transport accidents, not elsewhere classified**
Injury from machinery on aircraft
Excludes: aircraft accident NOS (V95.9)
exposure to changes in air pressure during ascent or
descent (W94.–)

Other and unspecified transport accidents (V98–V99)

Excludes: vehicle accident, type of vehicle unspecified (V89.–)

V98 Other specified transport accidents

Includes: accident to, on or involving:
- cable-car, not on rails
- ice-yacht
- land-yacht
- ski chair-lift
- ski-lift with gondola

caught or dragged by
fall or jump from } cable-car, not on rails
object thrown from or in

V99 Unspecified transport accident

Other external causes of accidental injury (W00–X59)

Falls
(W00–W19)

[See pages 1013–1017 for fourth-character subdivisions]

Excludes: assault (Y01–Y02)
fall (in)(from):
- animal (V80.–)
- burning building (X00.–)
- into fire (X00–X04, X08–X09)
- into water (with drowning or submersion) (W65–W74)
- machinery (in operation) (W28–W31)
- transport vehicle (V01–V99)
intentional self-harm (X80–X81)

W00   **Fall on same level involving ice and snow**
Excludes: fall with mention of:
- ice-skates and skis (W02.–)
- stairs and steps (W10.–)

W01   **Fall on same level from slipping, tripping and stumbling**
Excludes: fall involving ice or snow (W00.–)

W02   **Fall involving ice-skates, skis, roller-skates or skateboards**

W03 Other fall on same level due to collision with, or pushing by, another person

Includes: fall due to collision of pedestrian (conveyance) with another pedestrian (conveyance)

Excludes: crushed or pushed by crowd or human stampede (W52.–)

fall involving ice or snow (W00.–)

W04 Fall while being carried or supported by other persons

Includes: accidentally dropped while being carried

W05 Fall involving wheelchair

W06 Fall involving bed

W07 Fall involving chair

W08 Fall involving other furniture

W09 Fall involving playground equipment

Excludes: fall involving recreational machinery (W31.–)

W10 Fall on and from stairs and steps

Includes: fall (on)(from):
- escalator
- incline
- involving ice or snow on stairs and steps
- ramp

W11 Fall on and from ladder

W12 Fall on and from scaffolding

1059

W13 Fall from, out of or through building or structure

Includes: fall from, out of or through:
- balcony
- bridge
- building
- flag-pole
- floor
- railing
- roof
- tower
- turret
- viaduct
- wall
- window

Excludes: collapse of a building or structure (W20.–)
fall or jump from burning building (X00.–)

W14 Fall from tree

W15 Fall from cliff

W16 Diving or jumping into water causing injury other than drowning or submersion

Includes: striking or hitting:
- against bottom when jumping or diving into shallow water
- wall or diving board of swimming-pool
- water surface

Excludes: accidental drowning and submersion (W65–W74)
diving with insufficient air supply (W81.–)
effects of air pressure from diving (W94.–)

W17 Other fall from one level to another

Includes: fall from or into:
- cavity
- dock
- haystack
- hole
- pit
- quarry
- shaft
- tank
- well

W18 Other fall on same level

Includes: fall:
- from bumping against object
- from or off toilet
- on same level NOS

W19 Unspecified fall

Includes: accidental fall NOS

Exposure to inanimate mechanical forces (W20–W49)

[See pages 1013–1017 for fourth-character subdivisions]

Excludes: assault (X85–Y09)
contact or collision with animals or persons (W50–W64)
intentional self-harm (X60–X84)

W20 Struck by thrown, projected or falling object

Includes: cave-in without asphyxiation or suffocation
collapse of building, except on fire
falling:
- rock
- stone
- tree

Excludes: collapse of burning building (X00.–)
falling object in:
- cataclysm (X34–X39)
- machinery accident (W24.–, W28–W31)
- transport accident (V01–V99)
object set in motion by:
- explosion (W35–W40)
- firearm (W32–W34)
sports equipment (W21.–)

W21 Striking against or struck by sports equipment

Includes: struck by:
- hit or thrown ball
- hockey stick or puck

W22 Striking against or struck by other objects

Includes: walked into wall

W23 Caught, crushed, jammed or pinched in or between objects

Includes: caught, crushed, jammed or pinched:

- between:
  - moving objects
  - stationary and moving objects
- in object

such as

folding object
sliding door and door-frame
packing crate and floor, after losing grip
washing-machine wringer

Excludes: injury caused by:
- cutting or piercing instruments (W25–W27)
- lifting and transmission devices (W24.–)
- machinery (W28–W31)
- nonpowered hand tools (W27.–)
- transport vehicle (V01–V99)

struck by thrown, projected or falling object (W20.–)

W24 Contact with lifting and transmission devices, not elsewhere classified

Includes: chain hoist
drive belt
pulley (block)
rope
transmission belt or cable
winch
wire

Excludes: transport accidents (V01–V99)

W25 Contact with sharp glass

Excludes: fall involving glass (W00–W19)
flying glass due to explosion or firearm discharge (W32–W40)

W26 Contact with knife, sword or dagger

W27 Contact with nonpowered hand tool

Includes: axe
can-opener NOS
chisel
fork
handsaw
hoe
ice-pick
needle
paper-cutter
pitchfork
rake
scissors
screwdriver
sewing-machine, nonpowered
shovel

W28 Contact with powered lawnmower

Excludes: exposure to electric current (W86.–)

W29 Contact with other powered hand tools and household machinery

Includes: blender
powered:
- can-opener
- chain-saw
- do-it-yourself tool
- garden tool
- hedge-trimmer
- knife
- sewing-machine
- spin-drier
washing-machine

Excludes: exposure to electric current (W86.–)

W30 Contact with agricultural machinery

Includes: animal-powered farm machine
combine harvester
derrick, hay
farm machinery NOS
reaper
thresher

Excludes: contact with agricultural machinery in transport under
own power or being towed by a vehicle (V01–V99)
exposure to electric current (W86.–)

W31 Contact with other and unspecified machinery

Includes: machine NOS
recreational machinery

Excludes: contact with machinery in transport under own power
or being towed by a vehicle (V01–V99)
exposure to electric current (W86.–)

W32 Handgun discharge

Includes: gun for single hand use
pistol
revolver

Excludes: Very pistol (W34.–)

W33 Rifle, shotgun and larger firearm discharge

Includes: army rifle
hunting rifle
machine gun

Excludes: airgun (W34.–)

W34 Discharge from other and unspecified firearms

Includes: airgun
BB gun
gunshot wound NOS
shot NOS
Very pistol [flare]

1065

W35 **Explosion and rupture of boiler**

W36 **Explosion and rupture of gas cylinder**

Includes: aerosol can
air tank
pressurized-gas tank

W37 **Explosion and rupture of pressurized tyre, pipe or hose**

W38 **Explosion and rupture of other specified pressurized devices**

W39 **Discharge of firework**

W40 **Explosion of other materials**

Includes: blasting material
explosion (in):
• NOS
• dump
• factory
• grain store
• munitions
explosive gas

W41 **Exposure to high-pressure jet**

Includes: hydraulic jet
pneumatic jet

W42 **Exposure to noise**

Includes: sound waves
supersonic waves

W43 Exposure to vibration

Includes: infrasound waves

W44 Foreign body entering into or through eye or natural orifice

Excludes: corrosive fluid (X49.–)
inhalation or ingestion of foreign body with
obstruction of respiratory tract (W78–W80)

W45 Foreign body or object entering through skin

Includes: edge of stiff paper
nail
splinter
tin-can lid
Excludes: contact with:
• hand tools (nonpowered)(powered) (W27–W29)
• knife, sword or dagger (W26.–)
• sharp glass (W25.–)
struck by objects (W20–W22)

W49 Exposure to other and unspecified inanimate mechanical forces

Includes: abnormal gravitational [G] forces

Exposure to animate mechanical forces (W50–W64)

[See pages 1013–1017 for fourth-character subdivisions]

Excludes: bites, venomous (X20–X29)
stings (venomous) (X20–X29)

W50 Hit, struck, kicked, twisted, bitten or scratched by another person

Excludes: assault (X85–Y09)
struck by objects (W20–W22)

W51 **Striking against or bumped into by another person**

Excludes: fall due to collision of pedestrian (conveyance) with another pedestrian (conveyance) (W03.–)

W52 **Crushed, pushed or stepped on by crowd or human stampede**

W53 **Bitten by rat**

W54 **Bitten or struck by dog**

W55 **Bitten or struck by other mammals**

Excludes: contact with marine mammal (W56.–)

W56 **Contact with marine animal**

Bitten or struck by marine animal

W57 **Bitten or stung by nonvenomous insect and other nonvenomous arthropods**

W58 **Bitten or struck by crocodile or alligator**

W59 **Bitten or crushed by other reptiles**

Includes: lizard
snake, nonvenomous

W60 **Contact with plant thorns and spines and sharp leaves**

W64 **Exposure to other and unspecified animate mechanical forces**

Accidental drowning and submersion (W65–W74)

[See pages 1013–1017 for fourth-character subdivisions]

Excludes: drowning and submersion due to:
- cataclysm (X34–X39)
- transport accidents (V01–V99)
- water transport accident (V90.–, V92.–)

W65 **Drowning and submersion while in bath-tub**

W66 **Drowning and submersion following fall into bath-tub**

W67 **Drowning and submersion while in swimming-pool**

W68 **Drowning and submersion following fall into swimming-pool**

W69 **Drowning and submersion while in natural water**
Includes: lake
open sea
river
stream

W70 **Drowning and submersion following fall into natural water**

W73 **Other specified drowning and submersion**
Includes: quenching tank
reservoir

W74 **Unspecified drowning and submersion**
Includes: drowning NOS
fall into water NOS

Other accidental threats to breathing (W75–W84)

[See pages 1013–1017 for fourth-character subdivisions]

W75 **Accidental suffocation and strangulation in bed**
Includes: suffocation and strangulation due to:
• bed linen
• mother's body
• pillow

W76 **Other accidental hanging and strangulation**

W77 **Threat to breathing due to cave-in, falling earth and other substances**
Includes: cave-in NOS
Excludes: cave-in caused by cataclysm (X34–X39)
cave-in without asphyxiation or suffocation (W20.–)

W78   Inhalation of gastric contents

Includes: asphyxia by ⎱
              choked on ⎬ vomitus [regurgitated food]
              suffocation by ⎰
              aspiration and inhalation of vomitus (into respiratory
                 tract) NOS
              compression of trachea ⎱
              interruption of respiration ⎬ by vomitus in
              obstruction of respiration ⎰   oesophagus

Excludes: injury, except asphyxia or obstruction of respiratory
                 tract, caused by vomitus (W44.–)
              obstruction of oesophagus by vomitus without
                 mention of asphyxia or obstruction of respiratory
                 tract (W44.–)

W79   Inhalation and ingestion of food causing obstruction of respiratory tract

Includes: asphyxia by ⎱
              choked on ⎬ food [including bone or seed]
              suffocation by ⎰
              aspiration and inhalation of food [any] (into respiratory
                 tract) NOS
              compression of trachea ⎱
              interruption of respiration ⎬ by food in oesophagus
              obstruction of respiration ⎰
              obstruction of pharynx by food (bolus)

Excludes: inhalation of vomitus (W78.–)
              injury, except asphyxia or obstruction of respiratory
                 tract, caused by food (W44.–)
              obstruction of oesophagus by food without mention
                 of asphyxia or obstruction of respiratory tract
                 (W44.–)

W80 Inhalation and ingestion of other objects causing obstruction of respiratory tract

Includes: asphyxia by ⎫ any object, except food or
choked on ⎬ vomitus, entering by nose or
suffocation by ⎭ mouth
aspiration and inhalation of foreign body, except food or vomitus (into respiratory tract), NOS
compression of trachea ⎫
interruption of respiration ⎬ by foreign body in oesophagus
obstruction of respiration ⎭
foreign object in nose
obstruction of pharynx by foreign body

Excludes: inhalation of vomitus or food (W78–W79)
injury, except asphyxia or obstruction of respiratory tract, caused by foreign body (W44.–)
obstruction of oesophagus by foreign body without mention of asphyxia or obstruction of respiratory tract (W44.–)

W81 Confined to or trapped in a low-oxygen environment

Includes: accidentally shut in refrigerator or other airtight space
diving with insufficient air supply

Excludes: suffocation by plastic bag (W83.–)

W83 Other specified threats to breathing

Includes: suffocation by plastic bag

W84 Unspecified threat to breathing

Includes: asphyxiation NOS
aspiration NOS
suffocation NOS

Exposure to electric current, radiation and extreme ambient air temperature and pressure (W85–W99)

[See pages 1013–1017 for fourth-character subdivisions]

Excludes: exposure to:
- natural:
  - cold (X31.–)
  - heat (X30.–)
  - radiation NOS (X39.–)
- sunlight (X32.–)
victim of lightning (X33.–)

W85 Exposure to electric transmission lines

W86 Exposure to other specified electric current

W87 Exposure to unspecified electric current
Includes: burns or other injury from electric current NOS
electric shock NOS
electrocution NOS

W88 Exposure to ionizing radiation
Includes: radioactive isotopes
X-rays

W89 Exposure to man-made visible and ultraviolet light
Includes: welding light (arc)

W90 Exposure to other nonionizing radiation
Includes: infrared ⎫
laser ⎬ radiation
radiofrequency ⎭

W91 Exposure to unspecified type of radiation

W92 Exposure to excessive heat of man-made origin

W93 Exposure to excessive cold of man-made origin

Includes: contact with or inhalation of:
- dry ice
- liquid:
  - air
  - hydrogen
  - nitrogen

prolonged exposure in deep-freeze unit

W94 Exposure to high and low air pressure and changes in air pressure

Includes: high air pressure from rapid descent in water
reduction in atmospheric pressure while surfacing from:
- deep-water diving
- underground

residence or prolonged visit at high altitude as the cause of:
- anoxia
- barodontalgia
- barotitis
- hypoxia
- mountain sickness

sudden change in air pressure in aircraft during ascent or descent

W99 Exposure to other and unspecified man-made environmental factors

Exposure to smoke, fire and flames (X00–X09)

[See pages 1013–1017 for fourth-character subdivisions]

Includes: fire caused by lightning
Excludes: arson (X97.–)
secondary fire resulting from explosion (W35–W40)
transport accidents (V01–V99)

X00 Exposure to uncontrolled fire in building or structure

collapse of
fall from
hit by object falling from ⎫ burning building or
jump from ⎬ structure
conflagration ⎭

fire
melting ⎫ of ⎰ fittings
smouldering ⎭ ⎱ furniture

X01 Exposure to uncontrolled fire, not in building or structure

Includes: forest fire

X02 Exposure to controlled fire in building or structure

Includes: fire in:
- fireplace
- stove

X03 Exposure to controlled fire, not in building or structure

Includes: camp-fire

X04 **Exposure to ignition of highly flammable material**

Includes: ignition of:
- gasoline
- kerosene
- petrol

X05 **Exposure to ignition or melting of nightwear**

X06 **Exposure to ignition or melting of other clothing and apparel**

Includes: ignition } of plastic jewellery
melting

X08 **Exposure to other specified smoke, fire and flames**

X09 **Exposure to unspecified smoke, fire and flames**

Includes: burning NOS
incineration NOS

Contact with heat and hot substances (X10–X19)

[See pages 1013–1017 for fourth-character subdivisions]

Excludes: exposure to:
- excessive natural heat (X30.–)
- fire and flames (X00–X09)

X10 **Contact with hot drinks, food, fats and cooking oils**

X11 Contact with hot tap-water

Includes: hot water in:
- bath
- bucket
- tub

hot water running out of:
- hose
- tap

X12 Contact with other hot fluids

Includes: water heated on stove
Excludes: hot (liquid) metals (X18.–)

X13 Contact with steam and hot vapours

X14 Contact with hot air and gases

Includes: inhalation of hot air and gases

X15 Contact with hot household appliances

Includes: cooker
hotplate
kettle
saucepan (glass)(metal)
stove (kitchen)
toaster
Excludes: heating appliances (X16.–)

X16 Contact with hot heating appliances, radiators and pipes

X17 Contact with hot engines, machinery and tools

Excludes: hot heating appliances, radiators and pipes (X16.–)
hot household appliances (X15.–)

X18 Contact with other hot metals
Includes: liquid metal

X19 Contact with other and unspecified heat and hot substances
Excludes: objects that are not normally hot, e.g., an object
made hot by a house fire (X00–X09)

Contact with venomous animals and plants (X20–X29)

[See pages 1013–1017 for fourth-character subdivisions]

Includes: chemical released by:
  • animal
  • insect
  release of venom through fangs, hairs, spines, tentacles and
    other venom apparatus
  venomous bites and stings
Excludes: ingestion of poisonous animals or plants (X49.–)

X20 Contact with venomous snakes and lizards
Includes: cobra
fer de lance
Gila monster
krait
rattlesnake
sea snake
snake (venomous)
viper
Excludes: lizard (nonvenomous) (W59.–)
snake, nonvenomous (W59.–)

X21 Contact with venomous spiders
Includes: black widow spider
tarantula

X22   Contact with scorpions

X23   Contact with hornets, wasps and bees

Includes: yellow jacket

X24   Contact with centipedes and venomous millipedes (tropical)

X25   Contact with other specified venomous arthropods

Includes: ant
          caterpillar

X26   Contact with venomous marine animals and plants

Includes: coral
          jellyfish
          nematocysts
          sea:
          • anemone
          • cucumber
          • urchin

Excludes: nonvenomous marine animals (W56.–)
          sea snakes (X20.–)

X27   Contact with other specified venomous animals

X28   Contact with other specified venomous plants

Includes: injection of poisons or toxins into or through skin by plant thorns, spines or other mechanisms

Excludes: ingestion of poisonous plants (X49.–)
          puncture wound NOS caused by plant thorns or spines (W60.–)

X29 Contact with unspecified venomous animal or plant

Includes: sting (venomous) NOS
venomous bite NOS

Exposure to forces of nature (X30–X39)

[See pages 1013–1017 for fourth-character subdivisions]

X30 Exposure to excessive natural heat

Includes: excessive heat as the cause of sunstroke
exposure to heat NOS
Excludes: excessive heat of man-made origin (W92.–)

X31 Exposure to excessive natural cold

Includes: excessive cold as the cause of:
• chilblains NOS
• immersion foot or hand
exposure to:
• cold NOS
• weather conditions
Excludes: cold of man-made origin (W93.–)
contact with or inhalation of:
• dry ice (W93.–)
• liquefied gas (W93.–)

X32 Exposure to sunlight

X33 Victim of lightning

Excludes: fire caused by lightning (X00–X09)
injury from fall of tree or other object caused by
lightning (W20.–)

X34 Victim of earthquake

X35 Victim of volcanic eruption

X36 Victim of avalanche, landslide and other earth movements

Includes: mudslide of cataclysmic nature

Excludes: earthquake (X34.–)

transport accident involving collision with avalanche or landslide not in motion (V01–V99)

X37 Victim of cataclysmic storm

Includes: blizzard

cloudburst

cyclone

hurricane

tidal wave caused by storm

tornado

torrential rain

transport vehicle washed off road by storm

Excludes: collapse of dam or man-made structure causing earth movement (X36.–)

transport accident occurring after storm (V01–V99)

X38 Victim of flood

Includes: flood:
- arising from remote storm
- of cataclysmic nature arising from melting snow
- resulting directly from storm

Excludes: collapse of dam or man-made structure causing earth movement (X36.–)

tidal wave:
- NOS (X39.–)
- caused by storm (X37.–)

X39 Exposure to other and unspecified forces of nature

Includes: natural radiation NOS

tidal wave NOS

Excludes: exposure NOS (X59.–)

Accidental poisoning by and exposure to noxious substances
(X40–X49)

[See pages 1013–1017 for fourth-character subdivisions]

Note: For list of specific drugs and other substances classified under the three-character categories, see Table of drugs and chemicals in Alphabetical Index. Evidence of alcohol involvement in combination with substances specified below may be identified by using the supplementary codes Y90–Y91.

Includes: accidental overdose of drug, wrong drug given or taken in error, and drug taken inadvertently

accidents in the use of drugs, medicaments and biological substances in medical and surgical procedures

poisoning, when not specified whether accidental or with intent to harm

Excludes: administration with suicidal or homicidal intent, or intent to harm, or in other circumstances classifiable to X60–X69, X85–X90, Y10–Y19

correct drug properly administered in therapeutic or prophylactic dosage as the cause of any adverse effect (Y40–Y59)

X40 Accidental poisoning by and exposure to nonopioid analgesics, antipyretics and antirheumatics

Includes: 4-aminophenol derivatives
nonsteroidal anti-inflammatory drugs [NSAID]
pyrazolone derivatives
salicylates

X41 Accidental poisoning by and exposure to antiepileptic, sedative–hypnotic, antiparkinsonism and psychotropic drugs, not elsewhere classified

Includes: antidepressants
barbiturates
hydantoin derivatives
iminostilbenes
methaqualone compounds
neuroleptics
psychostimulants
succinimides and oxazolidinediones
tranquillizers

X42 Accidental poisoning by and exposure to narcotics and psychodysleptics [hallucinogens], not elsewhere classified

Includes: cannabis (derivatives)
cocaine
codeine
heroin
lysergide [LSD]
mescaline
methadone
morphine
opium (alkaloids)

X43 Accidental poisoning by and exposure to other drugs acting on the autonomic nervous system

Includes: parasympatholytics [anticholinergics and
antimuscarinics] and spasmolytics
parasympathomimetics [cholinergics]
sympatholytics [antiadrenergics]
sympathomimetics [adrenergics]

X44 Accidental poisoning by and exposure to other and unspecified drugs, medicaments and biological substances

Includes: agents primarily acting on smooth and skeletal
muscles and the respiratory system
anaesthetics (general)(local)
drugs affecting the:
• cardiovascular system
• gastrointestinal system
hormones and synthetic substitutes
systemic and haematological agents
systemic antibiotics and other anti-infectives
therapeutic gases
topical preparations
vaccines
water-balance agents and drugs affecting mineral and
uric acid metabolism

X45 Accidental poisoning by and exposure to alcohol

Includes: alcohol:
• NOS
• butyl [1-butanol]
• ethyl [ethanol]
• isopropyl [2-propanol]
• methyl [methanol]
• propyl [1-propanol]
fusel oil

X46 Accidental poisoning by and exposure to organic solvents and halogenated hydrocarbons and their vapours

Includes: benzene and homologues
carbon tetrachloride [tetrachloromethane]
chlorofluorocarbons
petroleum (derivatives)

X47 Accidental poisoning by and exposure to other gases and vapours

Includes: carbon monoxide
lacrimogenic gas [tear gas]
motor (vehicle) exhaust gas
nitrogen oxides
sulfur dioxide
utility gas

Excludes: metal fumes and vapours (X49.–)

X48 Accidental poisoning by and exposure to pesticides

Includes: fumigants
fungicides
herbicides
insecticides
rodenticides
wood preservatives

Excludes: plant foods and fertilizers (X49.–)

X49 Accidental poisoning by and exposure to other and unspecified chemicals and noxious substances

Includes: corrosive aromatics, acids and caustic alkalis
glues and adhesives
metals including fumes and vapours
paints and dyes
plant foods and fertilizers
poisoning NOS
poisonous foodstuffs and poisonous plants
soaps and detergents

Excludes: contact with venomous animals and plants
(X20–X29)

Overexertion, travel and privation (X50–X57)

[See pages 1013–1017 for fourth-character subdivisions]

Excludes: assault (X85–Y09)
transport accidents (V01–V99)

X50 Overexertion and strenuous or repetitive movements
Includes: lifting:
  • heavy objects
  • weights
  marathon running
  rowing

X51 Travel and motion

X52 Prolonged stay in weightless environment
Includes: weightlessness in spacecraft (simulator)

X53 Lack of food
Includes: lack of food as the cause of:
  • inanition
  • insufficient nourishment
  • starvation
Excludes: neglect or abandonment (Y06.–)

X54 Lack of water
Includes: lack of water as the cause of:
  • dehydration
  • inanition
Excludes: neglect or abandonment (Y06.–)

X57 Unspecified privation
Includes: destitution

Accidental exposure to other and unspecified factors (X58–X59)

[See pages 1013–1017 for fourth-character subdivisions]

X58 **Exposure to other specified factors**

X59 **Exposure to unspecified factor**
Includes: accident NOS
exposure NOS

Intentional self-harm (X60–X84)

[See pages 1013–1017 for fourth-character subdivisions]

Includes: purposely self-inflicted poisoning or injury
suicide (attempted)

X60 **Intentional self-poisoning by and exposure to nonopioid analgesics, antipyretics and antirheumatics**
Includes: 4-aminophenol derivatives
nonsteroidal anti-inflammatory drugs [NSAID]
pyrazolone derivatives
salicylates

X61 **Intentional self-poisoning by and exposure to antiepileptic, sedative–hypnotic, antiparkinsonism and psychotropic drugs, not elsewhere classified**

Includes: antidepressants
barbiturates
hydantoin derivatives
iminostilbenes
methaqualone compounds
neuroleptics
psychostimulants
succinimides and oxazolidinediones
tranquillizers

X62 **Intentional self-poisoning by and exposure to narcotics and psychodysleptics [hallucinogens], not elsewhere classified**

Includes: cannabis (derivatives)
cocaine
codeine
heroin
lysergide [LSD]
mescaline
methadone
morphine
opium (alkaloids)

X63 **Intentional self-poisoning by and exposure to other drugs acting on the autonomic nervous system**

Includes: parasympatholytics [anticholinergics and antimuscarinics] and spasmolytics
parasympathomimetics [cholinergics]
sympatholytics [antiadrenergics]
sympathomimetics [adrenergics]

X64 Intentional self-poisoning by and exposure to other and unspecified drugs, medicaments and biological substances

Includes: agents primarily acting on smooth and skeletal
muscles and the respiratory system
anaesthetics (general)(local)
drugs affecting the:
• cardiovascular system
• gastrointestinal system
hormones and synthetic substitutes
systemic and haematological agents
systemic antibiotics and other anti-infectives
therapeutic gases
topical preparations
vaccines
water-balance agents and drugs affecting mineral and
uric acid metabolism

X65 Intentional self-poisoning by and exposure to alcohol

Includes: alcohol:
• NOS
• butyl [1-butanol]
• ethyl [ethanol]
• isopropyl [2-propanol]
• methyl [methanol]
• propyl [1-propanol]
fusel oil

X66 Intentional self-poisoning by and exposure to organic solvents and halogenated hydrocarbons and their vapours

Includes: benzene and homologues
carbon tetrachloride [tetrachloromethane]
chlorofluorocarbons
petroleum (derivatives)

X67 Intentional self-poisoning by and exposure to other gases and vapours

Includes: carbon monoxide
lacrimogenic gas [tear gas]
motor (vehicle) exhaust gas
nitrogen oxides
sulfur dioxide
utility gas
Excludes: metal fumes and vapours (X69.–)

X68 Intentional self-poisoning by and exposure to pesticides

Includes: fumigants
fungicides
herbicides
insecticides
rodenticides
wood preservatives
Excludes: plant foods and fertilizers (X69.–)

X69 Intentional self-poisoning by and exposure to other and unspecified chemicals and noxious substances

Includes: corrosive aromatics, acids and caustic alkalis
glues and adhesives
metals including fumes and vapours
paints and dyes
plant foods and fertilizers
poisonous foodstuffs and poisonous plants
soaps and detergents

X70 Intentional self-harm by hanging, strangulation and suffocation

X71 Intentional self-harm by drowning and submersion

X72 Intentional self-harm by handgun discharge

X73 Intentional self-harm by rifle, shotgun and larger firearm discharge

X74 Intentional self-harm by other and unspecified firearm discharge

X75 Intentional self-harm by explosive material

X76 Intentional self-harm by smoke, fire and flames

X77 Intentional self-harm by steam, hot vapours and hot objects

X78 Intentional self-harm by sharp object

X79 Intentional self-harm by blunt object

X80 Intentional self-harm by jumping from a high place
Includes: intentional fall from one level to another

X81 Intentional self-harm by jumping or lying before moving object

X82 Intentional self-harm by crashing of motor vehicle
Includes: intentional collision with:
- motor vehicle
- train
- tram (streetcar)

Excludes: crashing of aircraft (X83.–)

X83   Intentional self-harm by other specified means

Includes: intentional self-harm by:
- caustic substances, except poisoning
- crashing of aircraft
- electrocution

X84   Intentional self-harm by unspecified means

Assault
(X85–Y09)

[See pages 1013–1017 for fourth-character subdivisions]

Includes: homicide
          injuries inflicted by another person with intent to injure or kill, by any means

Excludes: injuries due to:
- legal intervention (Y35.–)
- operations of war (Y36.–)

X85   Assault by drugs, medicaments and biological substances

Includes: homicidal poisoning by (any):
- biological substance
- drug
- medicament

X86   Assault by corrosive substance

Excludes: corrosive gas (X88.–)

X87   Assault by pesticides

Includes: wood preservatives
Excludes: plant food and fertilizers (X89.–)

X88   Assault by gases and vapours

X89 **Assault by other specified chemicals and noxious substances**

Includes: plant food and fertilizers

X90 **Assault by unspecified chemical or noxious substance**

Includes: homicidal poisoning NOS

X91 **Assault by hanging, strangulation and suffocation**

X92 **Assault by drowning and submersion**

X93 **Assault by handgun discharge**

X94 **Assault by rifle, shotgun and larger firearm discharge**

X95 **Assault by other and unspecified firearm discharge**

X96 **Assault by explosive material**

Excludes: incendiary device (X97.–)

X97 **Assault by smoke, fire and flames**

Includes: arson
cigarettes
incendiary device

X98 **Assault by steam, hot vapours and hot objects**

X99 **Assault by sharp object**

Includes: stabbed NOS

Y00   Assault by blunt object

Y01   Assault by pushing from high place

Y02   Assault by pushing or placing victim before moving object

Y03   Assault by crashing of motor vehicle

Includes: deliberately hitting or running over with motor vehicle

Y04   Assault by bodily force

Includes: unarmed brawl or fight

Excludes: assault by:
- strangulation (X91.–)
- submersion (X92.–)
- use of weapon (X93–X95, X99.–, Y00.–)

sexual assault by bodily force (Y05.–)

Y05   Sexual assault by bodily force

Includes: rape (attempted)
sodomy (attempted)

Y06   Neglect and abandonment

Y06.0   By spouse or partner

Y06.1   By parent

Y06.2   By acquaintance or friend

Y06.8   By other specified persons

Y06.9   By unspecified person

Y07 Other maltreatment syndromes

Includes: mental cruelty
            physical abuse
            sexual abuse
            torture

Excludes: neglect and abandonment (Y06.–)
            sexual assault by bodily force (Y05.–)

Y07.0	By spouse or partner
Y07.1	By parent
Y07.2	By acquaintance or friend
Y07.3	By official authorities
Y07.8	By other specified persons
Y07.9	By unspecified person

Y08 Assault by other specified means

Y09 Assault by unspecified means

Includes: assassination (attempt) NOS
            homicide (attempt) NOS
            manslaughter (nonaccidental)
            murder (attempt) NOS

Event of undetermined intent (Y10–Y34)

[See pages 1013–1017 for fourth-character subdivisions]

Note: This section covers events where available information is insufficient to enable a medical or legal authority to make a distinction between accident, self-harm and assault. It includes self-inflicted injuries, but not poisoning, when not specified whether accidental or with intent to harm.

Y10 Poisoning by and exposure to nonopioid analgesics, antipyretics and antirheumatics, undetermined intent

Includes: 4-aminophenol derivatives
nonsteroidal anti-inflammatory drugs [NSAID]
pyrazolone derivatives
salicylates

Y11 Poisoning by and exposure to antiepileptic, sedative–hypnotic, antiparkinsonism and psychotropic drugs, not elsewhere classified, undetermined intent

Includes: antidepressants
barbiturates
hydantoin derivatives
iminostilbenes
methaqualone compounds
neuroleptics
psychostimulants
succinimides and oxazolidinediones
tranquillizers

Y12 Poisoning by and exposure to narcotics and psychodysleptics [hallucinogens], not elsewhere classified, undetermined intent

Includes: cannabis (derivatives)
cocaine
codeine
heroin
lysergide [LSD]
mescaline
methadone
morphine
opium (alkaloids)

Y13 Poisoning by and exposure to other drugs acting on the autonomic nervous system, undetermined intent

Includes: parasympatholytics [anticholinergics and antimuscarinics] and spasmolytics
parasympathomimetics [cholinergics]
sympatholytics [antiadrenergics]
sympathomimetics [adrenergics]

Y14 Poisoning by and exposure to other and unspecified drugs, medicaments and biological substances, undetermined intent

Includes: agents primarily acting on smooth and skeletal muscles and the respiratory system
anaesthetics (general)(local)
drugs affecting the:
• cardiovascular system
• gastrointestinal system
hormones and synthetic substitutes
systemic and haematological agents
systemic antibiotics and other anti-infectives
therapeutic gases
topical preparations
vaccines
water-balance agents and drugs affecting mineral and uric acid metabolism

Y15 Poisoning by and exposure to alcohol, undetermined intent

Includes: alcohol:
• NOS
• butyl [1-butanol]
• ethyl [ethanol]
• isopropyl [2-propanol]
• methyl [methanol]
• propyl [1-propanol]
fusel oil

1097

Y16 Poisoning by and exposure to organic solvents and halogenated hydrocarbons and their vapours, undetermined intent

Includes: benzene and homologues
carbon tetrachloride [tetrachloromethane]
chlorofluorocarbons
petroleum (derivatives)

Y17 Poisoning by and exposure to other gases and vapours, undetermined intent

Includes: carbon monoxide
lacrimogenic gas [tear gas]
motor (vehicle) exhaust gas
nitrogen oxides
sulfur dioxide
utility gas

Excludes: metal fumes and vapours (Y19.–)

Y18 Poisoning by and exposure to pesticides, undetermined intent

Includes: fumigants
fungicides
herbicides
insecticides
rodenticides
wood preservatives

Excludes: plant foods and fertilizers (Y19.–)

Y19 Poisoning by and exposure to other and unspecified chemicals and noxious substances, undetermined intent

Includes: corrosive aromatics, acids and caustic alkalis
glues and adhesives
metals including fumes and vapours
paints and dyes
plant foods and fertilizers
poisonous foodstuffs and poisonous plants
soaps and detergents

Y20 Hanging, strangulation and suffocation, undetermined intent

Y21 Drowning and submersion, undetermined intent

Y22 Handgun discharge, undetermined intent

Y23 Rifle, shotgun and larger firearm discharge, undetermined intent

Y24 Other and unspecified firearm discharge, undetermined intent

Y25 Contact with explosive material, undetermined intent

Y26 Exposure to smoke, fire and flames, undetermined intent

Y27 Contact with steam, hot vapours and hot objects, undetermined intent

Y28 Contact with sharp object, undetermined intent

Y29 Contact with blunt object, undetermined intent

Y30 Falling, jumping or pushed from a high place, undetermined intent
   Includes: victim falling from one level to another, undetermined intent

Y31 Falling, lying or running before or into moving object, undetermined intent

Y32 Crashing of motor vehicle, undetermined intent

Y33 Other specified events, undetermined intent

Y34 Unspecified event, undetermined intent

Legal intervention and operations of war (Y35–Y36)

Y35 Legal intervention

Y35.0 **Legal intervention involving firearm discharge**
Gunshot wound
Injury by:
• machine gun
• revolver
• rifle pellet or rubber bullet
Shot NOS

Y35.1 **Legal intervention involving explosives**
Injury by:
• dynamite
• explosive shell
• grenade
• mortar bomb

Y35.2 **Legal intervention involving gas**
Asphyxiation by gas
Injury by tear gas
Poisoning by gas

Y35.3 **Legal intervention involving blunt objects**
Hit, struck by:
• baton
• blunt object
• stave

Y35.4   Legal intervention involving sharp objects
Cut
Injured by bayonet
Stabbed

Y35.5   Legal execution
Any execution performed at the behest of the judiciary or ruling
    authority [whether permanent or temporary], such as:
- asphyxiation by gas
- beheading, decapitation (by guillotine)
- capital punishment
- electrocution
- hanging
- poisoning
- shooting

Y35.6   Legal intervention involving other specified means
Manhandling

Y35.7   Legal intervention, means unspecified

Y36 Operations of war

Note: Injuries due to operations of war occurring after
        cessation of hostilities are classified to Y36.8.

Includes: injuries to military personnel and civilians caused by
        war and civil insurrection

Y36.0   War operations involving explosion of marine weapons
Depth-charge
Marine mine
Mine NOS, at sea or in harbour
Sea-based artillery shell
Torpedo
Underwater blast

Y36.1   War operations involving destruction of aircraft
Aircraft:
- burned
- exploded
- shot down
Crushed by falling aircraft

Y36.2   **War operations involving other explosions and fragments**
Accidental explosion of:
• munitions being used in war
• own weapons
Antipersonnel bomb (fragments)
Blast NOS
Explosion (of):
• NOS
• artillery shell
• breech-block
• cannon block
• mortar bomb
Fragments from:
• artillery shell
• bomb
• grenade
• guided missile
• land-mine
• rocket
• shell
• shrapnel
Mine NOS

Y36.3   **War operations involving fires, conflagrations and hot substances**
Asphyxia ⎫ originating from fire caused directly by a fire-
Burns ⎬ producing device or indirectly by any
Other injury ⎭ conventional weapon
Petrol bomb

Y36.4   **War operations involving firearm discharge and other forms of conventional warfare**
Battle wounds
Bayonet injury
Bullet:
• carbine
• machine gun
• pistol
• rifle
• rubber (rifle)
Drowned in war operations NOS
Pellets (shotgun)

Y36.5 **War operations involving nuclear weapons**
Blast effects
Exposure to ionizing radiation from nuclear weapon
Fireball effects
Heat
Other direct and secondary effects of nuclear weapons

Y36.6 **War operations involving biological weapons**

Y36.7 **War operations involving chemical weapons and other forms of unconventional warfare**
Gases, fumes and chemicals
Lasers

Y36.8 **War operations occurring after cessation of hostilities**
Injuries by explosion of bombs or mines placed in the course of operations of war, if the explosion occurred after cessation of hostilities
Injuries due to operations of war and classifiable to Y36.0–Y36.7 or Y36.9 but occurring after cessation of hostilities

Y36.9 **War operations, unspecified**

Complications of medical and surgical care (Y40–Y84)

Includes: complications of medical devices
correct drug properly administered in therapeutic or prophylactic dosage as the cause of any adverse effect
misadventures to patients during surgical and medical care
surgical and medical procedures as the cause of abnormal reaction of the patient, or of later complication, without mention of misadventure at the time of the procedure
Excludes: accidental overdose of drug or wrong drug given or taken in error (X40–X44)

Drugs, medicaments and biological substances causing adverse effects in therapeutic use (Y40–Y59)

Note: For list of specific drugs classified under the fourth-character subdivisions, see Table of drugs and chemicals in Alphabetical Index.

Excludes: accidents in the technique of administration of drugs, medicaments and biological substances in medical and surgical procedures (Y60–Y69)

Y40   Systemic antibiotics

Excludes: antibiotics, topically used (Y56.–)
antineoplastic antibiotics (Y43.3)

Y40.0   **Penicillins**

Y40.1   **Cefalosporins and other β-lactam antibiotics**

Y40.2   **Chloramphenicol group**

Y40.3   **Macrolides**

Y40.4   **Tetracyclines**

Y40.5   **Aminoglycosides**
Streptomycin

Y40.6   **Rifamycins**

Y40.7   **Antifungal antibiotics, systemically used**

Y40.8   **Other systemic antibiotics**

Y40.9   **Systemic antibiotic, unspecified**

Y41   Other systemic anti-infectives and antiparasitics

Excludes: anti-infectives, topically used (Y56.–)

Y41.0   **Sulfonamides**

Y41.1   **Antimycobacterial drugs**
Excludes: rifamycins (Y40.6)
streptomycin (Y40.5)

Y41.2   **Antimalarials and drugs acting on other blood protozoa**
Excludes: hydroxyquinoline derivatives (Y41.8)

Y41.3   **Other antiprotozoal drugs**

Y41.4   **Anthelminthics**

Y41.5   **Antiviral drugs**
Excludes: amantadine (Y46.7)
           cytarabine (Y43.1)

Y41.8   **Other specified systemic anti-infectives and antiparasitics**
Hydroxyquinoline derivatives
Excludes: antimalarial drugs (Y41.2)

Y41.9   **Systemic anti-infective and antiparasitic, unspecified**

Y42   Hormones and their synthetic substitutes and antagonists, not elsewhere classified

Excludes: mineralocorticoids and their antagonists
           (Y54.0–Y54.1)
           oxytocic hormones (Y55.0)
           parathyroid hormones and derivatives (Y54.7)

Y42.0   **Glucocorticoids and synthetic analogues**
Excludes: glucocorticoids, topically used (Y56.–)

Y42.1   **Thyroid hormones and substitutes**

Y42.2   **Antithyroid drugs**

Y42.3   **Insulin and oral hypoglycaemic [antidiabetic] drugs**

Y42.4   **Oral contraceptives**
Multiple- and single-ingredient preparations

Y42.5   **Other estrogens and progestogens**
Mixtures and substitutes

Y42.6   **Antigonadotrophins, antiestrogens, antiandrogens, not elsewhere classified**
Tamoxifen

Y42.7   **Androgens and anabolic congeners**

Y42.8   **Other and unspecified hormones and their synthetic substitutes**
Anterior pituitary [adenohypophyseal] hormones

Y42.9   **Other and unspecified hormone antagonists**

Y43 Primarily systemic agents
Excludes: vitamins NEC (Y57.7)

Y43.0 **Antiallergic and antiemetic drugs**
Excludes: phenothiazine-based neuroleptics (Y49.3)

Y43.1 **Antineoplastic antimetabolites**
Cytarabine

Y43.2 **Antineoplastic natural products**

Y43.3 **Other antineoplastic drugs**
Antineoplastic antibiotics
Excludes: tamoxifen (Y42.6)

Y43.4 **Immunosuppressive agents**

Y43.5 **Acidifying and alkalizing agents**

Y43.6 **Enzymes, not elsewhere classified**

Y43.8 **Other primarily systemic agents, not elsewhere classified**
Heavy-metal antagonists

Y43.9 **Primarily systemic agent, unspecified**

Y44 Agents primarily affecting blood constituents

Y44.0 **Iron preparations and other anti-hypochromic-anaemia preparations**

Y44.1 **Vitamin B$_{12}$, folic acid and other anti-megaloblastic-anaemia preparations**

Y44.2 **Anticoagulants**

Y44.3 **Anticoagulant antagonists, vitamin K and other coagulants**

Y44.4 **Antithrombotic drugs [platelet-aggregation inhibitors]**
Excludes: acetylsalicylic acid (Y45.1)
dipyridamole (Y52.3)

Y44.5 **Thrombolytic drugs**

Y44.6 **Natural blood and blood products**
Excludes: immunoglobulin (Y59.3)

Y44.7 **Plasma substitutes**

Y44.9 **Other and unspecified agents affecting blood constituents**

Y45   Analgesics, antipyretics and anti-inflammatory drugs

Y45.0   **Opioids and related analgesics**

Y45.1   **Salicylates**

Y45.2   **Propionic acid derivatives**
Propanoic acid derivatives

Y45.3   **Other nonsteroidal anti-inflammatory drugs [NSAID]**

Y45.4   **Antirheumatics**
Excludes: chloroquine (Y41.2)
glucocorticoids (Y42.0)
salicylates (Y45.1)

Y45.5   **4-Aminophenol derivatives**

Y45.8   **Other analgesics, antipyretics and anti-inflammatory drugs**

Y45.9   **Analgesic, antipyretic and anti-inflammatory drug, unspecified**

Y46   Antiepileptics and antiparkinsonism drugs
Excludes: acetazolamide (Y54.2)
barbiturates NEC (Y47.0)
benzodiazepines (Y47.1)
paraldehyde (Y47.3)

Y46.0   **Succinimides**

Y46.1   **Oxazolidinediones**

Y46.2   **Hydantoin derivatives**

Y46.3   **Deoxybarbiturates**

Y46.4   **Iminostilbenes**
Carbamazepine

Y46.5   **Valproic acid**

Y46.6   **Other and unspecified antiepileptics**

Y46.7   **Antiparkinsonism drugs**
Amantadine

Y46.8   **Antispasticity drugs**
Excludes: benzodiazepines (Y47.1)

Y47 Sedatives, hypnotics and antianxiety drugs

Y47.0 **Barbiturates, not elsewhere classified**
Excludes: deoxybarbiturates (Y46.3)
thiobarbiturates (Y48.1)

Y47.1 **Benzodiazepines**

Y47.2 **Cloral derivatives**

Y47.3 **Paraldehyde**

Y47.4 **Bromine compounds**

Y47.5 **Mixed sedatives and hypnotics, not elsewhere classified**

Y47.8 **Other sedatives, hypnotics and antianxiety drugs**
Methaqualone

Y47.9 **Sedative, hypnotic and antianxiety drug, unspecified**
Sleeping:
• draught ⎤
• drug ⎬ NOS
• tablet ⎦

Y48 Anaesthetics and therapeutic gases

Y48.0 **Inhaled anaesthetics**

Y48.1 **Parenteral anaesthetics**
Thiobarbiturates

Y48.2 **Other and unspecified general anaesthetics**

Y48.3 **Local anaesthetics**

Y48.4 **Anaesthetic, unspecified**

Y48.5 **Therapeutic gases**

Y49 Psychotropic drugs, not elsewhere classified
Excludes: appetite depressants [anorectics] (Y57.0)
barbiturates NEC (Y47.0)
benzodiazepines (Y47.1)
caffeine (Y50.2)
cocaine (Y48.3)
methaqualone (Y47.8)

Y49.0	Tricyclic and tetracyclic antidepressants
Y49.1	Monoamine-oxidase-inhibitor antidepressants
Y49.2	Other and unspecified antidepressants
Y49.3	Phenothiazine antipsychotics and neuroleptics
Y49.4	Butyrophenone and thioxanthene neuroleptics
Y49.5	Other antipsychotics and neuroleptics

Excludes: rauwolfia (Y52.5)

Y49.6	Psychodysleptics [hallucinogens]
Y49.7	Psychostimulants with abuse potential
Y49.8	Other psychotropic drugs, not elsewhere classified
Y49.9	Psychotropic drug, unspecified

Y50 Central nervous system stimulants, not elsewhere classified

Y50.0	Analeptics
Y50.1	Opioid receptor antagonists
Y50.2	Methylxanthines, not elsewhere classified

Caffeine

Excludes: aminophylline (Y55.6)
theobromine (Y55.6)
theophylline (Y55.6)

Y50.8	Other central nervous system stimulants
Y50.9	Central nervous system stimulant, unspecified

Y51 Drugs primarily affecting the autonomic nervous system

Y51.0	Anticholinesterase agents
Y51.1	Other parasympathomimetics [cholinergics]
Y51.2	Ganglionic blocking drugs, not elsewhere classified
Y51.3	Other parasympatholytics [anticholinergics and antimuscarinics] and spasmolytics, not elsewhere classified

Papaverine

Y51.4   **Predominantly α-adrenoreceptor agonists, not elsewhere classified**
Metaraminol

Y51.5   **Predominantly β-adrenoreceptor agonists, not elsewhere classified**
Excludes: salbutamol (Y55.6)

Y51.6   **α-Adrenoreceptor antagonists, not elsewhere classified**
Excludes: ergot alkaloids (Y55.0)

Y51.7   **β-Adrenoreceptor antagonists, not elsewhere classified**

Y51.8   **Centrally acting and adrenergic-neuron-blocking agents, not elsewhere classified**
Excludes: clonidine (Y52.5)
                    guanethidine (Y52.5)

Y51.9   **Other and unspecified drugs primarily affecting the autonomic nervous system**
Drugs stimulating both α- and β-adrenoreceptors

Y52   Agents primarily affecting the cardiovascular system
Excludes: metaraminol (Y51.4)

Y52.0   **Cardiac-stimulant glycosides and drugs of similar action**

Y52.1   **Calcium-channel blockers**

Y52.2   **Other antidysrhythmic drugs, not elsewhere classified**
Excludes: β-adrenoreceptor antagonists (Y51.7)

Y52.3   **Coronary vasodilators, not elsewhere classified**
Dipyridamole
Excludes: β-adrenoreceptor antagonists (Y51.7)
                    calcium-channel blockers (Y52.1)

Y52.4   **Angiotensin-converting-enzyme inhibitors**

Y52.5   **Other antihypertensive drugs, not elsewhere classified**
Clonidine
Guanethidine
Rauwolfia
Excludes: β-adrenoreceptor antagonists (Y51.7)
                    calcium-channel blockers (Y52.1)
                    diuretics (Y54.0–Y54.5)

Y52.6   **Antihyperlipidaemic and antiarteriosclerotic drugs**

Y52.7   **Peripheral vasodilators**
Nicotinic acid (derivatives)
Excludes: papaverine (Y51.3)

Y52.8   **Antivaricose drugs, including sclerosing agents**

Y52.9   **Other and unspecified agents primarily affecting the cardiovascular system**

Y53   Agents primarily affecting the gastrointestinal system

Y53.0   **Histamine H$_2$-receptor antagonists**

Y53.1   **Other antacids and anti-gastric-secretion drugs**

Y53.2   **Stimulant laxatives**

Y53.3   **Saline and osmotic laxatives**

Y53.4   **Other laxatives**
Intestinal atonia drugs

Y53.5   **Digestants**

Y53.6   **Antidiarrhoeal drugs**
Excludes: systemic antibiotics and other anti-infectives
(Y40–Y41)

Y53.7   **Emetics**

Y53.8   **Other agents primarily affecting the gastrointestinal system**

Y53.9   **Agent primarily affecting the gastrointestinal system, unspecified**

Y54   Agents primarily affecting water-balance and mineral and uric acid metabolism

Y54.0   **Mineralocorticoids**

Y54.1   **Mineralocorticoid antagonists [aldosterone antagonists]**

Y54.2   **Carbonic-anhydrase inhibitors**
Acetazolamide

Y54.3   **Benzothiadiazine derivatives**

Y54.4   **Loop [high-ceiling] diuretics**

Y54.5   **Other diuretics**

Y54.6   **Electrolytic, caloric and water-balance agents**
Oral rehydration salts

Y54.7   **Agents affecting calcification**
Parathyroid hormones and derivatives
Vitamin D group

Y54.8   **Agents affecting uric acid metabolism**

Y54.9   **Mineral salts, not elsewhere classified**

Y55   Agents primarily acting on smooth and skeletal muscles and the respiratory system

Y55.0   **Oxytocic drugs**
Ergot alkaloids
Excludes: estrogens, progestogens and antagonists
(Y42.5–Y42.6)

Y55.1   **Skeletal muscle relaxants [neuromuscular blocking agents]**
Excludes: antispasticity drugs (Y46.8)

Y55.2   **Other and unspecified agents primarily acting on muscles**

Y55.3   **Antitussives**

Y55.4   **Expectorants**

Y55.5   **Anti-common-cold drugs**

Y55.6   **Antiasthmatics, not elsewhere classified**
Aminophylline
Salbutamol
Theobromine
Theophylline
Excludes: β-adrenoreceptor agonists (Y51.5)
anterior pituitary [adenohypophyseal] hormones
(Y42.8)

Y55.7   **Other and unspecified agents primarily acting on the respiratory system**

Y56 Topical agents primarily affecting skin and mucous membrane and ophthalmological, otorhinolaryngological and dental drugs

Includes: glucocorticoids, topically used

Y56.0 **Local antifungal, anti-infective and anti-inflammatory drugs, not elsewhere classified**

Y56.1 **Antipruritics**

Y56.2 **Local astringents and local detergents**

Y56.3 **Emollients, demulcents and protectants**

Y56.4 **Keratolytics, keratoplastics and other hair treatment drugs and preparations**

Y56.5 **Ophthalmological drugs and preparations**

Y56.6 **Otorhinolaryngological drugs and preparations**

Y56.7 **Dental drugs, topically applied**

Y56.8 **Other topical agents**
Spermicides

Y56.9 **Topical agent, unspecified**

Y57 Other and unspecified drugs and medicaments

Y57.0 **Appetite depressants [anorectics]**

Y57.1 **Lipotropic drugs**

Y57.2 **Antidotes and chelating agents, not elsewhere classified**

Y57.3 **Alcohol deterrents**

Y57.4 **Pharmaceutical excipients**

Y57.5 **X-ray contrast media**

Y57.6 **Other diagnostic agents**

Y57.7 **Vitamins, not elsewhere classified**
Excludes: nicotinic acid (Y52.7)
vitamin B_{12} (Y44.1)
vitamin D (Y54.7)
vitamin K (Y44.3)

Y57.8 **Other drugs and medicaments**

Y57.9 **Drug or medicament, unspecified**

Y58   Bacterial vaccines

Y58.0   BCG vaccine

Y58.1   Typhoid and paratyphoid vaccine

Y58.2   Cholera vaccine

Y58.3   Plague vaccine

Y58.4   Tetanus vaccine

Y58.5   Diphtheria vaccine

Y58.6   Pertussis vaccine, including combinations with a pertussis component

Y58.8   Mixed bacterial vaccines, except combinations with a pertussis component

Y58.9   Other and unspecified bacterial vaccines

Y59   Other and unspecified vaccines and biological substances

Y59.0   Viral vaccines

Y59.1   Rickettsial vaccines

Y59.2   Protozoal vaccines

Y59.3   Immunoglobulin

Y59.8   Other specified vaccines and biological substances

Y59.9   Vaccine or biological substance, unspecified

Misadventures to patients during surgical and medical care
(Y60–Y69)

Excludes: medical devices associated with adverse incidents in diagnostic
and therapeutic use (Y70–Y82)
surgical and medical procedures as the cause of abnormal
reaction of the patient, without mention of misadventure at
the time of the procedure (Y83–Y84)

Y60 Unintentional cut, puncture, perforation or haemorrhage during surgical and medical care

Y60.0   During surgical operation

Y60.1   During infusion or transfusion

Y60.2   During kidney dialysis or other perfusion

Y60.3   During injection or immunization

Y60.4   During endoscopic examination

Y60.5   During heart catheterization

Y60.6   During aspiration, puncture and other catheterization

Y60.7   During administration of enema

Y60.8   During other surgical and medical care

Y60.9   During unspecified surgical and medical care

Y61 Foreign object accidentally left in body during surgical and medical care

Y61.0   During surgical operation

Y61.1   During infusion or transfusion

Y61.2   During kidney dialysis or other perfusion

Y61.3   During injection or immunization

Y61.4   During endoscopic examination

Y61.5   During heart catheterization

Y61.6   During aspiration, puncture and other catheterization

Y61.7	During removal of catheter or packing
Y61.8	During other surgical and medical care
Y61.9	During unspecified surgical and medical care

Y62 Failure of sterile precautions during surgical and medical care

Y62.0	During surgical operation
Y62.1	During infusion or transfusion
Y62.2	During kidney dialysis or other perfusion
Y62.3	During injection or immunization
Y62.4	During endoscopic examination
Y62.5	During heart catheterization
Y62.6	During aspiration, puncture and other catheterization
Y62.8	During other surgical and medical care
Y62.9	During unspecified surgical and medical care

Y63 Failure in dosage during surgical and medical care

Excludes: accidental overdose of drug or wrong drug given in error (X40–X44)

Y63.0	Excessive amount of blood or other fluid given during transfusion or infusion
Y63.1	Incorrect dilution of fluid used during infusion
Y63.2	Overdose of radiation given during therapy
Y63.3	Inadvertent exposure of patient to radiation during medical care
Y63.4	Failure in dosage in electroshock or insulin-shock therapy
Y63.5	Inappropriate temperature in local application and packing
Y63.6	Nonadministration of necessary drug, medicament or biological substance
Y63.8	Failure in dosage during other surgical and medical care
Y63.9	Failure in dosage during unspecified surgical and medical care

Y64 Contaminated medical or biological substances

Y64.0 Contaminated medical or biological substance, transfused or infused

Y64.1 Contaminated medical or biological substance, injected or used for immunization

Y64.8 Contaminated medical or biological substance administered by other means

Y64.9 Contaminated medical or biological substance administered by unspecified means

Administered contaminated medical or biological substance NOS

Y65 Other misadventures during surgical and medical care

Y65.0 Mismatched blood used in transfusion

Y65.1 Wrong fluid used in infusion

Y65.2 Failure in suture or ligature during surgical operation

Y65.3 Endotracheal tube wrongly placed during anaesthetic procedure

Y65.4 Failure to introduce or to remove other tube or instrument

Y65.5 Performance of inappropriate operation

Y65.8 Other specified misadventures during surgical and medical care

Y66 Nonadministration of surgical and medical care

Premature cessation of surgical and medical care

Y69 Unspecified misadventure during surgical and medical care

Medical devices associated with adverse incidents in diagnostic and therapeutic use (Y70–Y82)

The following fourth-character subdivisions are for use with categories Y70–Y82:

.0   Diagnostic and monitoring devices
.1   Therapeutic (nonsurgical) and rehabilitative devices
.2   Prosthetic and other implants, materials and accessory devices
.3   Surgical instruments, materials and devices (including sutures)
.8   Miscellaneous devices, not elsewhere classified

Y70 **Anaesthesiology devices associated with adverse incidents**

Y71 **Cardiovascular devices associated with adverse incidents**

Y72 **Otorhinolaryngological devices associated with adverse incidents**

Y73 **Gastroenterology and urology devices associated with adverse incidents**

Y74 **General hospital and personal-use devices associated with adverse incidents**

Y75 **Neurological devices associated with adverse incidents**

Y76 **Obstetric and gynaecological devices associated with adverse incidents**

Y77 **Ophthalmic devices associated with adverse incidents**

Y78 Radiological devices associated with adverse incidents

Y79 Orthopaedic devices associated with adverse incidents

Y80 Physical medicine devices associated with adverse incidents

Y81 General- and plastic-surgery devices associated with adverse incidents

Y82 Other and unspecified medical devices associated with adverse incidents

Surgical and other medical procedures as the cause of abnormal reaction of the patient, or of later complication, without mention of misadventure at the time of the procedure
(Y83–Y84)

Y83 Surgical operation and other surgical procedures as the cause of abnormal reaction of the patient, or of later complication, without mention of misadventure at the time of the procedure

Y83.0 Surgical operation with transplant of whole organ

Y83.1 Surgical operation with implant of artificial internal device

Y83.2 Surgical operation with anastomosis, bypass or graft

Y83.3 Surgical operation with formation of external stoma

Y83.4 Other reconstructive surgery

Y83.5 Amputation of limb(s)

Y83.6	Removal of other organ (partial) (total)
Y83.8	Other surgical procedures
Y83.9	Surgical procedure, unspecified

Y84 Other medical procedures as the cause of abnormal reaction of the patient, or of later complication, without mention of misadventure at the time of the procedure

Y84.0	Cardiac catheterization
Y84.1	Kidney dialysis
Y84.2	Radiological procedure and radiotherapy
Y84.3	Shock therapy
Y84.4	Aspiration of fluid
Y84.5	Insertion of gastric or duodenal sound
Y84.6	Urinary catheterization
Y84.7	Blood-sampling
Y84.8	Other medical procedures
Y84.9	Medical procedure, unspecified

Sequelae of external causes of morbidity and mortality
(Y85–Y89)

Note: Categories Y85–Y89 are to be used to indicate circumstances as the cause of death, impairment or disability from sequelae or "late effects", which are themselves classified elsewhere. The sequelae include conditions reported as such, or occurring as "late effects" one year or more after the originating event.

Y85 Sequelae of transport accidents

| Y85.0 | Sequelae of motor-vehicle accident |
| Y85.9 | Sequelae of other and unspecified transport accidents |

Y86 Sequelae of other accidents

Y87 Sequelae of intentional self-harm, assault and events of undetermined intent

Y87.0 Sequelae of intentional self-harm

Y87.1 Sequelae of assault

Y87.2 Sequelae of events of undetermined intent

Y88 Sequelae with surgical and medical care as external cause

Y88.0 Sequelae of adverse effects caused by drugs, medicaments and biological substances in therapeutic use

Y88.1 Sequelae of misadventures to patients during surgical and medical procedures

Y88.2 Sequelae of adverse incidents associated with medical devices in diagnostic and therapeutic use

Y88.3 Sequelae of surgical and medical procedures as the cause of abnormal reaction of the patient, or of later complication, without mention of misadventure at the time of the procedure

Y89 Sequelae of other external causes

Y89.0 Sequelae of legal intervention

Y89.1 Sequelae of war operations

Y89.9 Sequelae of unspecified external cause

Supplementary factors related to causes of morbidity and mortality classified elsewhere (Y90–Y98)

Note: These categories may be used, if desired, to provide supplementary information concerning causes of morbidity and mortality. They are not to be used for single-condition coding in morbidity or mortality.

Y90 Evidence of alcohol involvement determined by blood alcohol level

Y90.0 Blood alcohol level of less than 20 mg/100 ml

Y90.1 Blood alcohol level of 20–39 mg/100 ml

Y90.2 Blood alcohol level of 40–59 mg/100 ml

Y90.3 Blood alcohol level of 60–79 mg/100 ml

Y90.4 Blood alcohol level of 80–99 mg/100 ml

Y90.5 Blood alcohol level of 100–119 mg/100 ml

Y90.6 Blood alcohol level of 120–199 mg/100 ml

Y90.7 Blood alcohol level of 200–239 mg/100 ml

Y90.8 Blood alcohol level of 240 mg/100 ml or more

Y90.9 Presence of alcohol in blood, level not specified

Y91 Evidence of alcohol involvement determined by level of intoxication

Excludes: evidence of alcohol involvement determined by blood alcohol content (Y90.–)

Y91.0 **Mild alcohol intoxication**
Smell of alcohol on breath, slight behavioural disturbance in functions and responses, or slight difficulty in coordination.

Y91.1 **Moderate alcohol intoxication**
Smell of alcohol on breath, moderate behavioural disturbance in functions and responses, or moderate difficulty in coordination.

Y91.2 **Severe alcohol intoxication**
Severe disturbance in functions and responses, severe difficulty in coordination, or impaired ability to cooperate.

Y91.3   Very severe alcohol intoxication
Very severe disturbance in functions and responses, very severe difficulty in coordination, or loss of ability to cooperate.

Y91.9   Alcohol involvement, not otherwise specified
Suspected alcohol involvement NOS

Y95   Nosocomial condition

Y96   Work-related condition

Y97   Environmental-pollution-related condition

Y98   Lifestyle-related condition

CHAPTER XXI

Factors influencing health status and contact with health services (Z00–Z99)

Note: This chapter should not be used for international comparison or for primary mortality coding.

Categories Z00–Z99 are provided for occasions when circumstances other than a disease, injury or external cause classifiable to categories A00–Y89 are recorded as "diagnoses" or "problems". This can arise in two main ways:

(a) When a person who may or may not be sick encounters the health services for some specific purpose, such as to receive limited care or service for a current condition, to donate an organ or tissue, to receive prophylactic vaccination or to discuss a problem which is in itself not a disease or injury.

(b) When some circumstance or problem is present which influences the person's health status but is not in itself a current illness or injury. Such factors may be elicited during population surveys, when the person may or may not be currently sick, or be recorded as an additional factor to be borne in mind when the person is receiving care for some illness or injury.

This chapter contains the following blocks:

Z00–Z13   Persons encountering health services for examination and investigation

Z20–Z29   Persons with potential health hazards related to communicable diseases

Z30–Z39   Persons encountering health services in circumstances related to reproduction

Z40–Z54   Persons encountering health services for specific procedures and health care

Z55–Z65   Persons with potential health hazards related to socioeconomic and psychosocial circumstances

Z70–Z76   Persons encountering health services in other circumstances

Z80–Z99   Persons with potential health hazards related to family and personal history and certain conditions influencing health status

Persons encountering health services for examination and investigation (Z00–Z13)

Note: Nonspecific abnormal findings disclosed at the time of these examinations are classified to categories R70–R94.

Excludes: examinations related to pregnancy and reproduction (Z30–Z36, Z39.–)

Z00 General examination and investigation of persons without complaint or reported diagnosis
Excludes: examination for administrative purposes (Z02.–)
special screening examinations (Z11–Z13)

Z00.0 General medical examination
Health check-up NOS
Periodic examination (annual)(physical)
Excludes: general health check-up of:
- defined subpopulations (Z10.–)
- infant or child (Z00.1)

Z00.1 Routine child health examination
Development testing of infant or child
Excludes: health supervision of foundling or other healthy infant or child (Z76.1–Z76.2)

Z00.2 Examination for period of rapid growth in childhood

Z00.3 Examination for adolescent development state
Puberty development state

Z00.4 General psychiatric examination, not elsewhere classified
Excludes: examination requested for medicolegal reasons (Z04.6)

Z00.5 Examination of potential donor of organ and tissue

Z00.6 Examination for normal comparison and control in clinical research programme

Z00.8 Other general examinations
Health examination in population surveys

Z01 Other special examinations and investigations of persons without complaint or reported diagnosis

Includes: routine examination of specific system

Excludes: examination for:
- administrative purposes (Z02.–)
- suspected conditions, not proven (Z03.–)

special screening examinations (Z11–Z13)

Z01.0 Examination of eyes and vision

Excludes: examination for driving licence (Z02.4)

Z01.1 Examination of ears and hearing

Z01.2 Dental examination

Z01.3 Examination of blood pressure

Z01.4 Gynaecological examination (general)(routine)

Papanicolaou smear of cervix
Pelvic examination (annual)(periodic)

Excludes: pregnancy examination or test (Z32.–)
routine examination for contraceptive maintenance (Z30.4–Z30.5)

Z01.5 Diagnostic skin and sensitization tests

Allergy tests
Skin tests for:
- bacterial disease
- hypersensitivity

Z01.6 Radiological examination, not elsewhere classified

Routine:
- chest X-ray
- mammogram

Z01.7 Laboratory examination

Z01.8 Other specified special examinations

Z01.9 Special examination, unspecified

Z02 Examination and encounter for administrative purposes

Z02.0 Examination for admission to educational institution

Examination for admission to preschool (education)

Z02.1   **Pre-employment examination**
Excludes: occupational health examination (Z10.0)

Z02.2   **Examination for admission to residential institution**
Excludes: examination for admission to prison (Z02.8)
general health check-up of inhabitants of institutions (Z10.1)

Z02.3   **Examination for recruitment to armed forces**
Excludes: general health check-up of armed forces (Z10.2)

Z02.4   **Examination for driving licence**

Z02.5   **Examination for participation in sport**
Excludes: blood-alcohol and blood-drug test (Z04.0)
general health check-up of sports teams (Z10.3)

Z02.6   **Examination for insurance purposes**

Z02.7   **Issue of medical certificate**
Issue of medical certificate of:
• cause of death
• fitness
• incapacity
• invalidity
Excludes: encounter for general medical examination
(Z00–Z01, Z02.0–Z02.6, Z02.8–Z02.9, Z10.–)

Z02.8   **Other examinations for administrative purposes**
Examination (for):
• admission to:
  • prison
  • summer camp
• adoption
• immigration
• naturalization
• premarital
Excludes: health supervision of foundling or other healthy
infant or child (Z76.1–Z76.2)

Z02.9   **Examination for administrative purposes, unspecified**

Z03 Medical observation and evaluation for suspected diseases and conditions

Includes: persons who present some symptoms or evidence of an abnormal condition which requires study, but who, after examination and observation, show no need for further treatment or medical care

Excludes: person with feared complaint in whom no diagnosis is made (Z71.1)

Z03.0 Observation for suspected tuberculosis

Z03.1 Observation for suspected malignant neoplasm

Z03.2 Observation for suspected mental and behavioural disorders

Observation for:
- dissocial behaviour
- fire-setting
- gang activity
- shoplifting

} without manifest psychiatric disorder

Z03.3 Observation for suspected nervous system disorder

Z03.4 Observation for suspected myocardial infarction

Z03.5 Observation for other suspected cardiovascular diseases

Z03.6 Observation for suspected toxic effect from ingested substance

Observation for suspected:
- adverse effect from drug
- poisoning

Z03.8 Observation for other suspected diseases and conditions

Z03.9 Observation for suspected disease or condition, unspecified

Z04 Examination and observation for other reasons

Includes: examination for medicolegal reasons

Z04.0 Blood-alcohol and blood-drug test

Excludes: presence of:
- alcohol in blood (R78.0)
- drugs in blood (R78.–)

Z04.1 Examination and observation following transport accident

Excludes: following work accident (Z04.2)

Z04.2   **Examination and observation following work accident**

Z04.3   **Examination and observation following other accident**

Z04.4   **Examination and observation following alleged rape and seduction**
Examination of victim or culprit following alleged rape or
  seduction

Z04.5   **Examination and observation following other inflicted injury**
Examination of victim or culprit following other inflicted injury

Z04.6   **General psychiatric examination, requested by authority**

Z04.8   **Examination and observation for other specified reasons**
Request for expert evidence

Z04.9   **Examination and observation for unspecified reason**
Observation NOS

Z08   Follow-up examination after treatment for malignant neoplasm

Includes: medical surveillance following treatment
Excludes: follow-up medical care and convalescence (Z42–Z51,
  Z54.–)

Z08.0   **Follow-up examination after surgery for malignant neoplasm**

Z08.1   **Follow-up examination after radiotherapy for malignant neoplasm**
Excludes: radiotherapy session (Z51.0)

Z08.2   **Follow-up examination after chemotherapy for malignant neoplasm**
Excludes: chemotherapy session (Z51.1)

Z08.7   **Follow-up examination after combined treatment for malignant neoplasm**

Z08.8   **Follow-up examination after other treatment for malignant neoplasm**

Z08.9   **Follow-up examination after unspecified treatment for malignant neoplasm**

Z09 Follow-up examination after treatment for conditions other than malignant neoplasms

Includes: medical surveillance following treatment

Excludes: follow-up medical care and convalescence (Z42–Z51, Z54.–)

medical surveillance following treatment for malignant neoplasm (Z08.–)

surveillance of:
- contraception (Z30.4–Z30.5)
- prosthetic and other medical devices (Z44–Z46)

Z09.0 Follow-up examination after surgery for other conditions

Z09.1 Follow-up examination after radiotherapy for other conditions

Excludes: radiotherapy session (Z51.0)

Z09.2 Follow-up examination after chemotherapy for other conditions

Excludes: maintenance chemotherapy (Z51.1–Z51.2)

Z09.3 Follow-up examination after psychotherapy

Z09.4 Follow-up examination after treatment of fracture

Z09.7 Follow-up examination after combined treatment for other conditions

Z09.8 Follow-up examination after other treatment for other conditions

Z09.9 Follow-up examination after unspecified treatment for other conditions

Z10 Routine general health check-up of defined subpopulation

Excludes: medical examination for administrative purposes (Z02.–)

Z10.0 Occupational health examination

Excludes: pre-employment examination (Z02.1)

Z10.1 Routine general health check-up of inhabitants of institutions

Excludes: admission examination (Z02.2)

Z10.2   **Routine general health check-up of armed forces**
Excludes: recruitment examination (Z02.3)

Z10.3   **Routine general health check-up of sports teams**
Excludes: blood-alcohol and blood-drug test (Z04.0)
examination for participation in sport (Z02.5)

Z10.8   **Routine general health check-up of other defined subpopulations**
Schoolchildren
Students

Z11   Special screening examination for infectious and parasitic diseases

Z11.0   **Special screening examination for intestinal infectious diseases**

Z11.1   **Special screening examination for respiratory tuberculosis**

Z11.2   **Special screening examination for other bacterial diseases**

Z11.3   **Special screening examination for infections with a predominantly sexual mode of transmission**

Z11.4   **Special screening examination for human immunodeficiency virus [HIV]**

Z11.5   **Special screening examination for other viral diseases**
Excludes: viral intestinal disease (Z11.0)

Z11.6   **Special screening examination for other protozoal diseases and helminthiases**
Excludes: protozoal intestinal disease (Z11.0)

Z11.8   **Special screening examination for other infectious and parasitic diseases**
Chlamydial ⎫
Rickettsial ⎬ diseases
Spirochaetal ⎭
Mycoses

Z11.9   **Special screening examination for infectious and parasitic diseases, unspecified**

Z12   Special screening examination for neoplasms

Z12.0	Special screening examination for neoplasm of stomach
Z12.1	Special screening examination for neoplasm of intestinal tract
Z12.2	Special screening examination for neoplasm of respiratory organs
Z12.3	Special screening examination for neoplasm of breast

Z12.3   Special screening examination for neoplasm of breast

Excludes: routine mammogram (Z01.6)

Z12.4   Special screening examination for neoplasm of cervix

Excludes: when routine test or as part of general gynaecological examination (Z01.4)

Z12.5   Special screening examination for neoplasm of prostate

Z12.6   Special screening examination for neoplasm of bladder

Z12.8   Special screening examination for neoplasms of other sites

Z12.9   Special screening examination for neoplasm, unspecified

Z13   Special screening examination for other diseases and disorders

Z13.0   Special screening examination for diseases of the blood and blood-forming organs and certain disorders involving the immune mechanism

Z13.1   Special screening examination for diabetes mellitus

Z13.2   Special screening examination for nutritional disorders

Z13.3   Special screening examination for mental and behavioural disorders

Alcoholism
Depression
Mental retardation

Z13.4   Special screening examination for certain developmental disorders in childhood

Excludes: routine development testing of infant or child (Z00.1)

Z13.5   Special screening examination for eye and ear disorders

Z13.6   Special screening examination for cardiovascular disorders

Z13.7 **Special screening examination for congenital malformations, deformations and chromosomal abnormalities**

Z13.8 **Special screening examination for other specified diseases and disorders**
Dental disorder
Endocrine and metabolic disorders
Excludes: diabetes mellitus (Z13.1)

Z13.9 **Special screening examination, unspecified**

Persons with potential health hazards related to communicable diseases
(Z20–Z29)

Z20 Contact with and exposure to communicable diseases

Z20.0 **Contact with and exposure to intestinal infectious diseases**

Z20.1 **Contact with and exposure to tuberculosis**

Z20.2 **Contact with and exposure to infections with a predominantly sexual mode of transmission**

Z20.3 **Contact with and exposure to rabies**

Z20.4 **Contact with and exposure to rubella**

Z20.5 **Contact with and exposure to viral hepatitis**

Z20.6 **Contact with and exposure to human immunodeficiency virus [HIV]**
Excludes: asymptomatic human immunodeficiency virus [HIV] infection status (Z21)

Z20.7 **Contact with and exposure to pediculosis, acariasis and other infestations**

Z20.8 **Contact with and exposure to other communicable diseases**

Z20.9 **Contact with and exposure to unspecified communicable disease**

Z21 Asymptomatic human immunodeficiency virus [HIV] infection status

HIV positive NOS

Excludes: contact with or exposure to human immunodeficiency virus [HIV] (Z20.6)

human immunodeficiency virus [HIV] disease (B20–B24)

laboratory evidence of human immunodeficiency virus [HIV] (R75)

Z22 Carrier of infectious disease

Includes: suspected carrier

Z22.0 **Carrier of typhoid**

Z22.1 **Carrier of other intestinal infectious diseases**

Z22.2 **Carrier of diphtheria**

Z22.3 **Carrier of other specified bacterial diseases**

Carrier of bacterial disease due to:
- meningococci
- staphylococci
- streptococci

Z22.4 **Carrier of infections with a predominantly sexual mode of transmission**

Carrier of:
- gonorrhoea
- syphilis

Z22.5 **Carrier of viral hepatitis**

Hepatitis B surface antigen [HBsAg] carrier

Z22.6 **Carrier of human T-lymphotropic virus type 1 [HTLV-1] infection**

Z22.8 **Carrier of other infectious diseases**

Z22.9 **Carrier of infectious disease, unspecified**

Z23   Need for immunization against single bacterial diseases

Excludes: immunization:
- against combinations of diseases (Z27.–)
- not carried out (Z28.–)

Z23.0   **Need for immunization against cholera alone**

Z23.1   **Need for immunization against typhoid–paratyphoid alone [TAB]**

Z23.2   **Need for immunization against tuberculosis [BCG]**

Z23.3   **Need for immunization against plague**

Z23.4   **Need for immunization against tularaemia**

Z23.5   **Need for immunization against tetanus alone**

Z23.6   **Need for immunization against diphtheria alone**

Z23.7   **Need for immunization against pertussis alone**

Z23.8   **Need for immunization against other single bacterial diseases**

Z24   Need for immunization against certain single viral diseases

Excludes: immunization:
- against combinations of diseases (Z27.–)
- not carried out (Z28.–)

Z24.0   **Need for immunization against poliomyelitis**

Z24.1   **Need for immunization against arthropod-borne viral encephalitis**

Z24.2   **Need for immunization against rabies**

Z24.3   **Need for immunization against yellow fever**

Z24.4   **Need for immunization against measles alone**

Z24.5   **Need for immunization against rubella alone**

Z24.6   **Need for immunization against viral hepatitis**

Z25 Need for immunization against other single viral diseases

Excludes: immunization:
- against combinations of diseases (Z27.–)
- not carried out (Z28.–)

Z25.0 Need for immunization against mumps alone

Z25.1 Need for immunization against influenza

Z25.8 Need for immunization against other specified single viral diseases

Z26 Need for immunization against other single infectious diseases

Excludes: immunization:
- against combinations of diseases (Z27.–)
- not carried out (Z28.–)

Z26.0 Need for immunization against leishmaniasis

Z26.8 Need for immunization against other specified single infectious diseases

Z26.9 Need for immunization against unspecified infectious disease
Need for immunization NOS

Z27 Need for immunization against combinations of infectious diseases

Excludes: immunization not carried out (Z28.–)

Z27.0 Need for immunization against cholera with typhoid–paratyphoid [cholera + TAB]

Z27.1 Need for immunization against diphtheria–tetanus–pertussis, combined [DTP]

Z27.2 Need for immunization against diphtheria–tetanus–pertussis with typhoid–paratyphoid [DTP + TAB]

Z27.3 Need for immunization against diphtheria–tetanus–pertussis with poliomyelitis [DTP + polio]

Z27.4 Need for immunization against measles–mumps–rubella [MMR]

Z27.8   **Need for immunization against other combinations of infectious diseases**

Z27.9   **Need for immunization against unspecified combinations of infectious diseases**

Z28   Immunization not carried out

Z28.0   **Immunization not carried out because of contraindication**

Z28.1   **Immunization not carried out because of patient's decision for reasons of belief or group pressure**

Z28.2   **Immunization not carried out because of patient's decision for other and unspecified reasons**

Z28.8   **Immunization not carried out for other reasons**

Z28.9   **Immunization not carried out for unspecified reason**

Z29   Need for other prophylactic measures

Excludes: desensitization to allergens (Z51.6)
prophylactic surgery (Z40.–)

Z29.0   **Isolation**
Admission to protect the individual from his or her surroundings or for isolation of individual after contact with infectious disease

Z29.1   **Prophylactic immunotherapy**
Administration of immunoglobulin

Z29.2   **Other prophylactic chemotherapy**
Chemoprophylaxis
Prophylactic antibiotic therapy

Z29.8   **Other specified prophylactic measures**

Z29.9   **Prophylactic measure, unspecified**

Persons encountering health services in circumstances related to reproduction (Z30–Z39)

Z30 Contraceptive management

Z30.0 General counselling and advice on contraception
Family planning advice NOS
Initial prescription of contraceptives

Z30.1 Insertion of (intrauterine) contraceptive device

Z30.2 Sterilization
Admission for interruption of fallopian tubes or vasa deferentia

Z30.3 Menstrual extraction
Interception of pregnancy
Menstrual regulation

Z30.4 Surveillance of contraceptive drugs
Repeat prescription for contraceptive pill or other contraceptive
    drugs
Routine examination for contraceptive maintenance

Z30.5 Surveillance of (intrauterine) contraceptive device
Checking, reinsertion or removal of (intrauterine) contraceptive
    device

Z30.8 Other contraceptive management
Postvasectomy sperm count

Z30.9 Contraceptive management, unspecified

Z31 Procreative management
Excludes: complications associated with artificial fertilization
    (N98.–)

Z31.0 Tuboplasty or vasoplasty after previous sterilization

Z31.1 Artificial insemination

Z31.2 *In vitro* fertilization
Admission for harvesting or implantation of ova

Z31.3 Other assisted fertilization methods

Z31.4 **Procreative investigation and testing**
Fallopian insufflation
Sperm count
Excludes: postvasectomy sperm count (Z30.8)

Z31.5 **Genetic counselling**

Z31.6 **General counselling and advice on procreation**

Z31.8 **Other procreative management**

Z31.9 **Procreative management, unspecified**

Z32 Pregnancy examination and test

Z32.0 **Pregnancy, not (yet) confirmed**

Z32.1 **Pregnancy confirmed**

Z33 Pregnant state, incidental

Pregnant state NOS

Z34 Supervision of normal pregnancy

Z34.0 **Supervision of normal first pregnancy**

Z34.8 **Supervision of other normal pregnancy**

Z34.9 **Supervision of normal pregnancy, unspecified**

Z35 Supervision of high-risk pregnancy

Z35.0 **Supervision of pregnancy with history of infertility**

Z35.1 **Supervision of pregnancy with history of abortive outcome**
Supervision of pregnancy with history of:
• hydatidiform mole
• vesicular mole
Excludes: habitual aborter:
• care during pregnancy (O26.2)
• without current pregnancy (N96)

Z35.2 **Supervision of pregnancy with other poor reproductive or obstetric history**
Supervision of pregnancy with history of:
• conditions classifiable to O10–O92
• neonatal death
• stillbirth

Z35.3 **Supervision of pregnancy with history of insufficient antenatal care**
Pregnancy:
• concealed
• hidden

Z35.4 **Supervision of pregnancy with grand multiparity**
Excludes: multiparity without current pregnancy (Z64.1)

Z35.5 **Supervision of elderly primigravida**

Z35.6 **Supervision of very young primigravida**

Z35.7 **Supervision of high-risk pregnancy due to social problems**

Z35.8 **Supervision of other high-risk pregnancies**

Z35.9 **Supervision of high-risk pregnancy, unspecified**

Z36 Antenatal screening
Excludes: abnormal findings on antenatal screening of mother (O28.–)
routine prenatal care (Z34–Z35)

Z36.0 **Antenatal screening for chromosomal anomalies**
Amniocentesis
Placental sample (taken vaginally)

Z36.1 **Antenatal screening for raised alphafetoprotein level**

Z36.2 **Other antenatal screening based on amniocentesis**

Z36.3 **Antenatal screening for malformations using ultrasound and other physical methods**

Z36.4 **Antenatal screening for fetal growth retardation using ultrasound and other physical methods**

Z36.5 **Antenatal screening for isoimmunization**

Z36.8 **Other antenatal screening**
Screening for haemoglobinopathy

Z36.9 **Antenatal screening, unspecified**

Z37   Outcome of delivery

Note: This category is intended for use as an additional code to identify the outcome of delivery on the mother's record.

Z37.0	**Single live birth**
Z37.1	**Single stillbirth**
Z37.2	**Twins, both liveborn**
Z37.3	**Twins, one liveborn and one stillborn**
Z37.4	**Twins, both stillborn**
Z37.5	**Other multiple births, all liveborn**
Z37.6	**Other multiple births, some liveborn**
Z37.7	**Other multiple births, all stillborn**
Z37.9	**Outcome of delivery, unspecified** Multiple birth NOS Single birth NOS

Z38   Liveborn infants according to place of birth

Z38.0	**Singleton, born in hospital**
Z38.1	**Singleton, born outside hospital**
Z38.2	**Singleton, unspecified as to place of birth** Liveborn infant NOS
Z38.3	**Twin, born in hospital**
Z38.4	**Twin, born outside hospital**
Z38.5	**Twin, unspecified as to place of birth**
Z38.6	**Other multiple, born in hospital**
Z38.7	**Other multiple, born outside hospital**
Z38.8	**Other multiple, unspecified as to place of birth**

Z39   Postpartum care and examination

Z39.0	**Care and examination immediately after delivery** Care and observation in uncomplicated cases *Excludes:* care for postpartum complications—see Alphabetical Index

Z39.1   **Care and examination of lactating mother**
Supervision of lactation
Excludes: disorders of lactation (O92.–)

Z39.2   **Routine postpartum follow-up**

Persons encountering health services for specific procedures and health care (Z40–Z54)

Note: Categories Z40–Z54 are intended for use to indicate a reason for care. They may be used for patients who have already been treated for a disease or injury, but who are receiving follow-up or prophylactic care, convalescent care, or care to consolidate the treatment, to deal with residual states, to ensure that the condition has not recurred, or to prevent recurrence.

Excludes: follow-up examination for medical surveillance after treatment (Z08–Z09)

Z40   Prophylactic surgery

Z40.0   **Prophylactic surgery for risk-factors related to malignant neoplasms**
Admission for prophylactic organ removal

Z40.8   **Other prophylactic surgery**

Z40.9   **Prophylactic surgery, unspecified**

Z41   Procedures for purposes other than remedying health state

Z41.0   **Hair transplant**

Z41.1   **Other plastic surgery for unacceptable cosmetic appearance**
Breast implant
Excludes: plastic and reconstructive surgery following healed injury or operation (Z42.–)

Z41.2   **Routine and ritual circumcision**

Z41.3   **Ear piercing**

Z41.8   Other procedures for purposes other than remedying health state

Z41.9   Procedure for purposes other than remedying health state, unspecified

Z42   Follow-up care involving plastic surgery

Includes: plastic and reconstructive surgery following healed injury or operation
repair of scarred tissue

Excludes: plastic surgery:
* as treatment for current injury—code to relevant injury—see Alphabetical Index
* for unacceptable cosmetic appearance (Z41.1)

Z42.0   Follow-up care involving plastic surgery of head and neck

Z42.1   Follow-up care involving plastic surgery of breast

Z42.2   Follow-up care involving plastic surgery of other parts of trunk

Z42.3   Follow-up care involving plastic surgery of upper extremity

Z42.4   Follow-up care involving plastic surgery of lower extremity

Z42.8   Follow-up care involving plastic surgery of other body part

Z42.9   Follow-up care involving plastic surgery, unspecified

Z43   Attention to artificial openings

Includes: closure
passage of sounds or bougies
reforming
removal of catheter
toilet or cleansing

Excludes: artificial opening status only, without need for care (Z93.–)
complications of external stoma (J95.0, K91.4, N99.5)
fitting and adjustment of prosthetic and other devices (Z44–Z46)

Z43.0   Attention to tracheostomy

Z43.1   Attention to gastrostomy

Z43.2   **Attention to ileostomy**

Z43.3   **Attention to colostomy**

Z43.4   **Attention to other artificial openings of digestive tract**

Z43.5   **Attention to cystostomy**

Z43.6   **Attention to other artificial openings of urinary tract**
Nephrostomy
Ureterostomy
Urethrostomy

Z43.7   **Attention to artificial vagina**

Z43.8   **Attention to other artificial openings**

Z43.9   **Attention to unspecified artificial opening**

Z44   Fitting and adjustment of external prosthetic device

Excludes: presence of prosthetic device (Z97.–)

Z44.0   **Fitting and adjustment of artificial arm (complete)(partial)**

Z44.1   **Fitting and adjustment of artificial leg (complete)(partial)**

Z44.2   **Fitting and adjustment of artificial eye**
Excludes: mechanical complication of ocular prosthesis (T85.3)

Z44.3   **Fitting and adjustment of external breast prosthesis**

Z44.8   **Fitting and adjustment of other external prosthetic devices**

Z44.9   **Fitting and adjustment of unspecified external prosthetic device**

Z45   Adjustment and management of implanted device

Excludes: malfunction or other complications of device—see Alphabetical Index
presence of prosthetic and other devices (Z95–Z97)

Z45.0   **Adjustment and management of cardiac pacemaker**
Checking and testing of pulse generator [battery]

Z45.1   **Adjustment and management of infusion pump**

Z45.2   **Adjustment and management of vascular access device**

Z45.3 **Adjustment and management of implanted hearing device**
Bone conduction device
Cochlear device

Z45.8 **Adjustment and management of other implanted devices**

Z45.9 **Adjustment and management of unspecified implanted device**

Z46 Fitting and adjustment of other devices

Excludes: issue of repeat prescription only (Z76.0)
malfunction or other complications of device—see
Alphabetical Index
presence of prosthetic and other devices (Z95–Z97)

Z46.0 **Fitting and adjustment of spectacles and contact lenses**

Z46.1 **Fitting and adjustment of hearing aid**

Z46.2 **Fitting and adjustment of other devices related to nervous system and special senses**

Z46.3 **Fitting and adjustment of dental prosthetic device**

Z46.4 **Fitting and adjustment of orthodontic device**

Z46.5 **Fitting and adjustment of ileostomy and other intestinal appliances**

Z46.6 **Fitting and adjustment of urinary device**

Z46.7 **Fitting and adjustment of orthopaedic device**
Orthopaedic:
• brace
• cast
• corset
• shoes

Z46.8 **Fitting and adjustment of other specified devices**
Wheelchair

Z46.9 **Fitting and adjustment of unspecified device**

Z47 Other orthopaedic follow-up care

Excludes: care involving rehabilitation procedures (Z50.–)
complication of internal orthopaedic devices, implants and grafts (T84.–)
follow-up examination after treatment of fracture (Z09.4)

Z47.0 Follow-up care involving removal of fracture plate and other internal fixation device

Removal of:
- pins
- plates
- rods
- screws

Excludes: removal of external fixation device (Z47.8)

Z47.8 Other specified orthopaedic follow-up care

Change, checking or removal of:
- external fixation or traction device
- plaster cast

Z47.9 Orthopaedic follow-up care, unspecified

Z48 Other surgical follow-up care

Excludes: attention to artificial openings (Z43.–)
fitting and adjustment of prosthetic and other devices (Z44–Z46)
follow-up examination after:
- surgery (Z09.0)
- treatment of fracture (Z09.4)
orthopaedic follow-up care (Z47.–)

Z48.0 Attention to surgical dressings and sutures

Change of dressings
Removal of sutures

Z48.8 Other specified surgical follow-up care

Z48.9 Surgical follow-up care, unspecified

Z49 Care involving dialysis
Includes: dialysis preparation and treatment
Excludes: renal dialysis status (Z99.2)

Z49.0 Preparatory care for dialysis

Z49.1 Extracorporeal dialysis
Dialysis (renal) NOS

Z49.2 Other dialysis
Peritoneal dialysis

Z50 Care involving use of rehabilitation procedures
Excludes: counselling (Z70–Z71)

Z50.0 Cardiac rehabilitation

Z50.1 Other physical therapy
Therapeutic and remedial exercises

Z50.2 Alcohol rehabilitation

Z50.3 Drug rehabilitation

Z50.4 Psychotherapy, not elsewhere classified

Z50.5 Speech therapy

Z50.6 Orthoptic training

Z50.7 Occupational therapy and vocational rehabilitation, not elsewhere classified

Z50.8 Care involving use of other rehabilitation procedures
Tobacco rehabilitation
Training in activities of daily living [ADL] NEC

Z50.9 Care involving use of rehabilitation procedure, unspecified
Rehabilitation NOS

Z51 Other medical care
Excludes: follow-up examination after treatment (Z08–Z09)

Z51.0 Radiotherapy session

Z51.1 Chemotherapy session for neoplasm

Z51.2 **Other chemotherapy**
Maintenance chemotherapy NOS
Excludes: prophylactic chemotherapy for immunization
purposes (Z23–Z27, Z29.–)

Z51.3 **Blood transfusion without reported diagnosis**

Z51.4 **Preparatory care for subsequent treatment, not elsewhere classified**
Excludes: preparatory care for dialysis (Z49.0)

Z51.5 **Palliative care**

Z51.6 **Desensitization to allergens**

Z51.8 **Other specified medical care**
Excludes: holiday relief care (Z75.5)

Z51.9 **Medical care, unspecified**

Z52 Donors of organs and tissues
Excludes: examination of potential donor (Z00.5)

Z52.0 **Blood donor**

Z52.1 **Skin donor**

Z52.2 **Bone donor**

Z52.3 **Bone marrow donor**

Z52.4 **Kidney donor**

Z52.5 **Cornea donor**

Z52.8 **Donor of other organs and tissues**

Z52.9 **Donor of unspecified organ or tissue**
Donor NOS

Z53 Persons encountering health services for specific procedures, not carried out
Excludes: immunization not carried out (Z28.–)

Z53.0 **Procedure not carried out because of contraindication**

Z53.1 **Procedure not carried out because of patient's decision for reasons of belief or group pressure**

Z53.2 **Procedure not carried out because of patient's decision for other and unspecified reasons**

Z53.8   **Procedure not carried out for other reasons**

Z53.9   **Procedure not carried out, unspecified reason**

Z54   Convalescence

Z54.0   **Convalescence following surgery**

Z54.1   **Convalescence following radiotherapy**

Z54.2   **Convalescence following chemotherapy**

Z54.3   **Convalescence following psychotherapy**

Z54.4   **Convalescence following treatment of fracture**

Z54.7   **Convalescence following combined treatment**
Convalescence following any combination of treatments classified to Z54.0–Z54.4

Z54.8   **Convalescence following other treatment**

Z54.9   **Convalescence following unspecified treatment**

Persons with potential health hazards related to socioeconomic and psychosocial circumstances (Z55–Z65)

Z55   Problems related to education and literacy
Excludes: disorders of psychological development (F80–F89)

Z55.0   **Illiteracy and low-level literacy**

Z55.1   **Schooling unavailable and unattainable**

Z55.2   **Failed examinations**

Z55.3   **Underachievement in school**

Z55.4   **Educational maladjustment and discord with teachers and classmates**

Z55.8   **Other problems related to education and literacy**
Inadequate teaching

Z55.9   **Problem related to education and literacy, unspecified**

Z56 Problems related to employment and unemployment

Excludes: occupational exposure to risk-factors (Z57.–)
problems related to housing and economic
circumstances (Z59.–)

Z56.0 **Unemployment, unspecified**

Z56.1 **Change of job**

Z56.2 **Threat of job loss**

Z56.3 **Stressful work schedule**

Z56.4 **Discord with boss and workmates**

Z56.5 **Uncongenial work**
Difficult conditions at work

Z56.6 **Other physical and mental strain related to work**

Z56.7 **Other and unspecified problems related to employment**

Z57 Occupational exposure to risk-factors

Z57.0 **Occupational exposure to noise**

Z57.1 **Occupational exposure to radiation**

Z57.2 **Occupational exposure to dust**

Z57.3 **Occupational exposure to other air contaminants**

Z57.4 **Occupational exposure to toxic agents in agriculture**
Solids, liquids, gases or vapours

Z57.5 **Occupational exposure to toxic agents in other industries**
Solids, liquids, gases or vapours

Z57.6 **Occupational exposure to extreme temperature**

Z57.7 **Occupational exposure to vibration**

Z57.8 **Occupational exposure to other risk-factors**

Z57.9 **Occupational exposure to unspecified risk-factor**

Z58 Problems related to physical environment

Excludes: occupational exposure (Z57.–)

Z58.0 **Exposure to noise**

Z58.1	**Exposure to air pollution**
Z58.2	**Exposure to water pollution**
Z58.3	**Exposure to soil pollution**
Z58.4	**Exposure to radiation**
Z58.5	**Exposure to other pollution**
Z58.6	**Inadequate drinking-water supply**

Excludes: effects of thirst (T73.1)

Z58.8	**Other problems related to physical environment**
Z58.9	**Problem related to physical environment, unspecified**

Z59   Problems related to housing and economic circumstances

Excludes: inadequate drinking-water supply (Z58.6)

Z59.0   Homelessness

Z59.1   Inadequate housing
Lack of heating
Restriction of space
Technical defects in home preventing adequate care
Unsatisfactory surroundings
Excludes: problems related to physical environment (Z58.–)

Z59.2   Discord with neighbours, lodgers and landlord

Z59.3   Problems related to living in residential institution
Boarding-school resident
Excludes: institutional upbringing (Z62.2)

Z59.4   Lack of adequate food
Excludes: effects of hunger (T73.0)
inappropriate diet or eating habits (Z72.4)
malnutrition (E40–E46)

Z59.5   Extreme poverty

Z59.6   Low income

Z59.7   Insufficient social insurance and welfare support

Z59.8   Other problems related to housing and economic circumstances
Foreclosure on loan
Isolated dwelling
Problems with creditors

Z59.9   Problem related to housing and economic circumstances, unspecified

Z60   Problems related to social environment

Z60.0   Problems of adjustment to life-cycle transitions
Adjustment to retirement [pension]
Empty nest syndrome

Z60.1   Atypical parenting situation
Problems related to a parenting situation (rearing of children) with a single parent or other than that of two cohabiting biological parents.

Z60.2   Living alone

Z60.3   Acculturation difficulty
Migration
Social transplantation

Z60.4   Social exclusion and rejection
Exclusion and rejection on the basis of personal characteristics, such as unusual physical appearance, illness or behaviour.

Excludes: target of adverse discrimination such as for racial or religious reasons (Z60.5)

Z60.5   Target of perceived adverse discrimination and persecution
Persecution or discrimination, perceived or real, on the basis of membership of some group (as defined by skin colour, religion, ethnic origin, etc.) rather than personal characteristics.

Excludes: social exclusion and rejection (Z60.4)

Z60.8   Other problems related to social environment

Z60.9   Problem related to social environment, unspecified

Z61   Problems related to negative life events in childhood

Excludes: maltreatment syndromes (T74.–)

Z61.0   Loss of love relationship in childhood
Loss of an emotionally close relationship, such as of a parent, a sibling, a very special friend or a loved pet, by death or permanent departure or rejection.

Z61.1   Removal from home in childhood
Admission to a foster home, hospital or other institution causing psychosocial stress, or forced conscription into an activity away from home for a prolonged period.

Z61.2   **Altered pattern of family relationships in childhood**

Arrival of a new person into a family resulting in adverse change in child's relationships. May include new marriage by a parent or birth of a sibling.

Z61.3   **Events resulting in loss of self-esteem in childhood**

Events resulting in a negative self-reappraisal by the child such as failure in tasks with high personal investment; disclosure or discovery of a shameful or stigmatizing personal or family event; and other humiliating experiences.

Z61.4   **Problems related to alleged sexual abuse of child by person within primary support group**

Problems related to any form of physical contact or exposure between an adult member of the child's household and the child that has led to sexual arousal, whether or not the child has willingly engaged in the sexual acts (e.g. any genital contact or manipulation or deliberate exposure of breasts or genitals).

Z61.5   **Problems related to alleged sexual abuse of child by person outside primary support group**

Problems related to contact or attempted contact with the child's or the other person's breasts or genitals, sexual exposure in close confrontation or attempt to undress or seduce the child, by a substantially older person outside the child's family, either on the basis of this person's position or status or against the will of the child.

Z61.6   **Problems related to alleged physical abuse of child**

Problems related to incidents in which the child has been injured in the past by any adult in the household to a medically significant extent (e.g. fractures, marked bruising) or that involved abnormal forms of violence (e.g. hitting the child with hard or sharp implements, burning or tying up of the child).

Z61.7   **Personal frightening experience in childhood**

Experience carrying a threat for the child's future, such as a kidnapping, natural disaster with a threat to life, injury with a threat to self-image or security, or witnessing a severe trauma to a loved one.

Z61.8   **Other negative life events in childhood**

Z61.9   **Negative life event in childhood, unspecified**

Z62   Other problems related to upbringing

Excludes: maltreatment syndromes (T74.–)

Z62.0   **Inadequate parental supervision and control**

Lack of parental knowledge of what the child is doing or where the child is; poor control; lack of concern or lack of attempted intervention when the child is in risky situations.

Z62.1 Parental overprotection

Pattern of upbringing resulting in infantilization and prevention of independent behaviour.

Z62.2 Institutional upbringing

Group foster care in which parenting responsibilities are largely taken over by some form of institution (such as a residential nursery, orphanage, or children's home), or therapeutic care over a prolonged period in which the child is in a hospital, convalescent home or the like, without at least one parent living with the child.

Z62.3 Hostility towards and scapegoating of child

Negative parental behaviour specifically focused on the child as an individual, persistent over time and pervasive over several child behaviours (e.g. automatically blaming the child for any problems in the household or attributing negative characteristics to the child).

Z62.4 Emotional neglect of child

Parent talking to the child in a dismissive or insensitive way. Lack of interest in the child, of sympathy for the child's difficulties and of praise and encouragement. Irritated reaction to anxious behaviour and absence of sufficient physical comforting and emotional warmth.

Z62.5 Other problems related to neglect in upbringing

Lack of learning and play experience

Z62.6 Inappropriate parental pressure and other abnormal qualities of upbringing

Parents forcing the child to be different from the local norm, either sex-inappropriate (e.g. dressing a boy in girl's clothes), age-inappropriate (e.g. forcing a child to take on responsibilities above her or his own age) or otherwise inappropriate (e.g. pressing the child to engage in unwanted or too difficult activities).

Z62.8 Other specified problems related to upbringing

Z62.9 Problem related to upbringing, unspecified

Z63 Other problems related to primary support group, including family circumstances

Excludes: maltreatment syndromes (T74.–)

problems related to:

- negative life events in childhood (Z61.–)
- upbringing (Z62.–)

Z63.0 Problems in relationship with spouse or partner

Discord between partners resulting in severe or prolonged loss of control, in generalization of hostile or critical feelings or in a persisting atmosphere of severe interpersonal violence (hitting or striking).

Z63.1 Problems in relationship with parents and in-laws

Z63.2 **Inadequate family support**

Z63.3 **Absence of family member**

Z63.4 **Disappearance and death of family member**
Assumed death of family member

Z63.5 **Disruption of family by separation and divorce**
Estrangement

Z63.6 **Dependent relative needing care at home**

Z63.7 **Other stressful life events affecting family and household**
Anxiety (normal) about sick person in family
Health problems within family
Ill or disturbed family member
Isolated family

Z63.8 **Other specified problems related to primary support group**
Family discord NOS
High expressed emotional level within family
Inadequate or distorted communication within family

Z63.9 **Problem related to primary support group, unspecified**

Z64 Problems related to certain psychosocial circumstances

Z64.0 **Problems related to unwanted pregnancy**
Excludes: supervision of high-risk pregnancy due to social
problems (Z35.7)

Z64.1 **Problems related to multiparity**
Excludes: supervision of pregnancy with grand multiparity
(Z35.4)

Z64.2 **Seeking and accepting physical, nutritional and chemical interventions known to be hazardous and harmful**
Excludes: substance dependence—see Alphabetical Index

Z64.3 **Seeking and accepting behavioural and psychological interventions known to be hazardous and harmful**

Z64.4 **Discord with counsellors**
Discord with:
• probation officer
• social worker

Z65　Problems related to other psychosocial circumstances

Excludes: current injury—see Alphabetical Index

Z65.0　**Conviction in civil and criminal proceedings without imprisonment**

Z65.1　**Imprisonment and other incarceration**

Z65.2　**Problems related to release from prison**

Z65.3　**Problems related to other legal circumstances**
Arrest
Child custody or support proceedings
Litigation
Prosecution

Z65.4　**Victim of crime and terrorism**
Victim of torture

Z65.5　**Exposure to disaster, war and other hostilities**

Excludes: target of perceived discrimination or persecution (Z60.5)

Z65.8　**Other specified problems related to psychosocial circumstances**

Z65.9　**Problem related to unspecified psychosocial circumstances**

Persons encountering health services in other circumstances (Z70–Z76)

Z70　Counselling related to sexual attitude, behaviour and orientation

Excludes: contraceptive or procreative counselling (Z30–Z31)

Z70.0　**Counselling related to sexual attitude**
Person concerned regarding embarrassment, timidity or other negative response to sexual matters

Z70.1 **Counselling related to patient's sexual behaviour and orientation**
Patient concerned regarding:
- impotence
- non-responsiveness
- promiscuity
- sexual orientation

Z70.2 **Counselling related to sexual behaviour and orientation of third party**
Advice sought regarding sexual behaviour and orientation of:
- child
- partner
- spouse

Z70.3 **Counselling related to combined concerns regarding sexual attitude, behaviour and orientation**

Z70.8 **Other sex counselling**
Sex education

Z70.9 **Sex counselling, unspecified**

Z71 Persons encountering health services for other counselling and medical advice, not elsewhere classified

Excludes: contraceptive or procreation counselling (Z30–Z31)
sex counselling (Z70.–)

Z71.0 **Person consulting on behalf of another person**
Advice or treatment for non-attending third party
Excludes: anxiety (normal) about sick person in family (Z63.7)

Z71.1 **Person with feared complaint in whom no diagnosis is made**
Feared condition not demonstrated
Problem was normal state
"Worried well"
Excludes: medical observation and evaluation for suspected diseases and conditions (Z03.–)

Z71.2 **Person consulting for explanation of investigation findings**

Z71.3 **Dietary counselling and surveillance**
Dietary counselling and surveillance (for):
- NOS
- colitis
- diabetes mellitus
- food allergies or intolerance
- gastritis
- hypercholesterolaemia
- obesity

Z71.4 **Alcohol abuse counselling and surveillance**
Excludes: alcohol rehabilitation procedures (Z50.2)

Z71.5 **Drug abuse counselling and surveillance**
Excludes: drug rehabilitation procedures (Z50.3)

Z71.6 **Tobacco abuse counselling**
Excludes: tobacco rehabilitation procedures (Z50.8)

Z71.7 **Human immunodeficiency virus [HIV] counselling**

Z71.8 **Other specified counselling**
Consanguinity counselling

Z71.9 **Counselling, unspecified**
Medical advice NOS

Z72 Problems related to lifestyle
Excludes: problems related to:
- life-management difficulty (Z73.–)
- socioeconomic and psychosocial circumstances
  (Z55–Z65)

Z72.0 **Tobacco use**
Excludes: tobacco dependence (F17.2)

Z72.1 **Alcohol use**
Excludes: alcohol dependence (F10.2)

Z72.2 **Drug use**
Excludes: abuse of non-dependence-producing substances (F55)
drug dependence (F11–F16, F19 with common fourth
character .2)

Z72.3 **Lack of physical exercise**

Z72.4   Inappropriate diet and eating habits
Excludes: behavioural eating disorders of infancy or childhood
  (F98.2–F98.3)
  eating disorders (F50.–)
  lack of adequate food (Z59.4)
  malnutrition and other nutritional deficiencies
  (E40–E64)

Z72.5   High-risk sexual behaviour

Z72.6   Gambling and betting
Excludes: compulsive or pathological gambling (F63.0)

Z72.8   Other problems related to lifestyle
Self-damaging behaviour

Z72.9   Problem related to lifestyle, unspecified

Z73   Problems related to life-management difficulty
Excludes: problems related to socioeconomic and psychosocial
  circumstances (Z55–Z65)

Z73.0   Burn-out
State of vital exhaustion

Z73.1   Accentuation of personality traits
Type A behaviour pattern (characterized by unbridled ambition,
  a need for high achievement, impatience, competitiveness,
  and a sense of urgency)

Z73.2   Lack of relaxation and leisure

Z73.3   Stress, not elsewhere classified
Physical and mental strain NOS
Excludes: related to employment or unemployment (Z56.–)

Z73.4   Inadequate social skills, not elsewhere classified

Z73.5   Social role conflict, not elsewhere classified

Z73.6   Limitation of activities due to disability
Excludes: care-provider dependency (Z74.–)

Z73.8   Other problems related to life-management difficulty

Z73.9   Problem related to life-management difficulty, unspecified

Z74 Problems related to care-provider dependency

Excludes: dependence on enabling machines or devices NEC (Z99.–)

Z74.0 Reduced mobility
Bedfast
Chairfast

Z74.1 Need for assistance with personal care

Z74.2 Need for assistance at home and no other household member able to render care

Z74.3 Need for continuous supervision

Z74.8 Other problems related to care-provider dependency

Z74.9 Problem related to care-provider dependency, unspecified

Z75 Problems related to medical facilities and other health care

Z75.0 Medical services not available in home
Excludes: no other household member able to render care (Z74.2)

Z75.1 Person awaiting admission to adequate facility elsewhere

Z75.2 Other waiting period for investigation and treatment

Z75.3 Unavailability and inaccessibility of health-care facilities
Excludes: bed unavailable (Z75.1)

Z75.4 Unavailability and inaccessibility of other helping agencies

Z75.5 Holiday relief care
Provision of health-care facilities to a person normally cared for at home, in order to enable relatives to take a vacation.
Respite care

Z75.8 Other problems related to medical facilities and other health care

Z75.9 Unspecified problem related to medical facilities and other health care

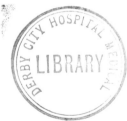

Z76 Persons encountering health services in other circumstances

Z76.0 **Issue of repeat prescription**

Issue of repeat prescription for:
- appliance
- medicaments
- spectacles

Excludes: issue of medical certificate (Z02.7)

repeat prescription for contraceptive (Z30.4)

Z76.1 **Health supervision and care of foundling**

Z76.2 **Health supervision and care of other healthy infant and child**

Medical or nursing care or supervision of healthy infant under circumstances such as:
- adverse socioeconomic conditions at home
- awaiting foster or adoptive placement
- maternal illness
- number of children at home preventing or interfering with normal care

Z76.3 **Healthy person accompanying sick person**

Z76.4 **Other boarder in health-care facility**

Excludes: homelessness (Z59.0)

Z76.5 **Malingerer [conscious simulation]**

Person feigning illness (with obvious motivation)

Excludes: factitious disorder (F68.1)

peregrinating patient (F68.1)

Z76.8 **Persons encountering health services in other specified circumstances**

Z76.9 **Person encountering health services in unspecified circumstances**

Persons with potential health hazards related to family and personal history and certain conditions influencing health status (Z80–Z99)

Excludes: follow-up examination (Z08–Z09)
follow-up medical care and convalescence (Z42–Z51, Z54.–)
when family or personal history is the reason for special
screening or other examination or investigation (Z00–Z13)
when the possibility that the fetus might be affected is the
reason for observation or action during pregnancy (O35.–)

Z80 Family history of malignant neoplasm

Z80.0 Family history of malignant neoplasm of digestive organs
Conditions classifiable to C15–C26

Z80.1 Family history of malignant neoplasm of trachea, bronchus and lung
Conditions classifiable to C33–C34

Z80.2 Family history of malignant neoplasm of other respiratory and intrathoracic organs
Conditions classifiable to C30–C32, C37–C39

Z80.3 Family history of malignant neoplasm of breast
Conditions classifiable to C50.–

Z80.4 Family history of malignant neoplasm of genital organs
Conditions classifiable to C51–C63

Z80.5 Family history of malignant neoplasm of urinary tract
Conditions classifiable to C64–C68

Z80.6 Family history of leukaemia
Conditions classifiable to C91–C95

Z80.7 Family history of other malignant neoplasms of lymphoid, haematopoietic and related tissues
Conditions classifiable to C81–C90, C96.–

Z80.8 Family history of malignant neoplasm of other organs or systems
Conditions classifiable to C00–C14, C40–C49, C69–C79, C97

Z80.9 Family history of malignant neoplasm, unspecified
Conditions classifiable to C80

Z81   Family history of mental and behavioural disorders

Z81.0   **Family history of mental retardation**
Conditions classifiable to F70–F79

Z81.1   **Family history of alcohol abuse**
Conditions classifiable to F10.–

Z81.2   **Family history of tobacco abuse**
Conditions classifiable to F17.–

Z81.3   **Family history of other psychoactive substance abuse**
Conditions classifiable to F11–F16, F18–F19

Z81.4   **Family history of other substance abuse**
Conditions classifiable to F55

Z81.8   **Family history of other mental and behavioural disorders**
Conditions classifiable elsewhere in F00–F99

Z82   Family history of certain disabilities and chronic diseases leading to disablement

Z82.0   **Family history of epilepsy and other diseases of the nervous system**
Conditions classifiable to G00–G99

Z82.1   **Family history of blindness and visual loss**
Conditions classifiable to H54.–

Z82.2   **Family history of deafness and hearing loss**
Conditions classifiable to H90–H91

Z82.3   **Family history of stroke**
Conditions classifiable to I60–I64

Z82.4   **Family history of ischaemic heart disease and other diseases of the circulatory system**
Conditions classifiable to I00–I52, I65–I99

Z82.5   **Family history of asthma and other chronic lower respiratory diseases**
Conditions classifiable to J40–J47

Z82.6   **Family history of arthritis and other diseases of the musculoskeletal system and connective tissue**
Conditions classifiable to M00–M99

Z82.7 **Family history of congenital malformations, deformations and chromosomal abnormalities**
Conditions classifiable to Q00–Q99

Z82.8 **Family history of other disabilities and chronic diseases leading to disablement, not elsewhere classified**

Z83 Family history of other specific disorders

Excludes: contact with or exposure to communicable disease in the family (Z20.–)

Z83.0 **Family history of human immunodeficiency virus [HIV] disease**
Conditions classifiable to B20–B24

Z83.1 **Family history of other infectious and parasitic diseases**
Conditions classifiable to A00–B19, B25–B94, B99

Z83.2 **Family history of diseases of the blood and blood-forming organs and certain disorders involving the immune mechanism**
Conditions classifiable to D50–D89

Z83.3 **Family history of diabetes mellitus**
Conditions classifiable to E10–E14

Z83.4 **Family history of other endocrine, nutritional and metabolic diseases**
Conditions classifiable to E00–E07, E15–E90

Z83.5 **Family history of eye and ear disorders**
Conditions classifiable to H00–H53, H55–H83, H92–H95
Excludes: family history of:
- blindness and visual loss (Z82.1)
- deafness and hearing loss (Z82.2)

Z83.6 **Family history of diseases of the respiratory system**
Conditions classifiable to J00–J39, J60–J99
Excludes: family history of chronic lower respiratory diseases (Z82.5)

Z83.7 **Family history of diseases of the digestive system**
Conditions classifiable to K00–K93

Z84 Family history of other conditions

Z84.0 **Family history of diseases of the skin and subcutaneous tissue**
Conditions classifiable to L00–L99

Z84.1 **Family history of disorders of kidney and ureter**
Conditions classifiable to N00–N29

Z84.2 **Family history of other diseases of the genitourinary system**
Conditions classifiable to N30–N99

Z84.3 **Family history of consanguinity**

Z84.8 **Family history of other specified conditions**

Z85 Personal history of malignant neoplasm

Excludes: follow-up medical care and convalescence (Z42–Z51, Z54.–)
follow-up examination after treatment of malignant neoplasm (Z08.–)

Z85.0 **Personal history of malignant neoplasm of digestive organs**
Conditions classifiable to C15–C26

Z85.1 **Personal history of malignant neoplasm of trachea, bronchus and lung**
Conditions classifiable to C33–C34

Z85.2 **Personal history of malignant neoplasm of other respiratory and intrathoracic organs**
Conditions classifiable to C30–C32, C37–C39

Z85.3 **Personal history of malignant neoplasm of breast**
Conditions classifiable to C50.–

Z85.4 **Personal history of malignant neoplasm of genital organs**
Conditions classifiable to C51–C63

Z85.5 **Personal history of malignant neoplasm of urinary tract**
Conditions classifiable to C64–C68

Z85.6 **Personal history of leukaemia**
Conditions classifiable to C91–C95

Z85.7 **Personal history of other malignant neoplasms of lymphoid, haematopoietic and related tissues**
Conditions classifiable to C81–C90, C96.–

Z85.8 **Personal history of malignant neoplasms of other organs and systems**
Conditions classifiable to C00–C14, C40–C49, C69–C79, C97

Z85.9 **Personal history of malignant neoplasm, unspecified**
Conditions classifiable to C80

Z86   Personal history of certain other diseases

Excludes: follow-up medical care and convalescence (Z42–Z51, Z54.–)

Z86.0 **Personal history of other neoplasms**
Conditions classifiable to D00–D48
Excludes: malignant neoplasms (Z85.–)

Z86.1 **Personal history of infectious and parasitic diseases**
Conditions classifiable to A00–B89, B99
Excludes: sequelae of infectious and parasitic diseases (B90–B94)

Z86.2 **Personal history of diseases of the blood and blood-forming organs and certain disorders involving the immune mechanism**
Conditions classifiable to D50–D89

Z86.3 **Personal history of endocrine, nutritional and metabolic diseases**
Conditions classifiable to E00–E90

Z86.4 **Personal history of psychoactive substance abuse**
Conditions classifiable to F10–F19
Excludes: current dependence (F10–F19 with common fourth character .2)
problems related to use of:
- alcohol (Z72.1)
- drug (Z72.2)
- tobacco (Z72.0)

Z86.5 **Personal history of other mental and behavioural disorders**
Conditions classifiable to F00–F09, F20–F99

Z86.6 **Personal history of diseases of the nervous system and sense organs**
Conditions classifiable to G00–G99, H00–H95

Z86.7   **Personal history of diseases of the circulatory system**
Conditions classifiable to I00–I99
Excludes: old myocardial infarction (I25.2)
postmyocardial infarction syndrome (I24.1)
sequelae of cerebrovascular disease (I69.–)

Z87   Personal history of other diseases and conditions
Excludes: follow-up medical care and convalescence (Z42–Z51,
Z54.–)

Z87.0   **Personal history of diseases of the respiratory system**
Conditions classifiable to J00–J99

Z87.1   **Personal history of diseases of the digestive system**
Conditions classifiable to K00–K93

Z87.2   **Personal history of diseases of the skin and subcutaneous tissue**
Conditions classifiable to L00–L99

Z87.3   **Personal history of diseases of the musculoskeletal system and connective tissue**
Conditions classifiable to M00–M99

Z87.4   **Personal history of diseases of the genitourinary system**
Conditions classifiable to N00–N99

Z87.5   **Personal history of complications of pregnancy, childbirth and the puerperium**
Conditions classifiable to O00–O99
Personal history of trophoblastic disease
Excludes: habitual aborter (N96)
supervision during current pregnancy of a woman
with poor obstetric history (Z35.–)

Z87.6   **Personal history of certain conditions arising in the perinatal period**
Conditions classifiable to P00–P96

Z87.7   **Personal history of congenital malformations, deformations and chromosomal abnormalities**
Conditions classifiable to Q00–Q99

Z87.8   **Personal history of other specified conditions**
Conditions classifiable to S00–T98

Z88   Personal history of allergy to drugs, medicaments and biological substances

Z88.0	**Personal history of allergy to penicillin**
Z88.1	**Personal history of allergy to other antibiotic agents**
Z88.2	**Personal history of allergy to sulfonamides**
Z88.3	**Personal history of allergy to other anti-infective agents**
Z88.4	**Personal history of allergy to anaesthetic agent**
Z88.5	**Personal history of allergy to narcotic agent**
Z88.6	**Personal history of allergy to analgesic agent**
Z88.7	**Personal history of allergy to serum and vaccine**
Z88.8	**Personal history of allergy to other drugs, medicaments and biological substances**
Z88.9	**Personal history of allergy to unspecified drugs, medicaments and biological substances**

Z89   Acquired absence of limb

Includes: loss of limb:
- postoperative
- post-traumatic

Excludes: acquired deformities of limbs (M20–M21)
congenital absence of limbs (Q71–Q73)

Z89.0	**Acquired absence of finger(s) [including thumb], unilateral**
Z89.1	**Acquired absence of hand and wrist**
Z89.2	**Acquired absence of upper limb above wrist** Arm NOS
Z89.3	**Acquired absence of both upper limbs [any level]** Acquired absence of finger(s), bilateral
Z89.4	**Acquired absence of foot and ankle** Toe(s)
Z89.5	**Acquired absence of leg at or below knee**
Z89.6	**Acquired absence of leg above knee** Leg NOS
Z89.7	**Acquired absence of both lower limbs [any level, except toes alone]**

Z89.8   Acquired absence of upper and lower limbs [any level]

Z89.9   Acquired absence of limb, unspecified

Z90 Acquired absence of organs, not elsewhere classified

Includes: postoperative or post-traumatic loss of body part NEC

Excludes: congenital absence—see Alphabetical Index
postoperative absence of:
• endocrine glands (E89.–)
• spleen (D73.0)

Z90.0   Acquired absence of part of head and neck
Eye
Larynx
Nose

Excludes: teeth (K08.1)

Z90.1   Acquired absence of breast(s)

Z90.2   Acquired absence of lung [part of]

Z90.3   Acquired absence of part of stomach

Z90.4   Acquired absence of other parts of digestive tract

Z90.5   Acquired absence of kidney

Z90.6   Acquired absence of other parts of urinary tract

Z90.7   Acquired absence of genital organ(s)

Z90.8   Acquired absence of other organs

Z91 Personal history of risk-factors, not elsewhere classified

Excludes: exposure to pollution and other problems related to physical environment (Z58.–)
occupational exposure to risk-factors (Z57.–)
personal history of psychoactive substance abuse (Z86.4)

Z91.0   Personal history of allergy, other than to drugs and biological substances

Excludes: personal history of allergy to drugs and biological substances (Z88.–)

Z91.1   **Personal history of noncompliance with medical treatment and regimen**

Z91.2   **Personal history of poor personal hygiene**

Z91.3   **Personal history of unhealthy sleep–wake schedule**
Excludes: sleep disorders (G47.–)

Z91.4   **Personal history of psychological trauma, not elsewhere classified**

Z91.5   **Personal history of self-harm**
Parasuicide
Self-poisoning
Suicide attempt

Z91.6   **Personal history of other physical trauma**

Z91.8   **Personal history of other specified risk-factors, not elsewhere classified**
Abuse NOS
Maltreatment NOS

Z92   Personal history of medical treatment

Z92.0   **Personal history of contraception**
Excludes: counselling or management of current contraceptive practices (Z30.–)
presence of (intrauterine) contraceptive device (Z97.5)

Z92.1   **Personal history of long-term (current) use of anticoagulants**

Z92.2   **Personal history of long-term (current) use of other medicaments**
Aspirin

Z92.3   **Personal history of irradiation**
Therapeutic radiation
Excludes: exposure to radiation in the physical environment (Z58.4)
occupational exposure to radiation (Z57.1)

Z92.4   **Personal history of major surgery, not elsewhere classified**
Excludes: artificial opening status (Z93.–)
postsurgical states (Z98.–)
presence of functional implants and grafts (Z95–Z96)
transplanted organ or tissue status (Z94.–)

Z92.5   **Personal history of rehabilitation measures**

Z92.8   **Personal history of other medical treatment**

Z92.9   **Personal history of medical treatment, unspecified**

Z93   Artificial opening status

> *Excludes:* artificial openings requiring attention or management
> (Z43.–)
> complications of external stoma (J95.0, K91.4, N99.5)

Z93.0   **Tracheostomy status**

Z93.1   **Gastrostomy status**

Z93.2   **Ileostomy status**

Z93.3   **Colostomy status**

Z93.4   **Other artificial openings of gastrointestinal tract status**

Z93.5   **Cystostomy status**

Z93.6   **Other artificial openings of urinary tract status**
Nephrostomy
Ureterostomy
Urethrostomy

Z93.8   **Other artificial opening status**

Z93.9   **Artificial opening status, unspecified**

Z94   Transplanted organ and tissue status

> *Includes:* organ or tissue replaced by heterogenous or
> homogenous transplant
> *Excludes:* complications of transplanted organ or tissue—see
> Alphabetical Index
> presence of:
> • vascular graft (Z95.–)
> • xenogenic heart valve (Z95.3)

Z94.0   **Kidney transplant status**

Z94.1   **Heart transplant status**

> *Excludes:* heart-valve replacement status (Z95.2–Z95.4)

Z94.2   **Lung transplant status**

Z94.3　　**Heart and lungs transplant status**

Z94.4　　**Liver transplant status**

Z94.5　　**Skin transplant status**
Autogenous skin transplant status

Z94.6　　**Bone transplant status**

Z94.7　　**Corneal transplant status**

Z94.8　　**Other transplanted organ and tissue status**
Bone marrow
Intestine
Pancreas

Z94.9　　**Transplanted organ and tissue status, unspecified**

Z95　Presence of cardiac and vascular implants and grafts

Excludes:　complications of cardiac and vascular devices,
　　　　　　implants and grafts (T82.–)

Z95.0　　**Presence of cardiac pacemaker**

Excludes:　adjustment or management of cardiac pacemaker
　　　　　　(Z45.0)

Z95.1　　**Presence of aortocoronary bypass graft**

Z95.2　　**Presence of prosthetic heart valve**

Z95.3　　**Presence of xenogenic heart valve**

Z95.4　　**Presence of other heart-valve replacement**

Z95.5　　**Presence of coronary angioplasty implant and graft**
Presence of coronary artery prosthesis
Status following coronary angioplasty NOS

Z95.8　　**Presence of other cardiac and vascular implants and grafts**
Presence of intravascular prosthesis NEC
Status following peripheral angioplasty NOS

Z95.9　　**Presence of cardiac and vascular implant and graft,
unspecified**

Z96 Presence of other functional implants

Excludes: complications of internal prosthetic devices, implants
and grafts (T82–T85)
fitting and adjustment of prosthetic and other devices
(Z44–Z46)

Z96.0 **Presence of urogenital implants**

Z96.1 **Presence of intraocular lens**
Pseudophakia

Z96.2 **Presence of otological and audiological implants**
Bone-conduction hearing device
Cochlear implant
Eustachian tube stent
Myringotomy tube(s)
Stapes replacement

Z96.3 **Presence of artificial larynx**

Z96.4 **Presence of endocrine implants**
Insulin pump

Z96.5 **Presence of tooth-root and mandibular implants**

Z96.6 **Presence of orthopaedic joint implants**
Finger-joint replacement
Hip-joint replacement (partial)(total)

Z96.7 **Presence of other bone and tendon implants**
Skull plate

Z96.8 **Presence of other specified functional implants**

Z96.9 **Presence of functional implant, unspecified**

Z97 Presence of other devices

Excludes: complications of internal prosthetic devices, implants
and grafts (T82–T85)
fitting and adjustment of prosthetic and other devices
(Z44–Z46)
presence of cerebrospinal fluid drainage device
(Z98.2)

Z97.0 **Presence of artificial eye**

Z97.1 **Presence of artificial limb (complete)(partial)**

Z97.2   Presence of dental prosthetic device (complete)(partial)

Z97.3   Presence of spectacles and contact lenses

Z97.4   Presence of external hearing-aid

Z97.5   Presence of (intrauterine) contraceptive device

Excludes: checking, reinsertion or removal of contraceptive device (Z30.5)

insertion of contraceptive device (Z30.1)

Z97.8   Presence of other specified devices

Z98 Other postsurgical states

Excludes: follow-up medical care and convalescence (Z42–Z51, Z54.–)

postprocedural or postoperative complication—see Alphabetical Index

Z98.0   Intestinal bypass and anastomosis status

Z98.1   Arthrodesis status

Z98.2   Presence of cerebrospinal fluid drainage device
CSF shunt

Z98.8   Other specified postsurgical states

Z99 Dependence on enabling machines and devices, not elsewhere classified

Z99.0   Dependence on aspirator

Z99.1   Dependence on respirator

Z99.2   Dependence on renal dialysis
Presence of arteriovenous shunt for dialysis
Renal dialysis status
Excludes: dialysis preparation, treatment or session (Z49.–)

Z99.3   Dependence on wheelchair

Z99.8   Dependence on other enabling machines and devices

Z99.9   Dependence on unspecified enabling machine and device

Morphology of neoplasms

Morphology of neoplasms

The second edition of the International Classification of Diseases for Oncology (ICD-O) was published in 1990. It contains a coded nomenclature for the morphology of neoplasms, which is reproduced here for those who wish to use it in conjunction with Chapter II.

The morphology code numbers consist of five digits; the first four identify the histological type of the neoplasm and the fifth, following a slash or solidus, indicates its behaviour. The one-digit behaviour code is as follows:

/0 Benign

/1 Uncertain whether benign or malignant
Borderline malignancy[1]
Low malignant potential[1]

/2 Carcinoma in situ
Intraepithelial
Noninfiltrating
Noninvasive

/3 Malignant, primary site

/6 Malignant, metastatic site
Malignant, secondary site

/9 Malignant, uncertain whether primary or metastatic site

In the nomenclature given here, the morphology code numbers include the behaviour code appropriate to the histological type of neoplasm; this behaviour code should be changed if the other reported information makes this appropriate. For example, chordoma is assumed to be malignant and is therefore assigned the code number M9370/3; the term "benign chordoma" should, however, be coded M9370/0. Similarly, superficial spreading adenocarcinoma (M8143/3) should be coded M8143/2 when described as "noninvasive", and melanoma (M8720/3), when described as "secondary",

---

[1] Except cystadenomas of ovary in M844–M849, which are considered to be malignant.

1179

should be coded M8720/6.

The following table shows the correspondence between the behaviour code and the different sections of Chapter II:

Behaviour code		Chapter II categories
/0	Benign neoplasms	D10–D36
/1	Neoplasms of uncertain or unknown behaviour	D37–D48
/2	In situ neoplasms	D00–D09
/3	Malignant neoplasms, stated or presumed to be primary	C00–C76 C80–C97
/6	Malignant neoplasms, stated or presumed to be secondary	C77–C79

The ICD-O behaviour digit /9 is not applicable in the ICD context, since all malignant neoplasms are presumed to be primary (/3) or secondary (/6), according to other information on the medical record.

Only the first-listed term of the full ICD-O morphology nomenclature appears against each code number in the list given here. The Alphabetical Index (Volume 3) however, includes all the ICD-O synonyms as well as a number of other morphological descriptions still likely to be encountered on medical records but omitted from ICD-O as outdated or otherwise undesirable.

Some types of neoplasm are specific to certain sites or types of tissue. For example, nephroblastoma (M8960/3), by definition, always arises in the kidney; hepatocellular carcinoma (M8170/3) is always primary in the liver; and basal cell carcinoma (M8090/3) usually arises in the skin. For such terms the appropriate code from Chapter II has been added in parentheses in the nomenclature. Thus nephroblastoma is followed by the code for malignant neoplasm of kidney (C64). For basal cell carcinoma the code for malignant neoplasm of skin (C44.–) is given with the fourth character left open. The appropriate fourth character for the reported site should be used. The Chapter II codes assigned to the morphologic terms should be used when the site of the neoplasm is not given in the diagnosis. Chapter II codes have not been assigned to many of the morphology terms because the histologic types can arise in more than one organ or type of tissue. For example, "Adenocarcinoma NOS" (M8140/3) has no assigned Chapter II code because it can be primary in many different organs.

Occasionally a problem arises when a site given in a diagnosis is different from the site indicated by the site-specific code. In such instances, the given Chapter II code should be ignored and the appropriate code for the site included in the diagnosis should be used. For example, C50.– (breast) is added to the morphologic term Infiltrating duct carcinoma (M8500/3), because this type of carcinoma usually arises in the breast. However, if the term "Infiltrating duct carcinoma" is used for a primary carcinoma arising in the pancreas, the correct code would be C25.9 (Pancreas, unspecified).

For neoplasms of lymphoid, haematopoietic and related tissue (M959–M998) the relevant codes from C81–C96 and D45–D47 are given. These Chapter II codes should be used irrespective of the stated site of the neoplasm.

A coding difficulty sometimes arises where a morphological diagnosis contains two qualifying adjectives that have different code numbers. An example is "transitional cell epidermoid carcinoma". "Transitional cell carcinoma NOS" is M8120/3 and "epidermoid carcinoma NOS" is M8070/3. In such circumstances, the higher number (M8120/3 in this example) should be used, as it is usually more specific. For other information about the coding of morphology see Volume 2.

Coded nomenclature for morphology of neoplasms

M800 Neoplasms NOS

M8000/0	Neoplasm, benign
M8000/1	Neoplasm, uncertain whether benign or malignant
M8000/3	Neoplasm, malignant
M8000/6	Neoplasm, metastatic
M8001/0	Tumour cells, benign
M8001/1	Tumour cells, uncertain whether benign or malignant
M8001/3	Tumour cells, malignant
M8002/3	Malignant tumour, small cell type
M8003/3	Malignant tumour, giant cell type
M8004/3	Malignant tumour, fusiform cell type

M801–M804 Epithelial neoplasms NOS

M8010/0	Epithelial tumour, benign
M8010/2	Carcinoma in situ NOS

M8010/3	Carcinoma NOS
M8010/6	Carcinoma, metastatic NOS
M8011/0	Epithelioma, benign
M8011/3	Epithelioma, malignant
M8012/3	Large cell carcinoma NOS
M8020/3	Carcinoma, undifferentiated NOS
M8021/3	Carcinoma, anaplastic NOS
M8022/3	Pleomorphic carcinoma
M8030/3	Giant cell and spindle cell carcinoma
M8031/3	Giant cell carcinoma
M8032/3	Spindle cell carcinoma
M8033/3	Pseudosarcomatous carcinoma
M8034/3	Polygonal cell carcinoma
M8040/1	Tumorlet
M8041/3	Small cell carcinoma NOS
M8042/3	Oat cell carcinoma (C34.–)
M8043/3	Small cell carcinoma, fusiform cell (C34.–)
M8044/3	Small cell carcinoma, intermediate cell (C34.–)
M8045/3	Small cell–large cell carcinoma (C34.–)

M805–M808 Squamous cell neoplasms

M8050/0	Papilloma NOS (except Papilloma of urinary bladder M8120/1)
M8050/2	Papillary carcinoma in situ
M8050/3	Papillary carcinoma NOS
M8051/0	Verrucous papilloma
M8051/3	Verrucous carcinoma NOS
M8052/0	Squamous cell papilloma
M8052/3	Papillary squamous cell carcinoma
M8053/0	Inverted papilloma
M8060/0	Papillomatosis NOS
M8070/2	Squamous cell carcinoma in situ NOS
M8070/3	Squamous cell carcinoma NOS
M8070/6	Squamous cell carcinoma, metastatic NOS
M8071/3	Squamous cell carcinoma, keratinizing NOS
M8072/3	Squamous cell carcinoma, large cell, nonkeratinizing
M8073/3	Squamous cell carcinoma, small cell, nonkeratinizing
M8074/3	Squamous cell carcinoma, spindle cell
M8075/3	Adenoid squamous cell carcinoma
M8076/2	Squamous cell carcinoma in situ with questionable stromal invasion (D06.–)
M8076/3	Squamous cell carcinoma, microinvasive (C53.–)
M8077/2	Intraepithelial neoplasia, grade III, of cervix, vulva and vagina

M8080/2	Queyrat's erythroplasia (D07.4)
M8081/2	Bowen's disease
M8082/3	Lymphoepithelial carcinoma

M809–M811 Basal cell neoplasms

M8090/1	Basal cell tumour (D48.5)
M8090/3	Basal cell carcinoma NOS (C44.–)
M8091/3	Multicentric basal cell carcinoma (C44.–)
M8092/3	Basal cell carcinoma, morphoea (C44.–)
M8093/3	Basal cell carcinoma, fibroepithelial (C44.–)
M8094/3	Basosquamous carcinoma (C44.–)
M8095/3	Metatypical carcinoma (C44.–)
M8096/0	Intraepidermal epithelioma of Jadassohn (D23.–)
M8100/0	Trichoepithelioma (D23.–)
M8101/0	Trichofolliculoma (D23.–)
M8102/0	Tricholemmoma (D23.–)
M8110/0	Pilomatrixoma NOS (D23.–)
M8110/3	Pilomatrix carcinoma (C44.–)

M812–M813 Transitional cell papillomas and carcinomas

M8120/0	Transitional cell papilloma NOS
M8120/1	Urothelial papilloma
M8120/2	Transitional cell carcinoma in situ
M8120/3	Transitional cell carcinoma NOS
M8121/0	Schneiderian papilloma
M8121/1	Transitional cell papilloma, inverted
M8121/3	Schneiderian carcinoma
M8122/3	Transitional cell carcinoma, spindle cell
M8123/3	Basaloid carcinoma (C21.1)
M8124/3	Cloacogenic carcinoma (C21.2)
M8130/3	Papillary transitional cell carcinoma

M814–M838 Adenomas and adenocarcinomas

M8140/0	Adenoma NOS
M8140/1	Bronchial adenoma NOS (D38.1)
M8140/2	Adenocarcinoma in situ NOS
M8140/3	Adenocarcinoma NOS
M8140/6	Adenocarcinoma, metastatic NOS
M8141/3	Scirrhous adenocarcinoma
M8142/3	Linitis plastica (C16.–)
M8143/3	Superficial spreading adenocarcinoma
M8144/3	Adenocarcinoma, intestinal type (C16.–)

M8145/3	Carcinoma, diffuse type (C16.–)
M8146/0	Monomorphic adenoma
M8147/0	Basal cell adenoma (D11.–)
M8147/3	Basal cell adenocarcinoma (C07.–, C08.–)
M8150/0	Islet cell adenoma (D13.7)
M8150/3	Islet cell carcinoma (C25.4)
M8151/0	Insulinoma NOS (D13.7)
M8151/3	Insulinoma, malignant (C25.4)
M8152/0	Glucagonoma NOS (D13.7)
M8152/3	Glucagonoma, malignant (C25.4)
M8153/1	Gastrinoma NOS
M8153/3	Gastrinoma, malignant
M8154/3	Mixed islet cell and exocrine adenocarcinoma (C25.–)
M8155/3	Vipoma
M8160/0	Bile duct adenoma (D13.4)
M8160/3	Cholangiocarcinoma (C22.1)
M8161/0	Bile duct cystadenoma
M8161/3	Bile duct cystadenocarcinoma
M8162/3	Klatskin's tumour (C22.1)
M8170/0	Liver cell adenoma (D13.4)
M8170/3	Hepatocellular carcinoma NOS (C22.0)
M8171/3	Hepatocellular carcinoma, fibrolamellar (C22.0)
M8180/3	Combined hepatocellular carcinoma and cholangiocarcinoma (C22.0)
M8190/0	Trabecular adenoma
M8190/3	Trabecular adenocarcinoma
M8191/0	Embryonal adenoma
M8200/0	Eccrine dermal cylindroma (D23.–)
M8200/3	Adenoid cystic carcinoma
M8201/3	Cribriform carcinoma
M8202/0	Microcystic adenoma (D13.7)
M8210/0	Adenomatous polyp NOS
M8210/2	Adenocarcinoma in situ in adenomatous polyp
M8210/3	Adenocarcinoma in adenomatous polyp
M8211/0	Tubular adenoma NOS
M8211/3	Tubular adenocarcinoma
M8220/0	Adenomatous polyposis coli (D12.–)
M8220/3	Adenocarcinoma in adenomatous polyposis coli (C18.–)
M8221/0	Multiple adenomatous polyps
M8221/3	Adenocarcinoma in multiple adenomatous polyps
M8230/3	Solid carcinoma NOS
M8231/3	Carcinoma simplex

M8240/1	Carcinoid tumour NOS, of appendix (D37.3)
M8240/3	Carcinoid tumour NOS (except of appendix M8240/1)
M8241/1	Carcinoid tumour, argentaffin NOS
M8241/3	Carcinoid tumour, argentaffin, malignant
M8243/3	Goblet cell carcinoid (C18.1)
M8244/3	Composite carcinoid
M8245/3	Adenocarcinoid tumour
M8246/3	Neuroendocrine carcinoma
M8247/3	Merkel cell carcinoma (C44.–)
M8248/1	Apudoma
M8250/1	Pulmonary adenomatosis (D38.1)
M8250/3	Bronchiolo-alveolar adenocarcinoma (C34.–)
M8251/0	Alveolar adenoma (D14.3)
M8251/3	Alveolar adenocarcinoma (C34.–)
M8260/0	Papillary adenoma NOS
M8260/3	Papillary adenocarcinoma NOS
M8261/1	Villous adenoma NOS
M8261/2	Adenocarcinoma in situ in villous adenoma
M8261/3	Adenocarcinoma in villous adenoma
M8262/3	Villous adenocarcinoma
M8263/0	Tubulovillous adenoma NOS
M8263/2	Adenocarcinoma in situ in tubulovillous adenoma
M8263/3	Adenocarcinoma in tubulovillous adenoma
M8270/0	Chromophobe adenoma (D35.2)
M8270/3	Chromophobe carcinoma (C75.1)
M8271/0	Prolactinoma (D35.2)
M8280/0	Acidophil adenoma (D35.2)
M8280/3	Acidophil carcinoma (C75.1)
M8281/0	Mixed acidophil-basophil adenoma (D35.2)
M8281/3	Mixed acidophil-basophil carcinoma (C75.1)
M8290/0	Oxyphilic adenoma
M8290/3	Oxyphilic adenocarcinoma
M8300/0	Basophil adenoma (D35.2)
M8300/3	Basophil carcinoma (C75.1)
M8310/0	Clear cell adenoma
M8310/3	Clear cell adenocarcinoma NOS
M8311/1	Hypernephroid tumour
M8312/3	Renal cell carcinoma (C64)
M8313/0	Clear cell adenofibroma
M8314/3	Lipid-rich carcinoma (C50.–)
M8315/3	Glycogen-rich carcinoma (C50.–)
M8320/3	Granular cell carcinoma

M8321/0	Chief cell adenoma (D35.1)
M8322/0	Water-clear cell adenoma (D35.1)
M8322/3	Water-clear cell adenocarcinoma (C75.0)
M8323/0	Mixed cell adenoma
M8323/3	Mixed cell adenocarcinoma
M8324/0	Lipoadenoma
M8330/0	Follicular adenoma (D34)
M8330/3	Follicular adenocarcinoma NOS (C73)
M8331/3	Follicular adenocarcinoma, well differentiated (C73)
M8332/3	Follicular adenocarcinoma, trabecular (C73)
M8333/0	Microfollicular adenoma (D34)
M8334/0	Macrofollicular adenoma (D34)
M8340/3	Papillary carcinoma, follicular variant (C73)
M8350/3	Nonencapsulated sclerosing carcinoma (C73)
M8360/1	Multiple endocrine adenomas
M8361/1	Juxtaglomerular tumour (D41.0)
M8370/0	Adrenal cortical adenoma NOS (D35.0)
M8370/3	Adrenal cortical carcinoma (C74.0)
M8371/0	Adrenal cortical adenoma, compact cell (D35.0)
M8372/0	Adrenal cortical adenoma, heavily pigmented variant (D35.0)
M8373/0	Adrenal cortical adenoma, clear cell (D35.0)
M8374/0	Adrenal cortical adenoma, glomerulosa cell (D35.0)
M8375/0	Adrenal cortical adenoma, mixed cell (D35.0)
M8380/0	Endometrioid adenoma NOS (D27)
M8380/1	Endometrioid adenoma, borderline malignancy (D39.1)
M8380/3	Endometrioid carcinoma (C56)
M8381/0	Endometrioid adenofibroma NOS (D27)
M8381/1	Endometrioid adenofibroma, borderline malignancy (D39.1)
M8381/3	Endometrioid adenofibroma, malignant (C56)

M839–M842 Adnexal and skin appendage neoplasms

M8390/0	Skin appendage adenoma (D23.–)
M8390/3	Skin appendage carcinoma (C44.–)
M8400/0	Sweat gland adenoma (D23.–)
M8400/1	Sweat gland tumour NOS (D48.5)
M8400/3	Sweat gland adenocarcinoma (C44.–)
M8401/0	Apocrine adenoma
M8401/3	Apocrine adenocarcinoma
M8402/0	Eccrine acrospiroma (D23.–)
M8403/0	Eccrine spiradenoma (D23.–)
M8404/0	Hidrocystoma (D23.–)
M8405/0	Papillary hidradenoma (D23.–)

M8406/0   Papillary syringadenoma (D23.–)
M8407/0   Syringoma NOS (D23.–)
M8408/0   Eccrine papillary adenoma (D23.–)
M8410/0   Sebaceous adenoma (D23.–)
M8410/3   Sebaceous adenocarcinoma (C44.–)
M8420/0   Ceruminous adenoma (D23.2)
M8420/3   Ceruminous adenocarcinoma (C44.2)

M843 Mucoepidermoid neoplasms
M8430/1   Mucoepidermoid tumour
M8430/3   Mucoepidermoid carcinoma

M844–M849 Cystic, mucinous and serous neoplasms
M8440/0   Cystadenoma NOS
M8440/3   Cystadenocarcinoma NOS
M8441/0   Serous cystadenoma NOS (D27)
M8441/3   Serous cystadenocarcinoma NOS (C56)
M8442/3   Serous cystadenoma, borderline malignancy (C56)
M8450/0   Papillary cystadenoma NOS (D27)
M8450/3   Papillary cystadenocarcinoma NOS (C56)
M8451/3   Papillary cystadenoma, borderline malignancy (C56)
M8452/1   Papillary cystic tumour (D37.7)
M8460/0   Papillary serous cystadenoma NOS (D27)
M8460/3   Papillary serous cystadenocarcinoma (C56)
M8461/0   Serous surface papilloma (D27)
M8461/3   Serous surface papillary carcinoma (C56)
M8462/3   Papillary serous cystadenoma, borderline malignancy (C56)
M8470/0   Mucinous cystadenoma NOS (D27)
M8470/3   Mucinous cystadenocarcinoma NOS (C56)
M8471/0   Papillary mucinous cystadenoma NOS (D27)
M8471/3   Papillary mucinous cystadenocarcinoma (C56)
M8472/3   Mucinous cystadenoma, borderline malignancy (C56)
M8473/3   Papillary mucinous cystadenoma, borderline malignancy (C56)
M8480/0   Mucinous adenoma
M8480/3   Mucinous adenocarcinoma
M8480/6   Pseudomyxoma peritonei (C78.6)
M8481/3   Mucin-producing adenocarcinoma
M8490/3   Signet ring cell carcinoma
M8490/6   Metastatic signet ring cell carcinoma

M850–M854 Ductal, lobular and medullary neoplasms
M8500/2   Intraductal carcinoma, noninfiltrating NOS

M8500/3	Infiltrating duct carcinoma (C50.–)
M8501/2	Comedocarcinoma, noninfiltrating (D05.–)
M8501/3	Comedocarcinoma NOS (C50.–)
M8502/3	Juvenile carcinoma of breast (C50.–)
M8503/0	Intraductal papilloma
M8503/2	Noninfiltrating intraductal papillary adenocarcinoma (D05.–)
M8503/3	Intraductal papillary adenocarcinoma with invasion (C50.–)
M8504/0	Intracystic papillary adenoma
M8504/2	Noninfiltrating intracystic carcinoma
M8504/3	Intracystic carcinoma NOS
M8505/0	Intraductal papillomatosis NOS
M8506/0	Adenoma of nipple (D24)
M8510/3	Medullary carcinoma NOS
M8511/3	Medullary carcinoma with amyloid stroma (C73)
M8512/3	Medullary carcinoma with lymphoid stroma (C50.–)
M8520/2	Lobular carcinoma in situ (D05.0)
M8520/3	Lobular carcinoma NOS (C50.–)
M8521/3	Infiltrating ductular carcinoma (C50.–)
M8522/2	Intraductal carcinoma and lobular carcinoma in situ (D05.1)
M8522/3	Infiltrating duct and lobular carcinoma (C50.–)
M8530/3	Inflammatory carcinoma (C50.–)
M8540/3	Paget's disease, mammary (C50.–)
M8541/3	Paget's disease and infiltrating duct carcinoma of breast (C50.–)
M8542/3	Paget's disease, extramammary (except Paget's disease of bone)
M8543/3	Paget's disease and intraductal carcinoma of breast (C50.–)

M855 Acinar cell neoplasms

M8550/0	Acinar cell adenoma
M8550/1	Acinar cell tumour
M8550/3	Acinar cell carcinoma

M856–M858 Complex epithelial neoplasms

M8560/3	Adenosquamous carcinoma
M8561/0	Adenolymphoma (D11.–)
M8562/3	Epithelial-myoepithelial carcinoma
M8570/3	Adenocarcinoma with squamous metaplasia
M8571/3	Adenocarcinoma with cartilaginous and osseous metaplasia
M8572/3	Adenocarcinoma with spindle cell metaplasia
M8573/3	Adenocarcinoma with apocrine metaplasia

| M8580/0 | Thymoma, benign (D15.0) |
| M8580/3 | Thymoma, malignant (C37) |

M859–M867 Specialized gonadal neoplasms

M8590/1	Sex cord–stromal tumour
M8600/0	Thecoma NOS (D27)
M8600/3	Thecoma, malignant (C56)
M8601/0	Thecoma, luteinized (D27)
M8602/0	Sclerosing stromal tumour (D27)
M8610/0	Luteoma NOS (D27)
M8620/1	Granulosa cell tumour NOS (D39.1)
M8620/3	Granulosa cell tumour, malignant (C56)
M8621/1	Granulosa cell–theca cell tumour (D39.1)
M8622/1	Juvenile granulosa cell tumour (D39.1)
M8623/1	Sex cord tumour with annular tubules (D39.1)
M8630/0	Androblastoma, benign
M8630/1	Androblastoma NOS
M8630/3	Androblastoma, malignant
M8631/0	Sertoli-Leydig cell tumour
M8632/1	Gynandroblastoma (D39.1)
M8640/0	Sertoli cell tumour NOS
M8640/3	Sertoli cell carcinoma (C62.–)
M8641/0	Sertoli cell tumour with lipid storage (D27)
M8650/0	Leydig cell tumour, benign (D29.2)
M8650/1	Leydig cell tumour NOS (D40.1)
M8650/3	Leydig cell tumour, malignant (C62.–)
M8660/0	Hilus cell tumour (D27)
M8670/0	Lipid cell tumour of ovary (D27)
M8671/0	Adrenal rest tumour

M868–M871 Paragangliomas and glomus tumours

M8680/1	Paraganglioma NOS
M8680/3	Paraganglioma, malignant
M8681/1	Sympathetic paraganglioma
M8682/1	Parasympathetic paraganglioma
M8683/0	Gangliocytic paraganglioma (D13.2)
M8690/1	Glomus jugulare tumour (D44.7)
M8691/1	Aortic body tumour (D44.7)
M8692/1	Carotid body tumour (D44.6)
M8693/1	Extra-adrenal paraganglioma NOS
M8693/3	Extra-adrenal paraganglioma, malignant
M8700/0	Phaeochromocytoma NOS (D35.0)

M8700/3	Phaeochromocytoma, malignant (C74.1)
M8710/3	Glomangiosarcoma
M8711/0	Glomus tumour
M8712/0	Glomangioma
M8713/0	Glomangiomyoma

M872–M879 Naevi and melanomas

M8720/0	Pigmented naevus NOS (D22.–)
M8720/2	Melanoma in situ (D03.–)
M8720/3	Malignant melanoma NOS
M8721/3	Nodular melanoma (C43.–)
M8722/0	Balloon cell naevus (D22.–)
M8722/3	Balloon cell melanoma (C43.–)
M8723/0	Halo naevus (D22.–)
M8723/3	Malignant melanoma, regressing (C43.–)
M8724/0	Fibrous papule of nose (D22.3)
M8725/0	Neuronaevus (D22.–)
M8726/0	Magnocellular naevus (D31.4)
M8727/0	Dysplastic naevus (D22.–)
M8730/0	Nonpigmented naevus (D22.–)
M8730/3	Amelanotic melanoma (C43.–)
M8740/0	Junctional naevus NOS (D22.–)
M8740/3	Malignant melanoma in junctional naevus (C43.–)
M8741/2	Precancerous melanosis NOS (D03.–)
M8741/3	Malignant melanoma in precancerous melanosis (C43.–)
M8742/2	Hutchinson's melanotic freckle NOS (D03.–)
M8742/3	Malignant melanoma in Hutchinson's melanotic freckle (C43.–)
M8743/3	Superficial spreading melanoma (C43.–)
M8744/3	Acral lentiginous melanoma, malignant (C43.–)
M8745/3	Desmoplastic melanoma, malignant (C43.–)
M8750/0	Intradermal naevus (D22.–)
M8760/0	Compound naevus (D22.–)
M8761/1	Giant pigmented naevus NOS (D22.–)
M8761/3	Malignant melanoma in giant pigmented naevus (C43.–)
M8770/0	Epithelioid and spindle cell naevus (D22.–)
M8770/3	Mixed epithelioid and spindle cell melanoma
M8771/0	Epithelioid cell naevus (D22.–)
M8771/3	Epithelioid cell melanoma
M8772/0	Spindle cell naevus (D22.–)
M8772/3	Spindle cell melanoma NOS
M8773/3	Spindle cell melanoma, type A (C69.–)
M8774/3	Spindle cell melanoma, type B (C69.–)

M8780/0	Blue naevus NOS (D22.–)
M8780/3	Blue naevus, malignant (C43.–)
M8790/0	Cellular blue naevus (D22.–)

M880 Soft tissue tumours and sarcomas NOS

M8800/0	Soft tissue tumour, benign
M8800/3	Sarcoma NOS
M8800/6	Sarcomatosis NOS
M8801/3	Spindle cell sarcoma
M8802/3	Giant cell sarcoma (except of bone M9250/3)
M8803/3	Small cell sarcoma
M8804/3	Epithelioid sarcoma

M881–M883 Fibromatous neoplasms

M8810/0	Fibroma NOS
M8810/3	Fibrosarcoma NOS
M8811/0	Fibromyxoma
M8811/3	Fibromyxosarcoma
M8812/0	Periosteal fibroma (D16.–)
M8812/3	Periosteal fibrosarcoma (C40.–, C41.–)
M8813/0	Fascial fibroma
M8813/3	Fascial fibrosarcoma
M8814/3	Infantile fibrosarcoma
M8820/0	Elastofibroma
M8821/1	Aggressive fibromatosis
M8822/1	Abdominal fibromatosis
M8823/1	Desmoplastic fibroma
M8824/1	Myofibromatosis
M8830/0	Fibrous histiocytoma NOS
M8830/1	Atypical fibrous histiocytoma
M8830/3	Fibrous histiocytoma, malignant
M8832/0	Dermatofibroma NOS (D23.–)
M8832/3	Dermatofibrosarcoma NOS (C44.–)
M8833/3	Pigmented dermatofibrosarcoma protuberans

M884 Myxomatous neoplasms

M8840/0	Myxoma NOS
M8840/3	Myxosarcoma
M8841/1	Angiomyxoma

M885–M888 Lipomatous neoplasms

M8850/0	Lipoma NOS (D17.–)

M8850/3	Liposarcoma NOS
M8851/0	Fibrolipoma (D17.–)
M8851/3	Liposarcoma, well differentiated
M8852/0	Fibromyxolipoma (D17.–)
M8852/3	Myxoid liposarcoma
M8853/3	Round cell liposarcoma
M8854/0	Pleomorphic lipoma (D17.–)
M8854/3	Pleomorphic liposarcoma
M8855/3	Mixed liposarcoma
M8856/0	Intramuscular lipoma (D17.–)
M8857/0	Spindle cell lipoma (D17.–)
M8858/3	Dedifferentiated liposarcoma
M8860/0	Angiomyolipoma (D17.–)
M8861/0	Angiolipoma NOS (D17.–)
M8870/0	Myelolipoma (D17.–)
M8880/0	Hibernoma (D17.–)
M8881/0	Lipoblastomatosis (D17.–)

M889–M892 Myomatous neoplasms

M8890/0	Leiomyoma NOS
M8890/1	Leiomyomatosis NOS
M8890/3	Leiomyosarcoma NOS
M8891/0	Epithelioid leiomyoma
M8891/3	Epithelioid leiomyosarcoma
M8892/0	Cellular leiomyoma
M8893/0	Bizarre leiomyoma
M8894/0	Angiomyoma
M8894/3	Angiomyosarcoma
M8895/0	Myoma
M8895/3	Myosarcoma
M8896/3	Myxoid leiomyosarcoma
M8897/1	Smooth muscle tumour NOS
M8900/0	Rhabdomyoma NOS
M8900/3	Rhabdomyosarcoma NOS
M8901/3	Pleomorphic rhabdomyosarcoma
M8902/3	Mixed type rhabdomyosarcoma
M8903/0	Fetal rhabdomyoma
M8904/0	Adult rhabdomyoma
M8910/3	Embryonal rhabdomyosarcoma
M8920/3	Alveolar rhabdomyosarcoma

M893–M899 Complex mixed and stromal neoplasms

M8930/0	Endometrial stromal nodule (D26.1)
M8930/3	Endometrial stromal sarcoma (C54.1)
M8931/1	Endolymphatic stromal myosis (D39.0)
M8932/0	Adenomyoma
M8933/3	Adenosarcoma
M8940/0	Pleomorphic adenoma
M8940/3	Mixed tumour, malignant NOS
M8941/3	Carcinoma in pleomorphic adenoma (C07.–, C08.–)
M8950/3	Müllerian mixed tumour (C54.–)
M8951/3	Mesodermal mixed tumour
M8960/1	Mesoblastic nephroma
M8960/3	Nephroblastoma NOS (C64)
M8963/3	Rhabdoid sarcoma
M8964/3	Clear cell sarcoma of kidney (C64)
M8970/3	Hepatoblastoma (C22.0)
M8971/3	Pancreatoblastoma (C25.–)
M8972/3	Pulmonary blastoma (C34.–)
M8980/3	Carcinosarcoma NOS
M8981/3	Carcinosarcoma, embryonal
M8982/0	Myoepithelioma
M8990/0	Mesenchymoma, benign
M8990/1	Mesenchymoma NOS
M8990/3	Mesenchymoma, malignant
M8991/3	Embryonal sarcoma

M900–M903 Fibroepithelial neoplasms

M9000/0	Brenner tumour NOS (D27)
M9000/1	Brenner tumour, borderline malignancy (D39.1)
M9000/3	Brenner tumour, malignant (C56)
M9010/0	Fibroadenoma NOS (D24)
M9011/0	Intracanalicular fibroadenoma (D24)
M9012/0	Pericanalicular fibroadenoma (D24)
M9013/0	Adenofibroma NOS (D27)
M9014/0	Serous adenofibroma (D27)
M9015/0	Mucinous adenofibroma (D27)
M9016/0	Giant fibroadenoma (D24)
M9020/0	Phyllodes tumour, benign (D24)
M9020/1	Phyllodes tumour NOS (D48.6)
M9020/3	Phyllodes tumour, malignant (C50.–)
M9030/0	Juvenile fibroadenoma (D24)

M904 Synovial-like neoplasms
M9040/0	Synovioma, benign
M9040/3	Synovial sarcoma NOS
M9041/3	Synovial sarcoma, spindle cell
M9042/3	Synovial sarcoma, epithelioid cell
M9043/3	Synovial sarcoma, biphasic
M9044/3	Clear cell sarcoma (except of kidney M8964/3)

M905 Mesothelial neoplasms
M9050/0	Mesothelioma, benign (D19.–)
M9050/3	Mesothelioma, malignant (C45.–)
M9051/0	Fibrous mesothelioma, benign (D19.–)
M9051/3	Fibrous mesothelioma, malignant (C45.–)
M9052/0	Epithelioid mesothelioma, benign (D19.–)
M9052/3	Epithelioid mesothelioma, malignant (C45.–)
M9053/0	Mesothelioma, biphasic, benign (D19.–)
M9053/3	Mesothelioma, biphasic, malignant (C45.–)
M9054/0	Adenomatoid tumour NOS (D19.–)
M9055/1	Cystic mesothelioma

M906–M909 Germ cell neoplasms
M9060/3	Dysgerminoma
M9061/3	Seminoma NOS (C62.–)
M9062/3	Seminoma, anaplastic (C62.–)
M9063/3	Spermatocytic seminoma (C62.–)
M9064/3	Germinoma
M9070/3	Embryonal carcinoma NOS
M9071/3	Endodermal sinus tumour
M9072/3	Polyembryoma
M9073/1	Gonadoblastoma
M9080/0	Teratoma, benign
M9080/1	Teratoma NOS
M9080/3	Teratoma, malignant NOS
M9081/3	Teratocarcinoma
M9082/3	Malignant teratoma, undifferentiated
M9083/3	Malignant teratoma, intermediate
M9084/0	Dermoid cyst NOS
M9084/3	Teratoma with malignant transformation
M9085/3	Mixed germ cell tumour
M9090/0	Struma ovarii NOS (D27)
M9090/3	Struma ovarii, malignant (C56)
M9091/1	Strumal carcinoid (D39.1)

M910 Trophoblastic neoplasms

M9100/0	Hydatidiform mole NOS (O01.9)
M9100/1	Invasive hydatidiform mole (D39.2)
M9100/3	Choriocarcinoma NOS
M9101/3	Choriocarcinoma combined with other germ cell elements
M9102/3	Malignant teratoma, trophoblastic (C62.–)
M9103/0	Partial hydatidiform mole (O01.1)
M9104/1	Placental site trophoblastic tumour (D39.2)

M911 Mesonephromas

M9110/0	Mesonephroma, benign
M9110/1	Mesonephric tumour
M9110/3	Mesonephroma, malignant

M912–M916 Blood vessel tumours

M9120/0	Haemangioma NOS (D18.0)
M9120/3	Haemangiosarcoma
M9121/0	Cavernous haemangioma (D18.0)
M9122/0	Venous haemangioma (D18.0)
M9123/0	Racemose haemangioma (D18.0)
M9124/3	Kupffer cell sarcoma (C22.0)
M9125/0	Epithelioid haemangioma (D18.0)
M9126/0	Histiocytoid haemangioma (D18.0)
M9130/0	Haemangioendothelioma, benign (D18.0)
M9130/1	Haemangioendothelioma NOS
M9130/3	Haemangioendothelioma, malignant
M9131/0	Capillary haemangioma (D18.0)
M9132/0	Intramuscular haemangioma (D18.0)
M9133/1	Epithelioid haemangioendothelioma NOS
M9133/3	Epithelioid haemangioendothelioma, malignant
M9134/1	Intravascular bronchial alveolar tumour (D38.1)
M9140/3	Kaposi's sarcoma (C46.–)
M9141/0	Angiokeratoma (D18.0)
M9142/0	Verrucous keratotic haemangioma (D18.0)
M9150/0	Haemangiopericytoma, benign (D18.0)
M9150/1	Haemangiopericytoma NOS
M9150/3	Haemangiopericytoma, malignant
M9160/0	Angiofibroma NOS (D18.0)
M9161/1	Haemangioblastoma

M917 Lymphatic vessel tumours

M9170/0	Lymphangioma NOS (D18.1)

M9170/3 Lymphangiosarcoma
M9171/0 Capillary lymphangioma (D18.1)
M9172/0 Cavernous lymphangioma (D18.1)
M9173/0 Cystic lymphangioma (D18.1)
M9174/0 Lymphangiomyoma (D18.1)
M9174/1 Lymphangiomyomatosis
M9175/0 Haemolymphangioma (D18.1)

M918–M924 Osseous and chondromatous neoplasms
M9180/0 Osteoma NOS (D16.–)
M9180/3 Osteosarcoma NOS (C40.–, C41.–)
M9181/3 Chondroblastic osteosarcoma (C40.–, C41.–)
M9182/3 Fibroblastic osteosarcoma (C40.–, C41.–)
M9183/3 Telangiectatic osteosarcoma (C40.–, C41.–)
M9184/3 Osteosarcoma in Paget's disease of bone (C40.–, C41.–)
M9185/3 Small cell osteosarcoma (C40.–, C41.–)
M9190/3 Juxtacortical osteosarcoma (C40.–, C41.–)
M9191/0 Osteoid osteoma NOS (D16.–)
M9200/0 Osteoblastoma NOS (D16.–)
M9200/1 Aggressive osteoblastoma (D48.0)
M9210/0 Osteochondroma (D16.–)
M9210/1 Osteochondromatosis NOS (D48.0)
M9220/0 Chondroma NOS (D16.–)
M9220/1 Chondromatosis NOS
M9220/3 Chondrosarcoma NOS (C40.–, C41.–)
M9221/0 Juxtacortical chondroma (D16.–)
M9221/3 Juxtacortical chondrosarcoma (C40.–, C41.–)
M9230/0 Chondroblastoma NOS (D16.–)
M9230/3 Chondroblastoma, malignant (C40.–, C41.–)
M9231/3 Myxoid chondrosarcoma
M9240/3 Mesenchymal chondrosarcoma
M9241/0 Chondromyxoid fibroma (D16.–)

M925 Giant cell tumours
M9250/1 Giant cell tumour of bone NOS (D48.0)
M9250/3 Giant cell tumour of bone, malignant (C40.–, C41.–)
M9251/1 Giant cell tumour of soft parts NOS
M9251/3 Malignant giant cell tumour of soft parts

M926 Miscellaneous bone tumours
M9260/3 Ewing's sarcoma (C40.–, C41.–)
M9261/3 Adamantinoma of long bones (C40.–, C41.–)
M9262/0 Ossifying fibroma (D16.–)

M927–M934 Odontogenic tumours

M9270/0	Odontogenic tumour, benign (D16.4, D16.5)
M9270/1	Odontogenic tumour NOS (D48.0)
M9270/3	Odontogenic tumour, malignant (C41.0, C41.1)
M9271/0	Dentinoma (D16.4, D16.5)
M9272/0	Cementoma NOS (D16.4, D16.5)
M9273/0	Cementoblastoma, benign (D16.4, D16.5)
M9274/0	Cementifying fibroma (D16.4, D16.5)
M9275/0	Gigantiform cementoma (D16.4, D16.5)
M9280/0	Odontoma NOS (D16.4, D16.5)
M9281/0	Compound odontoma (D16.4, D16.5)
M9282/0	Complex odontoma (D16.4, D16.5)
M9290/0	Ameloblastic fibro-odontoma (D16.4, D16.5)
M9290/3	Ameloblastic odontosarcoma (C41.0, C41.1)
M9300/0	Adenomatoid odontogenic tumour (D16.4, D16.5)
M9301/0	Calcifying odontogenic cyst (D16.4, D16.5)
M9302/0	Odontogenic ghost cell tumour (D16.4, D16.5)
M9310/0	Ameloblastoma NOS (D16.4, D16.5)
M9310/3	Ameloblastoma, malignant (C41.0, C41.1)
M9311/0	Odontoameloblastoma (D16.4, D16.5)
M9312/0	Squamous odontogenic tumour (D16.4, D16.5)
M9320/0	Odontogenic myxoma (D16.4, D16.5)
M9321/0	Central odontogenic fibroma (D16.4, D16.5)
M9322/0	Peripheral odontogenic fibroma (D16.4, D16.5)
M9330/0	Ameloblastic fibroma (D16.4, D16.5)
M9330/3	Ameloblastic fibrosarcoma (C41.0, C41.1)
M9340/0	Calcifying epithelial odontogenic tumour (D16.4, D16.5)

M935–M937 Miscellaneous tumours

M9350/1	Craniopharyngioma (D44.4)
M9360/1	Pinealoma (D44.5)
M9361/1	Pineocytoma (D44.5)
M9362/3	Pineoblastoma (C75.3)
M9363/0	Melanotic neuroectodermal tumour
M9364/3	Peripheral neuroectodermal tumour
M9370/3	Chordoma

M938–M948 Gliomas

M9380/3	Glioma, malignant (C71.–)
M9381/3	Gliomatosis cerebri (C71.–)
M9382/3	Mixed glioma (C71.–)
M9383/1	Subependymal glioma (D43.–)

M9384/1	Subependymal giant cell astrocytoma (D43.–)
M9390/0	Choroid plexus papilloma NOS (D33.0)
M9390/3	Choroid plexus papilloma, malignant (C71.5)
M9391/3	Ependymoma NOS (C71.–)
M9392/3	Ependymoma, anaplastic (C71.–)
M9393/1	Papillary ependymoma (D43.–)
M9394/1	Myxopapillary ependymoma (D43.–)
M9400/3	Astrocytoma NOS (C71.–)
M9401/3	Astrocytoma, anaplastic (C71.–)
M9410/3	Protoplasmic astrocytoma (C71.–)
M9411/3	Gemistocytic astrocytoma (C71.–)
M9420/3	Fibrillary astrocytoma (C71.–)
M9421/3	Pilocytic astrocytoma (C71.–)
M9422/3	Spongioblastoma NOS (C71.–)
M9423/3	Spongioblastoma polare (C71.–)
M9424/3	Pleomorphic xanthoastrocytoma (C71.–)
M9430/3	Astroblastoma (C71.–)
M9440/3	Glioblastoma NOS (C71.–)
M9441/3	Giant cell glioblastoma (C71.–)
M9442/3	Gliosarcoma (C71.–)
M9443/3	Primitive polar spongioblastoma (C71.–)
M9450/3	Oligodendroglioma NOS (C71.–)
M9451/3	Oligodendroglioma, anaplastic (C71.–)
M9460/3	Oligodendroblastoma (C71.–)
M9470/3	Medulloblastoma NOS (C71.6)
M9471/3	Desmoplastic medulloblastoma (C71.6)
M9472/3	Medullomyoblastoma (C71.6)
M9473/3	Primitive neuroectodermal tumour (C71.–)
M9480/3	Cerebellar sarcoma NOS (C71.6)
M9481/3	Monstrocellular sarcoma (C71.–)

M949–M952 Neuroepitheliomatous neoplasms

M9490/0	Ganglioneuroma
M9490/3	Ganglioneuroblastoma
M9491/0	Ganglioneuromatosis
M9500/3	Neuroblastoma NOS
M9501/3	Medulloepithelioma NOS
M9502/3	Teratoid medulloepithelioma
M9503/3	Neuroepithelioma NOS
M9504/3	Spongioneuroblastoma
M9505/1	Ganglioglioma
M9506/0	Neurocytoma

M9507/0	Pacinian tumour
M9510/3	Retinoblastoma NOS (C69.2)
M9511/3	Retinoblastoma, differentiated (C69.2)
M9512/3	Retinoblastoma, undifferentiated (C69.2)
M9520/3	Olfactory neurogenic tumour
M9521/3	Esthesioneurocytoma (C30.0)
M9522/3	Esthesioneuroblastoma (C30.0)
M9523/3	Esthesioneuroepithelioma (C30.0)

M953 Meningiomas

M9530/0	Meningioma NOS (D32.–)
M9530/1	Meningiomatosis NOS (D42.–)
M9530/3	Meningioma, malignant (C70.–)
M9531/0	Meningotheliomatous meningioma (D32.–)
M9532/0	Fibrous meningioma (D32.–)
M9533/0	Psammomatous meningioma (D32.–)
M9534/0	Angiomatous meningioma (D32.–)
M9535/0	Haemangioblastic meningioma (D32.–)
M9536/0	Haemangiopericytic meningioma (D32.–)
M9537/0	Transitional meningioma (D32.–)
M9538/1	Papillary meningioma (D42.–)
M9539/3	Meningeal sarcomatosis (C70.–)

M954–M957 Nerve sheath tumours

M9540/0	Neurofibroma NOS
M9540/1	Neurofibromatosis NOS (Q85.0)
M9540/3	Neurofibrosarcoma
M9541/0	Melanotic neurofibroma
M9550/0	Plexiform neurofibroma
M9560/0	Neurilemmoma NOS
M9560/1	Neurinomatosis
M9560/3	Neurilemmoma, malignant
M9561/3	Triton tumour, malignant
M9562/0	Neurothekeoma
M9570/0	Neuroma NOS

M958 Granular cell tumours and alveolar soft part sarcoma

M9580/0	Granular cell tumour NOS
M9580/3	Granular cell tumour, malignant
M9581/3	Alveolar soft part sarcoma

M959–M971 Hodgkin's and non-Hodgkin's lymphoma

M959 Malignant lymphomas NOS or diffuse
M9590/3   Malignant lymphoma NOS (C85.9)
M9591/3   Malignant lymphoma, non-Hodgkin's NOS (C85.9)
M9592/3   Lymphosarcoma NOS (C85.0)
M9593/3   Reticulosarcoma NOS (C83.9)
M9594/3   Microglioma (C85.7)
M9595/3   Malignant lymphoma, diffuse NOS (C83.9)

M965–M966 Hodgkin's disease
M9650/3   Hodgkin's disease NOS (C81.9)
M9652/3   Hodgkin's disease, mixed cellularity NOS (C81.2)
M9653/3   Hodgkin's disease, lymphocytic depletion NOS (C81.3)
M9654/3   Hodgkin's disease, lymphocytic depletion, diffuse fibrosis
             (C81.3)
M9655/3   Hodgkin's disease, lymphocytic depletion, reticular (C81.3)
M9657/3   Hodgkin's disease, lymphocytic predominance NOS (C81.0)
M9658/3   Hodgkin's disease, lymphocytic predominance, diffuse (C81.0)
M9659/3   Hodgkin's disease, lymphocytic predominance, nodular
             (C81.0)
M9660/3   Hodgkin's paragranuloma NOS (C81.7)
M9661/3   Hodgkin's granuloma (C81.7)
M9662/3   Hodgkin's sarcoma (C81.7)
M9663/3   Hodgkin's disease, nodular sclerosis NOS (C81.1)
M9664/3   Hodgkin's disease, nodular sclerosis, cellular phase (C81.1)
M9665/3   Hodgkin's disease, nodular sclerosis, lymphocytic
             predominance (C81.1)
M9666/3   Hodgkin's disease, nodular sclerosis, mixed cellularity (C81.1)
M9667/3   Hodgkin's disease, nodular sclerosis, lymphocytic depletion
             (C81.1)

M967–M968 Malignant lymphoma, diffuse or NOS, specified type
M9670/3   Malignant lymphoma, small lymphocytic NOS (C83.0)
M9671/3   Malignant lymphoma, lymphoplasmacytic (C83.8)
M9672/3   Malignant lymphoma, small cleaved cell, diffuse (C83.1)
M9673/3   Malignant lymphoma, lymphocytic, intermediate
             differentiation, diffuse (C83.8)
M9674/3   Malignant lymphoma, centrocytic (C83.8)
M9675/3   Malignant lymphoma, mixed small and large cell, diffuse
             (C83.2)
M9676/3   Malignant lymphoma, centroblastic-centrocytic, diffuse
             (C83.8)

M9677/3	Malignant lymphomatous polyposis (C83.8)
M9680/3	Malignant lymphoma, large cell, diffuse NOS (C83.3)
M9681/3	Malignant lymphoma, large cell, cleaved, diffuse (C83.3)
M9682/3	Malignant lymphoma, large cell, noncleaved, diffuse (C83.3)
M9683/3	Malignant lymphoma, centroblastic, diffuse (C83.8)
M9684/3	Malignant lymphoma, immunoblastic NOS (C83.4)
M9685/3	Malignant lymphoma, lymphoblastic (C83.5)
M9686/3	Malignant lymphoma, small cell, noncleaved, diffuse (C83.0)
M9687/3	Burkitt's lymphoma NOS (C83.7)

M969 Malignant lymphoma, follicular or nodular, with or without diffuse areas

M9690/3	Malignant lymphoma, follicular NOS (C82.9)
M9691/3	Malignant lymphoma, mixed small cleaved and large cell, follicular (C82.1)
M9692/3	Malignant lymphoma, centroblastic-centrocytic, follicular (C82.7)
M9693/3	Malignant lymphoma, lymphocytic, well differentiated, nodular (C82.7)
M9694/3	Malignant lymphoma, lymphocytic, intermediate differentiation, nodular (C82.7)
M9695/3	Malignant lymphoma, small cleaved cell, follicular (C82.0)
M9696/3	Malignant lymphoma, lymphocytic, poorly differentiated, nodular (C82.7)
M9697/3	Malignant lymphoma, centroblastic, follicular (C82.7)
M9698/3	Malignant lymphoma, large cell, follicular NOS (C82.2)

M970 Specified cutaneous and peripheral T-cell lymphomas

M9700/3	Mycosis fungoides (C84.0)
M9701/3	Sézary's disease (C84.1)
M9702/3	Peripheral T-cell lymphoma NOS (C84.4)
M9703/3	T-zone lymphoma (C84.2)
M9704/3	Lymphoepithelioid lymphoma (C84.3)
M9705/3	Peripheral T-cell lymphoma, AILD (angioimmunoblastic lymphadenopathy with dysproteinaemia) (C84.4)
M9706/3	Peripheral T-cell lymphoma, pleomorphic small cell (C84.4)
M9707/3	Peripheral T-cell lymphoma, pleomorphic medium and large cell (C84.4)
M9709/3	Cutaneous lymphoma (C84.5)

M971 Other specified non-Hodgkin's lymphomas

| M9711/3 | Monocytoid B-cell lymphoma (C85.7) |

M9712/3	Angioendotheliomatosis (C85.7)
M9713/3	Angiocentric T-cell lymphoma (C85.7)
M9714/3	Large cell (Ki-1+) lymphoma (C85.7)

M972 Other lymphoreticular neoplasms

M9720/3	Malignant histiocytosis (C96.1)
M9722/3	Letterer-Siwe disease (C96.0)
M9723/3	True histiocytic lymphoma (C96.3)

M973 Plasma cell tumours

| M9731/3 | Plasmacytoma NOS (C90.2) |
| M9732/3 | Multiple myeloma (C90.0) |

M974 Mast cell tumours

M9740/1	Mastocytoma NOS (D47.0)
M9740/3	Mast cell sarcoma (C96.2)
M9741/3	Malignant mastocytosis (C96.2)

M976 Immunoproliferative diseases

M9760/3	Immunoproliferative disease NOS (C88.9)
M9761/3	Waldenström's macroglobulinaemia (C88.0)
M9762/3	Alpha heavy chain disease (C88.1)
M9763/3	Gamma heavy chain disease (C88.2)
M9764/3	Immunoproliferative small intestinal disease (C88.3)
M9765/1	Monoclonal gammopathy (D47.2)
M9766/1	Angiocentric immunoproliferative lesion (D47.7)
M9767/1	Angioimmunoblastic lymphadenopathy (D47.7)
M9768/1	T-gamma lymphoproliferative disease (D47.7)

M980–M994 Leukaemias

M980 Leukaemias NOS

M9800/3	Leukaemia NOS (C95.9)
M9801/3	Acute leukaemia NOS (C95.0)
M9802/3	Subacute leukaemia NOS (C95.2)
M9803/3	Chronic leukaemia NOS (C95.1)
M9804/3	Aleukaemic leukaemia NOS (C95.7)

M982 Lymphoid leukaemias

M9820/3	Lymphoid leukaemia NOS (C91.9)
M9821/3	Acute lymphoblastic leukaemia NOS (C91.0)
M9822/3	Subacute lymphoid leukaemia (C91.2)

M9823/3   Chronic lymphocytic leukaemia (C91.1)
M9824/3   Aleukaemic lymphoid leukaemia (C91.7)
M9825/3   Prolymphocytic leukaemia (C91.3)
M9826/3   Burkitt's cell leukaemia (C91.7)
M9827/3   Adult T-cell leukaemia/lymphoma (C91.5)

M983 Plasma cell leukaemia
M9830/3   Plasma cell leukaemia (C90.1)

M984 Erythroleukaemias
M9840/3   Erythroleukaemia (C94.0)
M9841/3   Acute erythraemia (C94.0)
M9842/3   Chronic erythraemia (C94.1)

M985 Lymphosarcoma cell leukaemia
M9850/3   Lymphosarcoma cell leukaemia (C94.7)

M986 Myeloid (granulocytic) leukaemias
M9860/3   Myeloid leukaemia NOS (C92.9)
M9861/3   Acute myeloid leukaemia (C92.0)
M9862/3   Subacute myeloid leukaemia (C92.2)
M9863/3   Chronic myeloid leukaemia (C92.1)
M9864/3   Aleukaemic myeloid leukaemia (C92.7)
M9866/3   Acute promyelocytic leukaemia (C92.4)
M9867/3   Acute myelomonocytic leukaemia (C92.5)
M9868/3   Chronic myelomonocytic leukaemia (C92.7)

M987 Basophilic leukaemia
M9870/3   Basophilic leukaemia (C94.7)

M988 Eosinophilic leukaemia
M9880/3   Eosinophilic leukaemia (C94.7)

M989 Monocytic leukaemias
M9890/3   Monocytic leukaemia NOS (C93.9)
M9891/3   Acute monocytic leukaemia (C93.0)
M9892/3   Subacute monocytic leukaemia (C93.2)
M9893/3   Chronic monocytic leukaemia (C93.1)
M9894/3   Aleukaemic monocytic leukaemia (C93.7)

M990–M994 Other leukaemias
M9900/3   Mast cell leukaemia (C94.3)

M9910/3	Acute megakaryoblastic leukaemia (C94.2)
M9930/3	Myeloid sarcoma (C92.3)
M9931/3	Acute panmyelosis (C94.4)
M9932/3	Acute myelofibrosis (C94.5)
M9940/3	Hairy cell leukaemia (C91.4)
M9941/3	Leukaemic reticuloendotheliosis (C91.4)

M995–M997 Miscellaneous myeloproliferative and lymphoproliferative disorders

M9950/1	Polycythaemia vera (D45)
M9960/1	Chronic myeloproliferative disease (D47.1)
M9961/1	Myelosclerosis with myeloid metaplasia (D47.1)
M9962/1	Idiopathic thrombocythaemia (D47.3)
M9970/1	Lymphoproliferative disease NOS (D47.9)

M998 Myelodysplastic syndrome

M9980/1	Refractory anaemia NOS (D46.4)
M9981/1	Refractory anaemia without sideroblasts (D46.0)
M9982/1	Refractory anaemia with sideroblasts (D46.1)
M9983/1	Refractory anaemia with excess of blasts (D46.2)
M9984/1	Refractory anaemia with excess of blasts with transformation (D46.3)
M9989/1	Myelodysplastic syndrome NOS (D46.9)

Special tabulation lists
for mortality
and morbidity

Mortality tabulation lists

List 1—General mortality—condensed list (103 causes)
List 2—General mortality—selected list (80 causes)
List 3—Infant and child mortality—condensed list (67 causes)
List 4—Infant and child mortality—selected list (51 causes)

Tabulation list for morbidity (298 causes)

Special tabulation lists for mortality and morbidity

Note: These lists were adopted by the World Health Assembly in 1990 for the tabulation of data. They are described, and their use is explained, in Volume 2, the Instruction Manual.

Mortality tabulation list 1

General mortality
Condensed list

1–001	**Certain infectious and parasitic diseases**	**A00–B99**
1–002	Cholera	A00
1–003	Diarrhoea and gastroenteritis of presumed infectious origin	A09
1–004	Other intestinal infectious diseases	A01–A08
1–005	Respiratory tuberculosis	A15–A16
1–006	Other tuberculosis	A17–A19
1–007	Plague	A20
1–008	Tetanus	A33–A35
1–009	Diphtheria	A36
1–010	Whooping cough	A37
1–011	Meningococcal infection	A39
1–012	Septicaemia	A40–A41
1–013	Infections with a predominantly sexual mode of transmission	A50–A64
1–014	Acute poliomyelitis	A80
1–015	Rabies	A82
1–016	Yellow fever	A95
1–017	Other arthropod-borne viral fevers and viral haemorrhagic fevers	A90–A94, A96–A99
1–018	Measles	B05
1–019	Viral hepatitis	B15–B19
1–020	Human immunodeficiency virus [HIV] disease	B20–B24
1–021	Malaria	B50–B54
1–022	Leishmaniasis	B55

1–023	Trypanosomiasis	B56–B57
1–024	Schistosomiasis	B65
1–025	Remainder of certain infectious and parasitic diseases	A21–A32, A38, A42–A49, A65–A79, A81, A83–A89, B00–B04, B06–B09, B25–B49, B58–B64, B66–B94, B99
1–026	**Neoplasms**	**C00–D48**
1–027	Malignant neoplasm of lip, oral cavity and pharynx	C00–C14
1–028	Malignant neoplasm of oesophagus	C15
1–029	Malignant neoplasm of stomach	C16
1–030	Malignant neoplasm of colon, rectum and anus	C18–C21
1–031	Malignant neoplasm of liver and intrahepatic bile ducts	C22
1–032	Malignant neoplasm of pancreas	C25
1–033	Malignant neoplasm of larynx	C32
1–034	Malignant neoplasm of trachea, bronchus and lung	C33–C34
1–035	Malignant melanoma of skin	C43
1–036	Malignant neoplasm of breast	C50
1–037	Malignant neoplasm of cervix uteri	C53
1–038	Malignant neoplasm of other and unspecified parts of uterus	C54–C55
1–039	Malignant neoplasm of ovary	C56
1–040	Malignant neoplasm of prostate	C61
1–041	Malignant neoplasm of bladder	C67
1–042	Malignant neoplasm of meninges, brain and other parts of central nervous system	C70–C72
1–043	Non-Hodgkin's lymphoma	C82–C85
1–044	Multiple myeloma and malignant plasma cell neoplasms	C90
1–045	Leukaemia	C91–C95
1–046	Remainder of malignant neoplasms	C17, C23–C24, C26–C31, C37–C41, C44–C49, C51–C52, C57–C60, C62–C66, C68–C69, C73–C81, C88, C96–C97

1–047	Remainder of neoplasms	D00–D48
1–048	**Diseases of the blood and blood-forming organs and certain disorders involving the immune mechanism**	**D50–D89**
1–049	Anaemias	D50–D64
1–050	Remainder of diseases of the blood and blood-forming organs and certain disorders involving the immune mechanism	D65–D89
1–051	**Endocrine, nutritional and metabolic diseases**	**E00–E88**
1–052	Diabetes mellitus	E10–E14
1–053	Malnutrition	E40–E46
1–054	Remainder of endocrine, nutritional and metabolic diseases	E00–E07, E15–E34, E50–E88
1–055	**Mental and behavioural disorders**	**F01–F99**
1–056	Mental and behavioural disorders due to psychoactive substance use	F10–F19
1–057	Remainder of mental and behavioural disorders	F01–F09, F20–F99
1–058	**Diseases of the nervous system**	**G00–G98**
1–059	Meningitis	G00, G03
1–060	Alzheimer's disease	G30
1–061	Remainder of diseases of the nervous system	G04–G25, G31–G98
1–062	**Diseases of the eye and adnexa**	**H00–H57**
1–063	**Diseases of the ear and mastoid process**	**H60–H93**
1–064	**Diseases of the circulatory system**	**I00–I99**
1–065	Acute rheumatic fever and chronic rheumatic heart diseases	I00–I09
1–066	Hypertensive diseases	I10–I14
1–067	Ischaemic heart diseases	I20–I25
1–068	Other heart diseases	I26–I51
1–069	Cerebrovascular diseases	I60–I69
1–070	Atherosclerosis	I70
1–071	Remainder of diseases of the circulatory system	I71–I99
1–072	**Diseases of the respiratory system**	**J00–J98**
1–073	Influenza	J10–J11
1–074	Pneumonia	J12–J18
1–075	Other acute lower respiratory infections	J20–J22
1–076	Chronic lower respiratory diseases	J40–J47
1–077	Remainder of diseases of the respiratory system	J00–J06, J30–J39, J60–J98

1–078	**Diseases of the digestive system**	**K00–K92**
1–079	Gastric and duodenal ulcer	K25–K27
1–080	Diseases of the liver	K70–K76
1–081	Remainder of diseases of the digestive system	K00–K22, K28–K66, K80–K92
1–082	**Diseases of the skin and subcutaneous tissue**	**L00–L98**
1–083	**Diseases of the musculoskeletal system and connective tissue**	**M00–M99**
1–084	**Diseases of the genitourinary system**	**N00–N98**
1–085	Glomerular and renal tubulo-interstitial diseases	N00–N15
1–086	Remainder of diseases of the genitourinary system	N17–N98
1–087	**Pregnancy, childbirth and the puerperium**	**O00–O99**
1–088	Pregnancy with abortive outcome	O00–O07
1–089	Other direct obstetric deaths	O10–O92
1–090	Indirect obstetric deaths	O98–O99
1–091	Remainder of pregnancy, childbirth and the puerperium	O95–O97
1–092	**Certain conditions originating in the perinatal period**	**P00–P96**
1–093	**Congenital malformations, deformations and chromosomal abnormalities**	**Q00–Q99**
1–094	**Symptoms, signs and abnormal clinical and laboratory findings, not elsewhere classified**	**R00–R99**
1–095	**External causes of morbidity and mortality**	**V01–Y89**
1–096	Transport accidents	V01–V99
1–097	Falls	W00–W19
1–098	Accidental drowning and submersion	W65–W74
1–099	Exposure to smoke, fire and flames	X00–X09
1–100	Accidental poisoning by and exposure to noxious substances	X40–X49
1–101	Intentional self-harm	X60–X84
1–102	Assault	X85–Y09
1–103	All other external causes	W20–W64, W75–W99, X10–X39, X50–X59, Y10–Y89

Mortality tabulation list 2

General mortality
Selected list

2–001	Cholera	A00
2–002	Diarrhoea and gastroenteritis of presumed infectious origin	A09
2–003	Other intestinal infectious diseases	A01–A08
2–004	Respiratory tuberculosis	A15–A16
2–005	Other tuberculosis	A17–A19
2–006	Plague	A20
2–007	Tetanus	A33–A35
2–008	Diphtheria	A36
2–009	Whooping cough	A37
2–010	Meningococcal infection	A39
2–011	Septicaemia	A40–A41
2–012	Infections with a predominantly sexual mode of transmission	A50–A64
2–013	Acute poliomyelitis	A80
2–014	Rabies	A82
2–015	Yellow fever	A95
2–016	Other arthropod-borne viral fevers and viral haemorrhagic fevers	A90–A94, A96–A99
2–017	Measles	B05
2–018	Viral hepatitis	B15–B19
2–019	Human immunodeficiency virus [HIV] disease	B20–B24
2–020	Malaria	B50–B54
2–021	Leishmaniasis	B55
2–022	Trypanosomiasis	B56–B57
2–023	Schistosomiasis	B65
2–024	Remainder of certain infectious and parasitic diseases	A21–A32, A38, A42–A49, A65–A79, A81, A83–A89, B00–B04, B06–B09, B25–B49, B58–B64, B66–B94, B99
2–025	Malignant neoplasm of lip, oral cavity and pharynx	C00–C14
2–026	Malignant neoplasm of oesophagus	C15

2–027	Malignant neoplasm of stomach	C16
2–028	Malignant neoplasm of colon, rectum and anus	C18–C21
2–029	Malignant neoplasm of liver and intrahepatic bile ducts	C22
2–030	Malignant neoplasm of pancreas	C25
2–031	Malignant neoplasm of larynx	C32
2–032	Malignant neoplasm of trachea, bronchus and lung	C33–C34
2–033	Malignant melanoma of skin	C43
2–034	Malignant neoplasm of breast	C50
2–035	Malignant neoplasm of cervix uteri	C53
2–036	Malignant neoplasm of other and unspecified parts of uterus	C54–C55
2–037	Malignant neoplasm of ovary	C56
2–038	Malignant neoplasm of prostate	C61
2–039	Malignant neoplasm of bladder	C67
2–040	Malignant neoplasm of meninges, brain and other parts of central nervous system	C70–C72
2–041	Non-Hodgkin's lymphoma	C82–C85
2–042	Multiple myeloma and malignant plasma cell neoplasms	C90
2–043	Leukaemia	C91–C95
2–044	Remainder of malignant neoplasms	C17, C23–C24, C26–C31, C37–C41, C44–C49, C51–C52, C57–C60, C62–C66, C68–C69, C73–C81, C88, C96–C97
2–045	Anaemias	D50–D64
2–046	Diabetes mellitus	E10–E14
2–047	Malnutrition	E40–E46
2–048	Mental and behavioural disorders due to psychoactive substance use	F10–F19
2–049	Meningitis	G00, G03
2–050	Alzheimer's disease	G30
2–051	Acute rheumatic fever and chronic rheumatic heart diseases	I00–I09
2–052	Hypertensive diseases	I10–I14
2–053	Ischaemic heart diseases	I20–I25
2–054	Other heart diseases	I26–I51
2–055	Cerebrovascular diseases	I60–I69

2–056	Atherosclerosis	I70
2–057	Remainder of diseases of the circulatory system	I71–I99
2–058	Influenza	J10–J11
2–059	Pneumonia	J12–J18
2–060	Other acute lower respiratory infections	J20–J22
2–061	Chronic lower respiratory diseases	J40–J47
2–062	Remainder of diseases of the respiratory system	J00–J06, J30–J39, J60–J98
2–063	Gastric and duodenal ulcer	K25–K27
2–064	Diseases of the liver	K70–K76
2–065	Glomerular and renal tubulo-interstitial diseases	N00–N15
2–066	Pregnancy with abortive outcome	O00–O07
2–067	Other direct obstetric deaths	O10–O92
2–068	Indirect obstetric deaths	O98–O99
2–069	Certain conditions originating in the perinatal period	P00–P96
2–070	Congenital malformations, deformations and chromosomal abnormalities	Q00–Q99
2–071	Symptoms, signs and abnormal clinical and laboratory findings, not elsewhere classified	R00–R99
2–072	All other diseases	D00–D48, D65–D89, E00–E07, E15–E34, E50–E88, F01–F09, F20–F99, G04–G25, G31–G98, H00–H93, K00–K22, K28–K66, K80–K92, L00–L98, M00–M99, N17–N98, O95–O97
2–073	Transport accidents	V01–V99
2–074	Falls	W00–W19
2–075	Accidental drowning and submersion	W65–W74
2–076	Exposure to smoke, fire and flames	X00–X09
2–077	Accidental poisoning by and exposure to noxious substances	X40–X49
2–078	Intentional self-harm	X60–X84
2–079	Assault	X85–Y09

2–080   All other external causes

W20–W64, W75–W99, X10–X39, X50–X59, Y10–Y89

Mortality tabulation list 3

Infant and child mortality
Condensed list

3–001	**Certain infectious and parasitic diseases**	**A00–B99**
3–002	Diarrhoea and gastroenteritis of presumed infectious origin	A09
3–003	Other intestinal infectious diseases	A00–A08
3–004	Tuberculosis	A15–A19
3–005	Tetanus	A33, A35
3–006	Diphtheria	A36
3–007	Whooping cough	A37
3–008	Meningococcal infection	A39
3–009	Septicaemia	A40–A41
3–010	Acute poliomyelitis	A80
3–011	Measles	B05
3–012	Human immunodeficiency virus [HIV] disease	B20–B24
3–013	Other viral diseases	A81–B04, B06–B19, B25–B34
3–014	Malaria	B50–B54
3–015	Remainder of certain infectious and parasitic diseases	A20–A32, A38, A42–A79, B35–B49, B55–B94, B99
3–016	**Neoplasms**	**C00–D48**
3–017	Leukaemia	C91–C95
3–018	Remainder of malignant neoplasms	C00–C90, C96–C97
3–019	Remainder of neoplasms	D00–D48
3–020	**Diseases of the blood and blood-forming organs and certain disorders involving the immune mechanism**	**D50–D89**
3–021	Anaemias	D50–D64
3–022	Remainder of diseases of the blood and blood-forming organs and certain disorders involving the immune mechanism	D65–D89
3–023	**Endocrine, nutritional and metabolic diseases**	**E00–E88**
3–024	Malnutrition and other nutritional deficiencies	E40–E64
3–025	Remainder of endocrine, nutritional and metabolic diseases	E00–E34, E65–E88

3–056	**Symptoms, signs and abnormal clinical and laboratory findings, not elsewhere classified**	**R00–R99**
3–057	Sudden infant death syndrome	R95
3–058	Other symptoms, signs and abnormal clinical and laboratory findings, not elsewhere classified	R00–R94, R96–R99
3–059	**All other diseases**	**F01–F99, H00–H59, L00–L98, M00–M99**
3–060	**External causes of morbidity and mortality**	**V01–Y89**
3–061	Transport accidents	V01–V99
3–062	Accidental drowning and submersion	W65–W74
3–063	Other accidental threats to breathing	W75–W84
3–064	Exposure to smoke, fire and flames	X00–X09
3–065	Accidental poisoning by and exposure to noxious substances	X40–X49
3–066	Assault	X85–Y09
3–067	All other external causes	W00–W64, W85–W99, X10–X39, X50–X84, Y10–Y89

Mortality tabulation list 4

Infant and child mortality
Selected list

4–001	Diarrhoea and gastroenteritis of presumed infectious origin	A09
4–002	Other intestinal infectious diseases	A00–A08
4–003	Tuberculosis	A15–A19
4–004	Tetanus	A33, A35
4–005	Diphtheria	A36
4–006	Whooping cough	A37
4–007	Meningococcal infection	A39
4–008	Septicaemia	A40–A41
4–009	Acute poliomyelitis	A80
4–010	Measles	B05
4–011	Human immunodeficiency virus [HIV] disease	B20–B24
4–012	Other viral diseases	A81–B04, B06–B19, B25–B34
4–013	Malaria	B50–B54
4–014	Remainder of certain infectious and parasitic diseases	A20–A32, A38, A42–A79, B35–B49, B55–B94, B99
4–015	Leukaemia	C91–C95
4–016	Remainder of malignant neoplasms	C00–C90, C96–C97
4–017	Anaemias	D50–D64
4–018	Remainder of diseases of the blood and blood-forming organs and certain disorders involving the immune mechanism	D65–D89
4–019	Malnutrition and other nutritional deficiencies	E40–E64
4–020	Meningitis	G00, G03
4–021	Remainder of diseases of the nervous system	G04–G98
4–022	Pneumonia	J12–J18
4–023	Other acute respiratory infections	J00–J11, J20–J22
4–024	Diseases of the digestive system	K00–K92

4–025	Fetus and newborn affected by maternal factors and by complications of pregnancy, labour and delivery	P00–P04
4–026	Disorders relating to length of gestation and fetal growth	P05–P08
4–027	Birth trauma	P10–P15
4–028	Intrauterine hypoxia and birth asphyxia	P20–P21
4–029	Respiratory distress of newborn	P22
4–030	Congenital pneumonia	P23
4–031	Other respiratory conditions of newborn	P24–P28
4–032	Bacterial sepsis of newborn	P36
4–033	Omphalitis of newborn with or without mild haemorrhage	P38
4–034	Haemorrhagic and haematological disorders of fetus and newborn	P50–P61
4–035	Remainder of perinatal conditions	P29, P35, P37, P39, P70–P96
4–036	Congenital hydrocephalus and spina bifida	Q03, Q05
4–037	Other congenital malformations of the nervous system	Q00–Q02, Q04, Q06–Q07
4–038	Congenital malformations of the heart	Q20–Q24
4–039	Other congenital malformations of the circulatory system	Q25–Q28
4–040	Down's syndrome and other chromosomal abnormalities	Q90–Q99
4–041	Other congenital malformations	Q10–Q18, Q30–Q89
4–042	Sudden infant death syndrome	R95
4–043	Other symptoms, signs and abnormal clinical and laboratory findings, not elsewhere classified	R00–R94, R96–R99
4–044	All other diseases	D00–D48, E00–E34, E65–E88, F01–F99, H00–H95, I00–I99, J30–J98, L00–L98, M00–M99, N00–N98
4–045	Transport accidents	V01–V99
4–046	Accidental drowning and submersion	W65–W74
4–047	Other accidental threats to breathing	W75–W84
4–048	Exposure to smoke, fire and flames	X00–X09
4–049	Accidental poisoning by and exposure to noxious substances	X40–X49

| 4–050 | Assault | X85–Y09 |
| 4–051 | All other external causes | W00–W64, W85–W99, X10–X39, X50–X84, Y10–Y89 |

Tabulation list for morbidity

001	Cholera	A00
002	Typhoid and paratyphoid fevers	A01
003	Shigellosis	A03
004	Amoebiasis	A06
005	Diarrhoea and gastroenteritis of presumed infectious origin	A09
006	Other intestinal infectious diseases	A02, A04–A05, A07–A08
007	Respiratory tuberculosis	A15–A16
008	Other tuberculosis	A17–A19
009	Plague	A20
010	Brucellosis	A23
011	Leprosy	A30
012	Tetanus neonatorum	A33
013	Other tetanus	A34–A35
014	Diphtheria	A36
015	Whooping cough	A37
016	Meningococcal infection	A39
017	Septicaemia	A40–A41
018	Other bacterial diseases	A21–A22, A24–A28, A31–A32, A38, A42–A49
019	Congenital syphilis	A50
020	Early syphilis	A51
021	Other syphilis	A52–A53
022	Gonococcal infection	A54
023	Sexually transmitted chlamydial diseases	A55–A56
024	Other infections with a predominantly sexual mode of transmission	A57–A64
025	Relapsing fevers	A68
026	Trachoma	A71
027	Typhus fever	A75
028	Acute poliomyelitis	A80
029	Rabies	A82
030	Viral encephalitis	A83–A86
031	Yellow fever	A95
032	Other arthropod-borne viral fevers and viral haemorrhagic fevers	A90–A94, A96–A99
033	Herpesviral infections	B00
034	Varicella and zoster	B01–B02

035	Measles	B05
036	Rubella	B06
037	Acute hepatitis B	B16
038	Other viral hepatitis	B15, B17–B19
039	Human immunodeficiency virus [HIV] disease	B20–B24
040	Mumps	B26
041	Other viral diseases	A81, A87–A89, B03–B04, B07–B09, B25, B27–B34
042	Mycoses	B35–B49
043	Malaria	B50–B54
044	Leishmaniasis	B55
045	Trypanosomiasis	B56–B57
046	Schistosomiasis	B65
047	Other fluke infections	B66
048	Echinococcosis	B67
049	Dracunculiasis	B72
050	Onchocerciasis	B73
051	Filariasis	B74
052	Hookworm diseases	B76
053	Other helminthiases	B68–B71, B75, B77–B83
054	Sequelae of tuberculosis	B90
055	Sequelae of poliomyelitis	B91
056	Sequelae of leprosy	B92
057	Other infectious and parasitic diseases	A65–A67, A69–A70, A74, A77–A79, B58–B64, B85–B89, B94, B99
058	Malignant neoplasm of lip, oral cavity and pharynx	C00–C14
059	Malignant neoplasm of oesophagus	C15
060	Malignant neoplasm of stomach	C16
061	Malignant neoplasm of colon	C18
062	Malignant neoplasm of rectosigmoid junction, rectum, anus and anal canal	C19–C21
063	Malignant neoplasm of liver and intrahepatic bile ducts	C22
064	Malignant neoplasm of pancreas	C25

065	Other malignant neoplasms of digestive organs	C17, C23–C24, C26
066	Malignant neoplasms of larynx	C32
067	Malignant neoplasm of trachea, bronchus and lung	C33–C34
068	Other malignant neoplasms of respiratory and intrathoracic organs	C30–C31, C37–C39
069	Malignant neoplasm of bone and articular cartilage	C40–C41
070	Malignant melanoma of skin	C43
071	Other malignant neoplasms of skin	C44
072	Malignant neoplasms of mesothelial and soft tissue	C45–C49
073	Malignant neoplasm of breast	C50
074	Malignant neoplasm of cervix uteri	C53
075	Malignant neoplasm of other and unspecified parts of uterus	C54–C55
076	Other malignant neoplasms of female genital organs	C51–C52, C56–C58
077	Malignant neoplasm of prostate	C61
078	Other malignant neoplasms of male genital organs	C60, C62–C63
079	Malignant neoplasm of bladder	C67
080	Other malignant neoplasms of urinary tract	C64–C66, C68
081	Malignant neoplasm of eye and adnexa	C69
082	Malignant neoplasm of brain	C71
083	Malignant neoplasm of other parts of central nervous system	C70, C72
084	Malignant neoplasm of other, ill-defined, secondary, unspecified and multiple sites	C73–C80, C97
085	Hodgkin's disease	C81
086	Non-Hodgkin's lymphoma	C82–C85
087	Leukaemia	C91–C95
088	Other malignant neoplasms of lymphoid, haematopoietic and related tissue	C88–C90, C96
089	Carcinoma in situ of cervix uteri	D06
090	Benign neoplasm of skin	D22–D23
091	Benign neoplasm of breast	D24
092	Leiomyoma of uterus	D25
093	Benign neoplasm of ovary	D27
094	Benign neoplasm of urinary organs	D30
095	Benign neoplasm of brain and other parts of central nervous system	D33

096	Other in situ and benign neoplasms and neoplasms of uncertain and unknown behaviour	D00–D05, D07–D21, D26, D28–D29, D31–D32, D34–D48
097	Iron deficiency anaemia	D50
098	Other anaemias	D51–D64
099	Haemorrhagic conditions and other diseases of blood and blood-forming organs	D65–D77
100	Certain disorders involving the immune mechanism	D80–D89
101	Iodine-deficiency-related thyroid disorders	E00–E02
102	Thyrotoxicosis	E05
103	Other disorders of thyroid	E03–E04, E06–E07
104	Diabetes mellitus	E10–E14
105	Malnutrition	E40–E46
106	Vitamin A deficiency	E50
107	Other vitamin deficiencies	E51–E56
108	Sequelae of malnutrition and other nutritional deficiencies	E64
109	Obesity	E66
110	Volume depletion	E86
111	Other endocrine, nutritional and metabolic disorders	E15–E35, E58–E63, E65, E67–E85, E87–E90
112	Dementia	F00–F03
113	Mental and behavioural disorders due to use of alcohol	F10
114	Mental and behavioural disorders due to other psychoactive substance use	F11–F19
115	Schizophrenia, schizotypal, and delusional disorders	F20–F29
116	Mood [affective] disorders	F30–F39
117	Neurotic, stress-related, and somatoform disorders	F40–F48
118	Mental retardation	F70–F79
119	Other mental and behavioural disorders	F04–F09, F50–F69, F80–F99
120	Inflammatory diseases of the central nervous system	G00–G09
121	Parkinson's disease	G20
122	Alzheimer's disease	G30
123	Multiple sclerosis	G35
124	Epilepsy	G40–G41

125	Migraine and other headache syndromes	G43–G44
126	Transient cerebral ischaemic attacks and related syndromes	G45
127	Nerve, nerve root and plexus disorders	G50–G59
128	Cerebral palsy and other paralytic syndromes	G80–G83
129	Other diseases of the nervous system	G10–G13, G21–G26, G31–G32, G36–G37, G46–G47, G60–G73, G90–G99
130	Inflammation of eyelid	H00–H01
131	Conjunctivitis and other disorders of conjunctiva	H10–H13
132	Keratitis and other disorders of sclera and cornea	H15–H19
133	Cataract and other disorders of lens	H25–H28
134	Retinal detachments and breaks	H33
135	Glaucoma	H40–H42
136	Strabismus	H49–H50
137	Disorders of refraction and accommodation	H52
138	Blindness and low vision	H54
139	Other diseases of the eye and adnexa	H02–H06, H20–H22, H30–H32, H34–H36, H43–H48, H51, H53, H55–H59
140	Otitis media and other disorders of middle ear and mastoid	H65–H75
141	Hearing loss	H90–H91
142	Other diseases of the ear and mastoid process	H60–H62, H80–H83, H92–H95
143	Acute rheumatic fever	I00–I02
144	Chronic rheumatic heart disease	I05–I09
145	Essential (primary) hypertension	I10
146	Other hypertensive diseases	I11–I15
147	Acute myocardial infarction	I21–I22
148	Other ischaemic heart diseases	I20, I23–I25
149	Pulmonary embolism	I26
150	Conduction disorders and cardiac arrhythmias	I44–I49
151	Heart failure	I50
152	Other heart diseases	I27–I43, I51–I52
153	Intracranial haemorrhage	I60–I62
154	Cerebral infarction	I63

155	Stroke, not specified as haemorrhage or infarction	I64
156	Other cerebrovascular diseases	I65–I69
157	Atherosclerosis	I70
158	Other peripheral vascular diseases	I73
159	Arterial embolism and thrombosis	I74
160	Other diseases of arteries, arterioles and capillaries	I71–I72, I77–I79
161	Phlebitis, thrombophlebitis, venous embolism and thrombosis	I80–I82
162	Varicose veins of lower extremities	I83
163	Haemorrhoids	I84
164	Other diseases of the circulatory system	I85–I99
165	Acute pharyngitis and acute tonsillitis	J02–J03
166	Acute laryngitis and tracheitis	J04
167	Other acute upper respiratory infections	J00–J01, J05–J06
168	Influenza	J10–J11
169	Pneumonia	J12–J18
170	Acute bronchitis and acute bronchiolitis	J20–J21
171	Chronic sinusitis	J32
172	Other diseases of nose and nasal sinuses	J30–J31, J33–J34
173	Chronic disease of tonsils and adenoids	J35
174	Other diseases of upper respiratory tract	J36–J39
175	Bronchitis, emphysema and other chronic obstructive pulmonary diseases	J40–J44
176	Asthma	J45–J46
177	Bronchiectasis	J47
178	Pneumoconiosis	J60–J65
179	Other diseases of the respiratory system	J22, J66–J99
180	Dental caries	K02
181	Other disorders of teeth and supporting structures	K00–K01, K03–K08
182	Other diseases of the oral cavity, salivary glands and jaws	K09–K14
183	Gastric and duodenal ulcer	K25–K27
184	Gastritis and duodenitis	K29
185	Other diseases of oesophagus, stomach and duodenum	K20–K23, K28, K30–K31
186	Diseases of appendix	K35–K38
187	Inguinal hernia	K40
188	Other hernia	K41–K46
189	Crohn's disease and ulcerative colitis	K50–K51
190	Paralytic ileus and intestinal obstruction without hernia	K56

191	Diverticular disease of intestine	K57
192	Other diseases of intestines and peritoneum	K52–K55, K58–K67
193	Alcoholic liver disease	K70
194	Other diseases of liver	K71–K77
195	Cholelithiasis and cholecystitis	K80–K81
196	Acute pancreatitis and other diseases of the pancreas	K85–K86
197	Other diseases of the digestive system	K82–K83, K87–K93
198	Infections of the skin and subcutaneous tissue	L00–L08
199	Other diseases of the skin and subcutaneous tissue	L10–L99
200	Rheumatoid arthritis and other inflammatory polyarthropathies	M05–M14
201	Arthrosis	M15–M19
202	Acquired deformities of limbs	M20–M21
203	Other disorders of joints	M00–M03, M22–M25
204	Systemic connective tissue disorders	M30–M36
205	Cervical and other intervertebral disc disorders	M50–M51
206	Other dorsopathies	M40–M49, M53–M54
207	Soft tissue disorders	M60–M79
208	Disorders of bone density and structure	M80–M85
209	Osteomyelitis	M86
210	Other diseases of the musculoskeletal system and connective tissue	M87–M99
211	Acute and rapidly progressive nephritic syndromes	N00–N01
212	Other glomerular diseases	N02–N08
213	Renal tubulo-interstitial diseases	N10–N16
214	Renal failure	N17–N19
215	Urolithiasis	N20–N23
216	Cystitis	N30
217	Other diseases of the urinary system	N25–N29, N31–N39
218	Hyperplasia of prostate	N40
219	Other disorders of prostate	N41–N42
220	Hydrocele and spermatocele	N43
221	Redundant prepuce, phimosis and paraphimosis	N47

222	Other diseases of male genital organs	N44–N46, N48–N51
223	Disorders of breast	N60–N64
224	Salpingitis and oophoritis	N70
225	Inflammatory disease of cervix uteri	N72
226	Other inflammatory diseases of female pelvic organs	N71, N73–N77
227	Endometriosis	N80
228	Female genital prolapse	N81
229	Noninflammatory disorders of ovary, fallopian tube and broad ligament	N83
230	Disorders of menstruation	N91–N92
231	Menopausal and other perimenopausal disorders	N95
232	Female infertility	N97
233	Other disorders of genitourinary tract	N82, N84–N90, N93–N94, N96, N98–N99
234	Spontaneous abortion	O03
235	Medical abortion	O04
236	Other pregnancies with abortive outcome	O00–O02, O05–O08
237	Oedema, proteinuria and hypertensive disorders in pregnancy, childbirth and the puerperium	O10–O16
238	Placenta praevia, premature separation of placenta and antepartum haemorrhage	O44–O46
239	Other maternal care related to fetus and amniotic cavity and possible delivery problems	O30–O43, O47–O48
240	Obstructed labour	O64–O66
241	Postpartum haemorrhage	O72
242	Other complications of pregnancy and delivery	O20–O29, O60–O63, O67–O71, O73–O75, O81–O84
243	Single spontaneous delivery	O80
244	Complications predominantly related to the puerperium and other obstetric conditions, not elsewhere classified	O85–O99
245	Fetus and newborn affected by maternal factors and by complications of pregnancy, labour and delivery	P00–P04

246	Slow fetal growth, fetal malnutrition and disorders related to short gestation and low birth weight	P05–P07
247	Birth trauma	P10–P15
248	Intrauterine hypoxia and birth asphyxia	P20–P21
249	Other respiratory disorders originating in the perinatal period	P22–P28
250	Congenital infectious and parasitic diseases	P35–P37
251	Other infections specific to the perinatal period	P38–P39
252	Haemolytic disease of fetus and newborn	P55
253	Other conditions originating in the perinatal period	P08, P29, P50–P54, P56–P96
254	Spina bifida	Q05
255	Other congenital malformations of the nervous system	Q00–Q04, Q06–Q07
256	Congenital malformations of the circulatory system	Q20–Q28
257	Cleft lip and cleft palate	Q35–Q37
258	Absence, atresia and stenosis of small intestine	Q41
259	Other congenital malformations of the digestive system	Q38–Q40, Q42–Q45
260	Undescended testicle	Q53
261	Other malformations of the genitourinary system	Q50–Q52, Q54–Q64
262	Congenital deformities of hip	Q65
263	Congenital deformities of feet	Q66
264	Other congenital malformations and deformations of the musculoskeletal system	Q67–Q79
265	Other congenital malformations	Q10–Q18, Q30–Q34, Q80–Q89
266	Chromosomal abnormalities, not elsewhere classified	Q90–Q99
267	Abdominal and pelvic pain	R10
268	Fever of unknown origin	R50
269	Senility	R54
270	Other symptoms, signs and abnormal clinical and laboratory findings, not elsewhere classified	R00–R09, R11–R49, R51–R53, R55–R99
271	Fracture of skull and facial bones	S02
272	Fracture of neck, thorax or pelvis	S12, S22, S32, T08
273	Fracture of femur	S72

274	Fractures of other limb bones	S42, S52, S62, S82, S92, T10, T12
275	Fractures involving multiple body regions	T02
276	Dislocations, sprains and strains of specified and multiple body regions	S03, S13, S23, S33, S43, S53, S63, S73, S83, S93, T03
277	Injury of eye and orbit	S05
278	Intracranial injury	S06
279	Injury of other internal organs	S26–S27, S36–S37
280	Crushing injuries and traumatic amputations of specified and multiple body regions	S07–S08, S17–S18, S28, S38, S47–S48, S57–S58, S67–S68, S77–S78, S87–S88, S97–S98, T04–T05
281	Other injuries of specified, unspecified and multiple body regions	S00–S01, S04, S09–S11, S14–S16, S19–S21, S24–S25, S29–S31, S34–S35, S39–S41, S44–S46, S49–S51, S54–S56, S59–S61, S64–S66, S69–S71, S74–S76, S79–S81, S84–S86, S89–S91, S94–S96, S99, T00–T01, T06–T07, T09, T11, T13–T14
282	Effects of foreign body entering through natural orifice	T15–T19
283	Burns and corrosions	T20–T32
284	Poisoning by drugs and biological substances	T36–T50
285	Toxic effects of substances chiefly nonmedicinal as to source	T51–T65
286	Maltreatment syndromes	T74
287	Other and unspecified effects of external causes	T33–T35, T66–T73, T75–T78

288	Certain early complications of trauma and complications of surgical and medical care, not elsewhere classified	T79–T88
289	Sequelae of injuries, of poisoning and of other consequences of external causes	T90–T98
290	Persons encountering health services for examination and investigation	Z00–Z13
291	Asymptomatic human immunodeficiency virus [HIV] infection status	Z21
292	Other persons with potential health hazards related to communicable disease	Z20, Z22–Z29
293	Contraceptive management	Z30
294	Antenatal screening and other supervision of pregnancy	Z34–Z36
295	Liveborn infants according to place of birth	Z38
296	Postpartum care and examination	Z39
297	Persons encountering health services for specific procedures and health care	Z40–Z54
298	Persons encountering health services for other reasons	Z31–Z33, Z37, Z55–Z99

Definitions

Definitions

1. Causes of death

The causes of death to be entered on the medical certificate of cause of death are all those diseases, morbid conditions or injuries which either resulted in or contributed to death and the circumstances of the accident or violence which produced any such injuries.

2. Underlying cause of death

The underlying cause of death is (a) the disease or injury which initiated the train of events leading directly to death, or (b) the circumstances of the accident or violence which produced the fatal injury.

3. Definitions in relation to fetal, perinatal, neonatal and infant mortality

3.1 Live birth

Live birth is the complete expulsion or extraction from its mother of a product of conception, irrespective of the duration of the pregnancy, which, after such separation, breathes or shows any other evidence of life, such as beating of the heart, pulsation of the umbilical cord, or definite movement of voluntary muscles, whether or not the umbilical cord has been cut or the placenta is attached; each product of such a birth is considered liveborn.

3.2 Fetal death [deadborn fetus]

Fetal death is death prior to the complete expulsion or extraction from its mother of a product of conception, irrespective of the duration of pregnancy; the death is indicated by the fact that after such separation the fetus does not breathe or show any other evidence of life, such as beating of the heart, pulsation of the umbilical cord, or definite movement of voluntary muscles.

3.3 Birth weight
The first weight of the fetus or newborn obtained after birth.

3.4 Low birth weight
Less than 2500 g (up to, and including 2499 g).

3.5 Very low birth weight
Less than 1500 g (up to, and including 1499 g).

3.6 Extremely low birth weight
Less than 1000 g (up to, and including 999 g).

3.7 Gestational age
The duration of gestation is measured from the first day of the last normal menstrual period. Gestational age is expressed in completed days or completed weeks (e.g. events occurring 280 to 286 completed days after the onset of the last normal menstrual period are considered to have occurred at 40 weeks of gestation).

3.8 Pre-term
Less than 37 completed weeks (less than 259 days) of gestation.

3.9 Term
From 37 completed weeks to less than 42 completed weeks (259 to 293 days) of gestation.

3.10 Post-term
42 completed weeks or more (294 days or more) of gestation.

3.11 Perinatal period

The perinatal period commences at 22 completed weeks (154 days) of gestation (the time when birth weight is normally 500 g), and ends seven completed days after birth.

3.12 Neonatal period

The neonatal period commences at birth and ends 28 completed days after birth. Neonatal deaths (deaths among live births during the first 28 completed days of life) may be subdivided into *early neonatal deaths*, occurring during the first seven days of life, and *late neonatal deaths*, occurring after the seventh day but before 28 completed days of life.

Notes on definitions

i.   For live births, birth weight should preferably be measured within the first hour of life before significant postnatal weight loss has occurred. While statistical tabulations include 500 g groupings for birth weight, weights should not be recorded in those groupings. The actual weight should be recorded to the degree of accuracy to which it is measured.

ii. The definitions of "low", "very low", and "extremely low" birth weight do not constitute mutually exclusive categories. Below the set limits they are all-inclusive and therefore overlap (i.e. "low" includes "very low" and "extremely low", while "very low" includes "extremely low").

iii. Gestational age is frequently a source of confusion when calculations are based on menstrual dates. For the purposes of calculation of gestational age from the date of the first day of the last normal menstrual period and the date of delivery, it should be borne in mind that the first day is day zero and not day one; days 0–6 therefore correspond to "completed week zero", days 7–13 to "completed week one", and the 40th week of actual gestation is synonymous with "completed week 39". Where the date of the last normal menstrual period is not available, gestational age should be based on the best clinical estimate. In order to avoid misunderstanding, tabulations should indicate both weeks and days.

iv. Age at death during the first day of life (day zero) should be recorded in units of completed minutes or hours of life. For the second (day 1), third (day 2) and through 27 completed days of life, age at death should be recorded in days.

4. Definitions related to maternal mortality

4.1 Maternal death

A maternal death is the death of a woman while pregnant or within 42 days of termination of pregnancy, irrespective of the duration and the site of the pregnancy, from any cause related to or aggravated by the pregnancy or its management, but not from accidental or incidental causes.

4.2 Late maternal death

A late maternal death is the death of a woman from direct or indirect obstetric causes more than 42 days but less than one year after termination of pregnancy.

4.3 Pregnancy-related death

A pregnancy-related death is the death of a woman while pregnant or within 42 days of termination of pregnancy, irrespective of the cause of death.

Maternal deaths should be subdivided into two groups:

4.4 Direct obstetric deaths

Direct obstetric deaths are those resulting from obstetric complications of the pregnant state (pregnancy, labour and puerperium), from interventions, omissions, incorrect treatment, or from a chain of events resulting from any of the above.

4.5. Indirect obstetric deaths

Indirect obstetric deaths are those resulting from previous existing disease or disease that developed during pregnancy and which was not due to direct obstetric causes, but which was aggravated by physiologic effects of pregnancy.

Regulations regarding nomenclature

Regulations regarding nomenclature

(including the compilation and publication of statistics) with respect to diseases and causes of death

The Twentieth World Health Assembly,

Considering the importance of compiling and publishing statistics of mortality and morbidity in comparable form;

Having regard to Articles 2(s), 21(b), 22 and 64 of the Constitution of the World Health Organization,

ADOPTS, this twenty-second day of May 1967, the Nomenclature Regulations 1967; these Regulations may be cited as the WHO Nomenclature Regulations.

Article 1

Members of the World Health Organization for whom these Regulations shall come into force under Article 7 below shall be referred to hereinafter as Members.

Article 2

Members compiling mortality and morbidity statistics shall do so in accordance with the current revision of the International Statistical Classification of Diseases, Injuries and Causes of Death as adopted from time to time by the World Health Assembly. This Classification may be cited as the International Classification of Diseases.

Article 3

In compiling and publishing mortality and morbidity statistics, Members shall comply as far as possible with recommendations made by the World Health Assembly as to classification, coding procedure, age-grouping, territorial areas to be identified, and other relevant definitions and standards.

Article 4

Members shall compile and publish annually for each calendar year statistics of causes of death for the metropolitan (home) territory as a whole or for such part thereof as information is available, and shall indicate the area covered by the statistics.

Article 5

Members shall adopt a form of medical certificate of cause of death that provides for the statement of the morbid conditions or injuries resulting in or contributing to death, with a clear indication of the underlying cause.

Article 6

Each member shall, under Article 64 of the Constitution, provide the Organization on request with statistics prepared in accordance with these Regulations and not communicated under Article 63 of the Constitution.

Article 7

1. These Regulations shall come into force on the first day of January 1968.

2. Upon their entry into force these Regulations shall, subject to the exceptions hereinafter provided, replace as between the Members bound by these Regulations and as between these Members and the Organization, the provisions of the Nomenclature Regulations 1948 and subsequent revisions thereof.

3. Any revisions of the International Classification of Diseases adopted by the World Health Assembly pursuant to Article 2 of these Regulations shall enter into force on such date as is prescribed by the World Health Assembly and shall, subject to the exceptions hereinafter provided, replace any earlier classifications.

Article 8

1. The period provided in execution of Article 22 of the Constitution of the Organization for rejection or reservation shall be six months from the date

of the notification by the Director-General of the adoption of these Regulations by the World Health Assembly. Any rejection or reservation received by the Director-General after the expiry of this period shall have no effect.

2. The provisions of paragraph 1 of this Article shall likewise apply in respect of any subsequent revision of the International Classification of Diseases adopted by the World Health Assembly pursuant to Article 2 of these Regulations.

Article 9

A rejection, or the whole or part of any reservation, whether to these Regulations or to the International Classification of Diseases or any revision thereof, may at any time be withdrawn by notifying the Director-General.

Article 10

The Director-General shall notify all Members of the adoption of these Regulations, of the adoption of any revision of the International Classification of Diseases as well as of any notification received by him under Articles 8 and 9.

Article 11

The original texts of these Regulations shall be deposited in the Archives of the Organization. Certified true copies shall be sent by the Director-General to all Members. Upon the entry into force of these Regulations, certified true copies shall be delivered by the Director-General to the Secretary-General of the United Nations for registration in accordance with Article 102 of the Charter of the United Nations.

In faith whereof, we have set our hands at Geneva this twenty-second day of May 1967.

(signed) V.T.H. Gunaratne,
President of the World Health Assembly
(signed) M.G Candau
Director-General of the World Health
Organization